Medicinal Chemistry Lessons From Nature

(Volume 1)

Flavonoids and Phenolics

Edited By

Simone Carradori
Department of Pharmacy, G. d'Annunzio
University of Chieti-Pescara
Italy

Medicinal Chemistry Lessons From Nature

Volume # 1

Flavonoids and Phenolics

Editor: Simone Carradori

ISBN (Online): 978-981-5079-09-8

ISBN (Print): 978-981-5079-10-4

ISBN (Paperback): 978-981-5079-11-1

Published by Bentham Science Publishers Pte. Ltd. Singapore.

First published in 2022.

BENTHAM SCIENCE PUBLISHERS LTD.

End User License Agreement (for non-institutional, personal use)

This is an agreement between you and Bentham Science Publishers Ltd. Please read this License Agreement carefully before using the book/echapter/ejournal (**"Work"**). Your use of the Work constitutes your agreement to the terms and conditions set forth in this License Agreement. If you do not agree to these terms and conditions then you should not use the Work.

Bentham Science Publishers agrees to grant you a non-exclusive, non-transferable limited license to use the Work subject to and in accordance with the following terms and conditions. This License Agreement is for non-library, personal use only. For a library / institutional / multi user license in respect of the Work, please contact: permission@benthamscience.net.

Usage Rules:

1. All rights reserved: The Work is the subject of copyright and Bentham Science Publishers either owns the Work (and the copyright in it) or is licensed to distribute the Work. You shall not copy, reproduce, modify, remove, delete, augment, add to, publish, transmit, sell, resell, create derivative works from, or in any way exploit the Work or make the Work available for others to do any of the same, in any form or by any means, in whole or in part, in each case without the prior written permission of Bentham Science Publishers, unless stated otherwise in this License Agreement.
2. You may download a copy of the Work on one occasion to one personal computer (including tablet, laptop, desktop, or other such devices). You may make one back-up copy of the Work to avoid losing it.
3. The unauthorised use or distribution of copyrighted or other proprietary content is illegal and could subject you to liability for substantial money damages. You will be liable for any damage resulting from your misuse of the Work or any violation of this License Agreement, including any infringement by you of copyrights or proprietary rights.

Disclaimer:

Bentham Science Publishers does not guarantee that the information in the Work is error-free, or warrant that it will meet your requirements or that access to the Work will be uninterrupted or error-free. The Work is provided "as is" without warranty of any kind, either express or implied or statutory, including, without limitation, implied warranties of merchantability and fitness for a particular purpose. The entire risk as to the results and performance of the Work is assumed by you. No responsibility is assumed by Bentham Science Publishers, its staff, editors and/or authors for any injury and/or damage to persons or property as a matter of products liability, negligence or otherwise, or from any use or operation of any methods, products instruction, advertisements or ideas contained in the Work.

Limitation of Liability:

In no event will Bentham Science Publishers, its staff, editors and/or authors, be liable for any damages, including, without limitation, special, incidental and/or consequential damages and/or damages for lost data and/or profits arising out of (whether directly or indirectly) the use or inability to use the Work. The entire liability of Bentham Science Publishers shall be limited to the amount actually paid by you for the Work.

General:

1. Any dispute or claim arising out of or in connection with this License Agreement or the Work (including non-contractual disputes or claims) will be governed by and construed in accordance with the laws of Singapore. Each party agrees that the courts of the state of Singapore shall have exclusive jurisdiction to settle any dispute or claim arising out of or in connection with this License Agreement or the Work (including non-contractual disputes or claims).
2. Your rights under this License Agreement will automatically terminate without notice and without the

Bentham Science Publishers Pte. Ltd.
80 Robinson Road #02-00
Singapore 068898
Singapore
Email: subscriptions@benthamscience.net

BENTHAM
SCIENCE

CONTENTS

FOREWORD

The intention of this volume is to give an overview of the latest discoveries in the research on natural products-derived compounds, through a medicinal chemistry approach of the most exciting topics on flavonoids and (poly)phenolics derivatives. It is structured with innovative book setting outlines and a clear distinction between experimental and clinical results, in order to aid the reader to know at which step of the pipeline each compound is. Due to the scarcity of information of the other competing books, the Guest Editor wants to fulfil the gap of the acquired knowledge in the last few years with the aim to provide a guide for academic and professional researchers and clinicians.

The exploration of the chemical space ranges from flavonoids to phenolic compounds, covering all the aspects relevant for medicinal chemistry (drug design, structure-activity relationships, permeability data, cytotoxicity, appropriate statistical procedures, molecular modelling studies and technological formulations). Each chapter reviews on agents with common chemical features, considering them as scaffolds to obtain various derivatives aiming at the biological activity. The chemical modifications of these agents could increase their intrinsic properties, overcome limitations as drug candidates and introduce new properties. Thus, the volume is intended to be useful to researchers for more concrete applications in the natural product field. As far as I know, this is the first time these data are organized focusing on the synthetic methods and their strategies comprehending the last years.

KEY FEATURES

1. Updated information on synthetic/natural compounds;
2. In-depth analysis of novel findings and promising translational applications;
3. Use of organic reactions as a powerful tool in drug discovery to improve the biological activity or give new chemical and biological properties to the parent molecules;
4. Molecular mechanisms with innovative approaches for the readers to improve their own research investigations.

Rosa Amoroso
Department of Pharmacy
G. d'Annunzio University of Chieti-Pescara
Via dei Vestini 31, 66100 Chieti (Italy)

PREFACE

Natural products are often used in drug development due to their ability to provide unique and chemically diverse structures unmatched by any synthetic chemical collection. Medicinal Chemists have always been inspired by nature because natural products are often perceived as safer and for their capability to interact with biological targets. Indeed, in recent years, there has been emerging research on traditional herbal medicines based on their efficacy in the treatment of diseases for which they have been traditionally applied.

Conversely, natural compounds suffer from several issues such as scarce availability and seasonality, high differences in the production/extraction/isolation, low purity in commercial products from worldwide suppliers, and side effects. Moreover, due to their chemical complexity and the optional presence of different chiral centers, the total synthesis of a natural compound can be also challenging and expensive.

This book series would propose the latest discoveries in the field of compounds inspired by nature and obtained by chemical/enzymatic modification of a natural compound in the search for biologically active molecules for the treatment of human/animal ailments and permit the disposal of a wider arsenal for clinicians. The natural compounds are grouped into three clusters. The chapters are built in the following format: • General background on the (phyto)chemistry of the scaffold; • General background on the pharmacological profile of the scaffold; • Description of the proposed derivatives and their potentialities with respect to the parent compounds (with a particular emphasis on the synthetic approaches and structure-activity relationships); • *In silico* analysis of the crucial interactions with the biological target, when available; • Clinical studies and patent surveys (if available) on the new and proposed structures.

The readership of this book is represented primarily by Academies, Researchers, Specialists in the pharmaceutical field, Industry sector, Contract Research Organizations and hospitals dealing with clinical research.

Simone Carradori
Department of Pharmacy
G. d'Annunzio University of Chieti-Pescara
Italy

List of Contributors

Alessandra Ammazzalorso	Department of Pharmacy, Medicinal Chemistry Unit, G. d'Annunzio University of Chieti-Pescara, *Via* dei Vestini, 66100 Chieti, Italy
Alessandro Bonardi	Department of NEUROFARBA, Section of Pharmaceutical and Nutraceutical Sciences, Pharmaceutical and Nutraceutical Section, University of Florence, *Via* U, Schiff 6, 50019 Sesto Fiorentino, Firenze, Italy
Alessio Nocentini	Department of NEUROFARBA, Section of Pharmaceutical and Nutraceutical Sciences, Pharmaceutical and Nutraceutical Section, University of Florence, *Via* U, Schiff 6, 50019 Sesto Fiorentino, Firenze, Italy
Antonella Capperucci	Department of Chemistry "Ugo Schiff", University of Florence, *Via* della Lastruccia 13, I-50019 Sesto Fiorentino, Italy
Arafa Musa	Department of Pharmacognosy, College of Pharmacy, Jouf University, Sakaka, Al Jouf, 2014, Saudi Arabia
Atilla Akdemir	Computer-aided Drug Discovery Laboratory, Department of Pharmacology, Faculty of Pharmacy, Bezmialem Vakif University, Fatih, Istanbul 34093, Turkey
Barbara De Filippis	Department of Pharmacy, "G. d'Annunzio" University of Chieti-Pescara, *Via* dei Vestini 31, 66100 Chieti, Italy
Bijo Mathew	Department of Pharmaceutical Chemistry, Amrita School of Pharmacy, Amrita Vishwa Vidyapeetham, Amrita Health Science Campus, Kochi-682 041, India
Celeste De Monte	Department of Drug Chemistry and Technology, Sapienza, University of Rome, 00185 Rome, Italy
Claudio Ferrante	Department of Pharmacy, Medicinal Plant Unit (MPU), Botanic Garden Giardino dei Semplici, G. d'Annunzio University of Chieti-Pescara, *Via* dei Vestini, 66100 Chieti, Italy
Claudiu T. Supuran	Department of NEUROFARBA, Section of Pharmaceutical and Nutraceutical Sciences, Pharmaceutical and Nutraceutical Section, University of Florence, *Via* U. Schiff 6, 50019 Sesto Fiorentino, Firenze, Italy
Cristina Scarpecci	Department of Drug Chemistry and Technology, Sapienza, University of Rome, 00185 Rome, Italy
Damiano Tanini	Department of Chemistry "Ugo Schiff", University of Florence, *Via* della Lastruccia 13, I-50019 Sesto Fiorentino, Italy
Della Grace Thomas Parambi	Department of Pharmaceutical Chemistry, College of Pharmacy, Jouf University, Sakaka, Al Jouf, 2014, Saudi Arabia
Federico Appetecchia	Department of Drug Chemistry and Technology, Sapienza, University of Rome, 00185 Rome, Italy
Federico De Paolis	Department of Physiology and Pharmacology "V. Ersparmer", Sapienza University of Rome, P.le Aldo Moro 5, 00185 Rome, Italy
Francesco Cairone	Department of Drug Chemistry and Technology, Sapienza, University of Rome, 00185 Rome, Italy

Giovanna Poce	Department of Drug Chemistry and Technology, Sapienza, University of Rome, 00185 Rome, Italy
Heiko Lange	Department of Environmental and Earth Sciences, University of Milano-Bicocca, Milan, Italy
Leena K Pappachen	Department of Pharmaceutical Chemistry, Amrita School of Pharmacy, Amrita Vishwa Vidyapeetham, Amrita Health Science Campus, Kochi-682 041, India
Luc Zongo	Department of Pharmacy, University of Saint Dominic of West Africa (USDAO), Doulougou, Burkina Faso
Mohamed A. Abdelgawad	Department of Pharmaceutical Chemistry, College of Pharmacy, Jouf University, Sakaka, Al Jouf, 2014, Saudi Arabia
Manoj Kumar Sachidanandan	Department of Oral and maxillofacial surgery and diagnostics, College of Dentistry, Hail University, Hail Province, 2440, Saudi Arabia
Maria Antonietta Casadei	Department of Drug Chemistry and Technologies, Sapienza University of Rome, P.le A. Moro 5, 00185 Rome, Italy
Melissa D'Ascenzio	D'Arcy Thompson Unit, Biological and Biomedical Sciences Education, School of Life Sciences, University of Dundee, DD1 4HN, Dundee, UK
Mutairah Shaker Alshammari	Department of Pharmaceutical Analytical Chemistry, Faculty of science, Jouf University, Sakaka, Al Jouf, 2014, Saudi Arabia
Paolo Guglielmi	Department of Drug Chemistry and Technologies, Sapienza University of Rome, P.le A. Moro 5, 00185 Rome, Italy
Rania Bakr	Department of Pharmaceutical Chemistry, College of Pharmacy, Jouf University, Sakaka, Al Jouf, 2014, Saudi Arabia
Sara Consalvi	Department of Drug Chemistry and Technology, Sapienza, University of Rome, 00185 Rome, Italy
Stefania Cesa	Department of Drug Chemistry and Technology, Sapienza, University of Rome, 00185 Rome, Italy
Stefania Garzoli	Department of Drug Chemistry and Technologies, Sapienza University of Rome, P.le A. Moro 5, 00185 Rome, Italy
Stefania Petralito	Department of Drug Chemistry and Technologies, Sapienza University of Rome, P.le A. Moro 5, 00185 Rome, Italy
Trond Vidar Hansen	Department of Pharmacy, Section for Pharmaceutical Chemistry, University of Oslo, PO Box 1068 Blindern, N-0316 Oslo, Norway
Virginia Pontecorvi	Department of Drug Chemistry and Technologies, Sapienza University of Rome, P.le A. Moro 5, 00185 Rome, Italy
Vaishnav Bhaskar	Department of Pharmaceutical Chemistry, Amrita School of Pharmacy, Amrita Vishwa Vidyapeetham, Amrita Health Science Campus, Kochi-682 041, India

CHAPTER 1

Polyphenols and Flavonoids: Chemical, Pharmacological and Therapeutic Aspects

Stefania Cesa[1,*], **Francesco Cairone**[1] and **Celeste De Monte**[1]

[1] *Department of Drug Chemistry and Technology, Sapienza, University of Rome, 00185 Rome, Italy*

Abstract: Polyphenols and flavonoids represent a group of compounds characterized by a large assortment of phenolic structures, which can be naturally found in vegetables, roots, stems, flowers, grains, and fruits. Thanks to their biological activities, molecules belonging to these classes of compounds, besides their nutritional role, have found applications in several fields such as pharmaceutical, cosmetic, and nutraceutical. In fact, like many natural derivatives from plants, they possess several therapeutic properties, including antitumor, anti-oxidative, anti-neurodegenerative, antimicrobial and anti-inflammatory effects. Nowadays, the growing interest in polyphenolics and flavonoids translates into constant research to better define their pharmacological mechanism of action. Extraction studies in order to obtain pure compounds with a more defined biological activity, as well as pharmacokinetic studies to understand the bioavailability, the involved metabolic pathways and the related active metabolites, are carried out. Molecular docking studies are also continuously in progress to expand the field of application. Moreover, toxicity experiments to clarify their safety and studies about the interaction with other compounds to understand their selectivity of action are continuously forwarded and deepened. Consequently, many recent studies are aimed at introducing polyphenols, more specifically flavonoids, and their semi-synthetic derivatives, in the prevention, management and treatment of several diseases.

Keywords: Bioavailability, Biological properties, Chemical structures, Disease prevention, Flavonoids, Metabolism, Polyphenols, Semisynthetic derivatives.

INTRODUCTION

Polyphenols are the plant's secondary metabolites, contained in specialized cells in small quantities and not necessary for cell viability that vegetal organisms produce to perform different functions. They include several classes of chemical molecules characterized by the presence of aromatic rings bearing more than a hydroxylic function, up to complex polycyclic and polymeric compounds.

* **Corresponding author Stefania Cesa:** Department of Drug Chemistry and Technology, Sapienza, University of Rome, 00185 Rome, Italy; E-mail: stefania.cesa@uniroma1.it

Simone Carradori (Ed.)

All molecules presenting a simple phenolic group are theoretically able to act as anti-radical species since they could react with endogen radicals to undergo new and more stable radical residues, which tend to react by neutralizing rather than attacking macromolecules such as DNA or proteins causing damages up to mutagenesis or unfolding. Moreover, the presence of *ortho*-diphenol groups also allows the metals chelation, improving the antioxidant properties. Polyphenols are frequently classified in relation to their chemical structure into four principal molecules, represented by phenolic acids, flavonoids, stilbenes and lignans. Natural products have always been the subject of great interest thanks to their biological activities and pharmacological properties. The attention towards bioactive compounds is growing more and more over the years because they found applications in pharmaceutical, nutraceutical, cosmetic and medical fields [1]. By virtue of appropriate pharmacodynamic, pharmacokinetic, bioavailability and toxicity studies, they can potentially be included among dietary supplements and therapeutic tools for the prevention and treatment of many human diseases with important applications in phytotherapy and herbal medicine [2]. A recent review [3] reports the protection exerted by a polyphenol-rich diet, highlighting the potential ability of pure polyphenols and of phytocomplex to reverse oxidative stress-relative diseases and a "promising chemopreventive efficacy" through modulation of apoptosis and cellular growth, inhibition of DNA synthesis and modulation of signal transduction. Among the bioactive natural products, a preeminent position is occupied by flavonoids, plants and fungi secondary metabolites, of supreme interest both for their ubiquitous distribution in nature and for the wide structural diversification, to which is often correlated a specific bioactivity. They can be found in many parts of plants, including leaves, flowers (where flavonoids constitute the colored pigments of petals), roots, fruits, stems, seeds, rhizome, bark, gum and shell [4]. The reason for their ubiquitous location in many plant organs may be due to the flavonoids' important role in protecting them against oxidative stress and ultraviolet radiation, as well as in attracting pollinating animals [5].

Flavonoids have gained a special prominence among natural compounds of pharmaceutical and therapeutic interest, thanks to the wide range of chemical subclasses and their wide variety of pharmacological properties, such as the modulation of enzymatic activities by inhibiting lipid peroxidation and cyclo-oxygenase and lipoxygenase activity, anti-inflammatory, anti-mutagenic, antioxidative and antitumor effects [6].

In a recent review [7], authors underline the high interest, not only for polyphenols contained in several by-products of agroindustry processes but also for bound polyphenols, which could need hydrolytic treatment of the containing matrices, to make efficient their extraction yields. Analogously, Jablonsky *et al.*

[8] studied the bioactivity potential of phenolics extracted by softwood bark, emphasizing the extract complexity and the wide applications in the pharmacologic field as cytotoxic, antioxidant, fungicidal and antibacterial substances. Moreover, Cotas *et al.* [9] evaluated the potential applications of polyphenols, tannins and many others extracted from seaweed (Chlorophyta, Rhodophyta and Phaeophyceae). As polyphenols are one of the most represented classes of seaweed phytochemicals and seaweeds are one of the most available organic matrices in nature, they could be more exploited for large-scale production of polyphenolic compounds.

Healthy food containing polyphenols found also application in the prevention of skin aging and skin cancer, as functional foods or as sources of nutraceuticals to be used both in food supplements, cosmetic products or a topical formulation for dermatologic applications. This application field was also recently reviewed, but authors concluded that ingredients used with this aim, are often poorly characterised or represent part of complex mixtures by which it is difficult to establish the relationship between a single molecule and its biological effect [10].

The antioxidant and free radical scavenging activities were shown for many compounds of this class, as well as the cardioprotective, antidiabetic and antiviral potential. Most researchers are actually involved in the deepening of the mechanisms underlying the anti-cancer activity and the apoptosis induction, focusing the attention on the key enzyme involved in cellular proliferation, angiogenesis progression, and metastatic processes [11]. Anyway, most parts of these results were obtained by experiments performed *in vitro* or *ex vivo*, but the real potential of a molecule or of a class of compounds needs to be evaluated on the basis of its ability to be absorbed and metabolized while maintaining its biological effect, and finally its capability to reach the active site. As flavonoids generally display low water solubility and consequently low bioavailability, a topic of greatest interest for the scientific community is the application of several strategies aiming to solve this problem. So, a valent strategy for the polyphenolic fraction valorization is represented by the possibility of enhancing their efficacy, bioavailability and release to the action site, mediated by the exploitation of nanotechnologies capable of solving many and different problems [12] related to the specific structures, which could undergo low intestinal absorption, rapid metabolism and excretion, low plasmatic contents. This research field found application in the formulation based on many different systems, differently organized, such as liposomes, solid lipid nanoparticles, nanostructured lipid carriers, nanosuspensions, and nanoemulsions. These could be able to enhance the solubility of single nutraceuticals rather than solving problems inherent with the more or less complex nature of organic extracts obtained by food, non-edible by-products or waste of agricultural practices and, more generally, by biological resources [13, 14].

A number of different solutions were proposed, ranging among the use of adsorption enhancers, semisynthetic strategies, use of pro-drugs, transformation in more hydrophilic molecules by glycosylation, and the use of carrier systems as, among others, the just mentioned nanotechnologies. In a recent review by Zhao *et al.* [15], the advantages and limitations of the different applied solutions, together with an evaluation of their influence on dissolution rate, mucosal permeation and degradation during the passage throw the gastrointestinal tract are reported, and authors highlight a generally achieved great improvement of the pharmacokinetic behaviour of poorly absorbed flavonoids, significantly represented in nature and foods.

CHEMICAL STRUCTURES, CLASSIFICATION AND PROPERTIES OF FLAVONOIDS

Flavonoids are a wide group of polyphenolic natural, synthetic and semi-synthetic products with low molecular weight, whose name is due to their flavan nucleus that derives from 3,4-dihydro-2-phenyl-2*H*-1-benzopyran skeleton. They have a generic structure with C6-C3-C6 units, with a skeleton consisting of 15 carbons, organized in three rings, as reported in (Fig. **1**). two phenyl rings (A and B rings) with a six-carbons chain, and a pyran nucleus (C ring,) with a three-carbons chain [16].

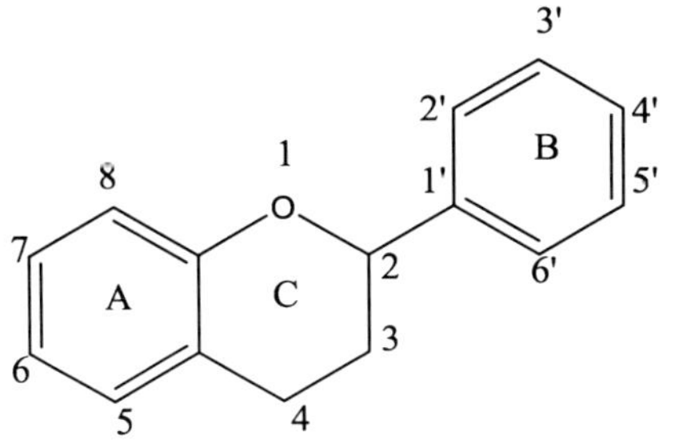

Fig. (1). Chemical skeleton of flavonoids consisting of C6-C3-C6 units.

The classification into which flavonoids are cataloged depends on the degree of oxidation and unsaturation of the C ring and also according to the position (the second, the third, or the fourth carbon atom) on which the B ring is attached to this heterocyclic ring. More frequently, the phenyl ring B is linked to the second position of the C ring and flavonoids are subdivided into many classes, such as flavones, flavonols, anthocyanidins, flavanones, flavanonols, flavanols or catechins. When the B ring is connected to the third position of the C ring, they are named isoflavonoids, as well as when the connection occurs at the fourth position, they are called neoflavonoids [17].Other kinds of phenolic compounds related to flavonoids are chalcones because they can be considered open-chain flavonoids [16]. According to Silva *et al.* [18], flavonoids represent about two thirds of the ingested polyphenols in the human diet and could be classified into seven classes, as shown by (Fig. **2**).

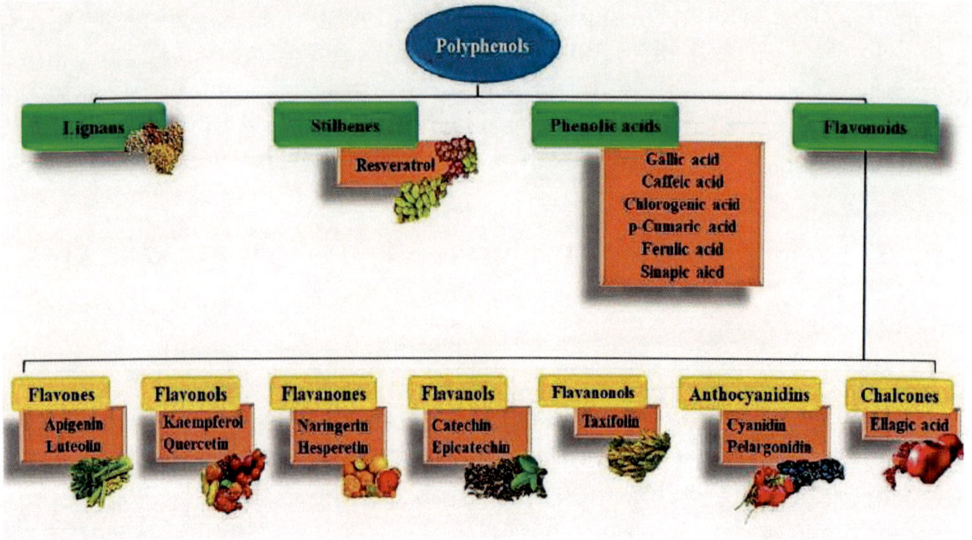

Fig. (2). Classification of polyphenols and flavonoids. For each class some molecules are mentioned.

Classes of Flavonoids with the B Ring on C_2

Flavones are characterized by a 2-phenyl-1-benzopyran-4-one skeleton, without substitution at the C3 position and a ketonic function at the C4 (Fig. **3**). Flavones derived from plants are generally conjugated with glycosides and can be *O*-glycosides or *C*-glycosides. Examples of *O*-glycosides are the 7-*O*-glycosides diosmin or the 7-*O*-rhamnosylglucoside diosmetin, as well as examples of *C*-glucosides, are the 6-*C*-glucosides vitexin or the 8-*C*-glucosides apigenin [19]. Flavonols, such as kaempferol, quercetin and myricetin, also possess a ketone moiety in C4 and can be glycosylated, but they also present a hydroxyl group at the C3 of the core structure [20]. Flavanols, also known as catechins when there is a hydroxyl group at C3 (flavan-3-ol structure), present the saturation of the double bond between C2 and C3, and there is not a carbonyl group at the C4 position, so they have two chiral carbons (C2 and C3) and four diastereomers [21]: (+)-catechin (2*R*,3*S*), (−)-catechin (2*S*,3*R*), (+)-epicatechin (2*R*,3*R*), and (−)-epicatechin (2*S*,3*S*). Moreover, when they are esterified with gallic acid, they give rise to gallate conjugates [22]. In addition, in the class of flavanols can be found: flavan-3,4-diols, which are called leucoanthocyanins, because by heating with aqueous acidic conditions, anthocyanidins can be obtained from them [23]; proanthocyanidins, that consist of dimers, trimers, or oligomers of flavan-3-ols [24]; and condensed tannins produced by the polymerization of flavan-3-ols [25]. Flavanones, or dihydroflavones, possess a ketone group at C4 and, such as flavanols, and they have no double bond between C2 and C3 of the C ring. Among this class, there is naringenin, which shows the 4'-hydroxy moiety on the B ring, and its 7-*O*-glycoside, naringin, and hesperetin, with 3'-OH and 4'-methoxy groups, from which derives its glycoside hesperidin [26]. Flavanonols are 3-hydroxyflavanone derivatives such as taxifolin or dihydroquercetin [27]. Conversely, anthocyanidins are characterized by a positive charge at the oxygen atom (forming oxonium ion) of the C-ring that, for this reason, is called flavylium (2-phenylchromenylium) ion. As anthocyanidins represent the aglycone form, anthocyanins are the glycoside forms representing the plants' blue, red and purple pigments. Anthocyanidins do not possess the ketone moiety at C4 of the heterocyclic core and, according to the hydroxy and methoxy groups at the B ring, they are named cyanidin, delphinidin, pelargonidin, peonidin, malvidin, and petunidin [28].

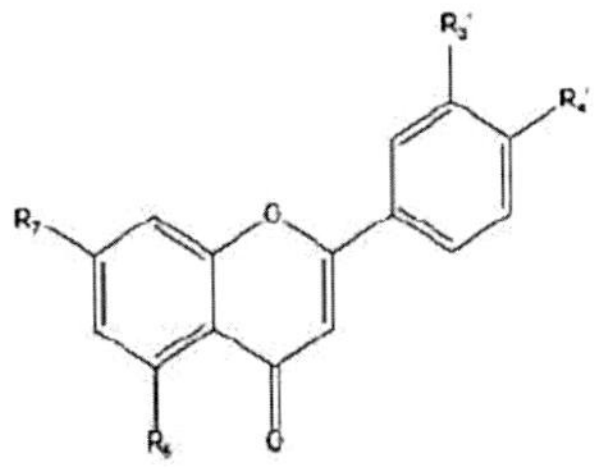

Flavones

$R_3 = R'_5 = H$ $R_5 = R_7 = OH$ $R'_4 = OH$ — Apigenin
$R_5 = R_7 = R'_3 = R'_4 = OH$ — Luteolin
$R_5 = R_7 = OH$ $R'_3 = R'_4 = H$ — Chrisin
$R_5 = R_6 = R_7 = OH$ $R'_3 = R'_4 = H$ — Baicalein

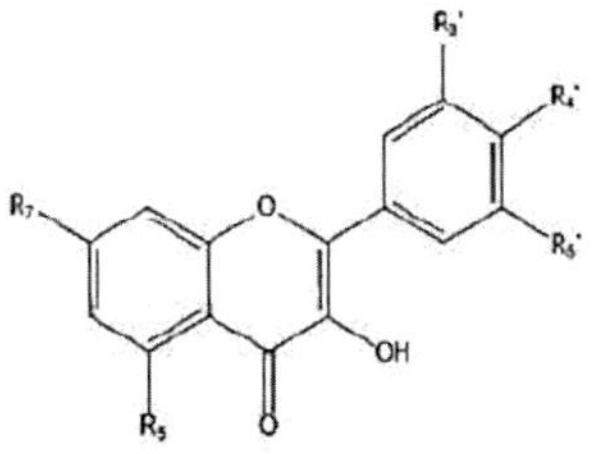

Flavonols

$R_5 = R_7 = R'_3 = R'_4 = OH$ $R'_5 = H$ — Quercetin
$R_5 = R_7 = R'_4 = OH$ $R'_3 = R'_5 = H$ — Kaempferol
$R_5 = R_7 = R'_3 = R'_4 = R'_5 = OH$ — Myricetin
$R_5 = R'_5 = H$ $R_7 = R'_3 = R'_4 = OH$ — Fisetin

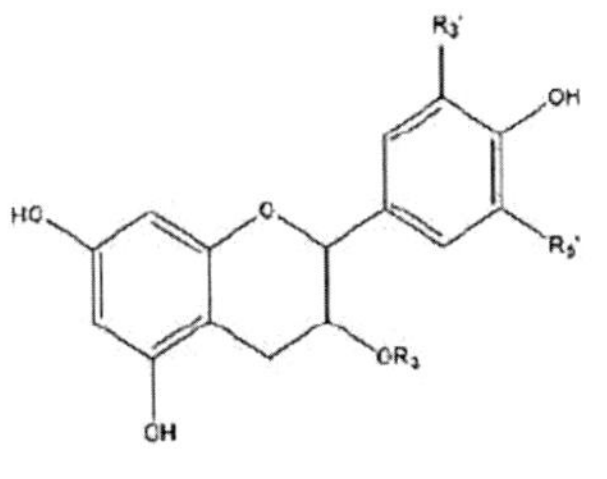

Flavanols

$R_3 = R'_5 = H$ $R'_3 = OH$ — Catechin
$R_3 = R'_5 = H$ $R'_3 = OH$ — Epicatechin
$R_3 =$ gallate $R'_3 = R'_5 = OH$ — Epigallocatechin gallate

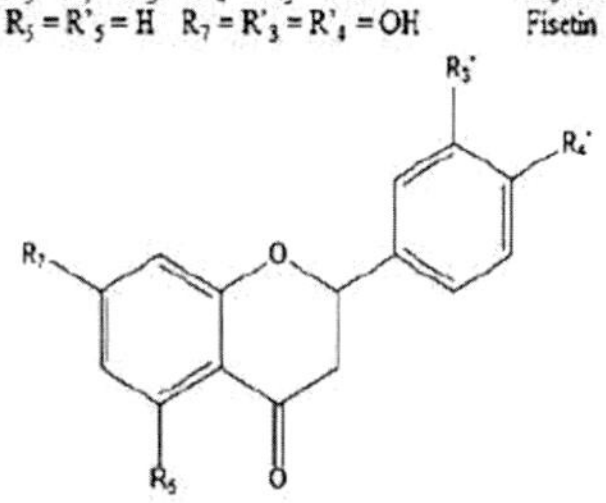

Flavanones

$R_5 = R_7 = R'_4 = OH$ $R'_3 = H$ — Naringenin
$R_5 = R_7 = R'_3 = OH$ $R'_4 = OCH3$ — Hesperetin

(Fig. 3) contd.....

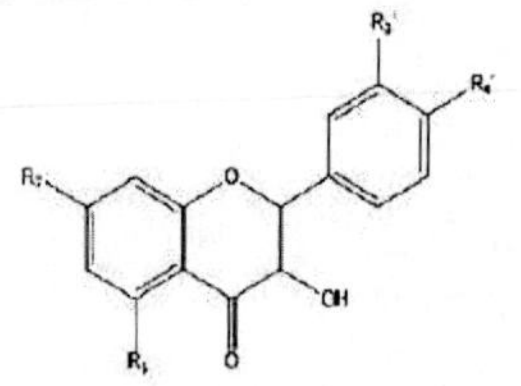

Flavanonols
$R_5 = R_7 = R'_3 = R'_4 = OH$ Taxifolin

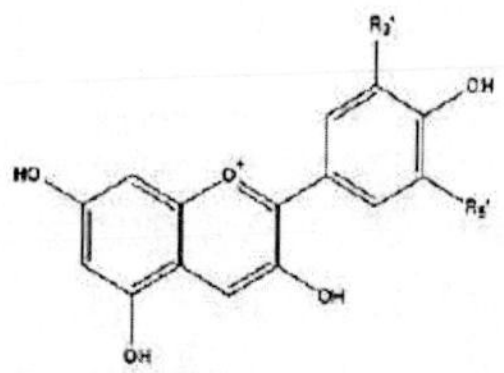

Anthocyanidins
$R'_3 = R'_5 = H$ Pelargonidin
$R'_3 = OH$ $R'_5 = H$ Cyanidin
$R'_3 = OH$ $R'_5 = OH$ Delphinidin
$R'_3 = R'_5 = OCH_3$ Malvidin

Fig. (3). Flavonoids with the B ring on C_2.

Classes of Flavonoids with the B Ring on C_3

Isoflavonoids have the 3-phenylchromen-4-one nucleus and are involved in the **phytoestrogens** pathway in **mammals** (Fig. **4**). They can be classified in isoflavones, such as genistein, found almost exclusively in Leguminosae and possess the 3-phenylchromen-4-one skeleton without the hydroxyl group at C2 in isoflavans, such as the nonsteroidal estrogen equol, when the skeleton is the 3-phenylchroman [29].

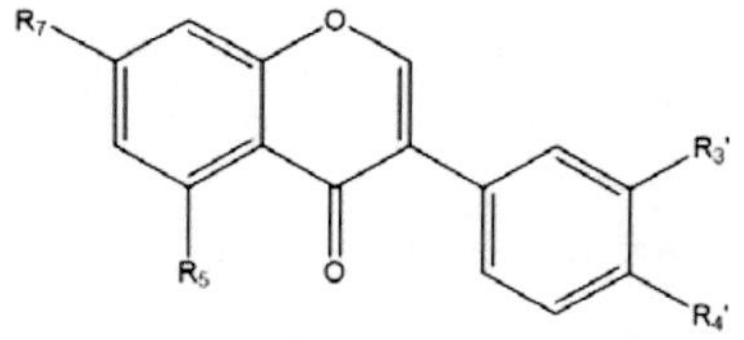

Isoflavones

$R_5 = R_7 = R'_4 = OH$	$R'_3 = H$	Genistein
$R_7 = R'_4 = OH$	$R_5 = R'_3 = H$	Daidzein

Fig. (4). Flavonoids with the B ring on C_3.

Classes of Flavonoids Where the B Ring is Connected to the C Ring Through the 4th Position

Neoflavonoids possess the 4-phenylchromen skeleton without the hydroxyl moiety at C2. Among the 4-arylcoumarin derivatives, called neoflavones, calophyllolide was isolated first [6], as well as dalbergichromene, and belongs to the 4-phenyl-2*H*-1-benzopyran derivatives called neoflavenes [30].

Classes of Open-Chain Flavonoids

Chalcones (Fig. **5**) or chalconoids, represent a subclass in which the C ring is absent [11]. Among chalconoids found in fruits and vegetables, there is phlorizin, that is, the glucosylated dihydrochalcone derived from the aglycone caphloretin [31], arbutin, glycosylated hydroquinone [32], chalconaringenin, from which spontaneous cyclization naringenin is obtained [33] and ellagic acid [34].

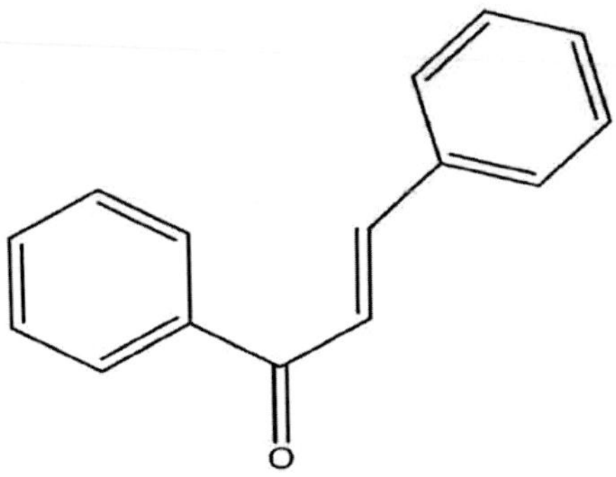

Chalcones

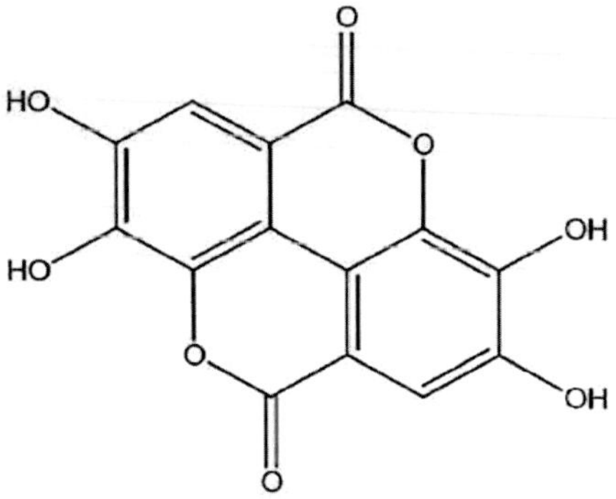

Ellagic acid

Fig. (5). Chalcones and chemical skeleton of ellagic acid.

PHARMACOLOGICAL ASPECTS OF POLYPHENOLS AND FLAVONOIDS

As described in the introduction section, the appropriate intake through the diet of polyphenolic compounds contained in fruits and vegetables could represent a valid approach in the prevention of the onset of chronic diseases, such as overweight and obesity, correlated inflammation, insulin resistance and diabetes, neurodegenerative and cardiovascular diseases and even various types of cancer [35 - 42]. These effects could be in part correlated with their inhibitive action on radical species of oxygen and nitrogen and with the ability to activate antioxidant enzymes, but it is also clear that each molecule could exerts more specific actions, not only attributable to its generic phenolic portion. A meta-analysis recently published [35] reports the correlation between flavonoid intake and life expectancy, with an evaluation of the associated total, cardiovascular and cancer risk. A lot of different factors were evaluated in the considered literature, among which age, sex and education level, body mass index and diabetes, habits such as smoking or physical activity, blood pressure, intake of healthy and non-healthy nutrients, such as vitamins and fibers or fatty acids, cholesterols and coffee, cardiovascular, cancer and other familiarities, and so on. The results of the meta-analysis indicated that flavonoid intake was inversely and significantly associated with total and cardiovascular risk but not with cancer mortality risk, a study whose reports are often contradictory. The conclusions support the potential protective role of polyphenols, also underlying the importance of the diet variety, including different flavonoid sources. But they also show the heterogenicity and different quality of the reviewed results. Effectively, many different aspects had to be evaluated with the aim of acquiring an overview of this complex issue. The specific character of every single molecule, as well as its capability to be absorbed and metabolized and give interaction with other nutrients or drugs, could also confer a specific activity connected to the interaction with complex biochemical pathways. The generical anti-inflammatory properties of flavonoids are probably connected to the inhibited formation of nitric oxide (NO) radicals, prostaglandin E_2, tumor necrosis factor alpha and specifically proinflammatory cytokines, such as the interleukins 1β and 6. A more specific action is shown by flavonone glucosides, acting as cyclooxygenase-2 (COX-2) inhibitors, or by quercetin in reducing cancer cells proliferation, inducing apoptosis and the expression of genes related to cyclin D1, involved in the cellular cycle, or finally by catechins supporting the immune system increasing antibody production [36]. The same authors reported that "the biologic potential of phenolic acids is as wide as their structural diversity", being able to act as antidepressant and neuroprotective as well as anticancer or antihyperglycemic, and even as enhancers of microbiota diversity with beneficium of cardiovascular and liver functionality. They conclude by asserting that clinical studies are needed to explore bioavailability, safety, and beneficial effects. One might also add that structure-activity relationship (SAR) studies, metabolism and toxicity need to be deepened to determine effective use of polyphenols as pharmaceutical compounds. Rolt & Cox [37] analysed polyphenols such as stilbenoids, flavonoids, and chalcones to support the molecular basis of inflammation and chronic disease prevention to provide a response to this strategy. Behind the scavenging action, these classes of compounds interact with transcription factors that regulate the oxidative status of cells. Resveratrol (Fig. **6**). and flavonoids represent molecules of particular interest due to their capacity to undergo highly stabilised radicals after reaction with superoxide anion or other oxygen radicals. The study of resveratrol isomers showed that molecules bearing *ortho* hydroxy groups were able to scavenge radicals at lower concentrations and molecules bearing hydroxy groups on both rings are more efficacious. Different derivatives, still retaining the resveratrol key features, provide or enhance the antiradical activity. The study conducted on flavonoids furtherly shows a more modulated activity connected with the different scaffolds. Flavones, isoflavones, flavanones, flavonols, and hydroxy flavanones were evaluated, showing that flavonols, having the best character of electron donors and the highest stabilization by resonance, represented the most potent antioxidant structures [37]. This is well shown by the comparison of the higher antiradical activity of quercetin with respect to luteolin, which only differs for the flavon (luteolin) and flavonols (quercetin) scaffold. Another important regulation key is represented by the transcription factor Nrf2 (nuclear factor erythroid 2-related factor 2), whose levels rise in the oxidized cells with the function of enhancing the antioxidant cellular mechanism. Consequently, the activation of Nrf2 signalling, induced by stilbenoids, flavonoids such as fisetin and its dihydroxy analogue in C_7, or chalcones, as well as other small molecules interfering by dithiol groups, ameliorates the age-related diseases. SAR studies have elucidated that the α,β-unsaturated carbonyl group is needed for this indirect antioxidant activity. In conclusion, the authors highlighted different polyvalent scaffolds, evidencing that compounds which simultaneously target multiple therapeutic pathways are more efficient in modulating and delaying age-related diseases, preventing oxidative stress, inflammation and cellular senescence. The ability of flavonoids to scavenge reactive species of oxygen and nitrogen, regardless of their sources, was also evaluated in another recent review as an effect on mitochondria activity, these organelles representing the main source of intracellular radical species [38]. Baicalein, silibinin, quercetin and catechins were found to protect several organs by the inhibition of the Fenton reaction and nitrosative stress, by increasing ATP levels and scavenging superoxide anion. Hippocampal, neuronal, heart, kidney and liver cells were protected against oxidative injuries through activation of antioxidant enzymes transcription in the nuclear factor erythroid 2-related factor 2 with a delay of all the relative associated chronic diseases, such as diabetes, cardiovascular and coronary heart, vasoconstriction, high blood pressure and stroke, Alzheimer's, Parkinson's and other chronic neurodegenerative and cardiac diseases [38]. Regarding dysmetabolic syndrome and obesity-related diseases, in the review by Sandoval *et al.* [39], the effect of the different groups of flavonoids on the liver and white and brown adipose tissue was evaluated, highlighting the involved molecular mechanism. According to the reported results, anthocyanins, catechins and proanthocyanidins activity in the liver is joined to the activation of adenosine monophosphate-activated protein kinase. This enzyme is involved in the metabolism of glucose and lipid oxidation, with the upregulation of glycolysis and fatty acid oxidation and downregulation of gluconeogenic and lipogenic genes. Flavonoids activity as SIRT1 (sirtuin 1) activators was discussed in the review by Sayed *et al.* [40]. SIRT1 is a member of the sirtuin protein implicated in the maintenance of health status and longevity, which in response to external and stress stimuli, regulates the gene expression and cell survival, decreasing the transcription nuclear factor kappa B (NF-kB) and cytokine release, through the inhibition of cyclooxygenase-2 and of inducible nitric oxide synthase enzymes. As counteract, downregulation of SIRT1 is correlated with increased acetylated NF-kB and the onset of the inflammatory cascade. Accordingly, many recent studies were reviewed about the potential of polyphenols, and particularly of flavonoids, alone or in combination, in the complex battle against cancer [34, 41 - 43]. Cancer onset, proliferation, migration and tumour cell dissemination, highly correlated with other diseases, such as obesity and inflammation, could be hindered by the appropriate use of a plethora of molecules, highly represented in vegetal, microbial and marine matrices, which could find application alone, or as phytocomplex, or better in combination with drugs usually adopted in cancer therapy. Many different polyphenolic molecules (some of which are reported in

Fig. **6**. were evaluated in the four cited reviews [34, 41 - 43], *e.g.,* the stilbene resveratrol, curcumin, coumaric acid, lignans as arctigenin, magnolol, honokiol; flavones, flavonols and flavonones as apigenin, luteolin and chrisin, quercetin, kaempferol, myricetin, taxifolin and fisetin, naringenin and hesperetin, as well as the corresponding glycosylated naringin, hesperidin and rutin; flavanols such as epigallocatechin gallate and catechin, isoflavones daidzein and genistein, the chalcone ellagic acid and the anthocyanin delphinidin.

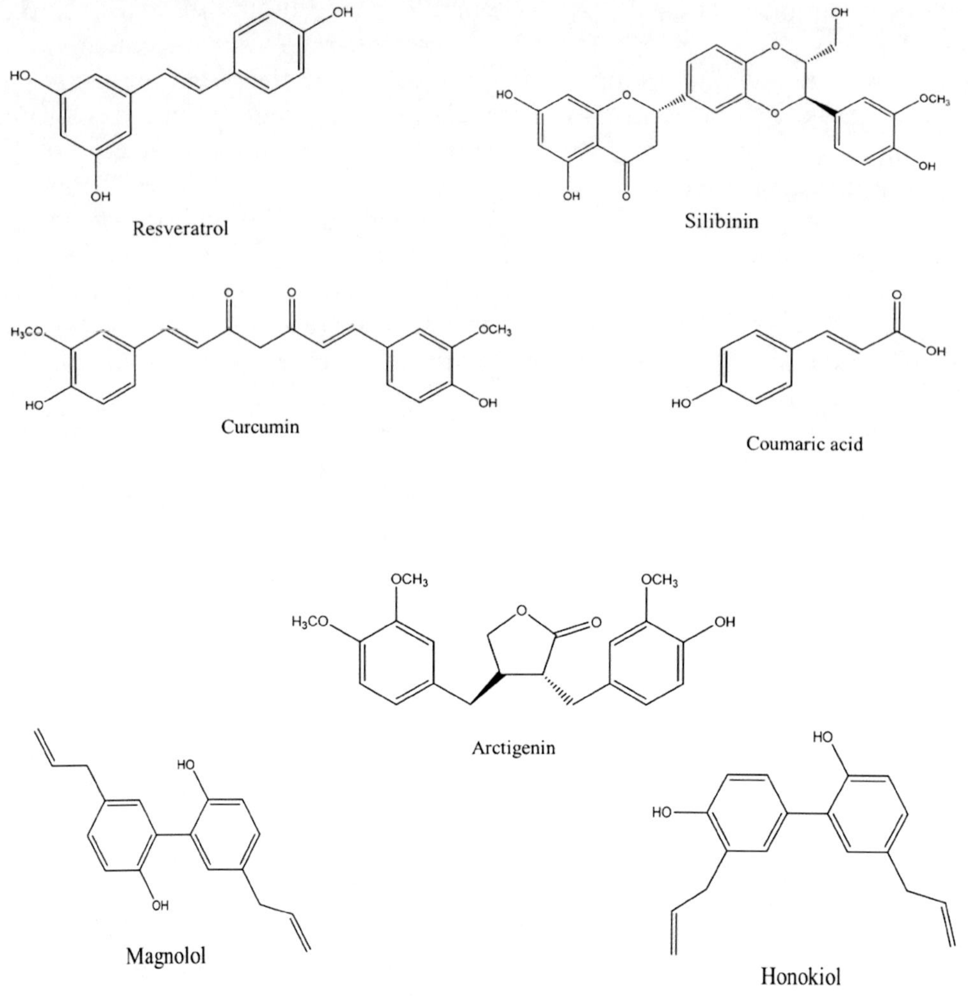

Fig. (6). Non-flavonoid polyphenols of pharmacological interest.

Many different action mechanisms, among which stand out the activity towards ROS and the inhibition of nitric oxide synthase, the activation of caspases, the inhibition of the transcription nuclear factor NF-kB and of the tumour nuclear factor TNF-α, the interleukins inhibition, the downregulation of COX-2, the modulation of p53 protein and of P-glycoprotein were evidenced. All these actions and many others explained in their role on specific signalling pathways, result, in turn, in DNA protection, inhibition of proliferation and promotion of apoptosis of cancer cells, inhibition of angiogenesis and metastatic processes, interference with other toxic drugs with an increase of cellular uptake, side effects reduction and amelioration of multidrug resistance. Highly correlated with the anti-inflammatory potential of these molecules are also the effects studied on rheumatoid arthritis [44] and neuropathic pain [45], the prevention of urinary tract infections [46], hyperuricemia [47], as well as the health effects shown on the prevention of chronic cardiovascular and neurodegenerative diseases [48 - 50]. In the review by Singh *et al.* [44], a series of 33 medicinal plants used against biomarkers of inflammation onset and progression was evaluated with the aim to show their efficacy against rheumatoid arthritis, an autoimmune disease characterized by rheumatic organ disease, as well as systemic implications. Conclusions indicate that polyphenols and flavonoids, such as gallic, vanillic and syringic acids, proanthocyanidins and tannins are active towards TNF-α, NF-kB and the correlated interleukins 1, 1a, 1b, 4, 6 and 17, as well as against COX-1 and -2, lipoperoxidase (LOX-1 and -2), inducible nitric oxide synthase (iNOS), prostaglandin E2 (PGE_2), mitogen-activated protein (MAP) kinase, preventing the joint damage, inflammation and pain, by targeting the inflammation mediators as a whole. Proinflammatory cytokines such as TNF-α and COX-2 are also produced in the case of nerve damage associated with neuropathic pain. Peripheral nerve injury causing sensitization and hyperexcitability, which lead to spontaneous, superficial, paroxysmal and finally neuropathic pain, is naturally counteracted by the γ-aminobutyric acid (GABA) activity. Two types of GABA receptors exist, GABA A and GABA B. GABA A receptor modulators, such as benzodiazepine drugs, were largely used in therapy. Flavonoids, with particular attention to 6-methoxy-flavones and flavanones, were widely studied for their activity as GABA A positive allosteric modulators [45]. Parkinson's disease and other neurodegenerative diseases are strictly associated with oxidative stress [49] because the degeneration of dopaminergic neurons of the substantia nigra could be induced by neurotoxic events highly correlated with the oxidative status, both in terms of radical oxygen species (ROS) production and of mitochondrial dysfunction, which could trigger downregulation of neurotrophic factors and promote protein aggregation. Besides Parkinson's, Alzheimer's and Huntington's diseases as well as multiple and amyotrophic lateral sclerosis, are induced by biochemical alterations strictly joined to cellular oxidative stress and ROS production. The phosphorylation of the nuclear erythroid 2-related factor 2/antioxidant response element (Nrf2/ARE) and its translocation in the cell nucleus is individuated as the key mechanism of flavonoid control of secondary oxidative stress. Many flavonoid structures such as flavanols catechin and epigallocatechin gallate, flavanones naringin, hesperetin and pinocembrin, flavononols as ampelopsin, flavones chrisin, baicalein, apigenin, luteolin, flavonols as quercetin, myricetin, fisetin, rutin, kaempferol, anthocyanidins as cyanidins and pelargonidins, isoflavones as genistein were all reported as anti-Parkinson bioactive molecules and deepened in their action mechanism [49]. As regards the isoflavones, well focused papers were also published in relation to their protective role as phytoestrogens in pregnancy, premenopausal and postmenopausal stages of a woman's life [51]. Besides isoflavones, dietary phytoestrogens were also recognized in coumestan and lignans structures, and relative studies indicate them as protective agents against osteoporosis progression, cardiometabolic and cognitive dysfunctions, breast and prostate cancer progression and menopausal symptoms. Among the modulating effects of the endocrine system, to these classes is recognized an action of thyroid stimulation, insulin-resistance amelioration and adiponectin activation, with overall positive effects on the prevention of the dysmetabolic syndrome [51]. Phytoestrogens can directly bind the estrogenic receptors, with different affinity for the α and β classes, which result in a modulated protection activity. Finally, in the last year, many studies were carried on in relation to the antiviral [52] and anti-COVID 19 (Coronavirus Disease 2019) potential [53]. Different flavonoids were already recognized for their antiviral activity. For example, apigenin, luteolin, quercetin, naringenin, and diosmetin were studied for their anti-HCV activity, epigallocatechin-3-gallate for anti-HCV (Hepatitis C virus), anti-HBV (Hepatitis B virus) and anti-HIV (Human immunodeficiency virus) activity, vitexin for anti-H1N1 (Hemagglutinin Type 1 and Neuraminidase Type 1 influenza virus) and anti-HAV (Hepatitis A virus) activity, myricetin for anti-HIV activity, vitexin and quercetin-3-rhamnoside against influenza virus, baicalin against Dengue virus, pinocembrin against Zika virus. The main antiviral mechanism is recognized in the inhibition of different enzymes essential for viral survival and replication, such as DNA/RNA polymerase, neuraminidase or proteases. Among flavonoids, a synergistic effect or absorption increase could be modulated by the same chemical compounds or by other metabolites present in the different phytocomplex [51]. In the last year, data were also collected to evaluate the potential capacity of specific known and less known flavonoid molecules to counteract COVID-19. Forty-seven molecules were well-known or very few widespread chalcones, flavans, flavanols, flavanons, flavanonols, flavones, isoflavones and procyanidins, were identified as lead compounds, mainly focusing the attention on their interference with 3-CL (3-chymotrypsi--like) and PL (papain-like) viral proteases. These represent, in fact, key targets involved in the genomic RNA replication and transcription within host cells. Deepened studies on the structure activity relations are reported, which seems to be very relevant for designing new potent drugs in this new challenge involving the scientific community.

BIOAVAILABILITY AND METABOLISM OF FLAVONOIDS, TOXICOLOGICAL ACTIVITY AND SEMI-SYNTHETIC STRATEGIES

The pharmacological effects of flavonoids are influenced not only by the great variety in the chemical structures but also by the natural source from which they are obtained, the concentration in the food intake, and the interaction with other dietary molecules. Therapeutic efficacy depends on the bioavailability and on metabolism of these bioactive phenolic derivatives [54, 55]. Furthermore, regarding their pharmacokinetic properties, absorption, distribution, metabolism and elimination (ADME), it is also important to consider the inter-individual differences and variability in the population [56, 57]. The bioavailability of flavonoids may actually differ from one individual to another and their metabolic pathway is influenced also by the microbiome in the intestinal tract. In fact, flavonoids are exposed to resident microorganisms reacting with them and converting these compounds into smaller aromatic and phenolic derivatives [58]. Another factor to be taken into consideration for the use of flavonoids as therapeutic tools, besides the bioavailability and metabolism, is represented by the problems related to their extraction. In fact, as flavonoids possess very similar chemical structures, the isolation and purification processes could be long and labor intensive. Therefore, research in recent years is also focusing on the study of new strategies in order to more easily obtain specific products. In particular, semi-synthetic natural flavonoids can be investigated from the point of view of the structure-activity relationship (SAR) to obtain specific information on the pharmacodynamics of these bioactive compounds [59].

ADME of Flavonoids

As reported in Fig. 7, flavonoids taken within the diet are mostly not absorbed in the small intestine and when they arrive in the colon tract, they interact with the local microbiota and are subjected to the action of hydrolysis. Flavonoids are metabolized in the epithelium and the derivatives are carried to the liver, metabolized again with phase I and phase II mechanisms and can return in the intestine through the biliary tract or reach systemic circulation and target tissues. Finally, flavonoid metabolites are excreted by kidneys and by the fecal route [55, 60].

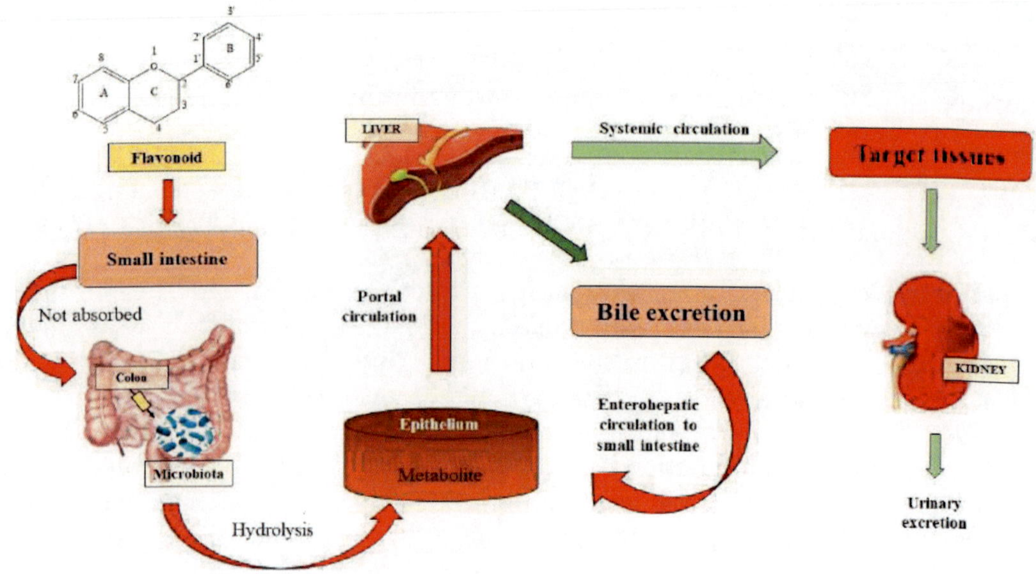

Fig. (7). Example scheme of flavonoids metabolism.

In detail, with the exception of anthocyanins, which arrive in plasma and urinary tract in the form of glycosides [43], flavonoid glycosides are generally hydrolyzed before absorption in two different ways. In the small intestine, they are subjected to the action of the transmembrane enzymatic protein lactase phlorizin hydrolase (LPH, lactase) and transformed into aglycones endowed with greater lipophilicity that allows them to enter the epithelium by passive diffusion. Otherwise, the glycoside forms are carried in the epithelial cells by sodium-dependent glucose transporter and then they are converted into aglycone thanks to intracellular *β*-glucosidases [61, 63]. The transcellular transport of flavonoids takes place thanks to membrane bound ATP binding cassette (ABC) transport proteins, such as P-glycoprotein and multidrug resistance proteins, that influence flavonoids' bioavailability by acting in two different ways. They could enhance bioavailability by allowing the flux of flavonoids from the intestinal cells into the portal bloodstream or, otherwise, decrease bioavailability by carrying the molecules back into the intestinal lumen [63]. In the liver, flavonoids are converted in the oxidated or *O*-demethylated forms, thanks to the activity of cytochrome P450 (CYP) monooxygenases such as CYP3A4 and CYP2C9 isoforms [64]. Flavonoids, not absorbed by the small intestine, undergo the action of the enzymes produced by microflora in the large intestine, resulting in the formation of aglycones and phenolic acid derivatives [65]. All these aglycone metabolites are available for conjugation by phase II metabolism with the reactions of methylation, glucuronidation, or sulphation by catechol-*O*-

methyltransferases (COMTs, whose reaction concerns the catecholic flavonoids like catechins, epicatechins, and epigallocatechins), urine-5'-diphosphate glucuronosyltransferases (UGTs), and sulphotransferases. By these reactions occurring in the intestine or in the liver, the resulting conjugated derivatives reach the bloodstream and are distributed in tissues [66]. Finally, a portion of metabolites is collected in the renal tubules through organic anion transporters and eliminated through the urine [67], whereas some of the metabolites are excreted through the biliary duct, and, thanks to enterohepatic recirculation, they come back in the intestine and undergo fecal elimination [68]. On the other hand, as regards the polymeric forms such as proanthocyanidins, only a few pharmacokinetic data are available and the *in vitro* and *in vivo* experiments show that their absorption is much lower than flavonoid monomers. Proanthocyanidins were detected in plasma with a degree of polymerization not higher than the dimer forms [65], maybe because they are hydrolyzed in the stomach by acid [69], even if the buffering effect of a specific food may differ from another and this could influence the stomach acidity necessary for their hydrolysis. So, as a result, there is also evidence of oligomer stability during gastric transit [70].

Factors that Could Affect ADME of Flavonoids

Flavonoids are taken within the diet together with other components present in foods such as proteins, carbohydrates, fats and ethanol. Even if the consumption of milk has no significant impact on the absorption of flavanols [69], quercetin and kaempferol present in green or black tea [72] reduce the bioavailability of epicatechin from dark chocolate [73]. Several studies have shown that bread and sugar can improve the bioavailability of catechin and epicatechin thanks to the enhanced secretions and motility in the stomach. Furthermore, it has been detected that ethanol in red wine considerably improves the elimination of catechins in urine, probably in relation to its diuretic action [65, 74]. An example of how fats taken with diet can affect the permanence in the gastrointestinal tract is given by a study on human patients in which it was proven that, when strawberries are eaten with cream, the excretion of anthocyanin metabolites is delayed even if without changes in AUC [75]. Another clinical experiment explained that the AUC of quercetin in plasma was elevated when a fat-rich breakfast was eaten in comparison to its bioavailability in subjects who consumed a fat-free breakfast [76]. With regard to the influence of sex and age on the human metabolism and bioavailability of flavonoids, there are restricted studies that demonstrate a correlation between age or sex with the activity of phase I and phase II enzymes on these molecules. Some experiments have shown that in females, the expression and activity of glucuronidation enzymes are higher than those of the male population [77], and some data claim that the metabolism of these bioactive compounds is reduced with age because of age-related metabolic ability [78]. However, at the moment, it is not possible to draw appropriate conclusions and more studies are needed. Other experiments are also required to investigate the impact of the genetic variability on phase I and phase II enzymes on the inter-individual differences in flavonoid pharmacokinetics [56]. Regarding the drug-drug interactions with natural compounds, the impact of the assumption of drugs in flavonoid metabolism and activity is plausible, even if more studies are necessary. For example, some data have been collected on silymarin, an extract from milk thistle which contains flavonolignan silibinin (Fig. **6**). which possesses anti-inflammatory, anti-oxidant, anti-diabetic and anti-neurodegenerative effects. In fact, silymarin finds applications against diseases affecting the liver, pancreas, central nervous system, kidney, and heart. The experiments show that the administration of silymarin enhances the bioavailability of the β-blocker talinolol and of the anti-sickness drug domperidone, whereas it reduces the bioavailability of the antimicrobic metronidazole and of the antiviral indinavir. Silybin also influences the pharmacokinetics of antihypertensive losartan, reducing its conversion into the active form [79]. Among the many factors that can influence the bioavailability of flavonoids, their interaction with the efflux transporter P-glycoprotein must be taken into consideration, although the specific mechanisms of interaction are still unknown. P-glycoprotein is an ATP-dependent efflux pump [80], which affects the flux of drugs and could reduce the access of flavonoids into the systemic circulation and into the blood-brain barrier (BBB), limiting the bioavailability and the neuroprotection explained by some flavonoids. Indeed, depending on the type of binding/interactions of the flavonoids with the steroid-interacting regions and ATP binding sites in the P-glycoprotein nucleotide binding domains, the permeability of flavonoids or their circulating metabolites, and so their efficacy, could be reduced or enhanced. Regarding the ability of some flavonoids and their metabolites to cross the blood-brain barrier, recent findings have shown that hesperetin, naringenin, their glucuronidated metabolites, cyanidin-3-rutinoside and pelargonidin-3-glucoside, permeated *in vitro* the blood-brain barrier, according to their lipophilicity [81]. In a comparison of the permeability of sucrose, which is a marker of paracellular transport, the permeability of the more lipophilic hesperetin and naringenin was higher than that of the sucrose, suggesting their transcellular flux, while the permeabilities of the glucuronide conjugates of hesperetin and naringenin and the permeability of the anthocyanins were poorer than that of sucrose. However, further investigations are needed to better understand the pharmacokinetic profiles of flavonoids, which also means better identifying their localization in the central nervous system and the correlation with neuroprotective effects and pharmacological activity against neurodegenerative diseases [82].

Toxicity of Flavonoids

Due to the beneficial effects of flavonoids for human health, it is worth taking into account their possible toxic effects, which may be due to their chemical properties, the interactions with other molecules and the concentration after consumption. In fact, evidence has demonstrated that when administered at high doses, phenolic bioactive compounds could produce reactive oxygen species (pro-oxidant activity); moreover, they could be involved in negatively regulating the expression of chaperones and antioxidant enzymes, they could have hepatotoxic and nephrotoxic effects and worsen some pathologies of the digestive system like colitis and colon tumor [83]. Conversely, in an experiment carried out on rats, Cladis *et al.* [84] observed that the oral administration of blueberry polyphenols, at a range of concentration from 0 to 1000 mg total polyphenols/kg bw/day for three months, did not cause changes in behavior, body weight, consumption of food, development of pathologies at the maximum concentration given. The toxic action of flavonoids is influenced also by way of assumption and the resulting biotransformation that occurs in the body. In fact, Zheleva-Dimitrova *et al.* [85] established that the toxicity levels of *Clinopodium vulgare* L. aqueous extract, which is a source of flavonoids, in mice and rats depended on the route of administration because the LD_{50} (Lethal Dose 50) in acute intraperitoneal administration reached at lower concentrations (675 mg/kg for mice and 500 mg/kg for rats, with central nervous system toxicity) than those of the oral administration for which LD_{50} was major than 2000 mg/kg. This evidence demonstrates the importance of *in vivo* experiments and clinical trials to assess the safe doses of flavonoids taken with a daily diet [36].

Strategies for a Better Investigation of Flavonoids Properties

Since it is not easy to obtain information from a specific natural compound due to the difficulty of separation and purification from complex matrices during the extraction processes, in order to evaluate the structure-activity relationship and the mechanism of action of the natural products, in recent years, research has also focused on the study of new semisynthetic strategies regarding natural bioactive compounds [86]. Moreover, the use of polymers such as cyclodextrins and nanoparticles could modify the solubility and could regulate the metabolism of natural molecules, and more specifically flavonoids, with the aim of improving their bioavailability and the therapeutic efficacy for the prevention and the management of several human diseases [87]. Among the semi-synthetic approaches, reactions of acetylation, methylation, hydrogenation, and cyclization of several flavonoids isolated from *Eriosema* genus have been described and the resulting synthetic derivatives have shown to possess interesting pharmacological properties such as antifungal, antimicrobial, antioxidant effects and also activity against erectile dysfunctions [88]. Another example of a semi-synthetic approach is given by the use of xanthohumol, which is a prenylated chalconoid found in the female inflorescences of *Humulus lupulus* [89], for the production of the isomers 8-prenylnaringenin and 6-prenylnaringenin, which are two secondary metabolites in hops, endowed with estrogen-like, cytotoxic, and neuro-regenerative effects. Because of the poor yield reached from their extraction, these two flavonoids can be formed from the demethylation, with lithium chloride and dimethylformamide, of xanthohumol, obtainable from the extraction industry of lupulus. The problem of this traditional method is given by the presence of by-products and the low amount of the desirable products. To avoid this inconvenience, microwave-assisted demethylation of xanthohumol could be used to optimize the temperature and the time of the reaction, using lithium chloride and dimethylformamide as not-expensive reagents, in order to achieve a final yield of 76% of 8-prenylnaringenin and 6-prenylnaringenin without by-products [90]. These new methodologies to produce natural derivatives demonstrate the importance of obtaining pure bioactive compounds of therapeutic interest that can thus be better investigated from the pharmaceutical point of view as potential drugs for the prevention and treatment of several pathologies.

CONCLUSION

Phenolic compounds extracted from plants have been shown to possess a wide spectrum of biological activities and focusing on the many classes and subclasses of polyphenols and flavonoids, there is evidence of their pharmacological properties that make them of interest to the development of new drugs. In this context, several experiments and molecular docking studies have been carried out in order to better understand their mechanism of action. Many research works have been designed to obtain information on the pharmacokinetic, safety and toxicity profiles. Moreover, different extraction techniques and semisynthetic strategies are investigated with the aim of improving the purity profile of these molecules in order to better analyze them from the pharmaceutical point of view. In conclusion, the deepening of these studies together with the implementation of preclinical and clinical trials, allows defining polyphenols and flavonoids as potential therapeutic tools with applications in preventing and treating many human pathologies.

CONSENT FOR PUBLICATION

Not applicable.

CONFLICT OF INTEREST

The authors declare no conflict of interest, financial or otherwise.

ACKNOWLEDGEMENTS

Declared none.

REFERENCES

[1] Santini, A.; Novellino, E.; Armini, V.; Ritieni, A. State of the art of Ready-to-Use Therapeutic Food: A tool for nutraceuticals addition to foodstuff. *Food Chem.,* **2013**, *140*(4), 843-849. [http://dx.doi.org/10.1016/j.foodchem.2012.10.098] [PMID: 23692774]

[2] Falzon, C.C.; Balabanova, A. Phytotherapy. *Prim. Care,* **2017**, *44*(2), 217-227. [http://dx.doi.org/10.1016/j.pop.2017.02.001] [PMID: 28501226]

[3] Piccolella, S.; Crescente, G.; Candela, L.; Pacifico, S. Nutraceutical polyphenols: New analytical challenges and opportunities. *J. Pharm. Biomed. Anal.,* **2019**, *175*, 112774. [http://dx.doi.org/10.1016/j.jpba.2019.07.022] [PMID: 31336288]

[4] Chaudhari, R.T.M.; Gunjan, M. A Novel approach towards phytosomal flavonoids. *Pharma Sci. Monitor,* **2012**, *3*(3), 3947-3963.

[5] Vuolo, M.M.; Lima, V.S.; Marostica, M.R., Junior Woodhead Publishing: Sawston Cambridge, RU., **2019**. Phenolic compounds: structure, classification, and antioxidant power

[6] Panche, A.N.; Diwan, A.D.; Chandra, S.R. Flavonoids: an overview. *J. Nutr. Sci.,* **2016**, *5*(47), e47. [http://dx.doi.org/10.1017/jns.2016.41] [PMID: 28620474]

[7] Dzah, C.S.; Duan, Y.; Zhang, H.; Serwah Boateng, N.A.; Ma, H. Latest developments in polyphenol recovery and purification from plant by-products: A review. *Trends Food Sci. Technol.,* **2020**, *99*, 375-388. [http://dx.doi.org/10.1016/j.tifs.2020.03.003]

[8] Jablonsky, M.; Nosalova, J.; Sládková, A.; Haz, A.; Kreps, F.; Valka, J.; Miertus, S.; Frecer, V.; Ondrejovic, M.; Sima, J.; Surina, I. Valorisation of softwood bark through extraction of utilizable chemicals. A review. *Biotechnol. Adv.,* **2017**, *35*(6), 726-750. [http://dx.doi.org/10.1016/j.biotechadv.2017.07.007] [PMID: 28739505]

[9] Cotas, J.; Leandro, A.; Monteiro, P.; Pacheco, D.; Figueirinha, A.; Gonçalves, A.M.M.; da Silva, G.J.; Pereira, L. Seaweed Phenolics: From Extraction to Applications. *Mar. Drugs,* **2020**, *18*(8), 384. [http://dx.doi.org/10.3390/md18080384] [PMID: 32722220]

[10] Pérez-Sánchez, A.; Barrajón-Catalán, E.; Herranz López, M.; Micol, V. Nutraceuticals for skin care: A comprehensive review of human clinical studies. *Nutrients,* **2018**, *10*(4), 403. [http://dx.doi.org/10.3390/nu10040403] [PMID: 29587342]

[11] Karak, P. Biological activities of flavonoids: An overview. *Int. J. Pharm. Sci. Res.,* **2019**, *10*(4), 1567-1574.

[12] Assadpour, E.; Mahdi Jafari, S. A systematic review on nanoencapsulation of food bioactive ingredients and nutraceuticals by various nanocarriers. *Crit. Rev. Food Sci. Nutr.,* **2019**, *59*(19), 3129-3151. [http://dx.doi.org/10.1080/10408398.2018.1484687] [PMID: 29883187]

[13] Gonçalves, R.F.S.; Martins, J.T.; Duarte, C.M.M.; Vicente, A.A.; Pinheiro, A.C. Advances in nutraceutical delivery systems: From formulation design for bioavailability enhancement to efficacy and safety evaluation. *Trends Food Sci. Technol.,* **2018**, *78*, 270-291. [http://dx.doi.org/10.1016/j.tifs.2018.06.011]

[14] Braithwaite, M.C.; Tyagi, C.; Tomar, L.K.; Kumar, P.; Choonara, Y.E.; Pillay, V. Nutraceutical-based therapeutics and formulation strategies augmenting their efficiency to complement modern medicine: An overview. *J. Funct. Foods,* **2014**, *6*, 82-99. [http://dx.doi.org/10.1016/j.jff.2013.09.022]

[15] Zhao, J.; Yang, J.; Xie, Y. Improvement strategies for the oral bioavailability of poorly water-soluble flavonoids: An overview. *Int. J. Pharm.*, **2019**, *570*, 118642. [http://dx.doi.org/10.1016/j.ijpharm.2019.118642] [PMID: 31446024]

[16] Cook, N.; Samman, S. Flavonoids--Chemistry, metabolism, cardioprotective effects, and dietary sources. *J. Nutr. Biochem.*, **1996**, *7*(2), 66-76. [http://dx.doi.org/10.1016/0955-2863(95)00168-9]

[17] Wen, K.; Fang, X.; Yang, J.; Yao, Y.; Nandakumar, K.S.; Salem, M.L.; Cheng, K. Recent Research on Flavonoids and their Biomedical Applications. *Curr. Med. Chem.*, **2021**, *28*(5), 1042-1066. [http://dx.doi.org/10.2174/0929867327666200713184138] [PMID: 32660393]

[18] Silva, A.S.; Reboredo-Rodríguez, P.; Süntar, I.; Sureda, A.; Belwal, T.; Loizzo, M.R.; Tundis, R.; Sobarzo-Sanchez, E.; Rastrelli, L.; Forbes-Hernandez, T.Y.; Battino, M.; Filosa, R.; Daglia, M.; Nabavi, S.F.; Nabavi, S.M. Evaluation of the *status quo* of polyphenols analysis: Part I—phytochemistry, bioactivity, interactions, and industrial uses. *Compr. Rev. Food Sci. Food Saf.*, **2020**, *19*(6), 3191-3218. [http://dx.doi.org/10.1111/1541-4337.12629] [PMID: 33337062]

[19] Hostetler, G.L.; Ralston, R.A.; Schwartz, S.J. Flavones: Food sources, bioavailability, metabolism, and bioactivity. *Adv. Nutr.*, **2017**, *8*(3), 423-435. [http://dx.doi.org/10.3945/an.116.012948] [PMID: 28507008]

[20] Li, Y.; Yao, J.; Han, C.; Yang, J.; Chaudhry, M.; Wang, S.; Liu, H.; Yin, Y. Quercetin, inflammation and immunity. *Nutrients,* **2016**, *8*(3), 167. [http://dx.doi.org/10.3390/nu8030167] [PMID: 26999194]

[21] Murkovic, M. Phenolic Compounds: Occurrence, Classes, and Analysis.*The Encyclopedia of Food and Health,* 1st ed; Caballero, B.; Finglas, P.M.; Toldrá, F., Eds.; Academic Press: Kidlington/Oxford, UK, **2016**, pp. 346-351. [http://dx.doi.org/10.1016/B978-0-12-384947-2.00539-0]

[22] Bernatoniene, J.; Kopustinskiene, D. The role of catechins in cellular responses to oxidative stress. *Molecules,* **2018**, *23*(4), 965. [http://dx.doi.org/10.3390/molecules23040965] [PMID: 29677167]

[23] Nakajima, J.; Tanaka, Y.; Yamazaki, M.; Saito, K. Reaction mechanism from leucoanthocyanidin to anthocyanidin 3-glucoside, a key reaction for coloring in anthocyanin biosynthesis. *J. Biol. Chem.*, **2001**, *276*(28), 25797-25803. [http://dx.doi.org/10.1074/jbc.M100744200] [PMID: 11316805]

[24] Rauf, A.; Imran, M.; Abu-Izneid, T.; Iahtisham-Ul-Haq, ; Patel, S.; Pan, X.; Naz, S.; Sanches Silva, A.; Saeed, F.; Rasul Suleria, H.A. Proanthocyanidins: A comprehensive review. *Biomed. Pharmacother.*, **2019**, *116*, 108999. [http://dx.doi.org/10.1016/j.biopha.2019.108999] [PMID: 31146109]

[25] Das, A.B.; Goud, V.V.; Das, C. Phenolic compounds as functional ingredients in beverages. In: *Value-Added Ingredients and Enrichments of Beverages*; Grumezesco, A.M.; Holban, A.M., Eds.; Academic Press: Cambridge, Massachusetts, **2019**; pp. 285-323. [http://dx.doi.org/10.1016/B978-0-12-816687-1.00009-6]

[26] Lewinsohn, E.; Britsch, L.; Mazur, Y.; Gressel, J. Flavanone glycoside biosynthesis in Citrus: Chalcone synthase, UDP-glucose: Flavanone-7-O-glucosyl-transferase and-rhamnosyl-transferase activities in cell-free extracts. *Plant Physiol.*, **1989**, *91*(4), 1323-1328. [http://dx.doi.org/10.1104/pp.91.4.1323] [PMID: 16667183]

[27] Lee, S.B.; Cha, K.H.; Selenge, D.; Solongo, A.; Nho, C.W. The chemopreventive effect of taxifolin is exerted through ARE-dependent gene regulation. *Biol. Pharm. Bull.*, **2007**, *30*(6), 1074-1079. [http://dx.doi.org/10.1248/bpb.30.1074] [PMID: 17541156]

[28] Khoo, H.E.; Azlan, A.; Tang, S.T.; Lim, S.M. Anthocyanidins and anthocyanins: colored pigments as

food, pharmaceutical ingredients, and the potential health benefits. *Food Nutr. Res.,* **2017**, *61*(1), 1361779.
[http://dx.doi.org/10.1080/16546628.2017.1361779] [PMID: 28970777]

[29] Franke, A.A.; Lai, J.F.; Halm, B.M. Absorption, distribution, metabolism, and excretion of isoflavonoids after soy intake. *Arch. Biochem. Biophys.,* **2014**, *559*, 24-28.
[http://dx.doi.org/10.1016/j.abb.2014.06.007] [PMID: 24946051]

[30] Li, S.R.; Chen, L.Y.; Tsai, J.C.; Tzeng, J.Y.; Tsai, I.L.; Wang, E.C. New syntheses of dalbergichromene and dalbergin from vanillin *via* neoflavene intermediate. *Tetrahedron Lett.,* **2007**, *48*(12), 2139-2141.
[http://dx.doi.org/10.1016/j.tetlet.2007.01.117]

[31] Miyamoto, L.; Tsuchiya, K. Sodium-glucose transporters as a therapeutic target for diabetes from the viewpoint of drug discovery and pharmacotherapy. *Yakugaku zasshi. Yakugaku Zasshi,* **2018**, *138*(7), 933-938.
[http://dx.doi.org/10.1248/yakushi.17-00223-1] [PMID: 29962472]

[32] Zhou, H.; Zhao, J.; Li, A.; Reetz, M.T. Chemical and Biocatalytic Routes to Arbutin †. *Molecules,* **2019**, *24*(18), 3303.
[http://dx.doi.org/10.3390/molecules24183303] [PMID: 31514332]

[33] Yadav, V.R.; Prasad, S.; Sung, B.; Aggarwal, B.B. The role of chalcones in suppression of NF-κ--mediated inflammation and cancer. *Int. Immunopharmacol.,* **2011**, *11*(3), 295-309.
[http://dx.doi.org/10.1016/j.intimp.2010.12.006] [PMID: 21184860]

[34] Montané, X.; Kowalczyk, O.; Reig-Vano, B.; Bajek, A.; Roszkowski, K.; Tomczyk, R.; Pawliszak, W.; Giamberini, M.; Mocek-Płóciniak, A.; Tylkowski, B. Current perspectives of the applications of polyphenols and flavonoids in cancer therapy. *Molecules,* **2020**, *25*(15), 3342.
[http://dx.doi.org/10.3390/molecules25153342] [PMID: 32717865]

[35] Mazidi, M.; Katsiki, N.; Banach, M. A greater flavonoid intake is associated with lower total and cause-specific mortality: a meta-analysis of cohort studies. *Nutrients,* **2020**, *12*(8), 2350.
[http://dx.doi.org/10.3390/nu12082350] [PMID: 32781562]

[36] de Araújo, F.F.; de Paulo Farias, D.; Neri-Numa, I.A.; Pastore, G.M. Polyphenols and their applications: An approach in food chemistry and innovation potential. *Food Chem.,* **2020**, *127535*
[http://dx.doi.org/10.1016/j.foodchem.2020.127535] [PMID: 32798817]

[37] Rolt, A.; Cox, L.S. Structural basis of the anti-ageing effects of polyphenolics: mitigation of oxidative stress. *BMC Chem.,* **2020**, *14*(1), 50.
[http://dx.doi.org/10.1186/s13065-020-00696-0] [PMID: 32793891]

[38] Kicinska, A.; Jarmuszkiewicz, W. Flavonoids and Mitochondria: Activation of Cytoprotective Pathways? *Molecules,* **2020**, *25*(13), 3060.
[http://dx.doi.org/10.3390/molecules25133060] [PMID: 32635481]

[39] Sandoval, V.; Sanz-Lamora, H.; Arias, G.; Marrero, P.F.; Haro, D.; Relat, J. Metabolic impact of flavonoids consumption in obesity: From central to peripheral. *Nutrients,* **2020**, *12*(8), 2393.
[http://dx.doi.org/10.3390/nu12082393] [PMID: 32785059]

[40] Sayed, A.M.; Hassanein, E.H.M.; Salem, S.H.; Hussein, O.E.; Mahmoud, A.M. Flavonoids-mediated SIRT1 signaling activation in hepatic disorders. *Life Sci.,* **2020**, *259*, 118173.
[http://dx.doi.org/10.1016/j.lfs.2020.118173] [PMID: 32750437]

[41] Pourakbari, R.; Taher, S.M.; Mosayyebi, B.; Ayoubi-Joshaghani, M.H.; Ahmadi, H.; Aghebati-Maleki, L. Implications for glycosylated compounds and their anti-cancer effects. *Int. J. Biol. Macromol.,* **2020**, *163*, 1323-1332.
[http://dx.doi.org/10.1016/j.ijbiomac.2020.06.281] [PMID: 32622770]

[42] Siddiqui, S.S.; Rahman, S.; Rupasinghe, H.P.V.; Vazhappilly, C.G. Dietary Flavonoids in p53—Mediated Immune Dysfunctions Linking to Cancer Prevention. *Biomedicines,* **2020**, *8*(8), 286.

[http://dx.doi.org/10.3390/biomedicines8080286] [PMID: 32823757]

[43] Cao, G.; Muccitelli, H.U.; Sánchez-Moreno, C.; Prior, R.L. Anthocyanins are absorbed in glycated forms in elderly women: a pharmacokinetic study. *Am. J. Clin. Nutr.,* **2001**, *73*(5), 920-926. [http://dx.doi.org/10.1093/ajcn/73.5.920] [PMID: 11333846]

[44] Singh, S.; Singh, T.G.; Mahajan, K.; Dhiman, S. Medicinal plants used against various inflammatory biomarkers for the management of rheumatoid arthritis. *J. Pharm. Pharmacol.,* **2020**, *72*(10), 1306-1327. [http://dx.doi.org/10.1111/jphp.13326] [PMID: 32812250]

[45] Uddin, M.S.; Mamun, A.A.; Rahman, M.A.; Kabir, M.T.; Alkahtani, S.; Alanazi, I.S.; Perveen, A.; Ashraf, G.M.; Bin-Jumah, M.N.; Abdel-Daim, M.M. Exploring the promise of flavonoids to combat neuropathic pain: From molecular mechanisms to therapeutic implications. *Front. Neurosci.,* **2020**, *14*, 478. [http://dx.doi.org/10.3389/fnins.2020.00478] [PMID: 32587501]

[46] González de Llano, D.; Moreno-Arribas, M.V.; Bartolomé, B. Cranberry polyphenols and prevention against urinary tract infections: relevant considerations. *Molecules,* **2020**, *25*(15), 3523. [http://dx.doi.org/10.3390/molecules25153523] [PMID: 32752183]

[47] Jiang, L.L.; Gong, X.; Ji, M.Y.; Wang, C.C.; Wang, J.H.; Li, M.H. Bioactive compounds from plant-based functional foods: a promising choice for the prevention and management of hyperuricemia. *Foods,* **2020**, *9*(8), 973. [http://dx.doi.org/10.3390/foods9080973] [PMID: 32717824]

[48] Mattioli, R.; Francioso, A.; Mosca, L.; Silva, P. Anthocyanins: A comprehensive review of their chemical properties and health effects on cardiovascular and neurodegenerative diseases. *Molecules,* **2020**, *25*(17), 3809. [http://dx.doi.org/10.3390/molecules25173809] [PMID: 32825684]

[49] Kim, T.Y.; Leem, E.; Lee, J.M.; Kim, S.R. Control of reactive oxygen species for the prevention of Parkinson's disease: the possible application of flavonoids. *Antioxidants,* **2020**, *9*(7), 583. [http://dx.doi.org/10.3390/antiox9070583] [PMID: 32635299]

[50] Batiha, G.E.S.; Beshbishy, A.M.; Ikram, M.; Mulla, Z.S.; El-Hack, M.E.A.; Taha, A.E.; Algammal, A.M.; Elewa, Y.H.A. The pharmacological activity, biochemical properties, and pharmacokinetics of the major natural polyphenolic flavonoid: quercetin. *Foods,* **2020**, *9*(3), 374. [http://dx.doi.org/10.3390/foods9030374] [PMID: 32210182]

[51] Domínguez-López, I.; Yago-Aragón, M.; Salas-Huetos, A.; Tresserra-Rimbau, A.; Hurtado-Barroso, S. Effects of dietary phytoestrogens on hormones throughout a human lifespan: A review. *Nutrients,* **2020**, *12*(8), 2456. [http://dx.doi.org/10.3390/nu12082456] [PMID: 32824177]

[52] Ninfali, P.; Antonelli, A.; Magnani, M.; Scarpa, E.S. Antiviral properties of flavonoids and delivery strategies. *Nutrients,* **2020**, *12*(9), 2534. [http://dx.doi.org/10.3390/nu12092534] [PMID: 32825564]

[53] Solnier, J.; Fladerer, J.P. Flavonoids: A complementary approach to conventional therapy of COVID-19? *Phytochem. Rev.,* **2020**, •••, 1-23. [http://dx.doi.org/10.1007/s11101-020-09720-6] [PMID: 32982616]

[54] Iglesias-Carres, L.; Mas-Capdevila, A.; Bravo, F.I.; Aragonès, G.; Arola-Arnal, A.; Muguerza, B. A comparative study on the bioavailability of phenolic compounds from organic and nonorganic red grapes. *Food Chem.,* **2019**, *299*, 125092. [http://dx.doi.org/10.1016/j.foodchem.2019.125092] [PMID: 31280001]

[55] Cassidy, A.; Minihane, A.M. The role of metabolism (and the microbiome) in defining the clinical efficacy of dietary flavonoids. *Am. J. Clin. Nutr.,* **2017**, *105*(1), 10-22. [http://dx.doi.org/10.3945/ajcn.116.136051] [PMID: 27881391]

[56] Lampe, J.; Chang, J. Interindividual differences in phytochemical metabolism and disposition. *Semin. Cancer Biol.,* **2007**, *17*(5), 347-353.
[http://dx.doi.org/10.1016/j.semcancer.2007.05.003] [PMID: 17588771]

[57] Graefe, E.U.; Wittig, J.; Mueller, S.; Riethling, A.K.; Uehleke, B.; Drewelow, B.; Pforte, H.; Jacobasch, G.; Derendorf, H.; Veit, M. Pharmacokinetics and bioavailability of quercetin glycosides in humans. *J. Clin. Pharmacol.,* **2001**, *41*(5), 492-499.
[http://dx.doi.org/10.1177/00912700122010366] [PMID: 11361045]

[58] Williamson, G.; Clifford, M.N. Colonic metabolites of berry polyphenols: the missing link to biological activity? *Br. J. Nutr.,* **2010**, *104*(S3) Suppl. 3, S48-S66.
[http://dx.doi.org/10.1017/S0007114510003946] [PMID: 20955650]

[59] Yan, S.; Xie, M.; Wang, Y.; Xiao, Q.; Ding, N.; Li, Y. Semi-synthesis of a series natural flavonoids and flavonoid glycosides from scutellarin. *Tetrahedron,* **2020**, *76*(8), 130950.
[http://dx.doi.org/10.1016/j.tet.2020.130950]

[60] Hollman, P. C. Absorption, bioavailability, and metabolism of flavonoids *Pharmaceutical Biology,* **2004**, *42*(1), 74-83.

[61] Day, A.J.; Cañada, F.J.; Díaz, J.C.; Kroon, P.A.; Mclauchlan, R.; Faulds, C.B.; Plumb, G.W.; Morgan, M.R.A.; Williamson, G. Dietary flavonoid and isoflavone glycosides are hydrolysed by the lactase site of lactase phlorizin hydrolase. *FEBS Lett.,* **2000**, *468*(2-3), 166-170.
[http://dx.doi.org/10.1016/S0014-5793(00)01211-4] [PMID: 10692580]

[62] Day, A.J.; DuPont, M.S.; Ridley, S.; Rhodes, M.; Rhodes, M.J.C.; Morgan, M.R.A.; Williamson, G. Deglycosylation of flavonoid and isoflavonoid glycosides by human small intestine and liver β-glucosidase activity. *FEBS Lett.,* **1998**, *436*(1), 71-75.
[http://dx.doi.org/10.1016/S0014-5793(98)01101-6] [PMID: 9771896]

[63] Brand, W.; Schutte, M.E.; Williamson, G.; van Zanden, J.J.; Cnubben, N.H.P.; Groten, J.P.; van Bladeren, P.J.; Rietjens, I.M.C.M. Flavonoid-mediated inhibition of intestinal ABC transporters may affect the oral bioavailability of drugs, food-borne toxic compounds and bioactive ingredients. *Biomed. Pharmacother.,* **2006**, *60*(9), 508-519.
[http://dx.doi.org/10.1016/j.biopha.2006.07.081] [PMID: 16978825]

[64] Hodek, P.; Trefil, P.; Stiborová, M. Flavonoids-potent and versatile biologically active compounds interacting with cytochromes P450. *Chem. Biol. Interact.,* **2002**, *139*(1), 1-21.
[http://dx.doi.org/10.1016/S0009-2797(01)00285-X] [PMID: 11803026]

[65] Manach, C.; Donovan, J.L. Pharmacokinetics and metabolism of dietary flavonoids in humans. *Free Radic. Res.,* **2004**, *38*(8), 771-785.
[http://dx.doi.org/10.1080/10715760410001727858] [PMID: 15493450]

[66] Chen, Z.; Zheng, S.; Li, L.; Jiang, H. Metabolism of flavonoids in human: a comprehensive review. *Curr. Drug Metab.,* **2014**, *15*(1), 48-61.
[http://dx.doi.org/10.2174/138920021501140218125020] [PMID: 24588554]

[67] Nigam, S.K.; Bush, K.T.; Martovetsky, G.; Ahn, S.Y.; Liu, H.C.; Richard, E.; Bhatnagar, V.; Wu, W. The organic anion transporter (OAT) family: a systems biology perspective. *Physiol. Rev.,* **2015**, *95*(1), 83-123.
[http://dx.doi.org/10.1152/physrev.00025.2013] [PMID: 25540139]

[68] Arts, I.C.W.; Sesink, A.L.A.; Faassen-Peters, M.; Hollman, P.C.H. The type of sugar moiety is a major determinant of the small intestinal uptake and subsequent biliary excretion of dietary quercetin glycosides. *Br. J. Nutr.,* **2004**, *91*(6), 841-847.
[http://dx.doi.org/10.1079/BJN20041123] [PMID: 15182387]

[69] Spencer, J.P.E.; Chaudry, F.; Pannala, A.S.; Srai, S.K.; Debnam, E.; Rice-Evans, C. Decomposition of cocoa procyanidins in the gastric milieu. *Biochem. Biophys. Res. Commun.,* **2000**, *272*(1), 236-241.
[http://dx.doi.org/10.1006/bbrc.2000.2749] [PMID: 10872833]

[70] Rios, L.Y.; Bennett, R.N.; Lazarus, S.A.; Rémésy, C.; Scalbert, A.; Williamson, G. Cocoa procyanidins are stable during gastric transit in humans. *Am. J. Clin. Nutr.,* **2002**, *76*(5), 1106-1110. [http://dx.doi.org/10.1093/ajcn/76.5.1106] [PMID: 12399286]

[71] Schramm, D.D.; Karim, M.; Schrader, H.R.; Holt, R.R.; Kirkpatrick, N.J.; Polagruto, J.A.; Ensunsa, J.L.; Schmitz, H.H.; Keen, C.L. Food effects on the absorption and pharmacokinetics of cocoa flavanols. *Life Sci.,* **2003**, *73*(7), 857-869. [http://dx.doi.org/10.1016/S0024-3205(03)00373-4] [PMID: 12798412]

[72] Hollman, P.C.H.; Van Het Hof, K.H.; Tijburg, L.B.M.; Katan, M.B. Addition of milk does not affect the absorption of flavonols from tea in man. *Free Radic. Res.,* **2001**, *34*(3), 297-300. [http://dx.doi.org/10.1080/10715760100300261] [PMID: 11264903]

[73] Serafini, M.; Bugianesi, R.; Maiani, G.; Valtuena, S.; De Santis, S.; Crozier, A. Plasma antioxidants from chocolate. *Nature,* **2003**, *424*(6952), 1013-1013. [http://dx.doi.org/10.1038/4241013a] [PMID: 12944955]

[74] Donovan, J.L.; Kasim-Karakas, S.; German, J.B.; Waterhouse, A.L. Urinary excretion of catechin metabolites by human subjects after red wine consumption. *Br. J. Nutr.,* **2002**, *87*(1), 31-37. [http://dx.doi.org/10.1079/BJN2001482] [PMID: 11895312]

[75] Mullen, W.; Edwards, C.A.; Serafini, M.; Crozier, A. Bioavailability of pelargonidin-3-O-glucoside and its metabolites in humans following the ingestion of strawberries with and without cream. *J. Agric. Food Chem.,* **2008**, *56*(3), 713-719. [http://dx.doi.org/10.1021/jf072000p] [PMID: 18211024]

[76] Guo, Y.; Mah, E.; Davis, C.G.; Jalili, T.; Ferruzzi, M.G.; Chun, O.K.; Bruno, R.S. Dietary fat increases quercetin bioavailability in overweight adults. *Mol. Nutr. Food Res.,* **2013**, *57*(5), 896-905. [http://dx.doi.org/10.1002/mnfr.201200619] [PMID: 23319447]

[77] Dai, P.; Luo, F.; Wang, Y.; Jiang, H.; Wang, L.; Zhang, G.; Zhu, L.; Hu, M.; Wang, X.; Lu, L.; Liu, Z. Species- and gender-dependent differences in the glucuronidation of a flavonoid glucoside and its aglycone determined using expressed UGT enzymes and microsomes. *Biopharm. Drug Dispos.,* **2015**, *36*(9), 622-635. [http://dx.doi.org/10.1002/bdd.1989] [PMID: 26317684]

[78] Bolling, B.W.; Court, M.H.; Blumberg, J.B.; Chen, C.Y.O. The kinetic basis for age-associated changes in quercetin and genistein glucuronidation by rat liver microsomes. *J. Nutr. Biochem.,* **2010**, *21*(6), 498-503. [http://dx.doi.org/10.1016/j.jnutbio.2009.02.006] [PMID: 19446449]

[79] Xie, Y.; Zhang, D.; Zhang, J.; Yuan, J. Metabolism, transport and drug–drug interactions of silymarin. *Molecules,* **2019**, *24*(20), 3693. [http://dx.doi.org/10.3390/molecules24203693] [PMID: 31615114]

[80] Begley, D.J. Efflux mechanisms in the central nervous system: a powerful influence on drug distribution within the brain. In: *Blood-spinal cord and brain barriers in health and disease*; Sharma, H.S.; Westman, J., Eds.; Academic Press: Cambridge, Massachusetts, **2004**; pp. 83-97. [http://dx.doi.org/10.1016/B978-012639011-7/50013-9]

[81] Youdim, K.A.; Dobbie, M.S.; Kuhnle, G.; Proteggente, A.R.; Abbott, N.J.; Rice-Evans, C. Interaction between flavonoids and the blood-brain barrier: *in vitro* studies. *J. Neurochem.,* **2003**, *85*(1), 180-192. [http://dx.doi.org/10.1046/j.1471-4159.2003.01652.x] [PMID: 12641740]

[82] Youdim, K.A.; Shukitt-Hale, B.; Joseph, J.A. Serial Review: Flavonoids and Isoflavones (Phytoestrogens: Absorption, Metabolism, and Bioactivity). *Free Radic. Biol. Med.,* **2004**, *37*(11), 1683-1693. [http://dx.doi.org/10.1016/j.freeradbiomed.2004.08.002] [PMID: 15528027]

[83] Murakami, A. Dose-dependent functionality and toxicity of green tea polyphenols in experimental rodents. *Arch. Biochem. Biophys.,* **2014**, *557*, 3-10.

[http://dx.doi.org/10.1016/j.abb.2014.04.018] [PMID: 24814373]

[84] Cladis, D.P.; Li, S.; Reddivari, L.; Cox, A.; Ferruzzi, M.G.; Weaver, C.M. A 90 day oral toxicity study of blueberry polyphenols in ovariectomized sprague-dawley rats. *Food Chem. Toxicol.,* **2020**, *139*, 111254.
[http://dx.doi.org/10.1016/j.fct.2020.111254] [PMID: 32165232]

[85] Zheleva-Dimitrova, D.; Simeonova, R.; Gevrenova, R.; Savov, Y.; Balabanova, V.; Nasar-Eddin, G.; Bardarov, K.; Danchev, N. *In vivo* toxicity assessment of *Clinopodium vulgare* L. water extract characterized by UHPLC-HRMS. *Food Chem. Toxicol.,* **2019**, *134*, 110841.
[http://dx.doi.org/10.1016/j.fct.2019.110841] [PMID: 31568851]

[86] De Monte, C.; Bizzarri, B.; Gidaro, M.C.; Carradori, S.; Mollica, A.; Luisi, G.; Granese, A.; Alcaro, S.; Costa, G.; Basilico, N.; Parapini, S.; Scaltrito, M.M.; Masia, C.; Sisto, F. Bioactive compounds of *Crocus sativus* L. and their semi-synthetic derivatives as promising anti- *Helicobacter pylori*, anti-malarial and anti-leishmanial agents. *J. Enzyme Inhib. Med. Chem.,* **2015**, *30*(6), 1027-1033.
[http://dx.doi.org/10.3109/14756366.2014.1001755] [PMID: 25766747]

[87] Chen, L.; Gnanaraj, C.; Arulselvan, P.; El-Seedi, H.; Teng, H. A review on advanced microencapsulation technology to enhance bioavailability of phenolic compounds: Based on its activity in the treatment of Type 2 Diabetes. *Trends Food Sci. Technol.,* **2019**, *85*, 149-162.
[http://dx.doi.org/10.1016/j.tifs.2018.11.026]

[88] Awouafack, M.D.; Tane, P.; Spiteller, M.; Eloff, J.N. *Eriosema* (Fabaceae) species represent a rich source of flavonoids with interesting pharmacological activities. *Nat. Prod. Commun.,* **2015**, *10*(7), 1934578X1501000.
[http://dx.doi.org/10.1177/1934578X1501000749] [PMID: 26411043]

[89] Stevens, J.F.; Page, J.E. Xanthohumol and related prenylflavonoids from hops and beer: to your good health! *Phytochemistry,* **2004**, *65*(10), 1317-1330.
[http://dx.doi.org/10.1016/j.phytochem.2004.04.025] [PMID: 15231405]

[90] Urmann, C.; Riepl, H. Semi-Synthetic Approach Leading to 8-Prenylnaringenin and 6-Prenylnaringenin: Optimization of the Microwave-Assisted Demethylation of Xanthohumol Using Design of Experiments. *Molecules,* **2020**, *25*(17), 4007.
[http://dx.doi.org/10.3390/molecules25174007] [PMID: 32887388]

CHAPTER 2

Recent Development of Hybrids and Derivatives of Resveratrol in Neurodegenerative Diseases

Barbara De Filippis[1,*] and **Marialuigia Fantacuzzi**[1]

[1] *Department of Pharmacy, G. d'Annunzio University of Chieti-Pescara, via dei Vestini 31, 66100 Chieti, Italy*

Abstract: Neurodegenerative diseases (NDs) are characterized by the progressive loss of neurons in different regions of the nervous system, being Alzheimer's disease (AD) and Parkinson's disease (PD) the most common NDs. Despite their high incidence, the pharmacological treatments are mainly symptomatic. For this reason, in recent years, the research has been focused on the discovery of new molecules able to target neuropathological pathways involved in NDs. In the last decades, several researchers investigated the neuroprotective actions of naturally occurring polyphenols, such as resveratrol, that has attracted special interest since its ability to interact simultaneously with the multiple targets implicated in NDs. Thanks to the structural simplicity of the stilbene core, the broad spectrum of possible modifications, and the improved synthetic strategies, resveratrol is an attractive chemical starting point for the searching of new entities with extended therapeutic uses in NDs. In this review, a systematic update of the stilbene-based hybrids and derivatives, and SAR analysis were provided for the development of new drugs potentially useful as NDs multitarget directed ligands.

Keywords: Antioxidant, Molecular Hybrids, Neurodegeneration, Polyphenols, Resveratrol, Stilbene Derivatives.

INTRODUCTION

Neurodegenerative diseases (NDs) are characterized by progressive disorders and devastating damages of the structure and function of neurons. NDs etiology is still not clear, despite the increased current knowledge of their neurobiology, but different contributing factors, such as aging, lifestyle and genetic factors are involved. Despite the differences in clinical signs, among others, the pathological processes appear similar, suggesting common neurodegenerative pathways. The pathogenesis of several NDs, including Alzheimer's (AD), Parkinson's (PD),

* **Corresponding Author Barbara De Filippis:** Department of Pharmacy, G. d'Annunzio University of Chieti-Pescara, *via* dei Vestini 31, 66100 Chieti, Italy; E-mail: barbara.defilippis@unich.it

Simone Carradori (Ed.)

Huntington's (HD) and amyotrophic lateral sclerosis diseases are associated with multiple factor risks [1]. Neuroinflammation and oxidative stress represent the main causes of induction of NDs, but also excitotoxicity, mitochondrial dysfunction, and apoptosis [2]. The role of oxidative stress in neurodegeneration is well documented and is correlated to the progression of AD and PD [3]. Microglia cells are resident cells in the central nervous system (CNS), with immune function under normal conditions. The activation of brain microglia, and the subsequent extra production of inflammatory mediators, such as nitric oxide (NO), may result in uncontrolled neuroinflammation in NDs [4]. Lipoxygenase (LOX) and cyclooxygenase (COX) cascades are upregulated in chronic and age-related brain pathologies [5].

AD is the most common form of dementia and the most studied ND. It is characterized by two neuropathological hallmarks: deposition of extracellular β-amyloid (Aβ) plaques and intracellular neurofibrillary tangles, even if other factors as neuroinflammation play an important role in progression of AD [6]. Due to the complexity of the involved pathways, it is difficult to control the progression of this pathology. Current treatment for AD is only symptomatic; thus, the development of drugs with the potential to change the progression of the disease is a priority. One of the major pharmacological approaches of AD regards the inhibition of acetyl and butyryl cholinesterase (AChE and BuChE). They are key enzymes that play important roles in cholinergic transmission by hydrolyzing the acetylcholine (ACh) [7]. In AD, the AChE level in the brain decreases progressively, but BuChE activity remains or increases compared to the basal level. Some research studies reported that the peripheral anionic site (PAS) of AChE can locate with Aβ protein and enhances the formation of amyloid fibrils in the senile plaques indicating that inhibiting the AChE activity is a promising approach to prevent Aβ aggregation [8]. However, AChE inhibition may cause the classical cholinergic toxicity [9]. $A\beta_{1-42}$ is responsible for the initial self-aggregation of Aβ, and the resulting β-amyloid oligomers and fibrils are toxic to neurons [10]. Moreover, high concentrations of copper, zinc and iron ions accelerate amyloid deposits in AD patients [11, 12]. Although the mechanisms that underlie NDs pathophysiology are not completely clarified, a series of studies described the critical role of inflammation and oxidative stress in the degeneration of neurons [13, 14], promoting the Aβ aggregation [3].

Monoamine oxidases (MAOs) have been received increasing attention in recent years due to their roles in the treatment of AD and PD. MAOs are FAD-containing enzymes that bind tightly to the outer mitochondrial membrane in brain, liver, intestinal mucosa, and other organs and catalyze the oxidative deamination of biogenic and xenobiotic amines. There are two types of isoenzymes, MAO-A and MAO-B, which can be distinguished by their differential primary DNA sequences, tissue distribution, substrates, and inhibitor selectivity. MAO-A is situated predominantly in catecholaminergic neurons and especially oxidizes serotonin, adrenaline and noradrenaline, while MAO-B is placed in serotonergic neurons and glia where deaminates dopamine and 2-phenylethylamine (2-PEA). Therefore, the study of MAO inhibitors has attracted increasing interest in recent years for their therapeutic effect on NDs. Selective MAO-B inhibitors, such as rasagiline and selegiline, are used as adjuvant therapy in the treatment of PD and AD [15]. However, the high levels of MAO-B in neuronal tissue could lead to an increase in the levels of H_2O_2 and oxidative free radicals, which ultimately contribute to the etiology of NDs. Thus, selective inhibition of MAO-B becomes another valuable approach for the treatment of AD [16].

PD is the second most common neurodegenerative disorder caused by progressive loss of dopaminergic nigrostriatal neurons. The neuropathological hallmark of PD involves the disruption to mitochondria, the oxidative stress, alterations to the presynaptic protein α-synuclein, resulting in the accumulation of intracellular protein aggregates, Lewy bodies, and Lewy neurites, and neuroinflammatory processes [17]. Unfortunately, current drugs are mainly focused on symptomatic controls, and a long-term application leads to the loss of drug efficacy and important adverse effects. Since conventional therapeutics are not sufficient for the treatment of PD, the development of new agents is crucial [18].

Currently available drugs only provide symptomatic treatment, and has modest benefits, rather than preventing or curing neurodegeneration [19], and effective therapeutic agents are still far to success. In this contest, it is essential to develop novel therapeutic approaches to fight the NDs. Since the complexity of the involved pathways, a single biological target often proves ineffective in the treatment of diseases with a complex path mechanism. This fact inspired the research to design and develop a single drug containing structural features able to act on multiple biological targets [20]. In this way, the design of poly-pharmacophores represents a further modern approach that provides effective pharmacological responses for diverse receptors or enzymatic systems, and responds to the ADMET limits, showing antioxidant, neuroprotective, and brain permeable properties [21]. These multitarget-directed ligands (MTDLs) could contain a variety of scaffolds. During the past decades, many studies reported the positive effect of natural compounds against different diseases such as cardiovascular, diabetes, and cancer. On the other hand, natural products have emerged as potential neuroprotective agents for the treatment of NDs [22]. In this context, natural products have been used as structural models in the drug design of ligands against AD, as evidenced by the high number of published studies [23].

Natural products have intrinsic multi-target profile and could be selected for appropriate starting points for the development of new agents for NDs [24].

In recent years, the interest in the natural polyphenols has markedly increased, due to their therapeutic effects [25]. They are plant secondary metabolites, with two or more phenolic rings. Natural polyphenols, particularly concentrated in fruits, vegetables, beverages such as chocolate, tea, red wine, or in olive oil, are produced in response to exogenous stimuli such as excessive heat or ultraviolet exposures, insect attacks, and bacterial or fungal infections. Polyphenols are involved with a wide range of neuroprotective activities such as inhibition of neuroinflammation, and oxidative stress [26, 27], providing protection to neurons against neurotoxin-induced injury, and improving cognitive function, learning, and memory. The important role of polyphenols in antioxidant activity are due to the ability of the hydroxyl groups directly linked to the aromatic rings to remove free radicals and prevent tissue damage [23, 28]. These important characteristics make natural polyphenols good lead compounds for the design and synthesis of new molecules with potential application in several diseases as NDs [27, 29].

Resveratrol (RSV) is a 3,4,5-trihydroxystilbene (Fig. **1**) found in peanuts, pistachios, berries, grapes, and red wine [30, 31]. Daily use of RSV may have numerous preventive and therapeutic properties in a vast range of human diseases ranging from cardioprotection, anti-diabetic properties, depigmentation, anti-inflammation, cancer prevention and neuroprotection [32]. RSV demonstrated excellent antioxidant, anti-inflammatory, anticancer and antimicrobial activities and has been widely studied as potential treatment for several disorders [33]. Numerous pharmacological studies have demonstrated neuroprotective effects of RSV in *in vitro* and in animal models [34]. In AD, RSV interferes with the formation of Aβ, stabilizes microtubule associated protein function, inhibits inflammatory response, and improves antioxidant activity [35]. RSV has been evaluated for its usefulness for mild to moderate AD patients [36 - 38].

Therefore, the neuroprotective effects of glucuronate and sulfate metabolites of RSV (Fig. **1**) and its natural derivatives, as pterostilbene (PTR, Fig. **1**), have been studied evaluating the antioxidant and anti-inflammatory activities [39, 40]. PTR demonstrated inhibition of the self-induced Aβ aggregation and neuroprotective properties [34]. 2,3,5,4'-Tetrahydroxystilbene-2-*O*-β-D-glucoside (TSG, Fig. **1**) is one of the active components extracted from *Polygonum multiflorum* Thunb., a traditional Chinese medicinal herb, widely used in the Orient as a tonic and antiaging agent. A recent study proved the effectiveness of TSG in protecting dopaminergic neurons against LPS-induced neurotoxicity through dual modulation on glial cells by attenuating microglia-mediated neuroinflammation and enhancing astroglia-derived neurotrophic effects [41].

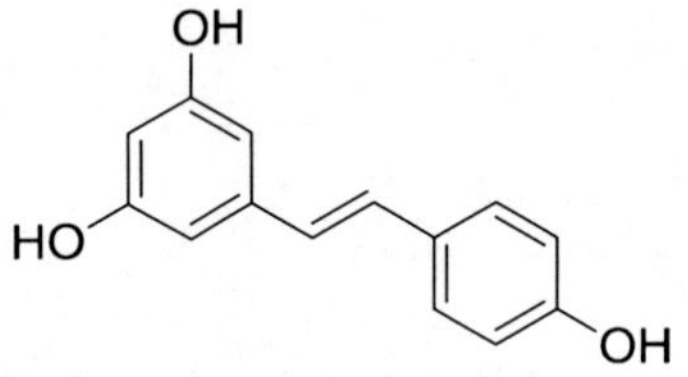

RSV

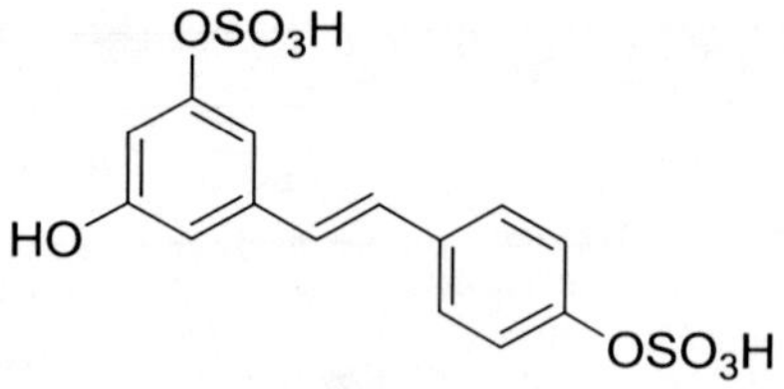

RSV-sulfated

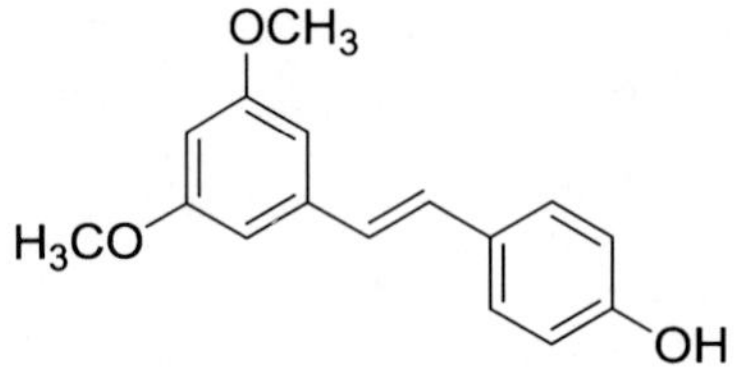

pterostilbene

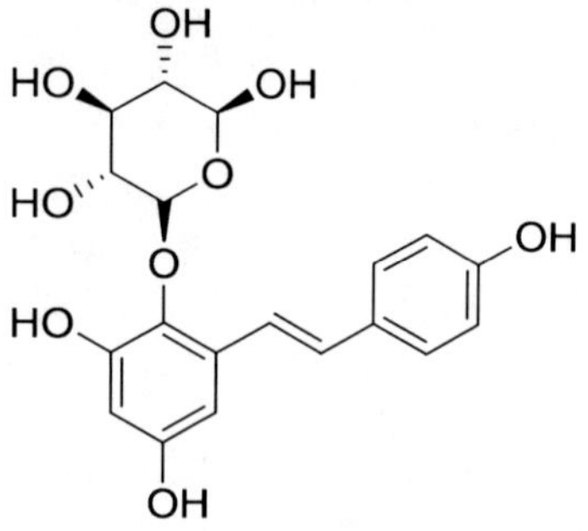

TSG

Fig. (1). Structures of resveratrol (RSV), sulfated metabolite of RSV, pterostilbene (PTR), and 2,3,5,4'-tetrahydroxystilbene-2-O-β-D-glucoside (TSG).

Even if RSV is known to be safe in humans, its poor solubility in water (less than 0.005 mg/mL) influences its drug-likeness. After oral administration, RSV is adsorbed at gastrointestinal level, but the extensive first pass effect reduces the bioavailability to less than 1% [42]. In order to improve the pharmacokinetic profile and enhance both the systemic and topical bioavailability, numerous strategies have been applied, such as chemical modification and complexation with bile acids, incorporation into liposomes, and formulation into nanoparticle delivery systems [43, 44].

The synthetic approach to the chemical modification of RSV deals with the building of hybrids or derivatives. Hybrids are conjugates of two or more different pharmacophores linked together with spacers or fused, depending upon the degree of overlap of the starting frameworks (Fig. **2**) [45]. Usually, the hybrid possesses improved drug-like features compared to the parent and this aspect is important especially for hybrids directed to the CNS, which improved permeability of BBB to exert its effects in NDs [46, 47].

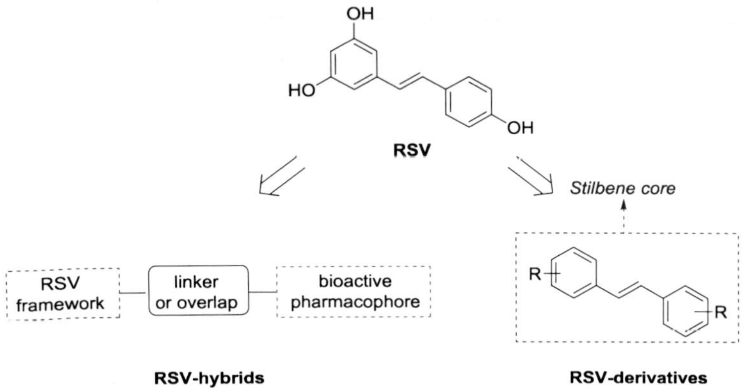

Fig. (2). General structures of hybrids and derivatives of RSV.

Derivatives (Fig. **2**) are designed by keeping the original stilbene skeleton and introducing different substituents on different rings position [48 - 51]. The synthesis of RSV derivatives is promoted by the multiple possible synthetic strategies to obtain substituted stilbene core, and the wide range of functionalization of phenols [52].

In this context, hybrids incorporating the stilbene core of RSV represent an efficacious way to obtain promising alternative to treat multifactorial and complex NDs. To date, many studies have been recommended and the number of publications concerning derivatives and hybrids of RSV are increasing in the last few years [53, 54]. Some reviews offer an interesting starting point to design RSV-based multi-target agents [55], useful in NDs [56, 57].

This review is centered on the description of hybrids and derivatives of RSV and explores the updated studies of the last three years. It focuses on the description of structural-activity relationships and highlights recent advances in the search of potential candidates for the treatment of NDs.

MULTITARGET ANALOGUES OF RSV

Hybrids of RSV

The most widely used strategy to design efficacious MTDL, useful in the treatment of NDs, is the molecular hybridization [45, 58]. Hybrids of RSV have been largely described in the field of cancer and other relevant diseases [59 - 61]. In this paragraph, the studies conducted on hybrids of RSV, useful in the neurodegenerative field is systematically described.

Lan and coworkers reported the study of hybrids obtained by the combination of two important pharmacophores: the *N*-alkyl-substituted indazole-5-carboxamide, a well-known scaffold with MAO inhibition property [62], and the stilbene core of RSV that demonstrated a good interaction with Aβ protein [63]. General structure of indazole-RSV hybrids and the pattern of substitutions are depicted in Fig. (**3**) [64]. They were tested for inhibitor activity of Aβ self-aggregation and inhibition of MAO. In general, most compounds showed a significant inhibition of self-induced Aβ aggregation and a good micromolar inhibition respect to iproniazid and rasagiline, used as references. The SAR of indazole-RSV hybrids was summarized in Fig. (**3**). The most potent MAO-B selective inhibitor was compound **1** (Fig. **3**) with the lowest IC_{50} of 1.14 μM. It demonstrated a reversible and competitive MAO-B inhibition, and its activity was explained by molecular modeling and docking study that established the exact interactions with the target protein. **1** exhibited an inhibition of Aβ self-aggregation of 58% at 20 μM, with an IC_{50} 19.5 μM calculated with fluorimetric assay [64].

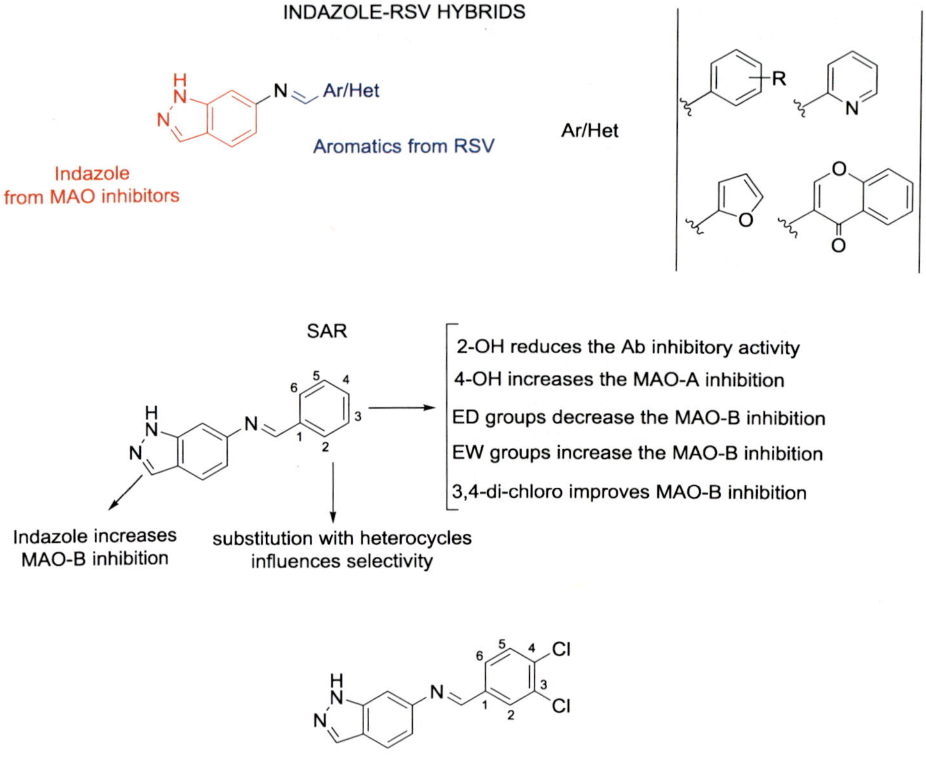

1

Fig. (3). Structures of imidazole-RSV hybrids and **1**.

The study of Liu Jiang *et al.* on hybrids of RSV and maltol [65] was enriched of a series of derivatives in which the aromatic ring was differently substituted (Fig. **4**) [66]. The study of antioxidant and inhibition of Aβ self-aggregation activities demonstrated that the substitution with hydroxyls is favorable for both the activity: compounds **2a** and **2b** (Fig. **4**) with 4-OH and 2-OH groups, respectively, were the best compounds: IC_{50}=7.20 and 8.29 μM for Aβ self-aggregation inhibition, and IC_{50}=1.94 and 1.18 μM for ABTS% scavenging activity, respectively. They also showed good metal chelating property and iron and copper ion-induced Aβ aggregation. It may be due to a multiple hydrogen formation at a surface region of Aβ that promotes the disruption of the intermolecular self-assembly process of Aβ.

MALTOL-RSV HYBRIDS

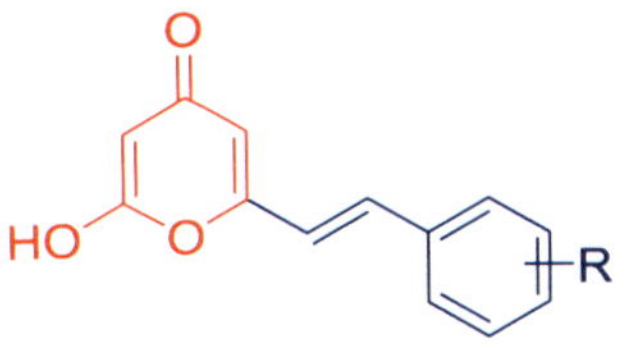

R	Antioxidant activity	Inhibition of Aβ self-aggregation
4-OH	↑	↑
2-OH	↑	↑
3,5-di-OH	↑	↑
3-F	↓	↑
$4-N(CH_3)_2$	↑	↑
$4-OCH_2CH_3$	↑	↑

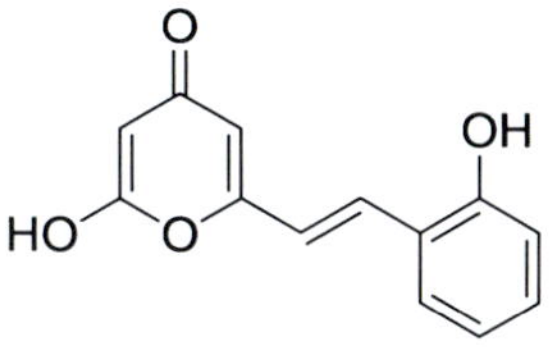

2a

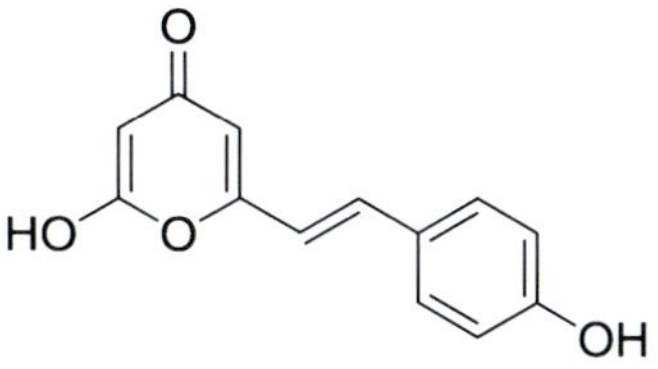

2b

Fig. (4). Structures of maltol-RSV hybrids and **2a** and 2**b**.

The pyridoxine, a 4,5-bis(hydroxymethyl)-2-methylpyridin-3-ol (Fig. **5**), possesses a well-known neuroprotective activity [66, 67]. As described, pyridoxine is an enzymatic regulatory cofactor for at least 140 enzymes. It is a natural antioxidant agent that inhibits the production of radicals and serves as quenchers for single oxygen [69]. To evaluate the synergistic effects of pyridoxine and RSV, a series of hybrids obtained combining these two pharmacophores have been designed and studied for antioxidant, inhibitory activity of AChE and metal chelating properties [70]. Their general structure is reported in Fig. **5**. They contain the ethenylbenzene scaffold of RSV substituted with hydroxyl group and an amino derivative in switching adjacent positions (compare **3a** with **3b** and **3c**, (Fig. **5**). In the **3a** and **3b** compounds the pyridinyl moiety is kept while in **3c** the methyl-hydroxyl group of the pyridoxine is cycled with the adjacent hydroxyl group. All these compounds are selective and potent inhibitor of AChE in micromolar range. The SAR of amine substituent affects the activity, as reported in Fig. (**5**). The best active inhibitors were compounds **3d** (Fig. **5**) with EC_{50} = 1.50 μM, and **3e** (Fig. **5**) with EC_{50} = 2.11 μM, lower than donepezil used as reference (EC_{50} = 23.0 μM). Kinetic study demonstrated a mixed-type inhibition of **3e** binding to both CAS and PAS of AChE. All compounds showed a selective MAO-B activity toward MAO-A. The introduction of Mannich base improved AChE inhibitory activity but decreased the MAO-B activity. The reduction of MAO inhibition activity is explained by molecular modelling study that highlighted how the intermediates without Mannich substituents reach the binding pocket of MAO-B in close proximity to the enzymatic cofactor FAD, reinforced with a π–π stacking interaction between the phenyl ring and Tyr398, while compounds substituted with Mannich base are positioned with completely opposite orientation. The best combination of substituents is represented by **3f** (Fig. **5**) with MAO-B EC_{50} = 2.68 μM, lower than clorgyline and iproniazid used as references (EC_{50} = 8.87 μM and 4.32 μM, respectively). All compounds exhibited good oxygen radical absorbance capacity (ORAC-FL) values of 1.52-2.63 μM of trolox equivalent, with best results for derivatives with a hydroxyl in 3' or 4' position.

Another important study conducted on hybrids of pyridinone led to an important consideration. This study started from the observation that RSV derivatives had a character of MAO-B inhibitor [71]. This fact is useful to manage PD because MAO-B activity increases in the human brain with age, and elderly PD patients have been proved to show a high MAO-B catalytic rate in their brain [72]. Moreover, selective MAO-B inhibitors are considered potential candidates for anti-AD drugs. This probably reduces the central dopamine (DA) supply and increases the production of hydrogen peroxide and aldehyde species, which may cause the neurodegeneration associated with PD. A new series of pyridoxine-RSV hybrids was synthesized and evaluated for their biological activities including inhibition of MAOs, reversibility study of MAO-B inhibition, molecular docking studies, anti-oxidative activities, neuroprotective activity, and the ability to cross the BBB [73]. This hybridization is described in Fig. (**6**). The hydroxyl groups of pyridoxine were cyclized to improve the lipophilicity, and amino groups were inserted on the RSV skeleton. The kind of substituents influences the activity, as described in Fig. (**6**). The results revealed that all pyridoxine-RSV hybrids had the most antioxidant activity and were selective MAO-B inhibitors with a weak activity against MAO-A. Some of them are MAO inhibitors in very low micromolar range (compounds **4a**, **4b**, **4c**, with IC_{50} 0.01 μM, 0.01 μM and 0.02 μM, respectively, (Fig. **6**), better than positive control drugs rasagiline (IC_{50} = 0.0437 μM) and iproniazid (IC_{50} = 4.32 μM) [73]. Their reversibility of MAO-B inhibition was evaluated by measuring the recovery of MAO-B activities after dialysis of enzyme-inhibitor mixtures and **4a** and **4c** resulted reversible inhibitors, while **4b** interacted with MAO-B irreversibly, like rasagiline. Probably, in this last case the presence of propargyl moiety induces a similar pattern of interactions with the active site. Molecular docking studies highlighted that the main interactions of **4a** with MAO-B active site involve a hydrogen bond between the hydroxyl group, a π-π stacking hydrophobic interactions and the hydrogen bond of the nitrogen atom on the pyridine ring, and these stronger interactions explained the higher potency of this molecule respect to the others. They are also able to penetrate the CNS with good BBB permeability, as demonstrated by the PAMPA-BBB model and are not cytotoxic at the concentration of 10 μM for PC-12 cell line, with or without H_2O_2-induced cell injury.

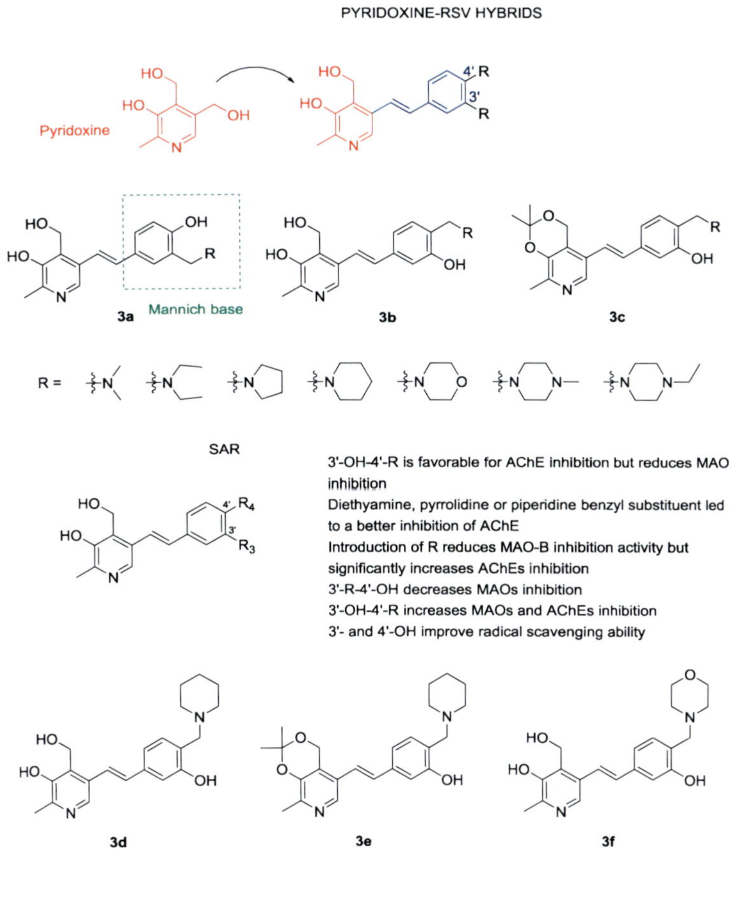

Fig. (5). Structures of pyridoxine-RSV hybrids and **3a**, **3b**, **3c**, **3d**, **3e**, **3f**.

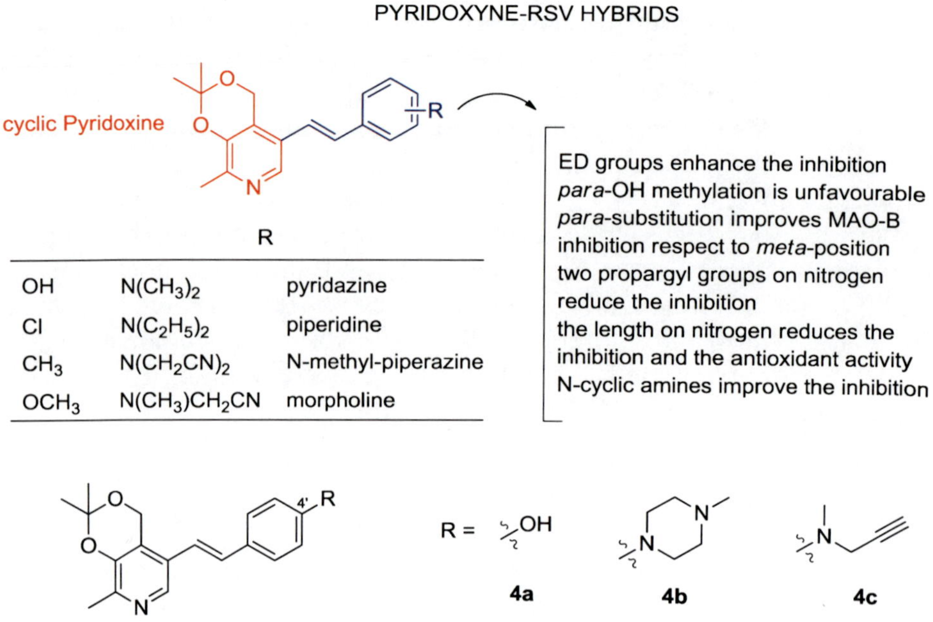

Fig. (6). Structures of pyridoxine-RSV hybrids and **4a**, **4b**, **4c**.

As a continuation of this research work, the introduction of the ethyl chain in position 2 of the pyridine ring (ethylpyridoxine-RSV hybrids **5**, (Fig. **7**) was evaluated. The presence of the ethyl radical led to a considerable increase of the DPPH antioxidant activity, in the presence of the 3',4'-*di*-hydroxy ring [74]. This fact is explained by the formation of a stable semiquinoid anion-radical structure stabilized by hydrogen bonds with the adjacent hydroxyls. The activity of mitochondria plays a key role in the development of oxidative stress [75]. A mitochondrial dysfunction is bound with an overproduction of superoxide radicals. For this reason, these ethylpyridoxine-RSV hybrids were studied also in the model of Fe^{2+}/ascorbate-induced mitochondrial membranes lipid peroxidation (LPO). It is reported the existence of antioxidant-binding sites in the hydrophobic core of the inner mitochondrial membrane or in the mitochondrial matrix and it suggests that hydrophobic compounds can modulate ROS associated with mitochondrial processes. The best result was obtained with derivatives with smaller number of hydroxyls already at low concentration of 15 μM, while for compounds with three hydroxyl groups the activity was measured only at a concentration of 40 μM. The activity is significantly reduced by the presence of three hydroxyl groups, because they reduce the intake through the cell lipid membrane by simple diffusion [74].

Semenov *et al.* reported important studies conducted on stilbazolic RSV analogues in which the RSV skeleton was combined with a derivative of pyridoxine (Fig. **7**) [68]. The importance of the nitrogen atom in *ortho*-position to the double bond (pyridine ring) and the number and the position of multiple hydroxyls on the adjacent aromatic ring were studied by the calculation of the energy of different rotamers. This study evidenced the importance of OH in 4' position that strongly stabilized semiquinone structure by resonance and the additional hydroxyl groups adjacent to the radical center (3' and 5' position) contribute to the delocalization and the radical stabilization by hydrogen bonds. The addition of the pyridine ring with its EW effect should increase the possibility to establish hydrogen bonds, even if the hydrogen bond in the pyridine fragment is slightly weaker than in the benzene ring and have the strength similar to the hydrogen bond of RSV, determining its antioxidant properties.

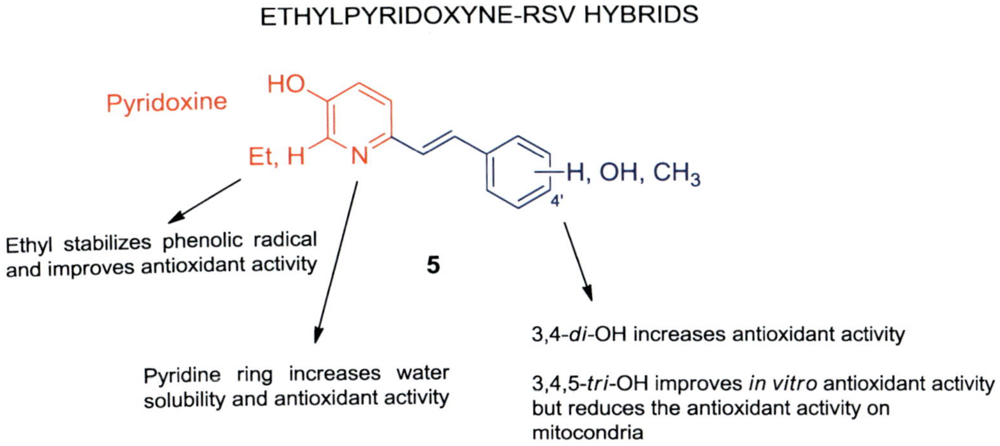

Fig. (7). Structure of ethylpyridoxine-RSV hybrids **5**.

Carbazole is a heterocycle present in phytochemicals with a documented biological activity. Many hybrids have been synthesized and tested as potential MTDLs agents [76]. Some authors proposed a study on RSV derivatives in which one of the aromatic rings of carbazole scaffold was fused with RSV and piperidine and pyrrolidine were attached on the RSV (R_1) or carbazole (R_2) side through a urea, thiourea or amide linker (Fig. **8**). They were tested for anti-AD activity as AChEs and Aβ-aggregation inhibitors, anti-oxidant and metal chelators [77]. The position of substituents does not affect the AChEs inhibition. Longer carbon chain (n = 4) induces a better AChE inhibitory activity (IC_{50} value of 1.84 μM) respect to compounds with chain where n = 3 and 2 (IC_{50} values of 3.54 and 4.59 μM, respectively). The amide linker reduces the AChEs inhibitory effect because there is a loss of a basic centers (urea and thiourea), indispensable for cation-π interaction with the enzymes and thiourea derivatives are most active than urea ones. All compounds showed good Aβ aggregation inhibition ranging from 38.9 to 55.79%. Compound with urea linker on the RSV side and piperidine ring showed the best Aβ aggregation inhibition (55.79%) at 25 μM concentration. Compound **6** (Fig. **8**) was found to be the most promising anti-Aβ agent thanks to its good inhibitory activities against AChE (IC_{50} 2.64 μM) and BuChE (IC_{50} 1.29 μM), significant inhibition of self-mediated Aβ aggregation (51.29% at 25 μM concentration), specific copper ion chelating property. Molecular docking studies indicated strong non-covalent interactions of **6** in the active sites of both the enzymes [77]. Furthermore, it respects the Lipinski's rule-of-five [78], making it as potential lead compound.

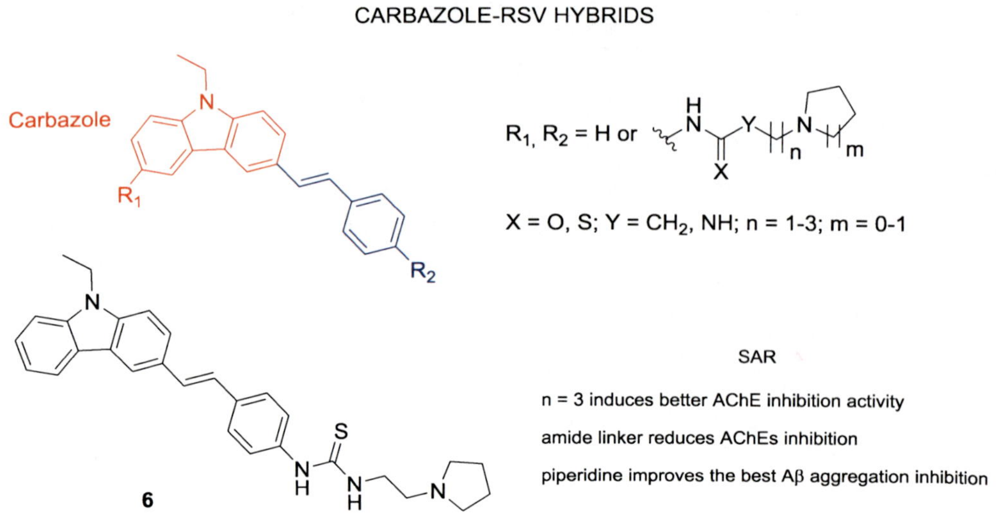

Fig. (8). Structures of carbazole-RSV hybrids and **6.**

Coumarin and some of its derivatives, such as furocoumarin, demonstrated a large variety of biological actions also in NDs thanks to their relatively low-molecular weights and high lipophilicity [79]. The way of interaction of coumarin into peripheral anionic site (PAS) of AChE was described [80]. Taking into account these statements, in a recent study, a series of hybrids of furocoumarin-PTR a natural *trans*-3,5-dimethoxy-4'-hydroxystilbene, were synthesized and evaluated for their ability to bind different targets involved in AD, as ChEs, β-secretase inhibitors, COX-2 and LOX-5 activities and for their free radical-scavenging properties [81]. The structure of coumarin-RSV hybrids is depicted in Fig. (**9**). They originate from the fusion of stilbene moiety of PTR and furocoumarin (**7**). A phenyl ring was added at the furyl ring. All compounds were found moderate to good inhibitors with a dual AChE and BChE inhibitory action, and SAR was defined. The introduction of the furan ring on coumarin improved the ChEs inhibition activity with IC_{50} values ranging from 1.8 to 21.6 μM (AChE) and 3.5-17.6 μM (BChE), respect to reference compounds donepezil (IC_{50} = 0.004 and 3.13 μM, respectively) and galantamine (IC_{50} = 1.17 and 2.05 μM, respectively). The lactone group promotes non-covalent interactions with the active site of the enzymes. Both the lactone moiety and the planar conjugated aromatic scaffolds favor the inhibitory effect compounds **7** against AChEs and β-secretase. The π-electron delocalizing Cl and F in *para* position of aromatic ring **A** and the 3,4-dimethoxy group exert a favorable effect on the AChE inhibition, probably due to additional non-covalent hydrogen bonding or dipole-dipole interactions, and/or increased van der Waals interactions with PAS of AChE. On the contrary, the 3,4-dimethoxy group is too much bulky to fit the BChE active site and this reduces its affinity but keeps the significant activity on β-secretase (IC_{50} 15.3 μM). These derivatives showed a moderate inhibition toward COX-2 (IC_{50} values range 8.6 μM to 28.6 μM) and LOX-5 (IC_{50} values range 13.9 μM to 27.1 μM), two targets implicated in the neuroinflammation [82], respect to references. They have moderate DPPH activity and ROS reduction in MCF7 and Hek293T cell lines. Above all, the best compound of this series, **7** (Fig. **9**), represents a good compromise for a potential lead compound, thanks to its 3,5-dimethoxy moiety that gives a good interaction with the enzymes, antioxidant activity and improves physico-chemical properties.

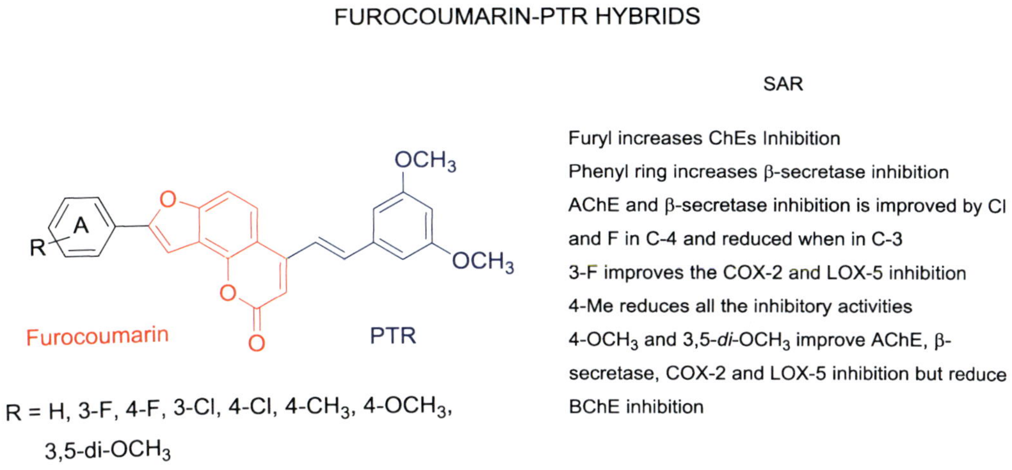

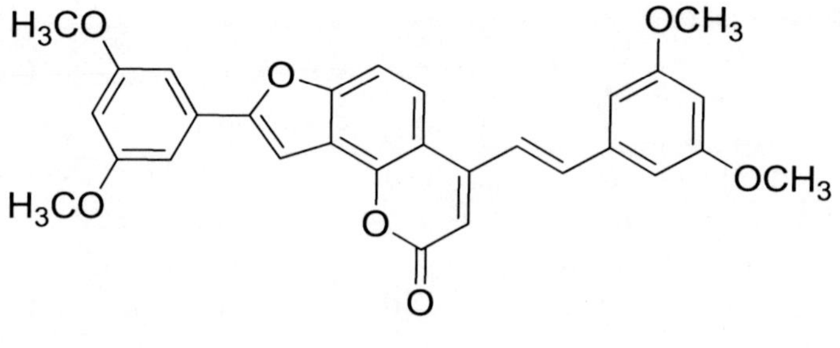

7

Fig. (9). Structures of furocoumarin-PTR hybrids and 7.

Another set of PTR hybrids was described by Zheng *et al.* in 2018 [83]. PTR was hybridized with tertiary amines through a 2-hydroxy propyl linker (Fig. **10**). They originate by important results obtained in a previous study in which PTR-alkylbenzylamines showed the ability to bind and modulate several targets involved in the AD [84]. They were tested for their inhibition of ChEs, anti--amyloid aggregation, neuroprotective on PC12 cell line injured by H_2O_2, and antioxidant properties. All the synthesized derivatives were moderate inhibitors of AChE but better than PTR, with IC_{50} values in the low micromolar range. The introduction of amine end on the side chain promotes the activity and it was noted that the aliphatic amines have better AChE inhibitory activity than the corresponding benzylamines. All compounds have a good protective effect on PC12 cell line when injured by H_2O_2, but methyl-ethylamine and diethyl-amine were the most neuroprotective ones. The amine derivatives are more potent respect the benzyl analogues even if benzyl amines demonstrated higher self-induced Aβ aggregation inhibition. Chirality does not influence in a remarkable way all the activity studied. An important result was that the ORAC-FL activity (*Oxygen Radical Absorbance Capacity by FLuorescein*) was reduced for all derivatives of PTR, confirming the crucial role of the hydroxyl group in 4-position that promotes the radical scavenging activity in a free form respect to the alkylated form. Compound **8** (Fig. **10**) resulted the best multiple inhibitor of this series of hybrids. It possesses moderate inhibitory effects with 40.23% at 25 μM on self-induced Aβ-aggregation and the tolerable antioxidant activity (1.20 *equivalent* of trolox), good neuroprotective effect against H_2O_2-induced PC12 cell injury with low toxicity in PC12 cells, high BBB permeability *in vitro* (P_e = 8.12 x 10^{-6} cm/s). Molecular docking conducted on **8** revealed that it binds both the catalytic and peripheral site of AChE. The hydroxyl interacts with a critical amino acid through a hydrogen bond.

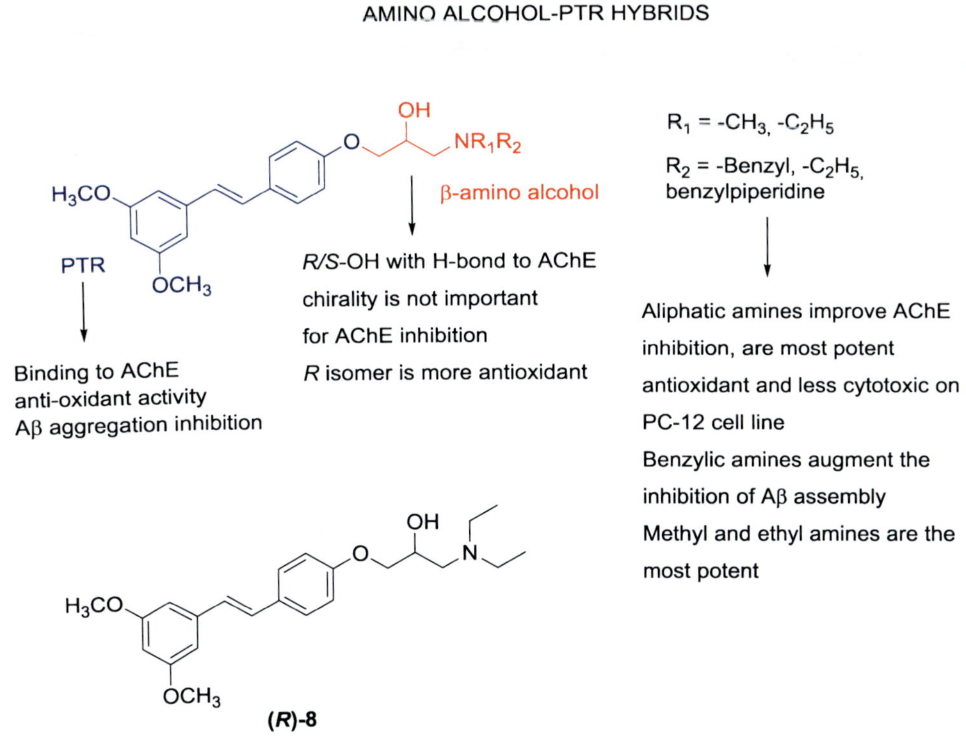

Fig. (10). Structures of β-amino alcohol-PTR hybrids and (*R*)-**8**.

In a similar study, a series of hybrids combining three different pharmacophores were investigated. They originate from the combination between the chromone scaffold with MAO-B inhibition activity [85], the clioquinol, a metal ion chelator useful in AD [86], and a Schiff base, named **L1**, with reported metal-induced Aβ aggregation, ROS production and neurotoxicity activity inhibition [87]. The structure of chromone-RSV hybrids is depicted in Fig. **11** [88]. Derivatives containing a Schiff base are also described in the section *2.2.1.* Most of these compounds are active in inhibiting MAOs with IC_{50} values in the micromolar range, ranging from 1.42 to 20.8 μM for MAO-A and 0.63-31.5 μM for MAO-B. The results were compared with those of rasagiline (IC_{50} = 49.7 μM for MAO-A and IC_{50} = 7.47 μM for MAO-B) and iproniazid, (IC_{50} = 6.46 μM for MAO-A and IC_{50} = 7.98 μM for MAO-B). The introduction of substituent with different steric hindrance to the chromone moiety or phenyl ring showed better MAO-B activity. A methyl group on chromone plus a 4-Cl on the phenyl ring, displayed the most potent inhibitory activity with an IC_{50} of 0.634 μM for MAO-B, about 12-fold more active than iproniazid (IC_{50} = 7.98 μM). **9a** was the strongest and more balanced MAOs inhibitor (IC_{50} = 5.12 μM for MAO-A and IC_{50} = 0.816 μM for MAO-B, (Fig. **11**). The selectivity of the most potent compound **9a** is explained with the different binding modes to the enzymes. **9a** interacts with a π–π stacking interaction of the aromatic ring of chromone moiety but with different amino acids (Tyr435 in MAO-B and Phe268 in MAO-A). The carbonyl of chromone ring engages an H-bonding with a glycine of MAO-A, while the benzene of phenol is involved in a second π–π stacking interaction with MAO-B. **9a** showed neuroprotective effects on neuroblastoma cells (PC12) and high inhibition of Cu^{2+}-induced Aβ aggregation. The pattern of substitutions does not influence dramatically to the Aβ self-induced aggregation inhibitory activity but in this case, compound **9b** (Fig. **11**) showed the best inhibitory activity (89.5%) compared to resveratrol (57.2%). The antioxidant activity was measured by the ORAC-FL method indicating that most of compounds have good ORAC-FL values of 1.82-3.62 trolox equivalents. Again, **9a** displayed most antioxidant activity (3.62 trolox equivalents), higher than other derivatives. Probably, the presence of two methyl groups on the two aromatics affects positively the antioxidant activity.

In 2017, Yang *et al.* described a study conducted on the chemical combination of RSV, the metal-chelator clioquinol [89] and benzyloxyl group of some MAO-B inhibitors [90]. These triple molecules are depicted in Fig. **12** [91]. Most of the studied compounds significantly inhibited self-induced Aβ aggregation determined by a thioflavin T (ThT) fluorescence assay. Electron-withdrawing substituents and the number of phenolic groups positively affected the inhibition activity with percentage superior (up to 53.4-88.5%) to RSV (65.1%) used as reference compound. All compounds showed a selective inhibition toward the MAO-B isoform in a micromolar range. Compounds with more than one or more hydroxyl group on aromatic ring had better but not statistically significant DPPH-scavenging activity (DPPH, IC_{50} = 13.3-43.4 μM) respect to RSV (DPPH, IC_{50} = 82.7 μM). Anyway, they showed strong protective capabilities on PC12 cell line, similar to RSV at the concentration of 25 μM. Above all, compound **10** (Fig. **12**) exhibited excellent potency for inhibition of self-induced Aβ aggregation (91.3 ± 2.1%, 25 μM), inhibition of MAO-B (IC_{50} 1.73 ± 0.39 μM), antioxidant effects (43.4 μM by DPPH method, 0.67 trolox equivalents by ABTS method), metal chelation (affinity order Cu^{2+} > Fe^{2+} > Fe^{3+}) and high BBB permeability, neuroprotective effects against ROS generation, H_2O_2-induced apoptosis, 6-OHDA-induced cell injury, and a significant *in vitro* anti-inflammatory activity with high inhibition of NO production in LPS-stimulated BV2 cells.

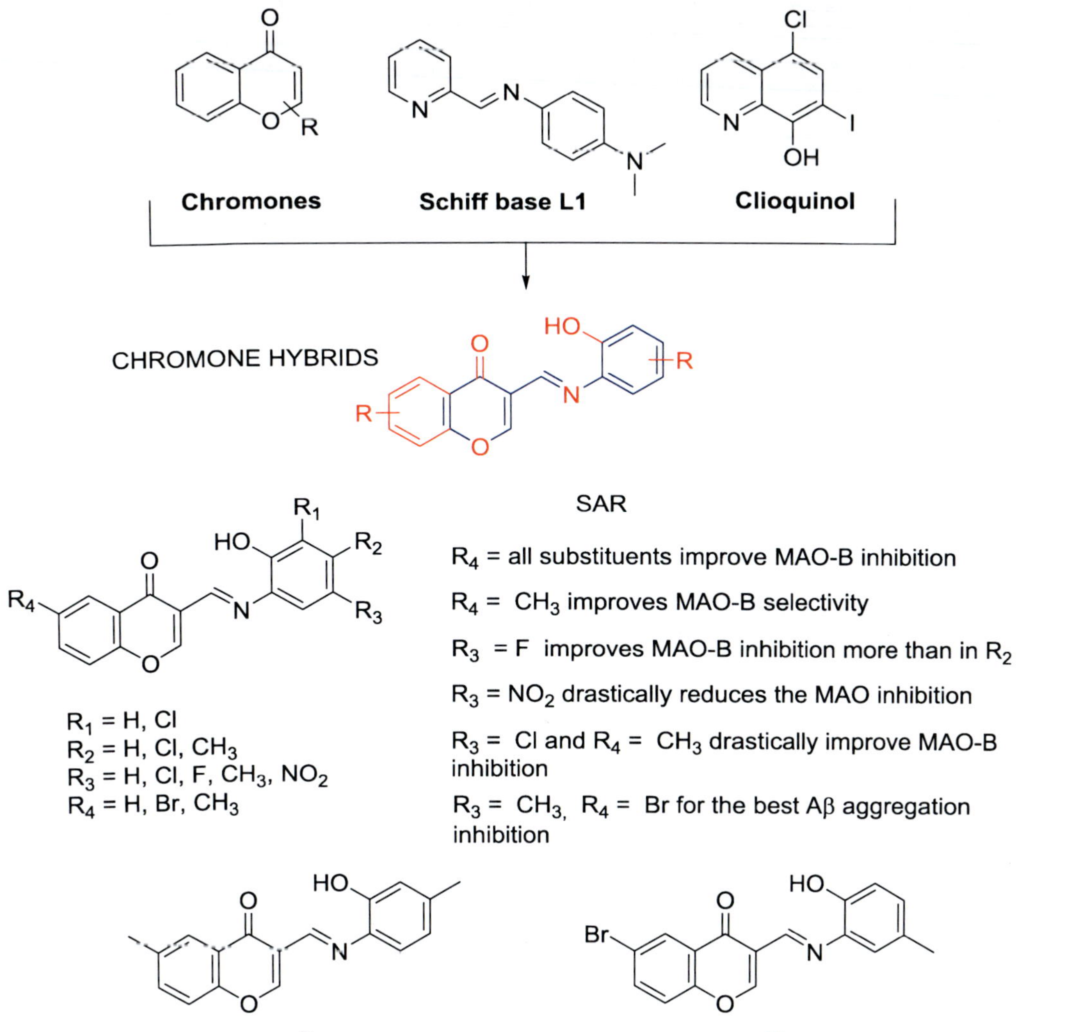

Fig. (11). Structures of chromone-RSV hydrids and **9a-b 9a**, **9b**.

Curcumin is a lipophilic polyphenol compound derived from the rhizome of the turmeric plant. It is recognized as one of the most promising anti-aging agents [92]. In 2018, de Freitas Silva *et al.* proposed the synthesis and the anticancer evaluation of some curcumin-RSV hybrids [93]. Starting from those results, recently the same research group studied the multifunctional antioxidant, anti-inflammatory, neuroprotective and AChE inhibitory properties [94]. They combine the *para*-hydroxy-*meta*-methoxy moiety of curcumin and the aromatic ring of RSV differently substituted, linked by an *N*-acylhydrazone 1,4-

disubstituted 1,2,3-triazole spacer (Fig. **13**). All tested compounds did not show relevant direct antioxidant activity but showed indirect antioxidant effects, in terms of increased neuronal resistance against the ROS formation. Among them, compound **11** (Fig. **13**) scavenged the DPPH radical in a similar manner to the trolox positive control (**11**, EC_{50} = 30.44 μM *vs* trolox, EC_{50} = 27.76 μM) and the best percentage of indirect antioxidant effect. The ability to modulate the intracellular GSH levels in SH-SY5Y cells, after 24 h of treatment using the fluorescent probe monochlorobimane (MCB), is dependent to the structural differences. Compounds with *para*-OH can relocate the radical from the phenolic hydroxyl to the N atom of the N-acylhydrazone group, due to the hydroxyl in *para* position in relation to the sp^2 carbon of N-acylhydrazone, the presence of *meta*-methoxy group increases the resonance, *meta* and *meta'* hydroxyls do not have the ability to relocate the free radical outside the aromatic ring or between the hydroxyls on the same aromatic ring. **11** remains the best free radical scavenger and protects the SH-SY5Y cells against the neurotoxicity elicited by Aβ peptide oligomers at 5 μM. Compound **11** was found to inhibit AChE in a potent manner (IC_{50} 26.30 μM) better than curcumin (IC_{50} 132.13 μM) and has acceptable predicted properties for oral absorption and permeation of BBB.

CLIOQUINOL-RSV HYBRIDS

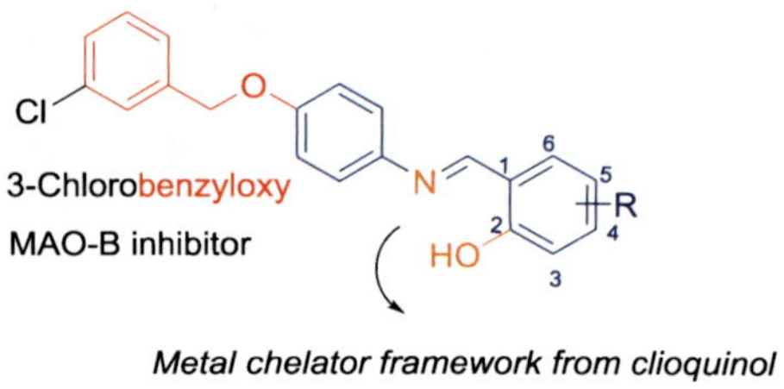

R = OH, OCH_3, F, Br, NO_2

SAR

5-F, 5-NO_2 and three hydroxyls increase the Aβ-aggregation inhibition

3,5-*di*-OH increases MAO-B inhibition and DPPH-scavenging activity

2,4-*di*-OH decreases MAO-B inhibition

different substituents are not favourable for DPPH-scavenging activity

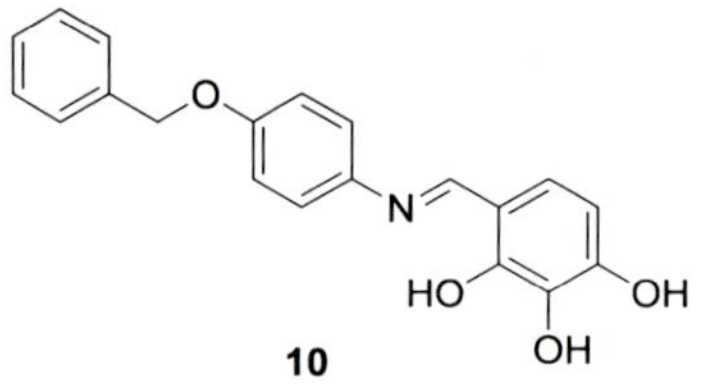

10

Fig. (12). Structures of clioquinol-RSV hybrids and **10**.

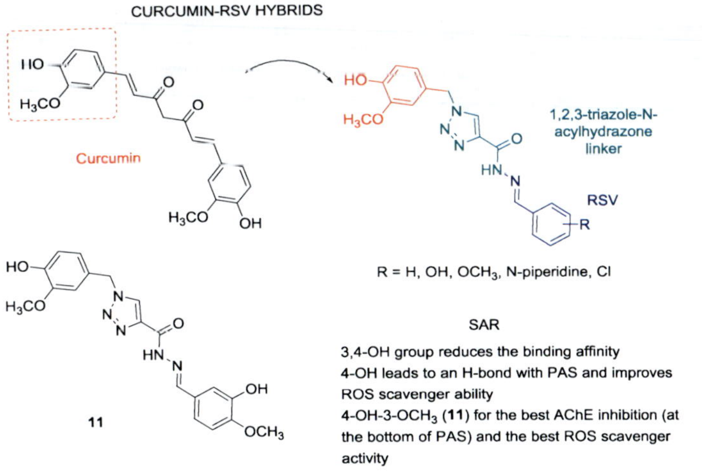

Fig. (13). Structures of curcumin-RSV hybrids and **11**.

Like previous studies on tacrine hybrids [95], a series of chloro/methoxy tacrine-RSV hybrids was studied for their antioxidant and anti-neuroinflammatory activities [96]. They combine the structure of RSV and tacrine (Fig. **14**), a well-known AChE inhibitor [19, 97]. Chlorine and methoxy substituents are inserted in specific positions, and the double bond of stilbene scaffold is reduced in some cases, as reported in Fig. **14**. The general effects of this modification are also reported. Generally, they are selective AChE inhibitors respect to BuChE. Compounds with the chlorine atom on tacrine fragment resulted more potent inhibitors of AChE (**12a**, AChE IC_{50} = 0.8 μM comparable to tacrine, IC_{50} 0.5 μM). This result was previously explained by the ability of the chloro-tacrine to establish van der Waals contacts with hydrophobic residues within the AChE active site and, decreasing also the electron density on the tacrine aromatic ring, and favoring π-electron interactions with nearby residues. The same fragment led to the best inhibition of Aβ self-aggregation, assessed through a thioflavin T-based fluorometric assay (**12b** and **12c**, 37.3% and 31.2%, respectively). In this last case, the kind of central bond does not seem to affect the activity, moreover the 2,4-di-hydroxyl moiety improves the Aβ self-aggregation inhibition [98] respect to 3,5-*di*-hydroxyl group of RSV, and the corresponding di-methoxy derivative. In contrast with reported information [26, 28], the free hydroxyl groups do not improve the antioxidant activity. **12c** (Fig. **14**) showed no neurotoxic effect on primary rat cerebellar granule neurons (CGNs) and interesting anti-inflammatory effects on astrocytes and microglia after treatment of 24 h at scalar concentrations (10-50 μM), after induction with LPS (lipopolysaccharide at 10 μg/mL) and it showed to effectively modulate the M1/M2 switch by positively decreasing inducible Nitric Oxide Synthases (*i*NOS) and slightly attenuating MRC1 expressions. The Nitric oxide (NO) free radical is a major signaling molecule in nervous systems and a close relationship with neurodegenerative diseases has been described. For this reason, the reduction of its production by a selective block of iNOS has been largely studied [99 - 101].

TACRINE-RSV HYBRIDS

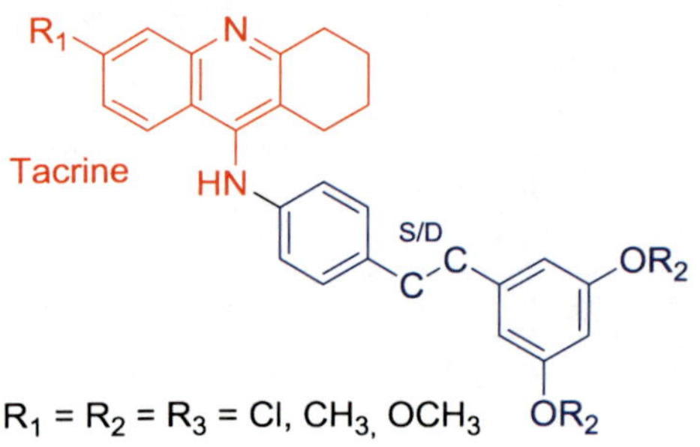

	R_1	R_2	C $\overset{S/D}{—}$ C
12a	Cl	CH_3	single
12b	Cl	H	single
12c	Cl	H	double

SAR

R_1 = Cl increases AChE and Aβ aggregation inhibition
Rigid double bond reduces AChE inhibition
More flexible single bond increases AChE inhibition
R_2 = OCH_3 augments AChE inhibition
R_2 = OH increases Aβ aggregation inhibition, but reduces antioxidant activity

Fig. (14). Structures of tacrine-RSV hybrids and **12a**, **12b**, **12c**.

Due to the role of activated microglia in the pathogenesis of AD, several piperazinyl pyrimidine hybrids of RSV were studied (Fig. **15**) as modulators of the inflammatory mediators including nitric oxide (NO), tumor necrosis factor α (TNF- α) and interleukin 1β (IL-1β) [102]. They incorporate the piperazinyl pyrimidine scaffold of some IL-1β inhibitors, as **GIBH-130** (IC_{50} = 3.4 nM in LPS-activated microglia, (Fig. **15**), approved by China Food and Drug Administration for clinical trials against AD [103]. The aromatic A was substituted with 4-F or 3-CF_3, while the aromatic B ring was substituted with F, Cl, OCH_3, OH, in different positions. Some of them are vinylogous of RSV, containing a second double bond (Fig. **15**). Their effects on NO production were tested in LPS-induced BV2 microglia cell lines comparing resulted with RSV, used as the positive control. The IC_{50} values (ranging from 1.0 μM to more than 50 μM) are function of the substituents on the aromatic rings. The addition of 4-F on aromatic A is favorable for NO inhibition (range IC_{50} 3.0-46.8 μM) respect to 3-CF_3 (range IC_{50} 6.5-42.6 μM). 4-CF_3 on B ring significantly increases the inhibition of NO release thanks to the stronger EW inductive effect. When on A ring there is no substituent, the effect of 4-Cl on ring B is detrimental for the NO inhibition, but better if in 2- or 3-position (>50, 10.1 and 12.6 μM, respectively). The double 2,5-substituents (2-OH, 5-OCH_3) reduce the inhibitory activity (IC_{50} > 40 μM *vs* RSV IC_{50} > 11.1 μM). The incorporation of the second double bond in **13** led to the most active compound on all the targets studied (NO-IC_{50} 1.0 μM, IL-1β-IC_{50} 0.5 μM and TNFα-IC_{50} 2.6 μM, respectively). **13** modulates the MAPK pathways through inhibiting the phosphorylation of JNK, ERK1/2, and p38 MAPK without disturbing NF-kB pathway.

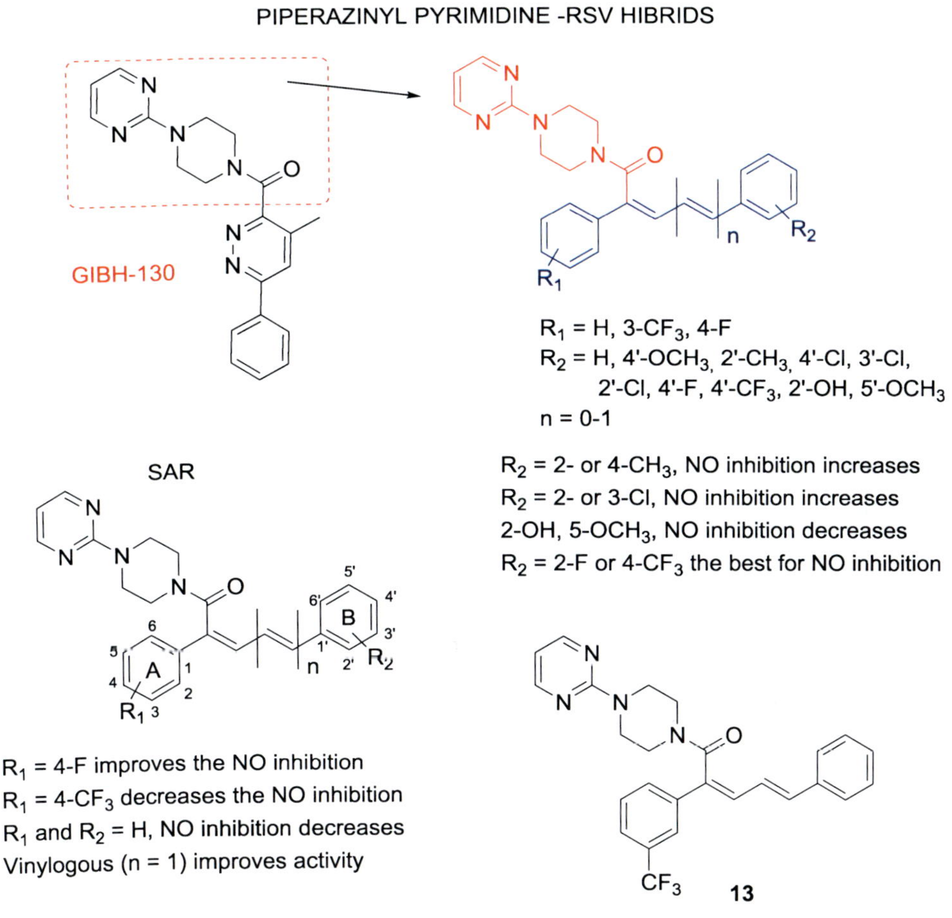

Fig. (15). Structures of piperazinyl pyrimidine-RSV hybrids and compound **13**.

Being the role of both iron and copper critical in the facilitating the aggregation of Aβ [104, 105], Xu *et al.* considered the positive effect of the substitution of one aromatic ring of RSV with deferiprone skeleton [106]. Deferiprone is an FDA approved iron chelator indicated for orally use to treat patients with trans-fusional iron overload due to thalassemia syndromes (Fig. **16**). It is a 3-hydroxy-1-2-dimethyl-4(*1H*)-pyridinone able to chelate the iron in a ratio 3:1 thanks to its bidentate structure. Recently, compounds incorporating its structure have been described as useful in NDs [107, 108]. These new compounds combine the pyridinone ring of deferiprone with the ethenyl benzene of RSV (Fig. **16**). Some different substituents have been introduced on aromatic ring to evaluate their effects on the activity against self-induced Aβ aggregation, antioxidant and metal chelating activity. Results revealed a good activity as antioxidant (ABTS IC_{50} 0.88-19.2 μM *vs* trolox IC_{50} 3.89 μM and RSV IC_{50} 0.76 μM), and Fe(III) chelator agents (pFe(III) values ranking 18.44-21.62 *vs* deferidone pFe(III) 20.60). The methyl group on *N*-pyridinone does not affect the antioxidant activity, otherwise the presence of two hydroxyl groups improves it. Most compounds showed an Aβ aggregation inhibition like RSV (51-65% and 64%, respectively). The 3,5-dihydroxy and 3,5-dimethoxy substituents lead to a decreased activity, while the 4-OH in **14a** and the 4-OEt in **14b** (Fig. **16**) lead to the best inhibitory activity (58.43% and 65.30%, respectively). ThT fluorescence and Transmission Electron Microscope (TEM) experiments revealed not only a marked reduction of ThT fluorescence to 62% and 64%, respectively, but also the ability of **14a** and **14b** to inhibit Fe(III) and Cu(II)-induced Aβ aggregation respect to reference RSV and an appreciable capability to disaggregate Fe(III)-induced fibrils, more than Cu(II)-induced one.

DEFERIPRONE-RSV HYBRIDS

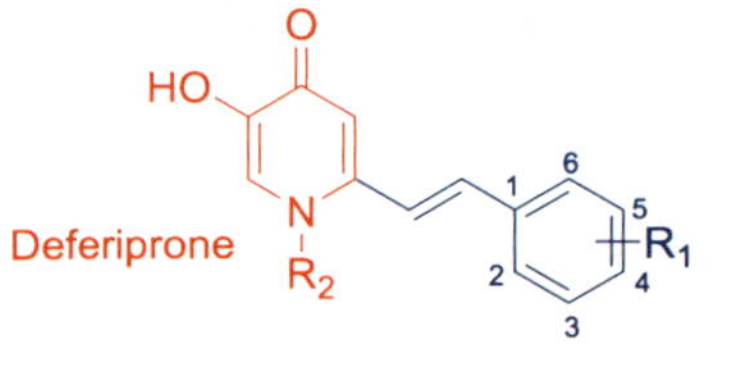

R_1 = H, Cl, F, $N(Me)_2$, NO_2, OEt, OMe, OH, 3,5-di-OH, 3,5-di-OMe

R_2 = H, CH_3

SAR

R_2= CH_3 improves antioxidant activity but does not affect the Aβ aggregation inhibition

3,5-*di*-OCH_3 improves Fe-chelator ability but reduces Aβ aggregation inhibition

3,5-*di*-OH improves antioxidant ability but reduces Aβ aggregation inhibition

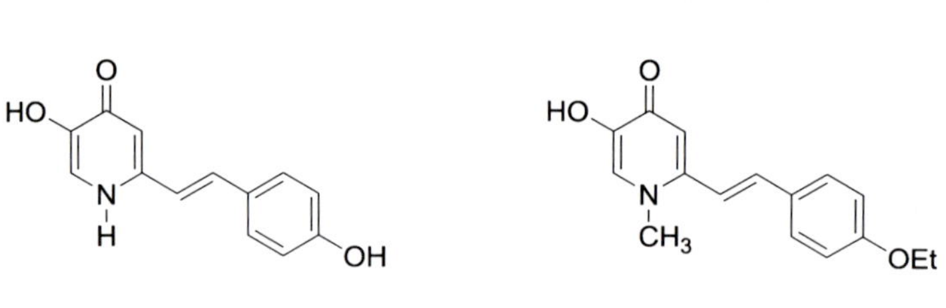

14a **14b**

Fig. (16). Structures of deferiprone-RSV hybrids and **14a** and **14b**.

It has been found that quinoline is a pharmacophore of many drugs candidate for AD [109, 110] and many researchers studied its derivatives and hybrids [111], also useful in AD [112]. Research works reported that the *N*-methylquinolinium increases the inhibitory activity of Aβ aggregation and ChE inhibition [113]. Based on these preliminary results, a series of RSV derivatives containing the *N*-methylquinolinium instead of one aromatic ring of RSV was synthesized (Fig. **17**) [114]. Many substituents in position 4 of pyridinium ring and in 4' of the benzene ring were added to explore the SAR. They contain piperazine or piperidine in 4-position and aminoaryl, methoxyaryl or heterocycles in 4'-position. Most of the compounds had moderate to strong inhibitor activity of Aβ self-aggregation (41.1-104.2% at 20 μM) compared to RSV (80.1% at 20 μM), used as reference. The Aβ self-aggregation inhibition is not influenced by the introduction of methylpiperazine, morpholine and hydroxyethylpiperazine group in 4 position on the quinoline ring while suffers of the 4-substituent in aromatic of RSV portion. In this position the introduction of dimethylamino, diethylamino, morpholinyl, and methylpiperazinyl groups increases the inhibition. In this position, the introduction of substituents with electronic effects reduces the activity in different entity: an EW substituent as chlorine induces a significant decrease of activity, but an ED as a methoxy group induces only a small decrease. Carbazolyl and indolyl instead of the aromatic of RSV improves the inhibition activity. The ORAC assay method with fluorescein highlighted that the introduction of an ED group on the benzene ring has better antioxidative activity than trolox and compounds with EW substituents. Most compounds had similar or weaker inhibitory activity toward AChE (IC_{50} ranging from 0.3 to 5 μM) than tacrine (IC_{50} 0.3 μM). They are less active on BuChE with a IC_{50} ranging from 1.1 to 5 μM than tacrine (IC_{50} 0.02 μM). Moreover, compounds unsubstituted in the 4-position in the quinoline ring have better AChE inhibitor activity than the corresponding substituted compounds. A 4-substituent on the benzene or pyridine ring has a positive effect on the inhibition of AChE. In Fig. **17** are depicted the structure of compound **15** that showed the best and specific inhibition of PAS of AChE, and the AChE-induced Aβ aggregation. It has a significant effect on the protection of neuronal cells against the glutamate-induced cytotoxicity in HT22 cells by preventing the ROS production and increasing the GSH level.

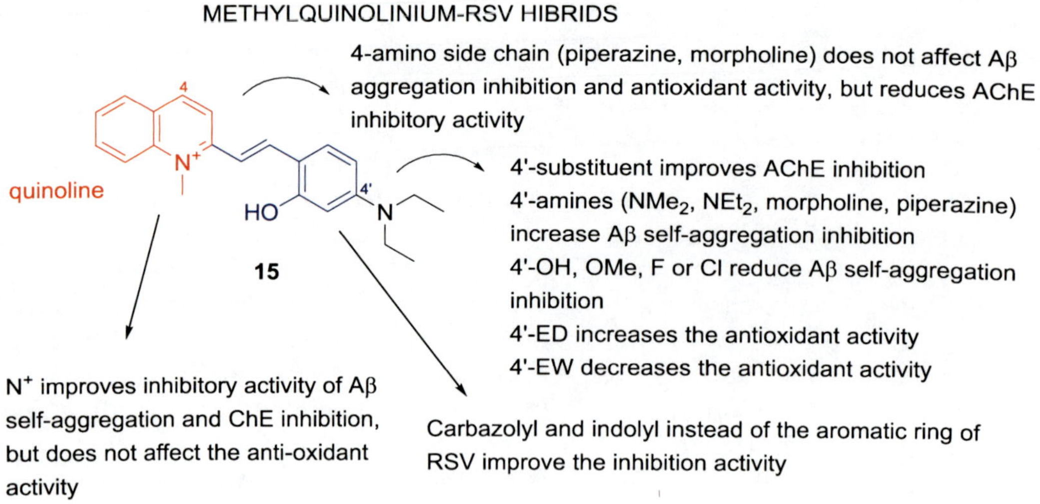

Fig. (17). Structures of methylquinolinium-RSV hybrid **15**.

PPARs (Peroxisome Proliferator-Activated Receptors) are a family of ligand-activated transcription factors; they play a critical role in many processes such as cell differentiation and metabolism [115, 116]. The pharmacological modulation of PPAR activity is useful in the control of neuropathological conditions, even if the mechanisms of action of PPAR ligands are so different. Recently, PPARγ agonists were shown to exert neuroprotective activity against oxidative damage, inflammation, and apoptosis in several neurodegenerative disorders. Many studies suggested that PPARγ ligands may be useful in the therapeutic management of patients with NDs [117, 118]. Considering the previous results reported in the literature, Giampietro *et al.* studied the biological behavior of some homemade hybrids that combine the stilbene core of RSV and the typical side chain of PPARγ ligands (Fig. **18**) [119]. Their work started from the observation that some RSV-fibrate hybrids showed interesting antioxidant activity [120], so they considered the best PPARγ agonists to evaluate their neuroprotective potential effect through the investigation of the cell viability, the catalase activity, the ROS production and the occurrence of apoptosis in an astrocyte cell line treated with these selected PPAR-γ agonists following the exposure to a PPAR-γ antagonist. In Fig. **18** are reported the structures of two compounds containing the RSV core bound to the tyrosine side chain, a framework presents in some selective PPARγ agonists (**16a** and **16b**, (Fig. **18**) [121]. **16a** and **16b** affect cell metabolism of CTX-TNA2 rat astrocyte cell line, at least after longer agonists exposure periods (96 h). They restored the catalase activity of CTX-TNA2 rat astrocytes disrupted by the treatment with a PPARγ antagonist, after 96 h of exposure, in a measure like the reference compound, rosiglitazone, a potent PPARγ agonist. The activity of this antioxidant enzyme is crucial in the physiological clearance of H_2O_2 in astrocytes [122]. Unfortunately, these two compounds resulted cytotoxic for CTX-TNA2 rat astrocytes.

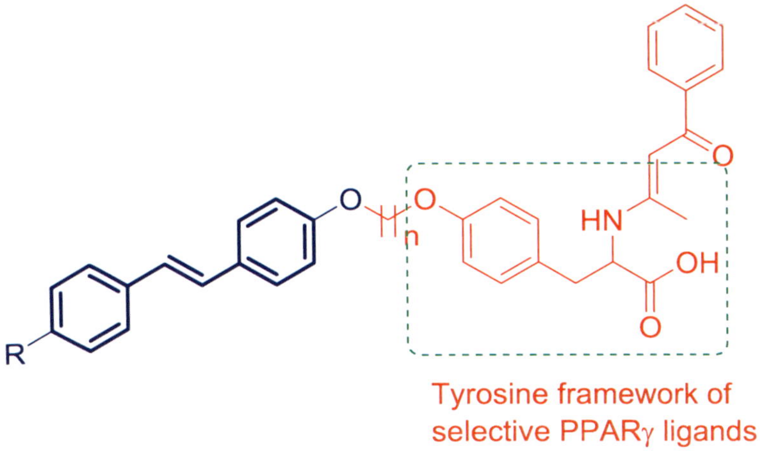

22a, n = 2, R = H

22b, n = 3, R = Cl

Fig. (18). Structures of tyrosine-RSV hybrids and **16a** and **16b**.

Derivatives of RSV

Derivatives of RSV comprise molecules in which the stilbene core is kept, and different substituents are introduced on the two aromatic rings. In some cases, the double bond is reduced, or one or two nitrogen atoms substitute the carbons.

In order to improve the efficacy and the bioavailability of RSV, a series of alkylated-RSV was prepared (Fig. **19**) and tested for their anti-oxidant and anti-inflammatory properties [123]. Since *O*- and *C*-alkylated and prenylated-RSV have been reported to be beneficial in NDs [124], these new compounds keep the skeleton of RSV, while the hydroxyl group are alkylated, sulfated or substituted with glucose or maltose (Fig. **19**). In some case, the glucose was monosubstituted with long chain esters. They were studied for their neuroprotection and anti-inflammatory activities. The selected alkylated RSV compounds showed higher inhibition of TNF-α production than RSV, and similar levels of IL-6 than RSV. The effect on SH-SY5Y neuroblastoma cells after oxidative stress challenge with hydrogen peroxide highlighted was positive for all compound at low dose of 10 μM, but at high dose of 100 μM they resulted toxic. The toxicity measured in a zebrafish embryonic model showed a quite toxicity for R1-monoalkylated derivatives but, above all, the free hydroxyl group led to lower toxicity in the studied system. Compound **17** (Fig. **19**) resulted to be the best in a model of HD and its anti-inflammatory activity better than RSV used as reference. The presence of octanoic acid chain plays an active role on attenuating the inflammation in the studied model.

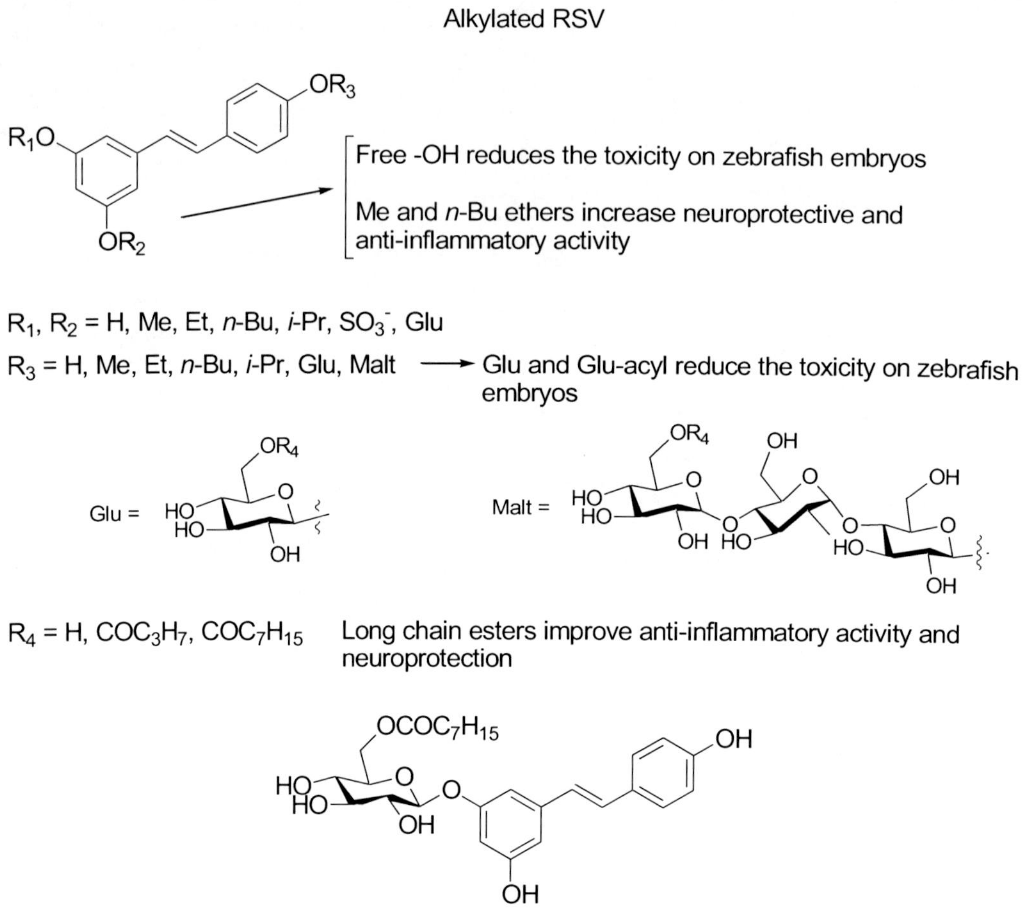

17

Fig. (19). Structures of alkylated RSV derivatives and compound **17**.

Like RSV, its natural oligomers show biological activities [125]. *trans*-Viniferin (Fig. **20**) is a dimer of RSV isolated from *Vitis vinifera*, that displays multiple effects [126]. *trans*-Viniferin and some of its isoprenylated derivatives were tested for their potential activity against AD (Fig. **20**) [127]. They combined the core of *trans*-Viniferin with an isoprenyl side chain natural and synthetic isoprenylated compounds have been described as anti-inflammatory, anti-oxidant and anti-tumor agents [128]. In Fig. **20** the structures of the most active prenylated derivative, **18a** and **18b**, are depicted. They displayed a moderate and selective inhibitory activity against MAO-B (IC_{50} = 3.91 ± 0.23 µM, 0.90 ± 0.01 µM), respectively. They also showed excellent antioxidant effects with different assay, after stress with H_2O_2, rotenone and oligomycin-A. They significantly inhibit cell PC-12 cell line death at concentrations ranging from 6.25 to 25 µM. They showed a significant *in vitro* anti-inflammatory and neuroprotective effects against LPS and H_2O_2 stimulated in BV2 microglia cells. The measure of their high permeability in the PAMPA-BBB assay indicated that the isoprenyl moieties have better penetrability, confirming the data. In general, **18a** was slightly better than **18b** and this is due to the presence of isoprenyl side chain.

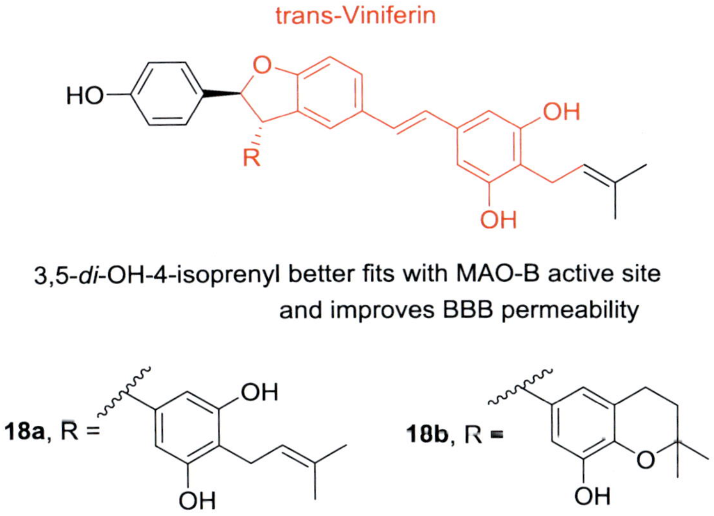

Fig. (20). Structures of isoprenylated *trans*-Viniferin derivatives and **18a** and **18b**.

Aging is a multifactorial phenomenon that alters the peroxisomal function with important consequences on the pathogenesis of a variety of diseases, including NDs. The atrophy of skeletal muscle fibers is a process to which the skeletal muscle tissue physiologically undergoes during aging. The effects of RSV on mouse skeletal muscle derived cells (C2C12 cells) in either undifferentiated (myoblasts) or differentiated state (myotubes) have been described [129]. RSV inhibits protein degradation and attenuates atrophy of skeletal muscle fibers [130]. C2C12 cell line represents one of the most used models for the study of skeletal muscle biology *in vitro* and is a useful preliminary analysis for more in-depth studies on CNS pathologies. In a recent study, a group of halogenated RSV derivatives was synthesized in order to explore their anti-oxidant effects on C2C12 cells [131]. In these molecules, the 4′-hydroxyl group was kept of RSV and chlorine atom was introduced in position 3′ and/or 2,4-position instead of the hydroxyls in 3,5 position of RSV and nitro or trifluoromethyl groups in 4-position were introduced (Fig. **21**). The colorimetric assay of 3-[4,5-dimethylthiazol-2-yl]-2,5-diphenyltetrazolium bromide (MTT), performed on C2C12 cell line, revealed that these molecules are not toxic respect to RSV at 1 and 10 μM. Of note, compound **19** (Fig. **21**) promotes an increase of the cell vitality at 1 and 10 μM, after 24 and 48 h of treatment. This effect is related to the high ability of compound **19** to scavenge the superoxide anion O_2^- in cells measured with both NBT (Nitro blue tetrazolium chloride) assay, with or without stress induced by hydrogen peroxide, and H_2DCFDA (2′,7′-dichlorodihydrofluorescein diacetate) assay. The cells, after the addition of 300 μM H_2O_2, reduce the ROS levels in the presence compound **19** at 10 μM, in a similar entity to RSV, used as reference. Noteworthy, the presence of the 3′-chlorine atom in **19** improves both the scavenger ability of the free 4′-hydroxyl and the lipophilicity.

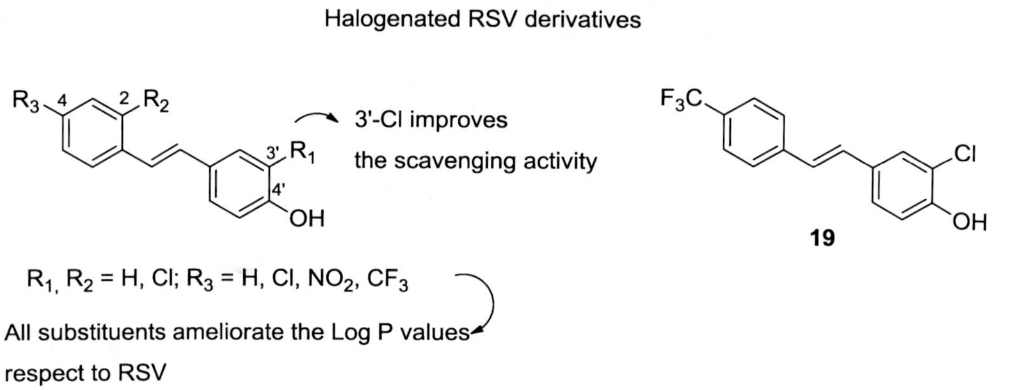

Fig. (21). Structure of halogenated RSV derivatives and **19**.

Schiff Base Derivatives of RSV

As introduced above, to improve the solubility and explore the biological potential of RSV, numerous chemical modifications have been carried out and some reviews collect these studies. One of the used strategies consists in the bioisomerism. In this case, the double bond of stilbene skeleton is replaced by the isosteric C=N or N=N bonds producing aza-stilbenes and azo-stilbenes [132]. Interestingly, the introduction of the imino bond induces a dissymmetry inside the stilbene double bond. In this case, the substituents on the two aromatics have different effects on the chemical and biological properties. For instance, the lone pair of the nitrogen atom plays a role in the stabilization of a phenoxyl radical or may allow an intramolecular hydrogen bond. Compounds containing an imino group are often presented as biologically active molecules [133] and the antioxidant and metal chelating properties have been described [134, 135].

Recently, Durgun *et al.* proposed a study on new Schiff base derivatives of RSV and relative amines, containing sulfonamide moiety (Fig. **22**) [136]. Sulfonamide-containing compounds are very important in medicinal chemistry and they are now extensively used drugs. Sulfonamide-based compounds have demonstrated biological properties as antimicrobial agents and useful against different diseases such as diabetes, psychosis, various cancers [137, 138], and anti-inflammatory, anticonvulsant, and antidepressant activities, as well as carbonic anhydrase inhibitors [139] and other central nervous system (CNS) disorders [140]. These compounds were assayed for their activity on human carbonic anhydrase (CA) I and II, and AChE enzyme activities and the antioxidant activity was determined using radical scavenging tests with ABTS, and DPPH and metal-reducing abilities with CUPRAC, and FRAP assays. CA is an enzyme containing a metal ion in active site. It catalyzes the reversible hydration of carbon dioxide (CO_2) to proton (H^+) and bicarbonate (HCO_3^-) [141]. The CA isoforms are grouped due to the properties such as catalytic activity, tissue and dispersion, subcellular location, expression levels, kinetic properties, and inhibitor sensitivity. To date, at least 16 variant CA isoforms were defined in mammalians. Pharmacological inhibitors of mitochondrial carbonic anhydrase have been reported to be useful in protecting against oxidative stress, with a positive effect on the progression of degenerative diseases [142]. All these new compounds showed high inhibition of CAs with major selectivity on CA I (K_i ranging from 32.1 to 100.6 nM) respect to CA II (K_i ranging from 10.1 to 79.3 nM) and acetazolamide, used as reference in this study (K_i 436.2 nM and 93.5 nM, respectively). All the amines showed better inhibitory effect (K_i values ranging from 32.1 ± 0.4 to 100.6 ± 1.9 nM). In fact, the reduced derivative **20a** (Fig. **22**) was the best inhibitor of CA I (K_i 32.1 nM) better than reference acetazolamide. Even if all tested compounds showed very good profile in nanomolar range, the imines showed more inhibitory effect on AChE enzyme activity respect to the amines (K_i 20.98-77.02 nM) and tacrine (K_i 109.75 nM). The imine **20b** (Fig. **22**) has the best inhibition profile (K_i 21.00 nM compared with K_i 109.75 nM of reference tacrine). The amines have also higher metal reduction capacity respect to the corresponding imines, probably because the amines contain an extra N-H bond compared to Schiff bases. They also showed better free radical scavenging activity (about 70% ABTS).

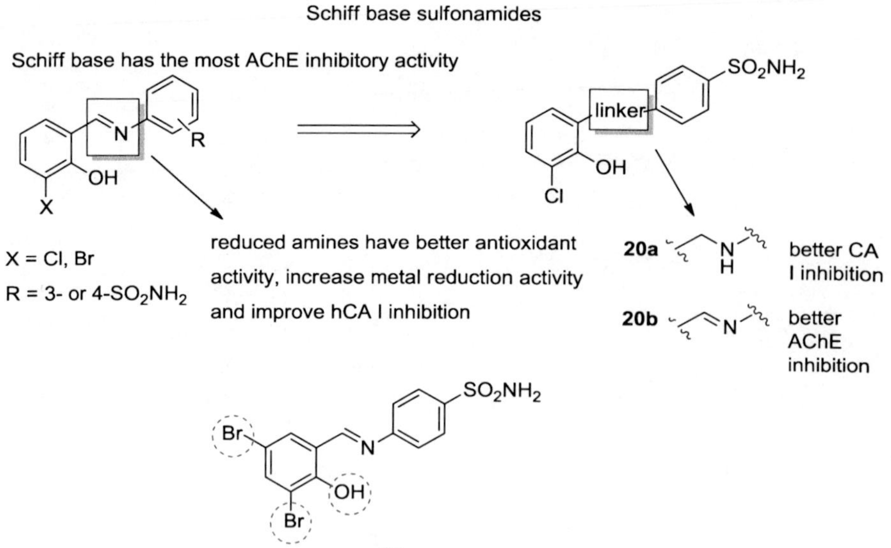

21

Fig. (22). Structures of Schiff base sulfonamides of RSV, **20a**, **20b** and **21**.

Starting from these results, a further study on the optimization of imines and amines was conducted introducing atoms of bromine and chlorine (Fig. **22**). These compounds were investigated for their cholinergic system regulatory effect [143]. The AChE inhibition ability was studied determining the K_i values: some of them showed a competitive inhibition effect, whereas others showed non-competitive inhibition. Among the non-competitive inhibitors, compound **21** (Fig. **22**) demonstrated the best inhibition activity on AChE (K_i 2.54 μM). Molecular modeling shed light the type of interaction with the targets, and two important hydrogen bonds between the amino group of the sulfonamide and two critical amino acids were observed, in addition to other important hydrogen and halogen bonds, making the affinity particularly remarkable. The higher inhibitory effect of **21** may be due to the bonding of the bound electronegative atoms present in the aromatic, that help the binding of the compounds to the active site of the enzyme. For compounds **21**, ADME studies were carried out, making them compounds with favorable physicochemical properties in line with Lipinski' rules [51].

Starting from the ability to inhibit the synthesis and release of several pro-inflammatory mediators, such as NO [144], some cytokines (as IL-1β, IL-6, IL-12 and TNF-α) and pro-inflammatory mediators [145], such as cyclooxygenase-1 (COX-1) and 2 (COX-2), Zimmermann-Franco *et al.* synthesized a series of imine and hydrazone analogues (Fig. **23**) and tested them for antioxidant, anti-inflammatory and immunomodulatory activities *in vitro* [146]. They contain the stilbene scaffold, but the double bond is substituted by an imine or hydrazone bridge. Substituents are in *meta* (R_1) and *para* (R_2) position on an aromatic ring and the 3,5-di-hydroxy moiety of RSV is substituted with a 2-hydroxy motif (Fig. **23**). At first, the cytotoxicity of RSV derivatives on RAW 264.7 cells, the popular murine macrophage cell line often used to initially screen natural products for bioactivity and to predict their potential effect *in vivo* or on primary cells [147], was measured and only the amines resulted not cytotoxic respect to hydrazones. The amines were selected for this study (structures of hydrazones were not shown). All the imines are more effective DPPH scavengers than RSV (IC_{50} range 34.1-49.1 μM *versus* RSV IC_{50} 65.6 μM). They reduce the production of pro-inflammatory cytokines IL-1β, IL-6, IL-12, CCL-2 and TNFα better than RSV and suppress *i*NOS and NF-kB. The influence on IL-12 production was particularly high for compound **22a** (Fig. **23**, IL-12 IC_{50} 4.7 pg/mL, RSV IC_{50} 1.03 mg/mL). These compounds have similar behaviour of RSV [148], then it may be hypothesized a similar mechanism of action. However, they have better bioavailability than RSV. This study revealed that all the substituents on aromatic ring improve the antioxidant and anti-inflammatory activity. Among all the imines, **22a** and **22b** (Fig. **23**) are the most active as anti-inflammatory agents and immunomodulators. Worth of note, the 4' position on the aromatic ring (methoxyl in **22a** and carboxyl in **22b**) are not involved in an intramolecular hydrogen bond, improving the ability to act. Thus, this characteristic seems to favour the anti-inflammatory activity. The hydrogen bond between the methoxyl group in the 4' position on the aromatic ring near to a 3'-OH reduces the activity. The same effect is noticeable when a carboxyl is positioned in 3' instead of 4' position.

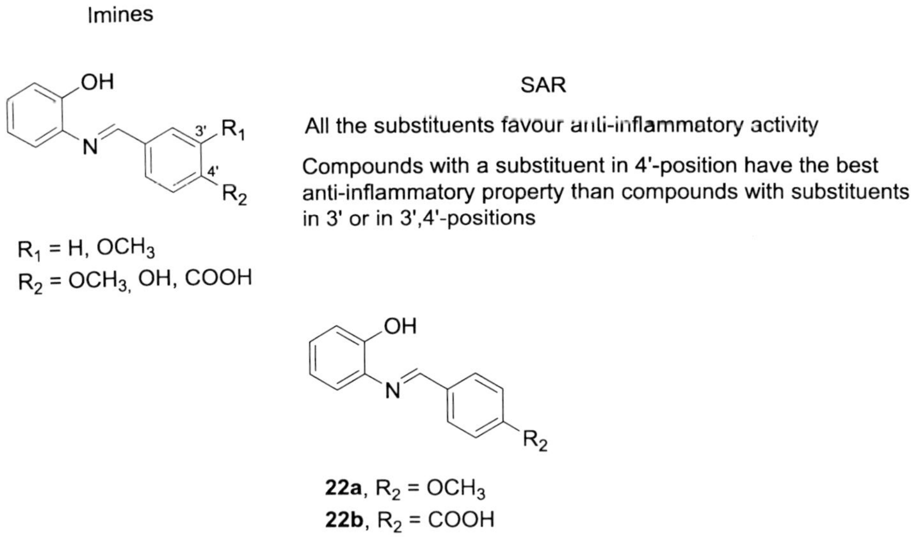

Fig. (23). Structures of imine derivatives of RSV and **22a** and **22b**.

The correlation between the position and number of hydroxyl groups in imino phenols (Fig. **24**) and efficiency of the radical scavenging ability was studied by Kotora *et al.* [149]. They assumed that compounds with three hydroxyl groups in the benzylidene part have the most effective antioxidant activity. These data were confirmed comparing the results obtained by study of DPPH, GOR and ABTS test expressed as SC_{50}, drug concentration eliciting 50% of the maximum stimulation calculated as the concentration of compound that causes a 50% decrease in absorbance at 517 nm, respect to reference RSV. In all cases, compound **23** (Fig. **24**) was the most active (SC_{50} 8.77 μmol/mL for DPPH, 15.39 μmol/mL for GOR and 1.98 μmol/mL for ABTS, *vs* corresponding values obtained for RSV used as reference of 26.37 μmol/mL, 72.66 μmol/mL and 1.43 μmol/mL, respectively). Very interesting was the correlation between the acidity of hydroxyls, measured by the chemical shift of NMR spectra of the compounds: high δ (12.25 to 14.19 ppm) corresponds to higher acidity and higher antioxidant activity. In particular, the compounds with the OH group in the *ortho* position of the ring A showed the most antioxidant activity because R_1 = OH could form intramolecular hydrogen bond with the nitrogen of imine group.

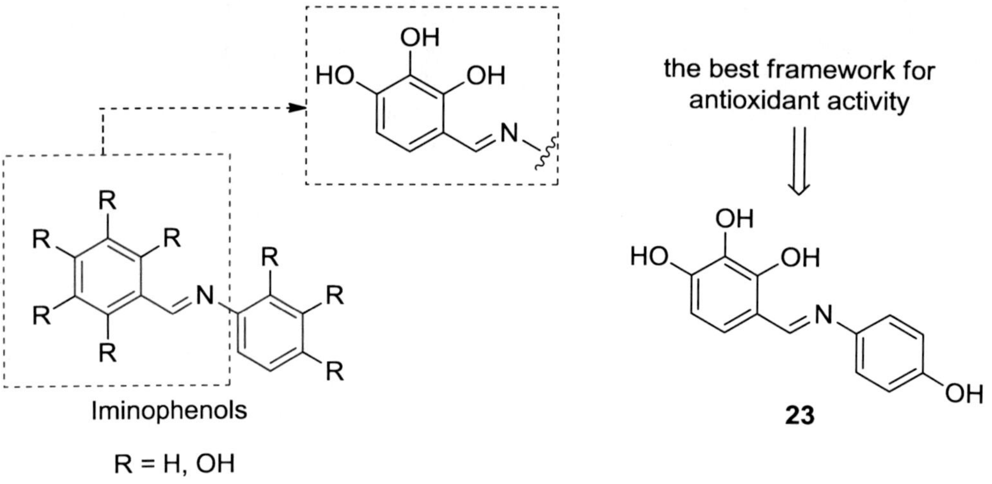

Fig. (24). Structure of iminophenol derivatives of RSV and **23**.

CONCLUDING REMARKS

NDs are complex neurodegenerative disorders causing multiple cellular changes and many pathways are involved in its pathogenesis. Neuroinflammation, metal dyshomeostasis, and oxidative stress have been described as common features in the progression of these pathologies. However, the exact cause of the disease is not known, and treatments are only symptomatic. Today, many efforts are directed toward the identification of new chemical entities able to modulate multiple targets such as AChEs, Aβ aggregation, MAOs inhibition, and many others.

Natural products exhibit promising health-promoting effects in NDs thanks to their multiple biological activity such as anti-inflammatory and antioxidant effects. Unfortunately, the low bioavailability and the reduced capability to cross the blood-brain barrier drastically reduce their clinical use. Anyway, they continue to be a useful source of new leads for the development of innovative agents. Therefore, many efforts have been directed to enhance the biological properties of natural compounds with chemical manipulation, developing MTDL based on natural templates.

RSV is a natural polyphenol with documented advantages in the control of the progression of NDs. Its stilbene core represents a "drug-likeness" scaffold, a privileged starting point for the new specific active agents. From a pharmaceutical point of view, synthetic analogues of RSV could be divided into hybrids and chemical derivatives. Molecular hybridization strategy consists in the combination of two or more pharmacophores in a single compound held together by a specific linker or by the overlapping of their structures. Derivatives of RSV originate from the addition of specific substituents with different electronic or lipophilic properties, such as halogens or methoxyl and hydroxyl groups, that improve the pharmacokinetic profiles and enlarge the activity and the selectivity. Taking it into account, many researchers have published reviews that cover the novel advances in the multi-target strategy for NDs therapy.

In the present chapter, the progression of recent hybrids and derivatives of RSV with particular attention to the use in NDs is explored. Due the NDs a multifactorial pathology, a general SAR cannot be deduced but the structural features and the SARs of the compounds have been reported in each figure.

Generally, the new derivatives of RSV showed potentiated ability to modulate important factors that contribute to the NDs simultaneously. Among the suggested modifications, the substitution or the overlap of one heterocycle with documented neuroprotection effect, instead of one aromatic ring of RSV, are useful to increase the inhibitory activity of AChE, Aβ aggregation, and for the anti-inflammatory and antioxidant activities. The introduction of different organic groups on the aromatic rings of RSV, such as fluoro, chloro, alkylamino, and hydroxyl groups, improve antioxidant and AChE inhibition activity. Moreover, the position and the number of the substituents are crucial for a specific inhibitory activity even if, in general, the 4'-position is beneficial to enhance the activity.

This review confirmed that the stilbene core could be considered a privileged scaffold in medicinal chemistry, with particular attention to NDs.

ABBREVIATIONS

Acetylcholine, ACh; Age-Related Macular Degeneration, AMD; Alzheimer's Disease, AD; Blood-Brain Barrier, BBB; C-C Motif Chemokine Ligand 2, CCL-2; Central Nervous System, CNS; Cyclooxygenase (COX); Electron-Donating, ED; Electron-Withdrawing, EW; Glucose Restriction, GR; Huntington's Disease, HD; Inducible Nitric Oxide Synthase, iNOS; Interleukin, IL; lipid peroxidation, LPO; Lipopolysaccharide, LPS; Monoamine Oxidases, MAOs; Multitarget-directed ligands, MTDLs; Nuclear Factor-κB, NF-κB; Neurodegenerative Diseases, NDs; Nitric Oxide, NO; Parallel Artificial Membrane Permeation Assay of the Blood-Brain Barrier, PAMPA-BBB; Parkinson's Disease, PD; peripheral anionic site, PAS; Pterostilbene, PTR; Reactive Oxygen Species, ROS; Resveratrol, RSV; Structure-Activity Relationship, SAR; 2,3,5,4'-Tetrahydroxystilbene-2-O-β-D-Glucoside, TSG; Tumor Necrosis Factor α, TNF-α; Type 2 Diabetes, T2D; Xanthine Oxidase, XO.

CONSENT FOR PUBLICATION

Not applicable.

CONFLICT OF INTEREST

The authors declare no conflict of interest, financial or otherwise.

ACKNOWLEDGEMENTS

Declared none.

REFERENCES

[1] Jellinger, K.A. General aspects of neurodegeneration. *J. Neural Transm. Suppl.,* **2003**, *65*(65), 101-144.
[http://dx.doi.org/10.1007/978-3-7091-0643-3_7] [PMID: 12946052]

[2] de A Boleti, A.P.; Almeida, J.A.; Migliolo, L. Impact of the metabolic syndrome on the evolution of neurodegenerative diseases. *Neural Regen. Res.,* **2021**, *16*(4), 688-689.
[http://dx.doi.org/10.4103/1673-5374.295329] [PMID: 33063727]

[3] Pisoschi, A.M.; Pop, A.; Iordache, F.; Stanca, L.; Predoi, G.; Serban, A.I. Oxidative stress mitigation by antioxidants - An overview on their chemistry and influences on health status. *Eur. J. Med. Chem.,* **2021**, *209*, 112891-112914.
[http://dx.doi.org/10.1016/j.ejmech.2020.112891] [PMID: 33032084]

[4] Wenjia, X.; Tianjiao, X.; Qingyun, Z.; Yujia, L.; Xiaoping, G. Role of microglia-mediated neuronal injury in neurodegenerative diseases. *Chinese Journal of Tissue Engineering Research,* **2021**, *25*, 1109-1115.
[http://dx.doi.org/10.3969/j.issn.2095-4344.2178]

[5] McGeer, P.L.; McGeer, E.G. NSAIDs and Alzheimer disease: Epidemiological, animal model and clinical studies. *Neurobiol. Aging,* **2007**, *28*(5), 639-647.
[http://dx.doi.org/10.1016/j.neurobiolaging.2006.03.013] [PMID: 16697488]

[6] Webers, A.; Heneka, M.T.; Gleeson, P.A. The role of innate immune responses and neuroinflammation in amyloid accumulation and progression of Alzheimer's disease. *Immunol. Cell Biol.*, **2020**, *98*(1), 28-41.
[http://dx.doi.org/10.1111/imcb.12301] [PMID: 31654430]

[7] Gamage, R.; Wagnon, I.; Rossetti, I.; Childs, R.; Niedermayer, G.; Chesworth, R.; Gyengesi, E. Cholinergic modulation of glial function during aging and chronic neuroinflammation. *Front. Cell. Neurosci.*, **2020**, *14*, 577912.
[http://dx.doi.org/10.3389/fncel.2020.577912] [PMID: 33192323]

[8] Sharma, P.; Tripathi, M.K.; Shrivastava, S.K. Cholinesterase as a target for drug development in alzheimer's disease. *Methods Mol. Biol.*, **2020**, *2089*, 257-286.
[http://dx.doi.org/10.1007/978-1-0716-0163-1_18] [PMID: 31773661]

[9] Moss, D.E. Improving anti-neurodegenerative benefits of acetylcholinesterase inhibitors in Alzheimer's disease: are irreversible inhibitors the future? *Int. J. Mol. Sci.*, **2020**, *21*(10), 3438-3456.
[http://dx.doi.org/10.3390/ijms21103438] [PMID: 32414155]

[10] Reitz, C. Alzheimer's disease and the amyloid cascade hypothesis: a critical review. *Int. J. Alzheimers Dis.*, **2012**, *2012*, 1-11.
[http://dx.doi.org/10.1155/2012/369808] [PMID: 22506132]

[11] Hider, R.C.; Ma, Y.; Molina-Holgado, F.; Gaeta, A.; Roy, S. Iron chelation as a potential therapy for neurodegenerative disease. *Biochem. Soc. Trans.*, **2008**, *36*(6), 1304-1308.
[http://dx.doi.org/10.1042/BST0361304] [PMID: 19021545]

[12] Santos, M.A.; Chand, K.; Chaves, S. Recent progress in multifunctional metal chelators as potential drugs for Alzheimer's disease. *Coord. Chem. Rev.*, **2016**, *327-328*, 287-303.
[http://dx.doi.org/10.1016/j.ccr.2016.04.013]

[13] Wang, X.; Wang, W.; Li, L.; Perry, G.; Lee, H.; Zhu, X. Oxidative stress and mitochondrial dysfunction in Alzheimer's disease. *Biochim. Biophys. Acta Mol. Basis Dis.*, **2014**, *1842*(8), 1240-1247.
[http://dx.doi.org/10.1016/j.bbadis.2013.10.015] [PMID: 24189435]

[14] Niranjan, R. The role of inflammatory and oxidative stress mechanisms in the pathogenesis of Parkinson's disease: focus on astrocytes. *Mol. Neurobiol.*, **2014**, *49*(1), 28-38.
[http://dx.doi.org/10.1007/s12035-013-8483-x] [PMID: 23783559]

[15] Dezsi, L.; Vecsei, L. Monoamine Oxidase B Inhibitors in Parkinson's Disease. *CNS Neurol. Disord. Drug Targets*, **2017**, *16*(4), 425-439.
[http://dx.doi.org/10.2174/1871527316666170124165222] [PMID: 28124620]

[16] Guglielmi, P.; Carradori, S.; Ammazzalorso, A.; Secci, D. Novel approaches to the discovery of selective human monoamine oxidase-B inhibitors: is there room for improvement? *Expert Opin. Drug Discov.*, **2019**, *14*(10), 995-1035.
[http://dx.doi.org/10.1080/17460441.2019.1637415] [PMID: 31268358]

[17] Balestrino, R.; Schapira, A.H.V. Parkinson disease. *Eur. J. Neurol.*, **2020**, *27*(1), 27-42.
[http://dx.doi.org/10.1111/ene.14108] [PMID: 31631455]

[18] d'Angelo, M.; Cimini, A.; Castelli, V.; Quintiliani, M.; Benedetti, E.; Cifone, M.G. The emerging role of probiotics in neurodegenerative diseases: new hope for Parkinson's disease? *Neural Regen. Res.*, **2021**, *16*(4), 628-634.
[http://dx.doi.org/10.4103/1673-5374.295270] [PMID: 33063712]

[19] Vaz, M.; Silvestre, S. Alzheimer's disease: Recent treatment strategies. *Eur. J. Pharmacol.*, **2020**, *887*, 173554.
[http://dx.doi.org/10.1016/j.ejphar.2020.173554] [PMID: 32941929]

[20] Simone Tranches Dias, K.; Viegas, C., Jr Simone Tranches Dias, K., Viegas, C., Dias, K.S.T., Viegas, C. Multi-target directed drugs: A modern approach for design of new drugs for the treatment of

Alzheimer's disease. *Curr. Neuropharmacol.,* **2014**, *12*(3), 239-255. [http://dx.doi.org/10.2174/1570159X1203140511153200] [PMID: 24851088]

[21] Gabr, M.T.; Ibrahim, M.M. Multitarget therapeutic strategies for Alzheimer's disease. *Neural Regen. Res.,* **2019**, *14*(3), 437-440. [http://dx.doi.org/10.4103/1673-5374.245463] [PMID: 30539809]

[22] Mohd Sairazi, N.S.; Sirajudeen, K.N.S. Natural products and their bioactive compounds: Neuroprotective potentials against neurodegenerative diseases. *Evid. Based Complement. Alternat. Med.,* **2020**, *2020*, 1-30. [http://dx.doi.org/10.1155/2020/6565396] [PMID: 32148547]

[23] Olajide, O.A.; Sarker, S.D. Alzheimer's disease: natural products as inhibitors of neuroinflammation. *Inflammopharmacology,* **2020**, *28*(6), 1439-1455. [http://dx.doi.org/10.1007/s10787-020-00751-1] [PMID: 32930914]

[24] Ji, H.; Zhang, H. Multipotent natural agents to combat Alzheimer's disease. Functional spectrum and structural features. *Acta Pharmacol. Sin.,* **2008**, *29*(2), 143-151. [http://dx.doi.org/10.1111/j.1745-7254.2008.00752.x] [PMID: 18215342]

[25] de Araújo, F.F.; de Paulo Farias, D.; Neri-Numa, I.A.; Pastore, G.M. Polyphenols and their applications: An approach in food chemistry and innovation potential. *Food Chem.,* **2021**, *338*, 127535. [http://dx.doi.org/10.1016/j.foodchem.2020.127535] [PMID: 32798817]

[26] Uddin, M.S.; Al Mamun, A.; Kabir, M.T.; Ahmad, J.; Jeandet, P.; Sarwar, M.S.; Ashraf, G.M.; Aleya, L. Neuroprotective role of polyphenols against oxidative stress-mediated neurodegeneration. *Eur. J. Pharmacol.,* **2020**, *886*, 173412. [http://dx.doi.org/10.1016/j.ejphar.2020.173412] [PMID: 32771668]

[27] Aryal, S.; Skinner, T.; Bridges, B.; Weber, J.T. The pathology of Parkinson's disease and potential benefit of dietary polyphenols. *Molecules,* **2020**, *25*(19), 4382-4409. [http://dx.doi.org/10.3390/molecules25194382] [PMID: 32987656]

[28] Blandini, F.; Giuliano, C.; Cerri, S. Potential therapeutic effects of polyphenols in Parkinson's disease: *in vivo* and *in vitro* pre-clinical studies. *Neural Regen. Res.,* **2021**, *16*(2), 234-241. [http://dx.doi.org/10.4103/1673-5374.290879] [PMID: 32859769]

[29] Almeida, A.F.; dos Santos, C.N.; Ventura, M.R. Polyphenols, their metabolites and derivatives as drug leads. *Curr. Pharm. Des.,* **2018**, *24*(19), 2188-2207. [http://dx.doi.org/10.2174/1381612824666180516103609] [PMID: 29766784]

[30] Shen, T.; Wang, X.N.; Lou, H.X. Natural stilbenes: an overview. *Nat. Prod. Rep.,* **2009**, *26*(7), 916-935. [http://dx.doi.org/10.1039/b905960a] [PMID: 19554241]

[31] Keylor, M.H.; Matsuura, B.S.; Stephenson, C.R.J. Chemistry and biology of resveratrol-derived natural products. *Chem. Rev.,* **2015**, *115*(17), 8976-9027. [http://dx.doi.org/10.1021/cr500689b] [PMID: 25835567]

[32] Akinwumi, B.; Bordun, K.A.; Anderson, H. Biological activities of stilbenoids. *Int. J. Mol. Sci.,* **2018**, *19*(3), 792. [http://dx.doi.org/10.3390/ijms19030792] [PMID: 29522491]

[33] Saad, N.M.; Sekar, M.; Gan, S.H.; Lum, P.T.; Vaijanathappa, J.; Ravi, S. Resveratrol: latest scientific evidences of its chemical, biological activities and therapeutic potentials. *Pharmacogn. J.,* **2020**, *12*(6s), 1779-1791. [http://dx.doi.org/10.5530/pj.2020.12.240]

[34] Rioux Bilan, A.; Freyssin, A.; Page, G.; Fauconneau, B. Natural stilbenes effects in animal models of Alzheimer's disease. *Neural Regen. Res.,* **2020**, *15*(5), 843-849. [http://dx.doi.org/10.4103/1673-5374.268970] [PMID: 31719245]

[35] Kulkarni, S.S.; Cantó, C. The molecular targets of resveratrol. *Biochim. Biophys. Acta Mol. Basis Dis.*, **2015**, *1852*(6), 1114-1123.
[http://dx.doi.org/10.1016/j.bbadis.2014.10.005] [PMID: 25315298]

[36] Turner, R.S.; Thomas, R.G.; Craft, S.; van Dyck, C.H.; Mintzer, J.; Reynolds, B.A.; Brewer, J.B.; Rissman, R.A.; Raman, R.; Aisen, P.S. A randomized, double-blind, placebo-controlled trial of resveratrol for Alzheimer disease. *Neurology,* **2015**, *85*(16), 1383-1391.
[http://dx.doi.org/10.1212/WNL.0000000000002035] [PMID: 26362286]

[37] http://www.clinicaltrials.gov/ct2/show/NCT01504854?term1/4resveratrol&rank1/442

[38] Moussa, C.; Hebron, M.; Huang, X.; Ahn, J.; Rissman, R.A.; Aisen, P.S.; Turner, R.S. Resveratrol regulates neuro-inflammation and induces adaptive immunity in Alzheimer's disease. *J. Neuroinflammation,* **2017**, *14*(1), 1-10.
[http://dx.doi.org/10.1186/s12974-016-0779-0] [PMID: 28086917]

[39] Peñalver, P.; Zodio, S.; Lucas, R.; de-Paz, M.V.; Morales, J.C. Neuroprotective and anti-inflammatory effects of pterostilbene metabolites in human neuroblastoma SH-SY5Y and RAW 264.7 macrophage cells. *J. Agric. Food Chem.,* **2020**, *68*(6), 1609-1620.
[http://dx.doi.org/10.1021/acs.jafc.9b07147] [PMID: 31957426]

[40] Chang, J.; Rimando, A.; Pallas, M.; Camins, A.; Porquet, D.; Reeves, J.; Shukitt-Hale, B.; Smith, M.A.; Joseph, J.A.; Casadesus, G. Low-dose pterostilbene, but not resveratrol, is a potent neuromodulator in aging and Alzheimer's disease. *Neurobiol. Aging,* **2012**, *33*(9), 2062-2071.
[http://dx.doi.org/10.1016/j.neurobiolaging.2011.08.015] [PMID: 21982274]

[41] Zhou, Y.; Wang, G.; Li, D.; Wang, Y.; Wu, Q.; Shi, J.; Zhang, F. Dual modulation on glial cells by tetrahydroxystilbene glucoside protects against dopamine neuronal loss. *J. Neuroinflammation,* **2018**, *15*(1), 161-176.
[http://dx.doi.org/10.1186/s12974-018-1194-5] [PMID: 29801454]

[42] Walle, T. Bioavailability of resveratrol. *Ann. N. Y. Acad. Sci.,* **2011**, *1215*(1), 9-15.
[http://dx.doi.org/10.1111/j.1749-6632.2010.05842.x] [PMID: 21261636]

[43] Intagliata, S.; Modica, M.N.; Santagati, L.M.; Montenegro, L. Strategies to improve resveratrol systemic and topical bioavailability: An update. *Antioxidants,* **2019**, *8*(8), 244-257.
[http://dx.doi.org/10.3390/antiox8080244] [PMID: 31349656]

[44] Fonseca-Santos, B.; Chorilli, M. The uses of resveratrol for neurological diseases treatment and insights for nanotechnology based-drug delivery systems. *Int. J. Pharm.,* **2020**, *589*, 119832.
[http://dx.doi.org/10.1016/j.ijpharm.2020.119832] [PMID: 32877730]

[45] Blaikie, L.; Kay, G.; Kong Thoo Lin, P. Current and emerging therapeutic targets of alzheimer's disease for the design of multi-target directed ligands. *MedChemComm,* **2019**, *10*(12), 2052-2072.
[http://dx.doi.org/10.1039/C9MD00337A] [PMID: 32206241]

[46] Rankovic, Z. CNS drug design: balancing physicochemical properties for optimal brain exposure. *J. Med. Chem.,* **2015**, *58*(6), 2584-2608.
[http://dx.doi.org/10.1021/jm501535r] [PMID: 25494650]

[47] Pardridge, W.M. Drug transport across the blood-brain barrier. *J. Cereb. Blood Flow Metab.,* **2012**, *32*(11), 1959-1972.
[http://dx.doi.org/10.1038/jcbfm.2012.126] [PMID: 22929442]

[48] Biasutto, L.; Mattarei, A.; Azzolini, M.; La Spina, M.; Sassi, N.; Romio, M.; Paradisi, C.; Zoratti, M. Resveratrol derivatives as a pharmacological tool. *Ann. N. Y. Acad. Sci.,* **2017**, *1403*(1), 27-37.
[http://dx.doi.org/10.1111/nyas.13401] [PMID: 28675763]

[49] Li, Q.S.; Li, Y.; Deora, G.S.; Ruan, B.F. Derivatives and analogues of resveratrol: recent advances in structural modification. *Mini Rev. Med. Chem.,* **2019**, *19*(10), 809-825.
[http://dx.doi.org/10.2174/1389557519666190128093840] [PMID: 30686253]

[50] Xiao, Y.; Chen, H.; Song, C.; Zeng, X.; Zheng, Q.; Zhang, Y.; Lei, X.; Zheng, X. Pharmacological activities and structure-modification of resveratrol analogues. *Pharmazie,* **2015**, *70*(12), 765-771. [PMID: 26817272]

[51] Liu, Y.; Liu, Y.; Chen, H.; Yao, X.; Xiao, Y.; Zeng, X.; Zheng, Q.; Wei, Y.; Song, C.; Zhang, Y.; Zhu, P.; Wang, J.; Zheng, X. Synthetic resveratrol derivatives and their biological activities: A review. *Open J. Med. Chem.,* **2015**, *5*(4), 97-105. [http://dx.doi.org/10.4236/ojmc.2015.54006]

[52] Giacomini, E.; Rupiani, S.; Guidotti, L.; Recanatini, M.; Roberti, M. The use of stilbene scaffold in medicinal chemistry and multi-target drug design. *Curr. Med. Chem.,* **2016**, *23*(23), 2439-2489. [http://dx.doi.org/10.2174/0929867323666160517121629] [PMID: 27183980]

[53] Arbo, B.D.; André-Miral, C.; Nasre-Nasser, R.G.; Schimith, L.E.; Santos, M.G.; Costa-Silva, D.; Muccillo-Baisch, A.L.; Hort, M.A. Resveratrol derivatives as potential treatments for Alzheimer's and Parkinson's disease. *Front. Aging Neurosci.,* **2020**, *12*, 103-118. [http://dx.doi.org/10.3389/fnagi.2020.00103] [PMID: 32362821]

[54] Pecyna, P.; Wargula, J.; Murias, M.; Kucinska, M. More than resveratrol: New insights into stilbene-based compounds. *Biomolecules,* **2020**, *10*(8), 1111-1151. [http://dx.doi.org/10.3390/biom10081111] [PMID: 32726968]

[55] Mishra, P.; Kumar, A.; Panda, G. Anti-cholinesterase hybrids as multi-target-directed ligands against Alzheimer's disease (1998–2018). *Bioorg. Med. Chem.,* **2019**, *27*(6), 895-930. [http://dx.doi.org/10.1016/j.bmc.2019.01.025] [PMID: 30744931]

[56] Wiciński, M.; Domanowska, A.; Wódkiewicz, E.; Malinowski, B. Neuroprotective properties of resveratrol and its derivatives-influence on potential mechanisms leading to the development of Alzheimer's disease. *Int. J. Mol. Sci.,* **2020**, *21*(8), 2749-2766. [http://dx.doi.org/10.3390/ijms21082749] [PMID: 32326620]

[57] Fantacuzzi, M.; Amoroso, R.; Carradori, S.; De Filippis, B. Resveratrol-based compounds and neurodegeneration: Recent insight in multitarget therapy. *Eur. J. Med. Chem.,* **2022**, *233*, 114242. [http://dx.doi.org/10.1016/j.ejmech.2022.114242] [PMID: 35276424]

[58] Singh, M.; Kaur, M.; Chadha, N.; Silakari, O. Hybrids: a new paradigm to treat Alzheimer's disease. *Mol. Divers.,* **2016**, *20*(1), 271-297. [http://dx.doi.org/10.1007/s11030-015-9628-9] [PMID: 26328942]

[59] Chen, L.Z.; Yao, L.; Jiao, M.M.; Shi, J.B.; Tan, Y.; Ruan, B.F.; Liu, X.H. Novel resveratrol-based flavonol derivatives: Synthesis and anti-inflammatory activity *in vitro* and *in vivo*. *Eur. J. Med. Chem.,* **2019**, *175*, 114-128. [http://dx.doi.org/10.1016/j.ejmech.2019.05.004] [PMID: 31077997]

[60] Decker, M. Hybrid molecules incorporating natural products: applications in cancer therapy, neurodegenerative disorders and beyond. *Curr. Med. Chem.,* **2011**, *18*(10), 1464-1475. [http://dx.doi.org/10.2174/092986711795328355] [PMID: 21428895]

[61] De Filippis, B.; Ammazzalorso, A.; Fantacuzzi, M.; Giampietro, L.; Maccallini, C.; Amoroso, R. Anticancer activity of stilbene-based derivatives. *ChemMedChem,* **2017**, *12*(8), 558-570. [http://dx.doi.org/10.1002/cmdc.201700045] [PMID: 28266812]

[62] Tzvetkov, N.T.; Stammler, H.G.; Neumann, B.; Hristova, S.; Antonov, L.; Gastreich, M. Crystal structures, binding interactions, and ADME evaluation of brain penetrant N -substituted indazole---carboxamides as subnanomolar, selective monoamine oxidase B and dual MAO-A/B inhibitors. *Eur. J. Med. Chem.,* **2017**, *127*, 470-492. [http://dx.doi.org/10.1016/j.ejmech.2017.01.011] [PMID: 28107736]

[63] Kung, H.F.; Lee, C.W.; Zhuang, Z.P.; Kung, M.P.; Hou, C.; Plössl, K. Novel stilbenes as probes for amyloid plaques. *J. Am. Chem. Soc.,* **2001**, *123*(50), 12740-12741. [http://dx.doi.org/10.1021/ja0167147] [PMID: 11741464]

[64] Lan, J.S.; Liu, Y.; Hou, J.; Yang, J.; Zhang, X.Y.; Zhao, Y.; Xie, S.S.; Ding, Y.; Zhang, T. Design, synthesis and evaluation of resveratrol-indazole hybrids as novel monoamine oxidases inhibitors with amyloid- β aggregation inhibition. *Bioorg. Chem.*, **2018**, *76*, 130-139. [http://dx.doi.org/10.1016/j.bioorg.2017.11.009] [PMID: 29172101]

[65] Jiang, L.; Zhang, M.; Tang, L.; Weng, Q.; Shen, Y.; Hu, Y.; Sheng, R. Identification of 2-subsituted benzothiazole derivatives as triple-functional agents with potential for AD therapy. *RSC Advances*, **2016**, *6*(21), 17318-17327. [http://dx.doi.org/10.1039/C5RA25788C]

[66] Cheng, G.; Xu, P.; Zhang, M.; Chen, J.; Sheng, R.; Ma, Y. Resveratrol-maltol hybrids as multi-targe--directed agents for Alzheimer's disease. *Bioorg. Med. Chem.*, **2018**, *26*(22), 5759-5765. [http://dx.doi.org/10.1016/j.bmc.2018.08.011] [PMID: 30360953]

[67] Calderón-Ospina, C.A.; Nava-Mesa, M.O. B Vitamins in the nervous system: Current knowledge of the biochemical modes of action and synergies of thiamine, pyridoxine, and cobalamin. *CNS Neurosci. Ther.*, **2020**, *26*(1), 5-13. [http://dx.doi.org/10.1111/cns.13207] [PMID: 31490017]

[68] Semenov, A.V.; Balakireva, O.I.; Tarasova, I.V.; Burtasov, A.A.; Semenova, E.V.; Petrov, P.S.; Minaeva, O.V.; Pyataev, N.A. Synthesis, theoretical, and experimental study of radical scavenging activity of 3-pyridinol containing trans-resveratrol analogs. *Med. Chem. Res.*, **2018**, *27*(4), 1298-1308. [http://dx.doi.org/10.1007/s00044-018-2150-8]

[69] Hashim, A.; Wang, L.; Juneja, K.; Ye, Y.; Zhao, Y.; Ming, L.J. Vitamin B6s inhibit oxidative stress caused by Alzheimer's disease-related CuII-β-amyloid complexes—cooperative action of phospho-moiety. *Bioorg. Med. Chem. Lett.*, **2011**, *21*(21), 6430-6432. [http://dx.doi.org/10.1016/j.bmcl.2011.08.123] [PMID: 21944860]

[70] Yang, X.; Qiang, X.; Li, Y.; Luo, L.; Xu, R.; Zheng, Y.; Cao, Z.; Tan, Z.; Deng, Y. Pyridoxine-resveratrol hybrids Mannich base derivatives as novel dual inhibitors of AChE and MAO-B with antioxidant and metal-chelating properties for the treatment of Alzheimer's disease. *Bioorg. Chem.*, **2017**, *71*, 305-314. [http://dx.doi.org/10.1016/j.bioorg.2017.02.016] [PMID: 28267984]

[71] Tripathi, A.C.; Upadhyay, S.; Paliwal, S.; Saraf, S.K. Privileged scaffolds as MAO inhibitors: Retrospect and prospects. *Eur. J. Med. Chem.*, **2018**, *145*, 445-497. [http://dx.doi.org/10.1016/j.ejmech.2018.01.003] [PMID: 29335210]

[72] Tripathi, R.K.P.; Ayyannan, S.R. Monoamine oxidase-B inhibitors as potential neurotherapeutic agents: An overview and update. *Med. Res. Rev.*, **2019**, *39*(5), 1603-1706. [http://dx.doi.org/10.1002/med.21561] [PMID: 30604512]

[73] Li, W.; Yang, X.; Song, Q.; Cao, Z.; Shi, Y.; Deng, Y.; Zhang, L. Pyridoxine-resveratrol hybrids as novel inhibitors of MAO-B with antioxidant and neuroprotective activities for the treatment of Parkinson's disease. *Bioorg. Chem.*, **2020**, *97*, 103707. [http://dx.doi.org/10.1016/j.bioorg.2020.103707] [PMID: 32146176]

[74] Semenov, A.V.; Balakireva, O.I.; Tarasova, I.V.; Semenova, E.V.; Zulfugarov, P.K. Synthesis, radical scavenging, and antioxidant activity of stilbazolic resveratrol analogs. *Med. Chem. Res.*, **2020**, *29*(9), 1590-1599. [http://dx.doi.org/10.1007/s00044-020-02585-6]

[75] Jardim, F.R.; de Rossi, F.T.; Nascimento, M.X.; da Silva Barros, R.G.; Borges, P.A.; Prescilio, I.C.; de Oliveira, M.R. Resveratrol and brain mitochondria: a review. *Mol. Neurobiol.*, **2018**, *55*(3), 2085-2101. [http://dx.doi.org/10.1007/s12035-017-0448-z] [PMID: 28283884]

[76] Makhaeva, G.F.; Shevtsova, E.F.; Boltneva, N.P.; Lushchekina, S.V.; Kovaleva, N.V.; Rudakova, E.V.; Bachurin, S.O.; Richardson, R.J. Overview of novel multifunctional agents based on conjugates of γ-carbolines, carbazoles, tetrahydrocarbazoles, phenothiazines, and aminoadamantanes for

treatment of Alzheimer's disease. *Chem. Biol. Interact.*, **2019**, *308*, 224-234. [http://dx.doi.org/10.1016/j.cbi.2019.05.020] [PMID: 31100279]

[77] Patel, D.V.; Patel, N.R.; Kanhed, A.M.; Teli, D.M.; Patel, K.B.; Joshi, P.D.; Patel, S.P.; Gandhi, P.M.; Chaudhary, B.N.; Prajapati, N.K.; Patel, K.V.; Yadav, M.R. Novel carbazole-stilbene hybrids as multifunctional anti-Alzheimer agents. *Bioorg. Chem.*, **2020**, *101*, 103977. [http://dx.doi.org/10.1016/j.bioorg.2020.103977] [PMID: 32485470]

[78] Lipinski, C.A.; Lombardo, F.; Dominy, B.W.; Feeney, P.J. Experimental and computational approaches to estimate solubility and permeability in drug discovery and development settings 1PII of original article: S0169-409X(96)00423-1. The article was originally published in Advanced Drug Delivery Reviews 23 (1997) 3–25. 1. *Adv. Drug Deliv. Rev.*, **2001**, *46*(1-3), 3-26. [http://dx.doi.org/10.1016/S0169-409X(00)00129-0] [PMID: 11259830]

[79] Marumoto, S.; Miyazawa, M. Structure–activity relationships for naturally occurring coumarins as β-secretase inhibitor. *Bioorg. Med. Chem.*, **2012**, *20*(2), 784-788. [http://dx.doi.org/10.1016/j.bmc.2011.12.002] [PMID: 22222157]

[80] Šinko, G. Assessment of scoring functions and in silico parameters for AChE-ligand interactions as a tool for predicting inhibition potency. *Chem. Biol. Interact.*, **2019**, *308*, 216-223. [http://dx.doi.org/10.1016/j.cbi.2019.05.047] [PMID: 31150627]

[81] Agbo, E.N.; Gildenhuys, S.; Choong, Y.S.; Mphahlele, M.J.; More, G.K. Synthesis of furocoumarin–stilbene hybrids as potential multifunctional drugs against multiple biochemical targets associated with Alzheimer's disease. *Bioorg. Chem.*, **2020**, *101*, 103997. [http://dx.doi.org/10.1016/j.bioorg.2020.103997] [PMID: 32554280]

[82] AlFadly, E.D.; Elzahhar, P.A.; Tramarin, A.; Elkazaz, S.; Shaltout, H.; Abu-Serie, M.M.; Janockova, J.; Soukup, O.; Ghareeb, D.A.; El-Yazbi, A.F.; Rafeh, R.W.; Bakkar, N.M.Z.; Kobeissy, F.; Iriepa, I.; Moraleda, I.; Saudi, M.N.S.; Bartolini, M.; Belal, A.S.F. Tackling neuroinflammation and cholinergic deficit in Alzheimer's disease: Multi-target inhibitors of cholinesterases, cyclooxygenase-2 and 15-lipoxygenase. *Eur. J. Med. Chem.*, **2019**, *167*, 161-186. [http://dx.doi.org/10.1016/j.ejmech.2019.02.012] [PMID: 30771604]

[83] Zheng, Y.; Qiang, X.; Xu, R.; Song, Q.; Tian, C.; Liu, H.; Li, W.; Tan, Z.; Deng, Y. Design, synthesis and evaluation of pterostilbene β-amino alcohol derivatives as multifunctional agents for Alzheimer's disease treatment. *Bioorg. Chem.*, **2018**, *78*, 298-306. [http://dx.doi.org/10.1016/j.bioorg.2018.03.016] [PMID: 29625269]

[84] Li, Y.; Qiang, X.; Li, Y.; Yang, X.; Luo, L.; Xiao, G.; Cao, Z.; Tan, Z.; Deng, Y. Pterostilbene---acetamidoalkylbenzylamines derivatives as novel dual inhibitors of cholinesterase with anti---amyloid aggregation and antioxidant properties for the treatment of Alzheimer's disease. *Bioorg. Med. Chem. Lett.*, **2016**, *26*(8), 2035-2039. [http://dx.doi.org/10.1016/j.bmcl.2016.02.079] [PMID: 26947607]

[85] Gaspar, A.; Silva, T.; Yáñez, M.; Vina, D.; Orallo, F.; Ortuso, F.; Uriarte, E.; Alcaro, S.; Borges, F. Chromone, a privileged scaffold for the development of monoamine oxidase inhibitors. *J. Med. Chem.*, **2011**, *54*(14), 5165-5173. [http://dx.doi.org/10.1021/jm2004267] [PMID: 21696156]

[86] Bareggi, S.R.; Cornelli, U. Clioquinol: review of its mechanisms of action and clinical uses in neurodegenerative disorders. *CNS Neurosci. Ther.*, **2012**, *18*(1), 41-46. [http://dx.doi.org/10.1111/j.1755-5949.2010.00231.x] [PMID: 21199452]

[87] Hindo, S.S.; Mancino, A.M.; Braymer, J.J.; Liu, Y.; Vivekanandan, S.; Ramamoorthy, A.; Lim, M.H. Small molecule modulators of copper-induced Abeta aggregation. *J. Am. Chem. Soc.*, **2009**, *131*(46), 16663-16665. [http://dx.doi.org/10.1021/ja907045h] [PMID: 19877631]

[88] Li, F.; Wu, J.J.; Wang, J.; Yang, X.L.; Cai, P.; Liu, Q.H.; Kong, L.Y.; Wang, X.B. Synthesis and pharmacological evaluation of novel chromone derivatives as balanced multifunctional agents against

Alzheimer's disease. *Bioorg. Med. Chem.*, **2017**, *25*(14), 3815-3826.
[http://dx.doi.org/10.1016/j.bmc.2017.05.027] [PMID: 28549891]

[89] Wang, Z.; Wang, Y.; Wang, B.; Li, W.; Huang, L.; Li, X. Li. X. Design, Synthesis, and Evaluation of Orally Available Clioquinol-Moracin M. Hybrids as multitarget-directed ligands for cognitive improvement in a rat model of neurodegeneration in Alzheimer's disease. *J. Med. Chem.*, **2015**, *58*(21), 8616-8637.
[http://dx.doi.org/10.1021/acs.jmedchem.5b01222] [PMID: 26473791]

[90] Wang, Z.; Wu, J.; Yang, X.; Cai, P.; Liu, Q.; Wang, K.D.G.; Kong, L.; Wang, X. Neuroprotective effects of benzyloxy substituted small molecule monoamine oxidase B inhibitors in Parkinson's disease. *Bioorg. Med. Chem.*, **2016**, *24*(22), 5929-5940.
[http://dx.doi.org/10.1016/j.bmc.2016.09.050] [PMID: 27692996]

[91] Yang, H.L.; Cai, P.; Liu, Q.H.; Yang, X.L.; Fang, S.Q.; Tang, Y.W.; Wang, C.; Wang, X.B.; Kong, L.Y. Design, synthesis, and evaluation of salicyladimine derivatives as multitarget-directed ligands against Alzheimer's disease. *Bioorg. Med. Chem.*, **2017**, *25*(21), 5917-5928.
[http://dx.doi.org/10.1016/j.bmc.2017.08.048] [PMID: 28988627]

[92] Vaiserman, A.; Koliada, A.; Zayachkivska, A.; Lushchak, O. Curcumin: A therapeutic potential in ageing-related disorders. *PharmaNutrition,* **2020**, *14*, 100226.
[http://dx.doi.org/10.1016/j.phanu.2020.100226]

[93] de Freitas Silva, M.; Coelho, L.F.; Guirelli, I.M.; Pereira, R.M.; Ferreira-Silva, G.Á.; Graravelli, G.Y.; Horvath, R.O.; Caixeta, E.S.; Ionta, M.; Viegas, C. Synthetic resveratrol-curcumin hybrid derivative inhibits mitosis progression in estrogen positive MCF-7 breast cancer cells. *Toxicol. In Vitro,* **2018**, *50*, 75-85.
[http://dx.doi.org/10.1016/j.tiv.2018.02.020] [PMID: 29501629]

[94] de Freitas Silva, M.; Tardelli Lima, E.; Pruccoli, L.; Castro, N.; Guimarães, M.; da Silva, F.; Fonseca Nadur, N.; de Azevedo, L.; Kümmerle, A.; Guedes, I.; Dardenne, L.; Gontijo, V.; Tarozzi, A.; Viegas, C., Jr Design, Synthesis and Biological Evaluation of Novel Triazole *N*-acylhydrazone Hybrids for Alzheimer's Disease. *Molecules,* **2020**, *25*(14), 3165.
[http://dx.doi.org/10.3390/molecules25143165] [PMID: 32664425]

[95] Minarini, A.; Milelli, A.; Simoni, E.; Rosini, M.; Bolognesi, M.; Marchetti, C.; Tumiatti, V. Multifunctional tacrine derivatives in Alzheimer's disease. *Curr. Top. Med. Chem.*, **2013**, *13*(15), 1771-1786.
[http://dx.doi.org/10.2174/15680266113139990136] [PMID: 23931443]

[96] Jeřábek, J., Uliassi, E.; Guidotti, L.; Korábečný, J.; Soukup, O.; Sepsova, V.; Hrabinova, M.; Kuča, K.; Bartolini, M.; Peña-Altamira, L.E.; Petralla, S.; Monti, B.; Roberti, M.; Bolognesi, M.L. Tacrine-resveratrol fused hybrids as multi-target-directed ligands against Alzheimer's disease. *Eur. J. Med. Chem.*, **2017**, *127*, 250-262.
[http://dx.doi.org/10.1016/j.ejmech.2016.12.048] [PMID: 28064079]

[97] Bartolini, M.; Marco-Contelles, J. Tacrines as therapeutic agents for Alzheimer's disease. IV. The tacripyrines and rRelated annulated tacrines. *Chem. Rec.*, **2019**, *19*(5), 927-937.
[http://dx.doi.org/10.1002/tcr.201800155] [PMID: 30489012]

[98] Simoni, E.; Serafini, M.M.; Bartolini, M.; Caporaso, R.; Pinto, A.; Necchi, D.; Fiori, J.; Andrisano, V.; Minarini, A.; Lanni, C.; Rosini, M. Nature-inspired multifunctional ligands: focusing on amyloid-based molecular mechanisms of Alzheimer's disease. *ChemMedChem,* **2016**, *11*(12), 1309-1317.
[http://dx.doi.org/10.1002/cmdc.201500422] [PMID: 26497622]

[99] Zhao, B. Nitric oxide in neurodegenerative diseases. *Front. Biosci.*, **2005**, *10*(1-3), 454-461.
[http://dx.doi.org/10.2741/1541] [PMID: 15574382]

[100] Fantacuzzi, M.; Maccallini, C.; Lannutti, F.; Patruno, A.; Masella, S.; Pesce, M.; Speranza, L.; Ammazzalorso, A.; De Filippis, B.; Giampietro, L.; Re, N.; Amoroso, R. Selective inhibition of iNOS by benzyl- and dibenzyl derivatives of N-(3-aminobenzyl)acetamidine. *ChemMedChem,* **2011**, *6*(7),

1203-1206.
[http://dx.doi.org/10.1002/cmdc.201100125] [PMID: 21567968]

[101] Fantacuzzi, M.; Maccallini, C.; Di Matteo, M.; Ammazzalorso, A.; Bruno, I.; De Filippis, B.; Giampietro, L.; Mollica, A.; Amoroso, R. Screening of NOS activity and selectivity of newly synthesized acetamidines using RP-HPLC. *J. Pharm. Biomed. Anal.,* **2016**, *120*, 419-424.
[http://dx.doi.org/10.1016/j.jpba.2015.11.045] [PMID: 26689740]

[102] Fang, Y.; Xia, W.; Cheng, B.; Hua, P.; Zhou, H.; Gu, Q.; Xu, J. Design, synthesis, and biological evaluation of compounds with a new scaffold as anti-neuroinflammatory agents for the treatment of Alzheimer's disease. *Eur. J. Med. Chem.,* **2018**, *149*, 129-138.
[http://dx.doi.org/10.1016/j.ejmech.2018.02.063] [PMID: 29499485]

[103] Gaeta, A.; Hider, R.C. The crucial role of metal ions in neurodegeneration: the basis for a promising therapeutic strategy. *Br. J. Pharmacol.,* **2005**, *146*(8), 1041-1059.
[http://dx.doi.org/10.1038/sj.bjp.0706416] [PMID: 16205720]

[104] Cicero, C.E.; Mostile, G.; Vasta, R.; Rapisarda, V.; Signorelli, S.S.; Ferrante, M.; Zappia, M.; Nicoletti, A. Metals and neurodegenerative diseases. A systematic review. *Environ. Res.,* **2017**, *159*, 82-94.
[http://dx.doi.org/10.1016/j.envres.2017.07.048] [PMID: 28777965]

[105] Greenough, M.A.; Camakaris, J.; Bush, A.I. Metal dyshomeostasis and oxidative stress in Alzheimer's disease. *Neurochem. Int.,* **2013**, *62*(5), 540-555.
[http://dx.doi.org/10.1016/j.neuint.2012.08.014] [PMID: 22982299]

[106] Xu, P.; Zhang, M.; Sheng, R.; Ma, Y. Synthesis and biological evaluation of deferiprone-resveratrol hybrids as antioxidants, Aβ $_{1\text{–}42}$ aggregation inhibitors and metal-chelating agents for Alzheimer's disease. *Eur. J. Med. Chem.,* **2017**, *127*, 174-186.
[http://dx.doi.org/10.1016/j.ejmech.2016.12.045] [PMID: 28061347]

[107] Zhang, C.; Yang, K.; Yu, S.; Su, J.; Yuan, S.; Han, J.; Chen, Y.; Gu, J.; Zhou, T.; Bai, R.; Xie, Y. Design, synthesis and biological evaluation of hydroxypyridinone-coumarin hybrids as multimodal monoamine oxidase B inhibitors and iron chelates against Alzheimer's disease. *Eur. J. Med. Chem.,* **2019**, *180*, 367-382.
[http://dx.doi.org/10.1016/j.ejmech.2019.07.031] [PMID: 31325784]

[108] Chand, K.; Rajeshwari, R.; Candeias, E.; Cardoso, S.M.; Chaves, S.; Santos, M.A. Tacrine–deferiprone hybrids as multi-target-directed metal chelators against Alzheimer's disease: a two-in-one drug. *Metallomics,* **2018**, *10*(10), 1460-1475.
[http://dx.doi.org/10.1039/C8MT00143J] [PMID: 30183790]

[109] Panda, P.; Chakroborty, S. Navigating the synthesis of quinoline hybrid molecules as promising anticancer agents. *ChemistrySelect,* **2020**, *5*(33), 10187-10199.
[http://dx.doi.org/10.1002/slct.202002790]

[110] Weyesa, A.; Mulugeta, E. Recent advances in the synthesis of biologically and pharmaceutically active quinoline and its analogues: a review. *RSC Advances,* **2020**, *10*(35), 20784-20793.
[http://dx.doi.org/10.1039/D0RA03763J] [PMID: 35517753]

[111] Fernández-Bachiller, M.I.; Pérez, C.; González-Muñoz, G.C.; Conde, S.; López, M.G.; Villarroya, M.; García, A.G.; Rodríguez-Franco, M.I. Novel tacrine-8-hydroxyquinoline hybrids as multifunctional agents for the treatment of Alzheimer's disease, with neuroprotective, cholinergic, antioxidant, and copper-complexing properties. *J. Med. Chem.,* **2010**, *53*(13), 4927-4937.
[http://dx.doi.org/10.1021/jm100329q] [PMID: 20545360]

[112] Wang, X.Q.; Xia, C.L.; Chen, S.B.; Tan, J.H.; Ou, T.M.; Huang, S.L.; Li, D.; Gu, L.Q.; Huang, Z.S. Design, synthesis, and biological evaluation of 2-arylethenylquinoline derivatives as multifunctional agents for the treatment of Alzheimer's disease. *Eur. J. Med. Chem.,* **2015**, *89*, 349-361.
[http://dx.doi.org/10.1016/j.ejmech.2014.10.018] [PMID: 25462251]

[113] Kapková, P.; Alptüzün, V.; Frey, P.; Erciyas, E.; Holzgrabe, U. Search for dual function inhibitors for

Alzheimer's disease: Synthesis and biological activity of acetylcholinesterase inhibitors of pyridinium-type and their Aβ fibril formation inhibition capacity. *Bioorg. Med. Chem.*, **2006**, *14*(2), 472-478.
[http://dx.doi.org/10.1016/j.bmc.2005.08.034] [PMID: 16198581]

[114] Xia, C.L.; Wang, N.; Guo, Q.L.; Liu, Z.Q.; Wu, J.Q.; Huang, S.L.; Ou, T.M.; Tan, J.H.; Wang, H.G.; Li, D.; Huang, Z.S. Design, synthesis and evaluation of 2-arylethenyl- N -methylquinolinium derivatives as effective multifunctional agents for Alzheimer's disease treatment. *Eur. J. Med. Chem.*, **2017**, *130*, 139-153.
[http://dx.doi.org/10.1016/j.ejmech.2017.02.042] [PMID: 28242549]

[115] Ammazzalorso, A.; D'Angelo, A.; Giancristofaro, A.; De Filippis, B.; Di Matteo, M.; Fantacuzzi, M.; Giampietro, L.; Linciano, P.; Maccallini, C.; Amoroso, R. Fibrate-derived N-(methylsulfonyl)amides with antagonistic properties on PPARα. *Eur. J. Med. Chem.*, **2012**, *58*, 317-322.
[http://dx.doi.org/10.1016/j.ejmech.2012.10.019] [PMID: 23137448]

[116] Giampietro, L.; Ammazzalorso, A.; Amoroso, R.; De Filippis, B. Development of fibrates as important scaffold in medicinal chemistry. *ChemMedChem,* **2019**, *14*(11), 1051-1066.
[http://dx.doi.org/10.1002/cmdc.201900128] [PMID: 30957432]

[117] Giampietro, L.; Laghezza, A.; Cerchia, C.; Florio, R.; Recinella, L.; Capone, F.; Ammazzalorso, A.; Bruno, I.; De Filippis, B.; Fantacuzzi, M.; Ferrante, C.; Maccallini, C.; Tortorella, P.; Verginelli, F.; Brunetti, L.; Cama, A.; Amoroso, R.; Loiodice, F.; Lavecchia, A. Novel Phenyldiazenyl Fibrate Analogues as PPAR α/γ/δ Pan-Agonists for the Amelioration of Metabolic Syndrome. *ACS Med. Chem. Lett.*, **2019**, *10*(4), 545-551.
[http://dx.doi.org/10.1021/acsmedchemlett.8b00574] [PMID: 30996794]

[118] Prashantha Kumar, B.R.; Kumar, A.P.; Jose, J.A.; Prabitha, P.; Yuvaraj, S.; Chipurupalli, S.; Jeyarani, V.; Manisha, C.; Banerjee, S.; Jeyabalan, J.B.; Mohankumar, S.K.; Dhanabal, S.P.; Justin, A. Minutes of PPAR-γ agonism and neuroprotection. *Neurochem. Int.*, **2020**, *140*, 104814.
[http://dx.doi.org/10.1016/j.neuint.2020.104814] [PMID: 32758586]

[119] Giampietro, L.; Gallorini, M.; De Filippis, B.; Amoroso, R.; Cataldi, A.; di Giacomo, V. PPAR-γ agonist GL516 reduces oxidative stress and apoptosis occurrence in a rat astrocyte cell line. *Neurochem. Int.*, **2019**, *126*, 239-245.
[http://dx.doi.org/10.1016/j.neuint.2019.03.021] [PMID: 30946848]

[120] Leporini, L.; Giampietro, L.; Amoroso, R.; Ammazzalorso, A.; Fantacuzzi, M.; Menghini, L.; Maccallini, C.; Ferrante, C.; Brunetti, L.; Orlando, G.; De Filippis, B. In vitro protective effects of resveratrol and stilbene alkanoic derivatives on induced oxidative stress on C2C12 and MCF7 cells. *J. Biol. Regul. Homeost. Agents,* **2017**, *31*(3), 589-601.
[PMID: 28889799]

[121] De Filippis, B.; Linciano, P.; Ammazzalorso, A.; Di Giovanni, C.; Fantacuzzi, M.; Giampietro, L.; Laghezza, A.; Maccallini, C.; Tortorella, P.; Lavecchia, A.; Loiodice, F.; Amoroso, R. Structural development studies of PPARs ligands based on tyrosine scaffold. *Eur. J. Med. Chem.*, **2015**, *89*, 817-825.
[http://dx.doi.org/10.1016/j.ejmech.2014.10.083] [PMID: 25462281]

[122] Dai, D.F.; Chiao, Y.A.; Martin, G.M.; Marcinek, D.J.; Basisty, N.; Quarles, E.K.; Rabinovitch, P.S. Mitochondrial-Targeted Catalase. *Prog. Mol. Biol. Transl. Sci.*, **2017**, *146*, 203-241.
[http://dx.doi.org/10.1016/bs.pmbts.2016.12.015] [PMID: 28253986]

[123] Peñalver, P.; Belmonte-Reche, E.; Adán, N.; Caro, M.; Mateos-Martín, M.L.; Delgado, M.; González-Rey, E.; Morales, J.C. Alkylated resveratrol prodrugs and metabolites as potential therapeutics for neurodegenerative diseases. *Eur. J. Med. Chem.*, **2018**, *146*, 123-138.
[http://dx.doi.org/10.1016/j.ejmech.2018.01.037] [PMID: 29407944]

[124] Puksasook, T.; Kimura, S.; Tadtong, S.; Jiaranaikulwanitch, J.; Pratuangdejkul, J.; Kitphati, W.; Suwanborirux, K.; Saito, N.; Nukoolkarn, V. Semisynthesis and biological evaluation of prenylated resveratrol derivatives as multi-targeted agents for Alzheimer's disease. *J. Nat. Med.*, **2017**, *71*(4),

665-682.
[http://dx.doi.org/10.1007/s11418-017-1097-2] [PMID: 28600778]

[125] Liu, S.; Li, Y.; Yi, F.; Liu, Q.; Chen, N.; He, X.; He, C.; Xiao, P. Resveratrol oligomers from Paeonia suffruticosa protect mice against cognitive dysfunction by regulating cholinergic, antioxidant and anti-inflammatory pathways. *J. Ethnopharmacol.*, **2020**, *260*, 112983.
[http://dx.doi.org/10.1016/j.jep.2020.112983] [PMID: 32442589]

[126] Wu, C.W.; Nakamoto, Y.; Hisatome, T.; Yoshida, S.; Miyazaki, H. Resveratrol and its dimers ε□viniferin and δ□viniferin in red wine protect vascular endothelial cells by a similar mechanism with different potency and efficacy. *Kaohsiung J. Med. Sci.*, **2020**, *36*(7), 535-542.
[http://dx.doi.org/10.1002/kjm2.12199] [PMID: 32118360]

[127] Tang, Y.W.; Shi, C.J.; Yang, H.L.; Cai, P.; Liu, Q.H.; Yang, X.L.; Kong, L.Y.; Wang, X.B. Synthesis and evaluation of isoprenylation-resveratrol dimer derivatives against Alzheimer's disease. *Eur. J. Med. Chem.*, **2019**, *163*, 307-319.
[http://dx.doi.org/10.1016/j.ejmech.2018.11.040] [PMID: 30529634]

[128] Yang, T.; Fang, L.; Nopo-Olazabal, C.; Condori, J.; Nopo-Olazabal, L.; Balmaceda, C.; Medina-Bolivar, F. Enhanced production of resveratrol, piceatannol, arachidin-1 and arachidin-3 in hairy root cultures of peanut co-treated with methyl jasmonate and cyclodextrin. *J. Agric. Food Chem.*, **2015**, *63*(15), 3942-3950.
[http://dx.doi.org/10.1021/jf5050266] [PMID: 25837778]

[129] Dugdale, H.F.; Hughes, D.C.; Allan, R.; Deane, C.S.; Coxon, C.R.; Morton, J.P.; Stewart, C.E.; Sharples, A.P. The role of resveratrol on skeletal muscle cell differentiation and myotube hypertrophy during glucose restriction. *Mol. Cell. Biochem.*, **2018**, *444*(1-2), 109-123.
[http://dx.doi.org/10.1007/s11010-017-3236-1] [PMID: 29189984]

[130] Salucci, S.; Falcieri, E. Polyphenols and their potential role in preventing skeletal muscle atrophy. *Nutr. Res.*, **2020**, *74*, 10-22.
[http://dx.doi.org/10.1016/j.nutres.2019.11.004] [PMID: 31895993]

[131] Di Filippo, E.S.; Giampietro, L.; De Filippis, B.; Balaha, M.; Ferrone, V.; Locatelli, M.; Pietrangelo, T.; Tartaglia, A.; Amoroso, R.; Fulle, S. Synthesis and biological evaluation of halogenated *E*-stilbenols as promising antiaging agents. *Molecules,* **2020**, *25*(23), 5770.
[http://dx.doi.org/10.3390/molecules25235770] [PMID: 33297520]

[132] Lizard, G.; Latruffe, N.; Vervandier-Fasseur, D. Aza- and azo-stilbenes: bio-isosteric analogs of resveratrol. *Molecules,* **2020**, *25*(3), 605-618.
[http://dx.doi.org/10.3390/molecules25030605] [PMID: 32019195]

[133] Hameed, A.; al-Rashida, M.; Uroos, M.; Abid Ali, S.; Khan, K.M. Schiff bases in medicinal chemistry: a patent review (2010-2015). *Expert Opin. Ther. Pat.*, **2017**, *27*(1), 63-79.
[http://dx.doi.org/10.1080/13543776.2017.1252752] [PMID: 27774821]

[134] Zhang, Y.; Zou, B.; Wang, K.; Pan, Y.; Liang, H.; Yi, X.; Wang, H. Antioxidant activities and transition metal ion chelating studies of some hydroxyl Schiff base derivatives. *Med. Chem. Res.*, **2012**, *21*(7), 1341-1346.
[http://dx.doi.org/10.1007/s00044-011-9648-7]

[135] Lu, J.; Li, C.; Chai, Y.F.; Yang, D.Y.; Sun, C.R. The antioxidant effect of imine resveratrol analogues. *Bioorg. Med. Chem. Lett.*, **2012**, *22*(17), 5744-5747.
[http://dx.doi.org/10.1016/j.bmcl.2012.06.026] [PMID: 22832313]

[136] Durgun, M.; Türkeş, C.; Işık, M.; Demir, Y.; Saklı, A.; Kuru, A.; Güzel, A.; Beydemir, Ş.; Akocak, S.; Osman, S.M.; AlOthman, Z.; Supuran, C.T. Synthesis, characterisation, biological evaluation and *in silico* studies of sulphonamide Schiff bases. *J. Enzyme Inhib. Med. Chem.*, **2020**, *35*(1), 950-962.
[http://dx.doi.org/10.1080/14756366.2020.1746784] [PMID: 32249705]

[137] Fantacuzzi, M.; De Filippis, B.; Gallorini, M.; Ammazzalorso, A.; Giampietro, L.; Maccallini, C.; Aturki, Z.; Donati, E.; Ibrahim, R.S.; Shawky, E.; Cataldi, A.; Amoroso, R. Synthesis, biological

evaluation, and docking study of indole aryl sulfonamides as aromatase inhibitors. *Eur. J. Med. Chem.*, **2020**, *185*, 111815.
[http://dx.doi.org/10.1016/j.ejmech.2019.111815] [PMID: 31732252]

[138] Fantacuzzi, M.; Gallorini, M.; Gambacorta, N.; Ammazzalorso, A.; Aturki, Z.; Balaha, M.; Carradori, S.; Giampietro, L.; Maccallini, C.; Cataldi, A.; Nicolotti, O.; Amoroso, R.; De Filippis, B. Design, Synthesis and Biological Evaluation of Aromatase Inhibitors Based on Sulfonates and Sulfonamides of Resveratrol. *Pharmaceuticals (Basel)*, **2021**, *14*(10), 984.
[http://dx.doi.org/10.3390/ph14100984] [PMID: 34681208]

[139] Mondal, S.; Malakar, S. Synthesis of sulfonamide and their synthetic and therapeutic applications: Recent advances. *Tetrahedron*, **2020**, *76*(48), 131662.
[http://dx.doi.org/10.1016/j.tet.2020.131662]

[140] de Souza, M.M.; Andreolla, M.C.; Ribeiro, T.C.; Gonçalves, A.E.; Medeiros, A.R.; de Souza, A.S.; Ferreira, L.L.G.; Andricopulo, A.D.; Yunes, R.A.; de Oliveira, A.S. Structure–activity relationships of sulfonamides derived from carvacrol and their potential for the treatment of Alzheimer's disease. *RSC Medicinal Chemistry*, **2020**, *11*(2), 307-316.
[http://dx.doi.org/10.1039/D0MD00009D] [PMID: 33479638]

[141] Angeli, A.; Carta, F.; Supuran, C.T. Carbonic anhydrases: Versatile and useful biocatalysts in chemistry and biochemistry. *Catalysts*, **2020**, *10*(9), 1008.
[http://dx.doi.org/10.3390/catal10091008]

[142] Solesio, M.E.; Peixoto, P.M.; Debure, L.; Madamba, S.M.; de Leon, M.J.; Wisniewski, T.; Pavlov, E.V.; Fossati, S. Carbonic anhydrase inhibition selectively prevents amyloid β neurovascular mitochondrial toxicity. *Aging Cell*, **2018**, *17*(4), e12787.
[http://dx.doi.org/10.1111/acel.12787] [PMID: 29873184]

[143] Işık, M.; Demir, Y.; Durgun, M.; Türkeş, C.; Necip, A.; Beydemir, Ş. Molecular docking and investigation of 4-(benzylideneamino)- and 4-(benzylamino)-benzenesulfonamide derivatives as potent AChE inhibitors. *Chem. Pap.*, **2020**, *74*(5), 1395-1405.
[http://dx.doi.org/10.1007/s11696-019-00988-3]

[144] Frombaum, M.; Le Clanche, S.; Bonnefont-Rousselot, D.; Borderie, D. Antioxidant effects of resveratrol and other stilbene derivatives on oxidative stress and NO bioavailability: Potential benefits to cardiovascular diseases. *Biochimie*, **2012**, *94*(2), 269-276.
[http://dx.doi.org/10.1016/j.biochi.2011.11.001] [PMID: 22133615]

[145] Das, S.; Das, D. Anti-inflammatory responses of resveratrol. *Inflamm. Allergy Drug Targets*, **2007**, *6*(3), 168-173.
[http://dx.doi.org/10.2174/187152807781696464] [PMID: 17897053]

[146] Zimmermann-Franco, D.C.; Esteves, B.; Lacerda, L.M.; Souza, I.O.; Santos, J.A.; Pinto, N.C.C.; Scio, E.; da Silva, A.D.; Macedo, G.C. In vitro and in vivo anti-inflammatory properties of imine resveratrol analogues. *Bioorg. Med. Chem.*, **2018**, *26*(17), 4898-4906.
[http://dx.doi.org/10.1016/j.bmc.2018.08.029] [PMID: 30193941]

[147] Merly, L.; Smith, S.L. Murine RAW 264.7 cell line as an immune target: are we missing something? *Immunopharmacol. Immunotoxicol.*, **2017**, *39*(2), 55-58.
[http://dx.doi.org/10.1080/08923973.2017.1282511] [PMID: 28152640]

[148] Qureshi, A.A.; Guan, X.; Reis, J.C.; Papasian, C.J.; Jabre, S.; Morrison, D.C.; Qureshi, N. Inhibition of nitric oxide and inflammatory cytokines in LPS-stimulated murine macrophages by resveratrol, a potent proteasome inhibitor. *Lipids Health Dis.*, **2012**, *11*(1), 76-93.
[http://dx.doi.org/10.1186/1476-511X-11-76] [PMID: 22698256]

[149] Kotora, P.; Šeršeň, F.; Filo, J.; Loos, D.; Gregáň, J.; Gregáň, F. The scavenging of DPPH, galvinoxyl and ABTS radicals by imine analogs of resveratrol. *Molecules*, **2016**, *21*(1), 127.
[http://dx.doi.org/10.3390/molecules21010127] [PMID: 26805801]

Medicinal Chemistry Lessons From Nature, 2022, *Vol. 1*, 73-111

CHAPTER 3

Biological Activities of Synthetic Derivatives of Xanthones: An Update (2016-2020)

Cristina Scarpecci[1] and **Sara Consalvi**[1,*]

[1] *Department of Chemistry and Technologies of Drug, Sapienza University of Rome, P.le A. Moro 5, 00185 Rome, Italy.*

Abstract: Natural xanthones are a class of secondary metabolites widely distributed in nature and with a broad spectrum of biological activities. Their scaffold is amenable to several modifications and has emerged as a "privileged structure" for drug development, representing a very attractive point for medicinal chemistry optimization. A combination of innovative synthetic methodologies and medicinal chemistry studies have provided several xanthone synthetic derivatives for different therapeutic purposes, including cancer, inflammation, Alzheimer's disease (AD), cardiovascular and infectious diseases. The aim of this chapter is to give an update on the significance of synthetic xanthones in medicinal chemistry over the last five years (2016-2020), with a focus on their biological activities and structure-activity relationship (SAR).

Keywords: anticancer, drug discovery, natural xanthones, synthetic xanthones, SAR analysis.

INTRODUCTION

Xanthones are a class of *O*-heterocycles symmetrical compounds characterized by a dibenzo-γ-pyrone scaffold (Fig. **1**) They can be extracted from different sources [1, 2] (fungi, lichens [3], higher plants [4] and marine organisms [5]) and are widely distributed in nature.

Natural xanthones have been a rich source for the discovery of novel therapeutic agents for many decades [4, 6]. One of the most representative examples is the polyprenylated xanthone gambogic acid (GA), isolated from *Garcinia hanburyi* (Clusiaceae), which entered clinical trials for the treatment of patients with advanced malignant tumors, including non-small cell lung cancer [7, 8]. Another well-known xanthone is mangosteen, isolated from *Garcinia mangostana* and sold worldwide as a nutritional supplement with anti- oxidant, anti- inflammatory

* **Corresponding author Sara Consalvi:** Department of Chemistry and Technologies of Drug, Sapienza University of Rome, P.le A. Moro 5, 00185 Rome, Italy; E-mail: sara.consalvi@uniroma1.it

and immunostimulating properties [9, 10]. Depending on their structures and position of substituents, natural xanthones have an incredibly broad spectrum of biological activities [11], such as cytotoxic [12], antiinfective [13], antioxidant [14], cardioprotective [15, 16], anti-inflammatory [17], and antihypertensive [18]. The xanthone scaffold has then emerged as a "privileged structure" for drug development and represents a very attractive point for medicinal chemistry optimization. The xanthone core is amenable to several modifications. However, even though natural sources offer a wide variety of differently substituted xanthones, the enzymes involved in their biosynthetic pathways could limit their structural diversity. Furthermore, some of them are difficult to obtain through conventional extraction methods and are present only at low concentrations. On the other hand, total synthesis can be a *via*ble strategy to easily obtain xanthones and explore the chemical space and the structure-activity relationship (SAR) around their scaffold [1, 12]. Therefore, combining novel synthetic methodologies and medicinal chemistry optimization is essential to allow the generation of libraries of xanthone synthetic derivatives with enhanced activities, improved safety profiles and acceptable drug-like properties. The importance of xanthone synthetic derivatives has been extensively reviewed [13, 19, 20]. The aim of this chapter is to give an update on the significance of synthetic xanthones in medicinal chemistry over the last five years (2016-2020), with a focus on their biological activities and SAR.

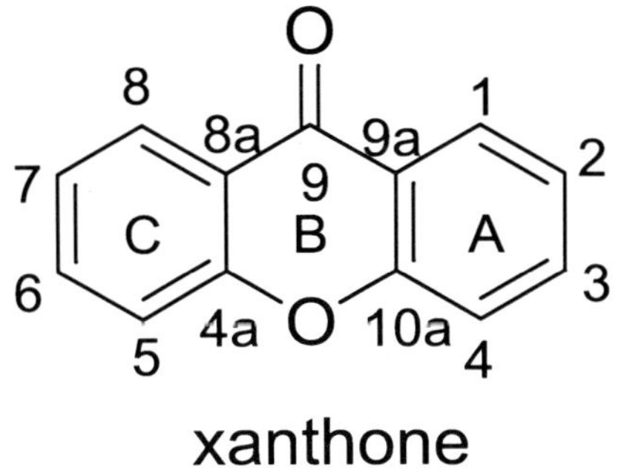

Fig. (1). General scaffold of xanthones.

XANTHONE SYNTHETIC DERIVATIVES FOR CANCER THERAPY

The anticancer properties of xanthones, such as gambogic acid (GA) [21], α-mangostin and 5,6-dimethylxanthenone-4-acetic acid (DMXAA), have been amply studied, and some of them underwent clinical trials [12]. Xanthones can inhibit tumor growth both *in vitro* and *in vivo*. As shown in Fig. **(2).,** they have several putative mechanisms of action, including apoptosis induction, cell cycle arrest, anti-angiogenesis and anti-metastatic effects, and antioxidant or reactive oxygen species (ROS)-stimulating activity. However, their exact molecular mechanism is yet to be clarified. The planar scaffold of xanthones, involving a three-ring system, might intercalate DNA and establish non-covalent DNA interactions [22]. Consequently, these promising activities prompted a continuous search for novel xanthone-based anticancer candidates.

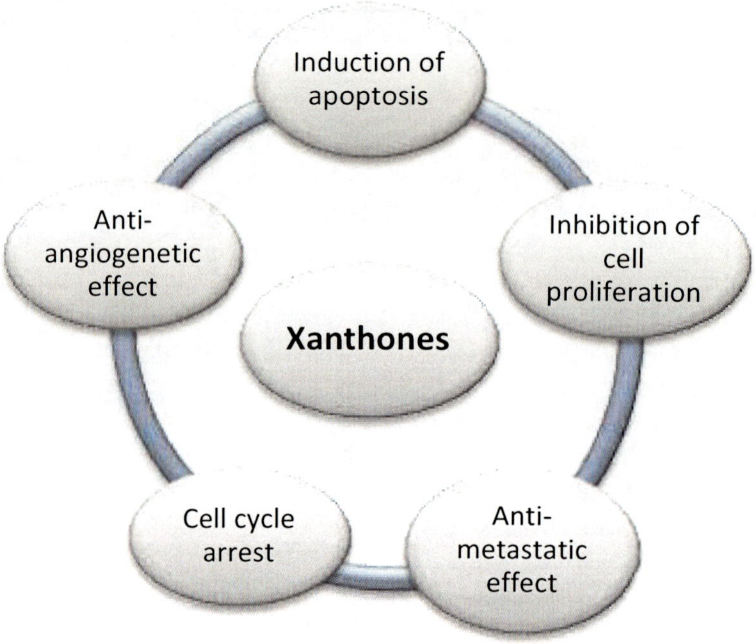

Fig. (2). Proposed Anticancer mechanisms for xanthones.

Caged Xanthones (CXs)

Gambogic acid (GA) represents the main bioactive natural product isolated from the gambogin resin secreted by the tropical trees of *Garcinia hanburyi.* GA has a unique prenylated caged xanthone structure and exhibits a wide range of biological activities, including anticancer. Notably, GA inhibits the growth of a broad panel of cancer cell lines *in vitro* and *in vivo* and entered clinical trials in China for the treatment of non-small cell lung, colon, and renal cancers. Several biological targets of GA are described in the literature, including transferrin receptor, nuclear factor kappa-light-chain-enhancer of activated B cells (NF-kB) pathway, inhibitory kappa B kinase-β (IKKβ), heat shock protein 90 (Hsp90) ATPase, p53-Mouse double minute 2 homolog (MDM2) interaction, B-cell lymphoma 2 (bcl-2) pathway [7]. However, as common setbacks of natural products, pharmacokinetic drawbacks such as poor aqueous solubility and a short half-life limited its use as an anticancer drug. Thus, structural modifications were made to improve its drug-like profile and obtain analogues as potential anticancer agents [12]. Recently, Zhang's research group identified SARs around the unique caged xanthone architecture. Previous molecular simplification studies had unveiled the minimum pharmacophore core for the CX family. As shown in Fig. (**3**)., the pharmacophore core (in red) is composed of the BCD rings planar system, including the α,ß-unsaturated ketone in the CD ring and a caged region involving the D ring. In light of this, Zhang's research group identified the hit **DDO-6101** [23]. This compound is characterized by a simple structure that maintained the antitumor activity of GA on different cancer cell lines (Fig. **3**). but exhibited limited physicochemical properties.

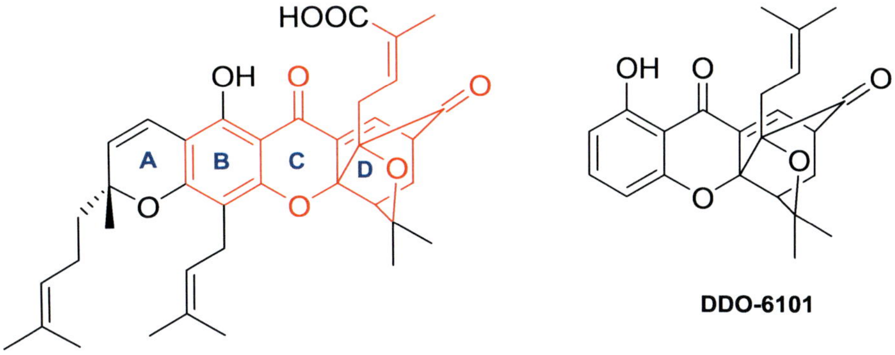

Fig. (3). Chemical structure of GA with the pharmacophore in red and its simplified analogue **DDO-6101**.

As part of a wide lead optimization program, preliminary attempts to increase solubility were made by inserting heteroatom-containing substituents at C14 (**DDO-6306**) or at C19 (**DDO-6267**) of the B ring. Unfortunately, such structural modifications did not provide the desired results and did not afford improved analogues (Fig. **4**).

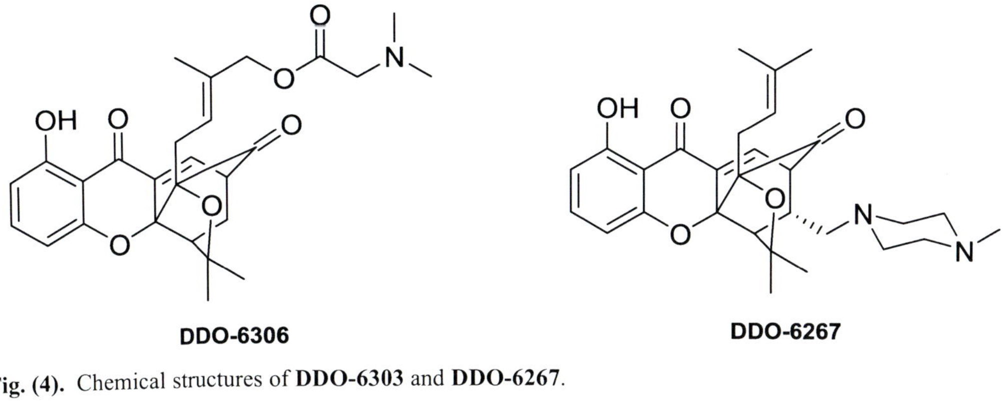

Fig. (4). Chemical structures of **DDO-6303** and **DDO-6267**.

In 2016 Xu *et al*. [24] focused on the design of novel caged xanthones CXs as potential Hsp90 inhibitors and conducted a systematic SAR study on the hit

DDO-6101 to examine the effects of several manipulations on the B ring:

- Hydroxyl group at C1 contributes to the activity but is not essential; its replacement with electron-withdrawing moieties, such as esters, is well tolerated. Indeed, these groups reduce the electron cloud density on the α,ß-unsaturated bond of ring D, making it more susceptible to the attack of target protein nucleophilic groups and thereby maintaining an inhibitory activity comparable to that of **DDO-6101**; electron-donating methoxy groups, alkoxy and carboxyl substituents with longer chains reduce the activity;
- Replacing C1–OH with substituted carbamates, particularly bipiperidine carbamates, furnishes the best activities, as the heteroatoms enhanced solubility and permeability *in vivo*.

These findings led to the development of **DDO-6337** (Fig. **5**) the most representative compound of the carbamate-bearing CXs series.

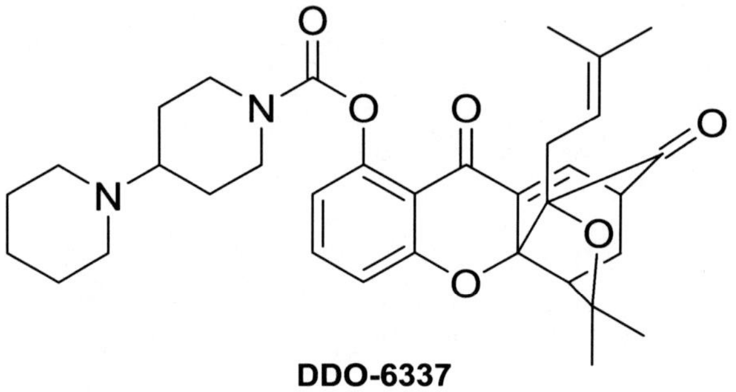

DDO-6337

Fig. (5). Chemical structure of **DDO-6337**.

DDO-6337 displayed a significantly improved antiproliferative activity evaluated against various cancer cell lines, including HepG2, HCT116, MDA-MB-231, taxol-resistant and cisplatin-resistant A549 cells Table **1**. The low solubility of **DDO-6337** (S = 0.08 mM) prompted the authors to synthesize its hydrochloride, which enhanced both solubility (S > 40 mM) and permeability. When administered intravenously (IV) twice daily in hepatoblastoma xenograft models to evaluate the *in vivo* efficacy, **HCl • DDO-6337** showed a better dose-dependent activity (inhibitory rates of 27.97%, 38.50% and 48.36% at 2.5, 5 and 10 mg/Kg, respectively), compared to the 36.81% growth inhibition provided by **DDO-6101** at 10 mg/kg twice daily. When administered orally at 50 mg/kg, **HCl • DDO-6337** exhibited enhanced potency, with a tumor growth inhibition of 30.12%.

Despite the advancement in terms of potency, *in vivo* **DDO-6337** still displayed moderate drug-like properties.

Therefore, the authors performed additional SAR studies on a novel set of CXs to increase the Hsp90 inhibitory activity, and results can be summarized as follows [25]:

• Substitutions at the C2, C3 and C4 retain the activity, but dihydroxyl derivatives with -OH at C1 and C3 exhibit higher IC_{50} values compared to monosubstituted compounds bearing –OH at C1;
• C17 gem-dimethyl group and bulky moieties (isopentene) at C2 or C4 reduce the affinity for Hsp90, probably due to a major steric hindrance;
• A C13 gem-dimethyl group is essential for activity. Analogues bearing hydroxyl or halogen substituents at C14 are the most active ones, while the introduction of C14 aldehyde is detrimental.

Among these compounds, compound **1** (Fig. **6**) proved to be the most potent Hsp90 inhibitor, with an IC_{50} value of 3.68 ± 0.18 µM and a K_D value of 38 ± 1.41 µM. Its antiproliferative activity was assessed in several cell lines Table **1**, proving that this candidate induced dose-dependent apoptosis of treated cancer cells *in vitro*. Interestingly, compound **1** presented the best growth inhibition property (IC_{50} = 1.92 ± 0.09 µM) on the SK-BR-3 cell line from breast carcinoma.

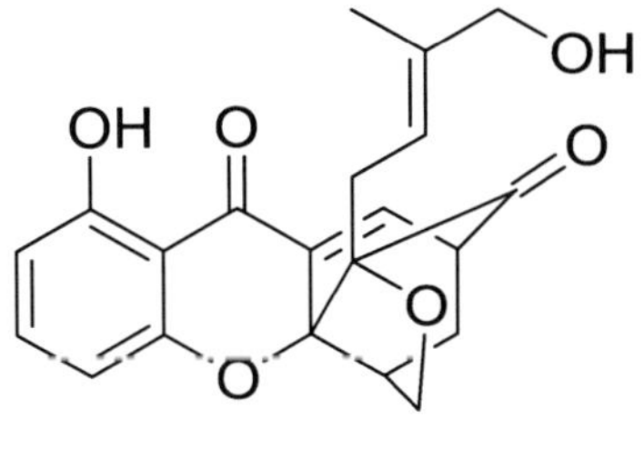

1

Fig. (6). Chemical structure of compound **1**.

In 2017 Li *et al.* speculated that the solubility and *in vivo* issues of **DDO-6306** and **DDO-6337** could be related to the unstable ester linkers [26]. Accordingly, the authors introduced a 1,2,3-triazole group as a stable linker between C1 of the B ring and diverse nitrogen-containing side chains. The ten triazole-bearing compounds synthesized in this work exhibited growth inhibitory activities in the micromolar against several cancer cell lines, comparable to those of **DDO-6101** Table **1**.

Table 1. Cytotoxicities of CXs in different cell lines.

Compounds	IC_{50} ± SD (μM)					
	HepG2[a]	HCT116[b]	MDA-MB-231[c]	A-549[d]	A-549/taxol[e]	A-549 /cisplatin[f]
DDO-6101	1.14 ± 0.09	0.71 ± 0.1	0.32 ± 0.09	2.59 ± 0.17	0.46 ± 0.03	2.11 ± 0.20
DDO-6337	0.34 ± 0.27	2.49 ± 0.33	0.88 ± 0.05	10.05 ± 2.1	0.61 ± 0.04	0.98 ± 0.13
DDO-6337 • HCl	1.32 ± 0.45	0.97 ± 0.12	1.20 ± 0.07	7.23 ± 0.56	1.90 ± 0.12	1.10 ±0.17
1	3.34 ± 0.37	-	-	3.25 ± 0.22	-	-
DDO-6318	3.79 ± 0.43	0.28 ± 0.03	-	0.31 ± 0.02	0.42 ± 0.05	0.33 ± 0.07

[a] Liver hepatocellular carcinoma cell line; [b] Human colorectal carcinoma cell line; [c] Triple-negative breast cancer cell line; [d] Lung carcinoma cell line; [e] Lung carcinoma cell line resistant to taxol treatment; [f] Lung carcinoma cell line resistant to cisplatin treatment

Further experimental studies to evaluate the drug-like properties showed that most of these compounds have a more favourable partition coefficient (logD from 0.7 to 2.7) than **DDO-6101** (logD = 2.9). Their improved solubility could be due not only to the introduction of heteroatoms but also to the disruption of the intramolecular hydrogen bond between C1-OH and the proximal carboxyl group. Surprisingly, an increment in permeability was also observed. Yet generally decreasing in an acidic environment, **DDO-6318** (Fig. **7**). demonstrated an acceptable permeability coefficient (Pe) even at pH 5, suggesting that this compound is properly absorbed and distributed *in vivo*. As expected, **DDO-6318** exhibited a more relevant dose-dependent antitumor activity against A54 cells when administered twice daily for two weeks in lung cancer A59 transplanted mice (growth inhibition rate = 30.88%, 52.21% and 71.32% at 5, 10 and 20 mg/Kg, respectively) than **DDO-6101** at the same regimen (growth inhibition rate = 34.56 at 20 mg/Kg). Furthermore, **DDO-6318** conserved a significant potency with oral administration of 50 mg/Kg daily dose for one week in the lung cancer A59 mouse model, showing a 66.43% inhibitory rate in comparison to 21.43% inhibitory rate of **DDO-6101** at the same regimen.

In conclusion, the extensive medicinal chemistry efforts to optimize GA elucidated CXs SARs (Fig. **8**) and led to **DDO-6318**, the best candidate of these series for further clinical studies.

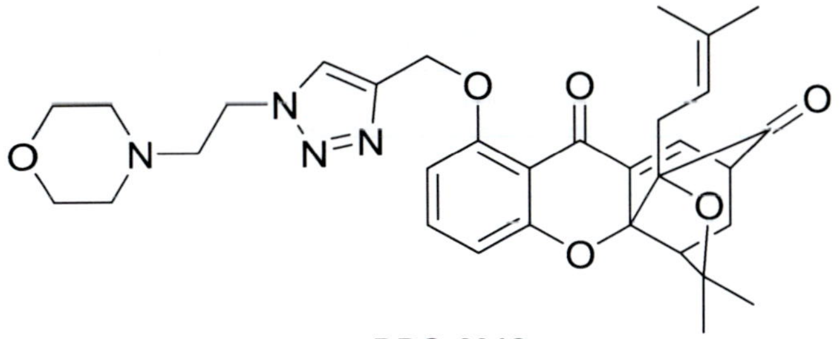

DDO-6318

Fig. (7). Chemical structure of **DDO-6318**.

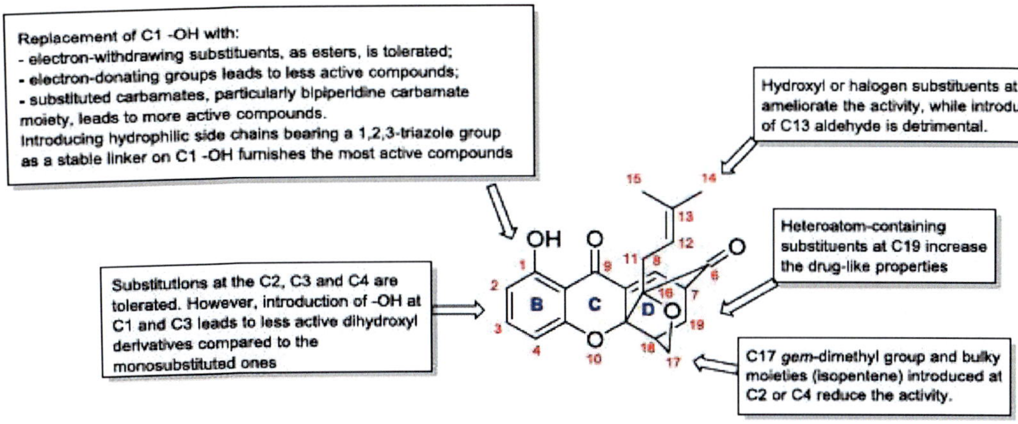

Fig. (8). SAR analysis of CXs.

These promising results inspired Chantarasriwong *et al.* to evaluate the pharmacological potential of CXs against inflammatory breast cancer (IBC) [21]. This extremely aggressive and mostly lethal variant of BC is characterized by lymphovascular invasion of tumour embolus and is resistant to conventional therapies. The need for new efficacious therapy against IBC persuaded the authors to explore additional SAR around the CXs pharmacophore by decorating the B ring:

- Any modification at C1 -OH drastically decreases the activity;
- Insertion of the free hydroxylic group at C3 reduces the activity while alkylating the same –OH enhances the activity;
- Oxidation of the B ring to furnish the corresponding quinone leads to completely inactive derivatives;
- Introduction of fluorine substituents at C1 and C3 retains the activity.

Compound **2** (Fig. **9**) bearing alkylated C3-OH, induced complete dissolution of spheroids^{MARY-X}, a common *in vitro* model of IBC. These findings correlated with the greatest cytotoxicity observed (IC_{50} = 0.38 μM). These promising preliminary results could pave the way to the development of effective therapeutics against IBC.

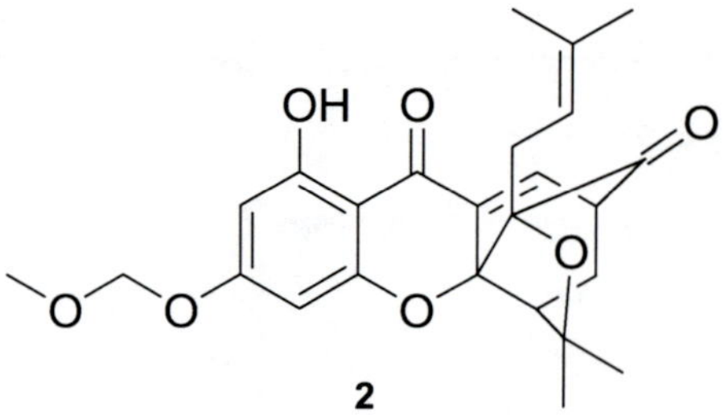

2

Fig. (9). Chemical structure of compound **2.**

Mangostin Analogs

The natural xanthone α-mangostin (Fig. **10**) is extracted from the pericarp of mangosteen fruit (*Garcinia mangostana*) and is endowed with a wide spectrum of pharmacological properties, including antitumor, antinflammatory and antibacterial. As extensively documented, α-mangostin prevents cancer growth both *in vitro* and *in vivo* by promoting apoptosis and regulating p21, p27 and (phosphatidylinositol 3-kinase) PI3K/Akt pathways involved in cell cycle arrest [27].

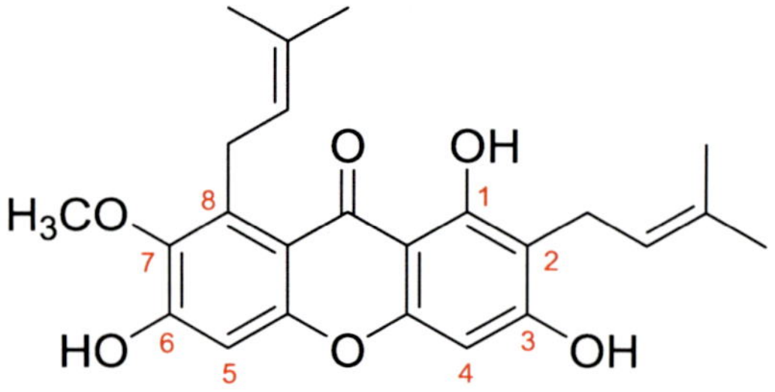

α-mangostin

Fig. (10). Chemical structure of α-mangostin.

Similar to GA, α-mangostin has poor drug-like properties and moderate bioavailability, and several strategies have been evaluated to overcome these drawbacks. Chi *et al.* designed a series of α-mangostin derivatives to investigate the SARs around this core [28]. Accordingly, diverse modifications were introduced on the isopentene groups at C2 and C8, the hydroxyl groups at C1, C3 and C6, and the available C4 and C5 positions of the benzene and the analogs were tested on several cancer cell lines. Moreover, the hydroxyl groups at C1, C3 and C6 were alkylated, acetylated, oxidized, or replaced by a carbon chain. Unfortunately, such modifications led to decreased or total loss of activity. The isopentene at C2 tolerates few modifications and only the reduction or the oxidation of the C2 isopentene to form a cyclic system with the C3 –OH retained the activity. Finally, halogenation at C4 and C5 with chlorine and bromine atoms slightly increases the cytotoxicity. Among these derivatives, compound **3** (Fig. **11**) exhibited the best cell growth inhibitory activity in all the treated cancer cell lines Table **2**.

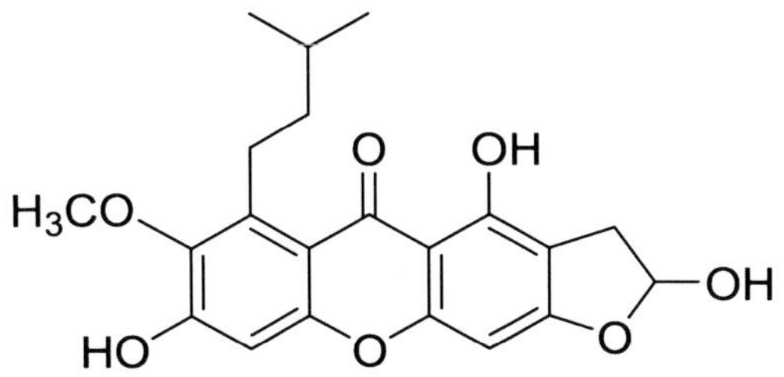

3

Fig. (11). Chemical structure of compound **3**.

In 2018 Shibata *et al.* proposed the synthetic α-mangostin dilaurate (**MGD**) as a potential therapeutic agent for metastatic tumors (Fig. **12**) [29]. Indeed, lauric acid (or dodecanoic acid) demonstrated a high affinity for lymphatic absorption and induced both apoptosis and cell cycle arrest. Therefore, its insertion on the α-mangostin scaffold could allow the xanthone to exert a proper anti-metastatic activity in the lymphatic system, which is the primary pathway for the initial diffusion of solid tumor metastasis.

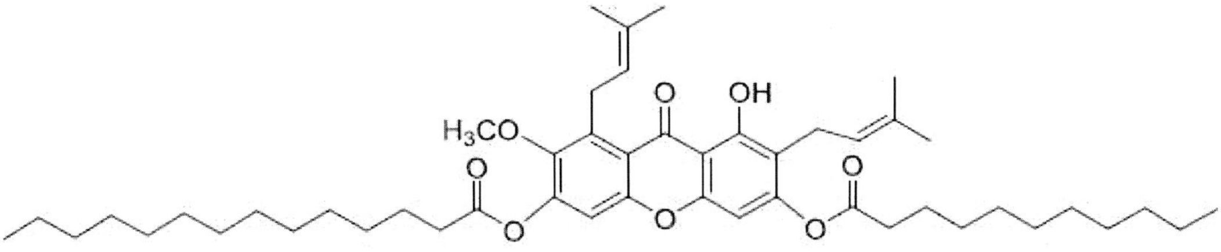

MGD

Fig. (12). Chemical structure of α-mangostin dilaurate (**MGD**).

In this study, a mouse model of breast cancer was obtained *via* inoculation of BJMC3879Luc2 breast cancer cells expressing a mutant p53 protein. A significant decrease in the number of metastasis-positive lymph nodes, the metastatic lung foci size and the overall number of organs with metastases were detected in

MGD-treated mice. **MGD** acts through the induction of apoptosis and the regulation of diverse cell cycle proteins, including p21, p27, PCNA, caspase-3 and phospo-Akt, and induces cell cycle arrest at G1. Altogether, these findings support the hypothesis that **MGD** is a promising anti-metastatic agent.

Carboxyxanthones

The growing interest in both natural and synthetic xanthones led to the discovery of Vadimexan (5,6-dimethylxanthone-4-acetic acid, DMXAA, ASA404), a small tumour vascular-disrupting agent characterized by a carboxyxanthone scaffold [30] (Fig. **13**) Vadimexan selectively disrupts the tumour vessels by inducing apoptosis of vascular endothelial cells without harming healthy vasculatures. Moreover, it hampers the tumour blood flow and promotes haemorrhagic tumour necrosis. Its mechanism of action can be related to the activation of innate-immune response through the stimulation of pro-inflammatory cytokines, chemokines and vasoactive factors and the regulation of several molecular signaling pathways implicated in cell cycle progression and apoptosis homeostasis. Vadimexan entered phase I/II clinical trials in combination with other anticancer drugs for the treatment of non-small cell lung cancer (NSCLC) and preliminary results were very encouraging. However, the synergistic effects in combination with paclitaxel were not confirmed in phase III clinical trials and several side effects were observed [31]. Intrigued by the great potential of Vadimexan, Liu *et al.* explored a multi-target-addressed ligand strategy by combining Vadimexan and pyranoxanthone, two potential synergistic xanthone derivatives, which both exert a plethora of anticancer mechanisms of action [32]. The hybrids were obtained by linking Vadimezan (DMAXX or **D**) and pyranoxanthone (**P**) units *via* a central carbon spacer with different lengths (Fig. **13**) The hybrids were then tested against MDA-MB-231, MCF-7, HepG2 and K562 cancer cell lines and showed significant activity, higher both than that of the single **D** and **P** units and the **D+P** equimolar mixture. Notably, the hybrids with longer carbon chains were the most active ones, suggesting that these spacers allow higher conformational flexibility and bind either different pockets or more than one target. The hybrid **D-P-4** (Fig. **13**) was the best candidate, with an improved inhibitory activity compared to the parent compound Vadimexan Table **2**.

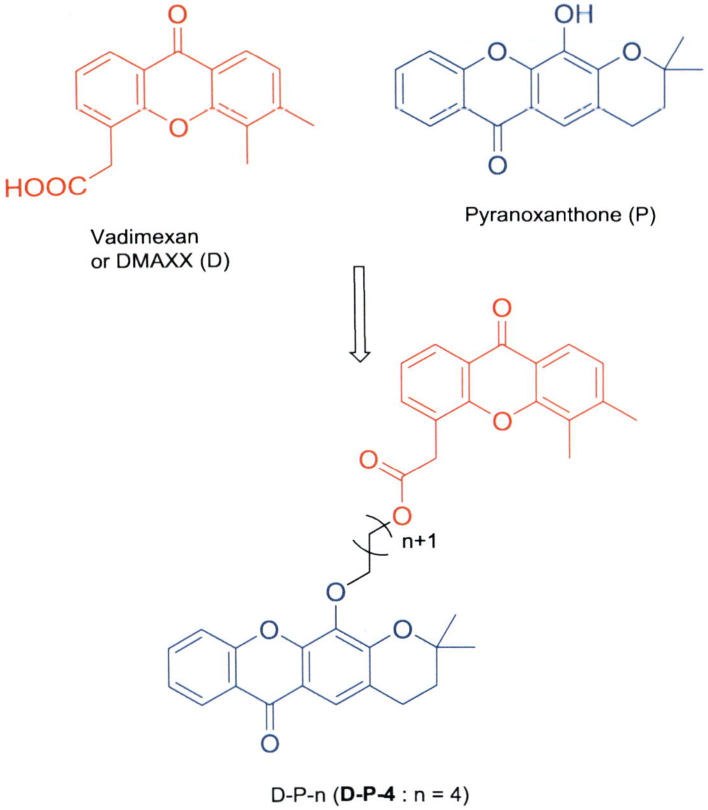

Fig. (13). Chemical structures of Vadimexan, pyranoxanthone and the **D-P-n** hybrids.

D-P-4 was also able to induce an 80% total apoptosis/necrosis rate at 0.2 μM in HepG-2 cells. The apoptotic mechanisms included arresting the cell cycle at S, regulation of caspase 3, caspase 9 and Poly (ADP-ribose) polymerase (PARP) levels. The same authors also assessed the activity of 33 newly synthesized 1,3-diihydroxyxanthones alone and in combination with Vadimexan [33]. SAR analysis highlighted the 1,3-dihydroxyl xanthones as the best candidates, while any variations in terms of position, number and methylations of the –OH groups of the C ring drastically reduced the activity. Introduction of electron-withdrawing moieties into the A ring increased the anticancer activity, whereas electron-donating groups were detrimental. 7-Bromo-1,3-dihydroxy-9*H*-xanthen-9-one compound **4**, (Fig. **14**) was the most active inhibitor in MDA-MB-231 cells, with an IC_{50} of 0.46 ± 0.03 μM.

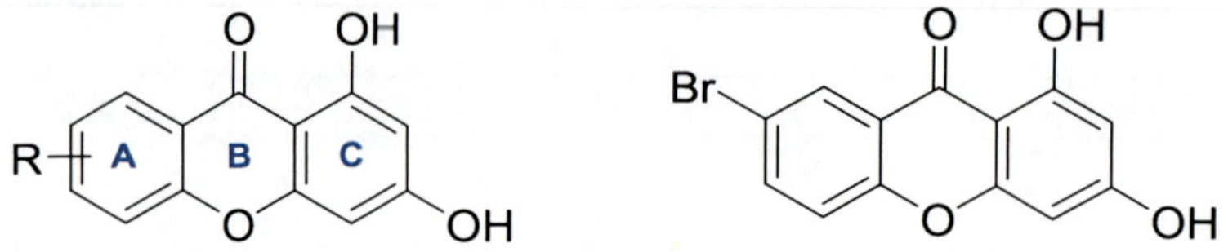

4

Fig. (14). General structure of 1,3-dihydroxyxanthones and chemical structure of compound **4**.

The synergistic effect was confirmed by testing Vadimexan and the most active derivatives in equimolar combinations. The association of compound **4** with Vadimexan greatly improved inhibitory activity, with an IC_{50} of 0.042 ± 0.005 μM against MDA-MB-231 cell line growth. The inhibitory effect of compound **4** alone and, in combination, induced 60.9% total apoptosis/necrosis of the treated cells related to the regulation of caspase 3, caspase 9, PARP and p53/MDM2 levels. These encouraging data suggest that xanthones derivatives are amenable both to a combination therapy and a multi-target strategy, representing an innovative and effective approach towards novel anticancer therapeutics.

Dihydroxyxanthones

The discovery of potential antitumor 1,3-dihydroxyxanthones, such as 1,3-diihydroxy-6-methoxyxanthone for the treatment of Multidrug Resistance-associated Protein 1 (MRP1)-positive cancers, led to exploring several manipulations around this scaffold. Zhou *et al.* introduced hydroxyl, chlorine, nitro and trifluoromethyl groups on the 1,3-diihydroxyxanthones scaffold [34]. Most of these compounds showed good activities in different cell lines Table **2.**, and 7-chloro-1,3-dihydroxyxanthone Compound **5**, (Fig. **15**) was the most active one.

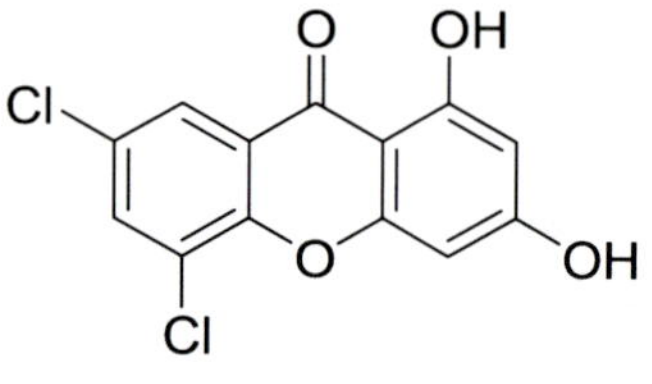

5

Fig. (15). Chemical structure of compound **5**.

Recently, inspired by the structural similarity between the polycyclic aromatic hydrocarbon pollutant benzo[*a*]pyrene (BaP) and the xanthone scaffold, Liu *et al.*

proposed new diihydroxyxanthones as potential aryl hydrocarbon receptor [35] (AhR) inhibitors for the treatment of hepatocellular carcinoma (HCC). The AhR is a transcription factor activated by toxic chemicals, including BaP. AhR is overexpressed in hepatocellular cancer and represents a potential target for the treatment of HCC. Accordingly, several diihydroxanthone analogues were synthesized as potential competitive AhR inhibitors and tested on four liver cancer cell lines. Most of them displayed good anticancer activities. In particular, the introduction of 3-methyl-2-butenyl substituents at diverse positions on the A and C rings provided the most active compounds. Compound **6**, depicted in Fig. **(16).**, emerged as the most promising anti-proliferative agent Table **2**.

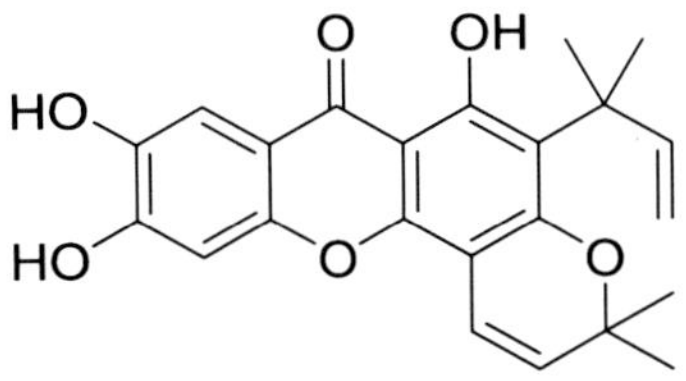

6

Fig. (16). Chemical structure of compound **6**.

Table 2. Cytotoxic activities of carboxyxanthones and dihydroxyxanthones in different cell lines.

Compounds	IC_{50} ± SD (μM)				
	HepG2[a]	MDA-MB-231[b]	A-549[c]	SMCC-7721[d]	MCF-7[e]
3	-	-	11.77 ± 0.13	6.92 ± 0.55	17.97 ± 0.23
D-P-4	0.216 ± 0.031	1.129 ± 0.13	-	-	0.534 ± 0.043
4	9.2 ± 1.0	0.46 ± 0.03	-	-	3.4 ± 0.1
5	-	-	-	6.14 ± 0.13	-
6	18.6 ± 2.31	-	-	52.8 ± 6.11	-

[a] Liver hepatocellular carcinoma cell line; [b] Triple-negative breast cancer cell line; [c] Lung carcinoma cell line [d] Hepatocellular carcinoma cell line; [e] Breast cancer cell line

N-Xanthone Benzensulphonamides

Zhou's research group developed **PGMI-004A** (Fig. **17**) a benzensulphonamide active against phosphoglycerate mutase 1 (PGAM1), an enzyme upregulated in several forms of cancers and involved in glycolysis and anabolic biosynthesis of macromolecules required for aberrant cell proliferation. PGAM1 acts by limiting the metabolic supplies of energy and building blocks for biosynthetic processes required by cancer cells, thus preventing tumor growth [36].

In 2018, Wang *et al.* designed a series of novel *N*-xanthone benzenesulfonamides by replacing the anthraquinone core with a xanthone scaffold and reversing the sulfonamide moiety [37]. The SAR studies demonstrated that the methylation of the hydroxyl groups decreased the activity. The D ring tolerated diverse substituents, suggesting that this ring accommodates a large cave of PGAM1. Larger substituents increased the activity, with the best results furnished by the insertion of a larger ring system (IC_{50} values in the range of 0.5–2.7 μM). When tested in the NSCLC cell line H2199, compound **7** (Fig. **17**) was more active than PGMI-004A (IC_{50} = 5.0 ± 0.9 μM *vs.* 26.0 ± 2.1 μM). As the *o*-dihydroxy phenols showed metabolic issues, the hydroxyl group at C2 was removed and different substituents were introduced at the A and D rings [38] (Fig. **17**) Consistent with the previous SAR findings, removal of the C2-OH was detrimental. However, increasing the overall compound lipophilicity *via* the insertion of iodine or di-halogen atoms at the D ring and the introduction of bulky (*tert*-butyl)phenyl, cyclohexylphenyl, biphenyl and naphthalenyl substituents restored the activity. Compound **8** (Fig. **17**)., bearing a biphenyl moiety, was more active against PGAM1 (IC_{50} = 5.5 ± 1.1 μM) than PGMI-004A (IC_{50} = 13 ± 0.1 μM), but less than compound **6** (IC_{50} = 2.7 ± 0.1 μM). The second series of *N*-xanthone benzenesulfonamides was designed by introducing halogens, methyl, methoxy, acetoxy and nitro moieties at C5 and C7. These analogs were more active than the parent compounds. Compound **9** (Fig. **17**) was the best PGAM1 inhibitor (IC_{50} = 2.1 μM). Molecular docking studies between compound **9** and PGAM1 suggested that additional hydrogen bonds formed by the nitro group and the hydrophobic interactions established by the biphenyl moiety might be responsible for the enhancement of activity.

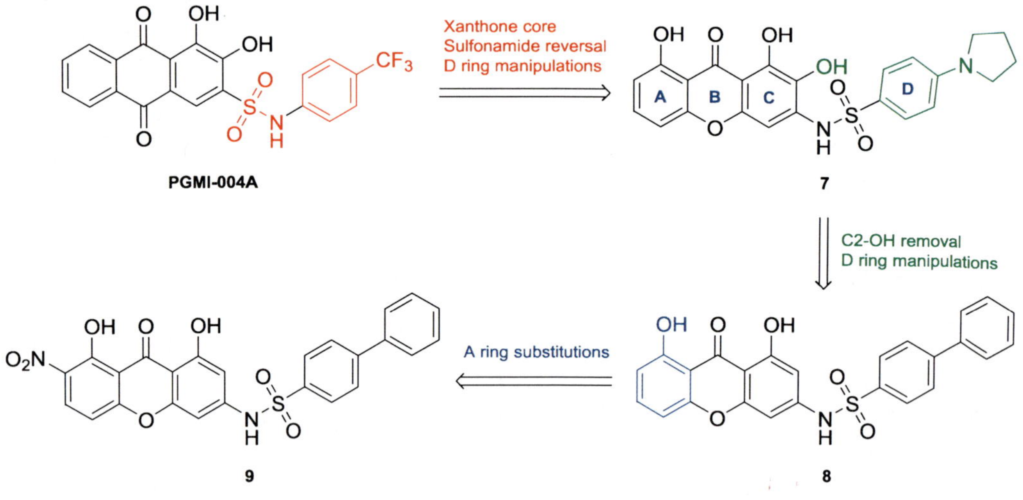

Fig. (17). Chemical structures of **PGMI-004A** and compounds **7**, **8** and **9**.

Dioxygenated Xanthones

In 2018, Gomes *et al.* reported the 1-carbaldehyde-3,4-dimethoxyxanthone **LEM2** (Fig. **18**) as a transcriptionally active p73 (TAp73) activating agent with potent antitumor activity. TAp73 is a tumor suppressor protein that regulates p53 target genes and modulates key cellular processes [39]. Its activation is also crucial in chemotherapy response and might represent a valuable alternative strategy to p53 activation in p53-impaired tumors, such as neuroblastoma (NBL). **LEM2** enhances TaP73 transcriptional activity by disrupting its interaction with mutated p53 and MDM2 and showed promising antitumor activity in patient derived NBL cells, both alone and in combination with conventional chemotherapeutics.

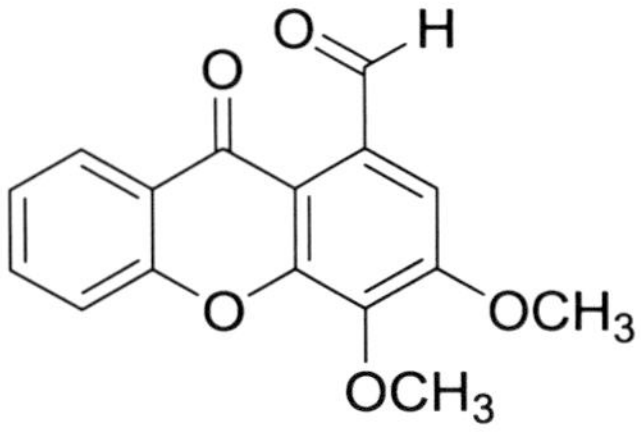

LEM2

Fig. (18). Chemical structure of **LEM2**.

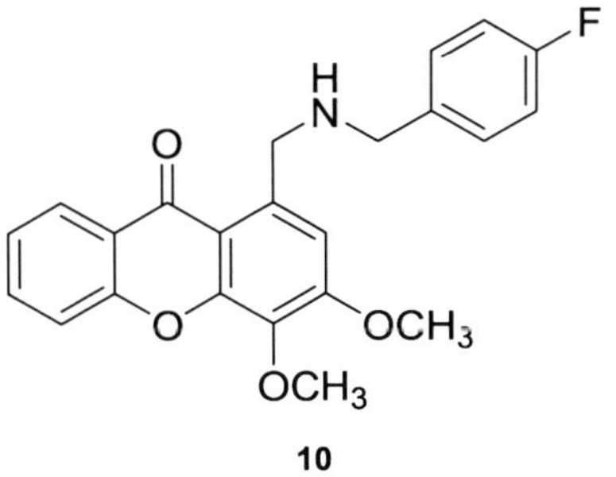

10

Fig. (19). Chemical structure of compound **10**.

LEM2 showed strong anti-proliferative activity in the assessed cell lines through G2/M-phase cell cycle arrest and apoptosis. Moreover, it has a potential antiangiogenic activity and can downregulate the vascular endothelial growth factor (VEGF). The scaffold of **LEM2** was used as a template to build a library of novel 3,4-dioxygenated xanthones as MDM2-p53 interaction disrupting agents [40]. Following a molecular hybridization approach, the authors synthesized a set of eleven aminated xanthones through the reductive amination of **LEM2** with amine precursors containing structural motifs of described MDM2-p53 disruptors.

Compound **10** (Fig. **19**) was the most active one of the series, with IC_{50} values in the micromolar range against both the colorectal carcinoma cell line HCT116 p53$^{+/+}$ and HepG2.

Compound **10** was posed into the p53-binding site of MDM2 to predict the possible interactions. As expected, the *p*-fluorobenzylamino moiety accommodates within the Trp23 pocket, establishing π-stacking interactions with Phe91, amide-π interactions with Leu57 and Gly58, and CH-π interactions with Leu54, Leu57, Gly58, Ile61, Val93, and Ile99. The methoxyl groups formed CH-CH interactions with Leu54, while the non-substituted benzene ring established π-stacking interactions with Phe55 and amide-π and CH-π interactions with Gln59.

Xanthones Bearing Long Side Chains

The insertion of different side chains in the xanthone core is a strategy explored by several research groups to enhance the anticancer activity. In 2016, Liu *et al.* proposed a series of xanthones bearing *N*-substituted aminocarbonylmethoxy side chains on both benzene rings at C3 and C6 positions and screened their anticancer activities on human cancer cell lines [41]. Compound **11** (Fig. **20**) was the hit of this series and exhibited promising cytotoxic activities in different cell lines exhibiting IC_{50} values in the micromolar in several cancer cell lines, including MDA- MB-231, A549, and HCT116. Preliminary results suggest that the cytotoxic effects could be exerted *via* a caspase-dependent pathway, but further studies are needed to elucidate the mechanism of action of this class of compounds.

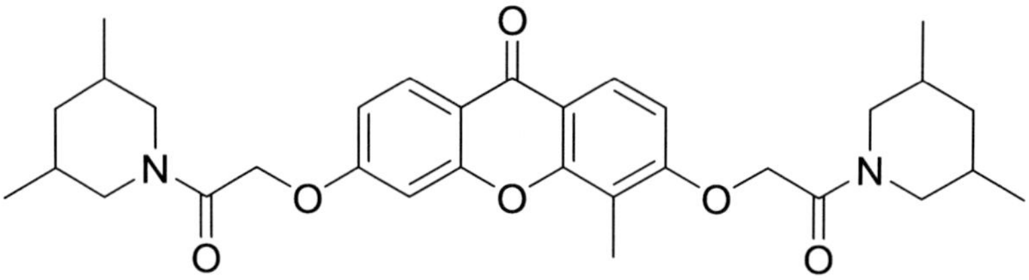

11

Fig. (20). Chemical structure of compound **11**.

In 2018, Sypniewski *et al.* examined the involvement of reactive oxygen species in the anticancer mechanism of a series of novel xanthones bearing aminoalkanol side chains [42] (Fig. **21**) In this study, A549 and T24 cell lines were exposed to aminoalkanol xanthones and the corresponding hydrochloride salts. Notably, the tested derivatives promoted oxidative stress, stimulated ROS-mediated apoptosis, and induced the expression of the antioxidant enzymes catalase (CAT), glutathione peroxidase (GPX), and superoxide dismutase (SOD) in the analyzed cell cultures. The natural xanthones GA and mangostin were included in this study. Consistent with previous findings, GA strongly promoted oxidative stress, while mangostin displayed antioxidative properties, confirming the importance of the nature and the position of substituents for the biological features of xanthones.

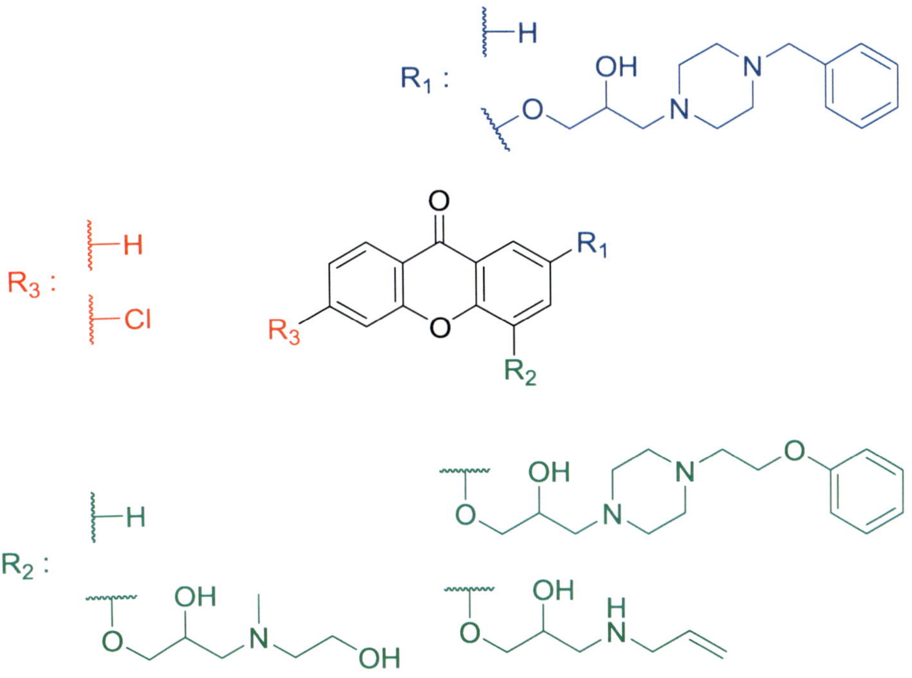

Fig. (21). General structures of a novel series of xanthones bearing aminoalkanol side chains at positions 2 and 4.

Wu *et al.* introduced on the xanthone scaffold a triazole ring, a heterocycle often used in drug design as an amide's bioisostere with the potential to interact with biological targets and DNA *via* hydrogen bonds [22]. The triazole was introduced at C3 and served as a linker between the xanthone core and diversely substituted benzyl rings. SAR studies proved that side chains incorporating benzyls decorated with weak electron-withdrawing groups, namely bromine atoms, provide the highest active analogues of the series, while electron-donating groups were detrimental for the activity. When screened against A549 cancer cells, compound **12** demonstrated the best antiproliferative activity (IC_{50} = 32.4 ± 2.2 μM), inducing apoptosis *via* the regulation of the expression of caspase 3, Bax, JNK and p53 in treated cells (Fig. **22**)

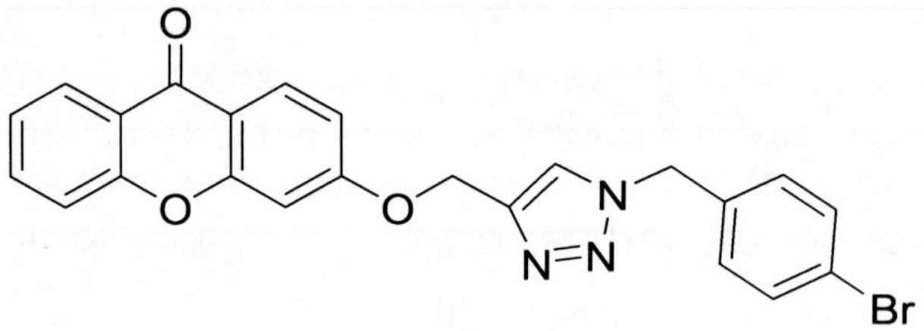

12

Fig. (22). Chemical structure of compound **12**.

C3 and C6 glycosylated xanthones were also developed as potential agents for the treatment of glioblastoma cancers [43] (Fig. **23**). Currently available therapeutics against glioblastoma are still ineffective due to the complexity of achieving a local drug activity by crossing the blood-brain barrier. Xanthone **13** was endowed with promising growth inhibitory activities against the tested glioblastoma cancer lines (IC_{50} values of 0.42 ± 0.02 and 0.42 ± 0.07 μM against U373 and U87-MG, respectively). To improve its blood-brain barrier permeability and prevent esterase hydrolysis, this candidate was encapsulated in a liposome and a proliposome. This formulation improved its ability to permeate the blood-brain barrier and retained *in vitro* activity, suggesting that exploring new xanthone formulations might be a valuable approach to finding novel treatments for glioblastoma.

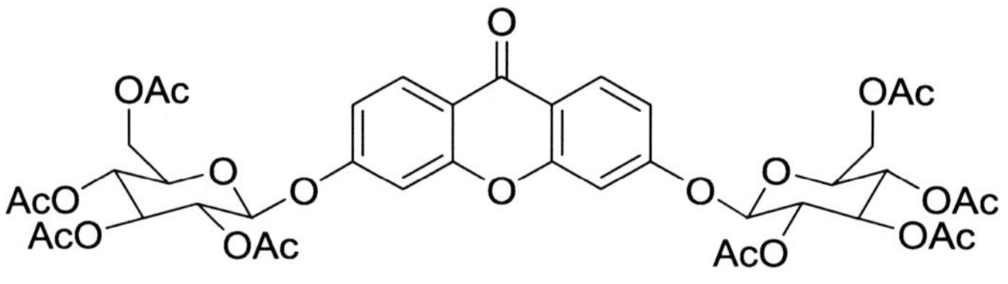

13

Fig. (23). Chemical structure of compound **13**.

ANTIBACTERIAL XANTHONE SYNTHETIC DERIVATIVES

Amphiphilic Xanthones

Small antimicrobial peptidomimetics (SAPs) were developed to address the poor pharmacokinetic properties and high toxicity of antimicrobial peptides (AMPs), a class of antibiotics able to penetrate the anionic bacterial membrane through hydrophobic interactions and disrupt membrane integrity. Despite their good antibacterial activities, SAPs often cause haemolysis and suffer from low membrane selectivity. Amphiphilic xanthones are a promising and thoroughly studied class of SAPs. These compounds are endowed with excellent antimicrobial properties, along with rapid killing, not species-specificity and a low tendency to generate resistance [44, 45]. Oligomerization strongly impacts their bactericidal activities: biophysical studies proved that in aqueous solution compound 14 (Fig. **24**) forms oligomers that first bind to the membrane-water interface and then insert into the bilayer membrane hydrophobic phase [46]. The oligomers increase in size within the membrane, causing membrane leakage and as oligomers further increase, they cause decreased membrane fluidity and cell death. These findings clearly indicate that physicochemical properties are crucial for the mechanism of action and antimicrobial activities of amphiphilic xanthones. To further explore the potential of this scaffold, Lin *et al.* designed and developed a novel generation of symmetric amphiphilic xanthones with outstanding antibacterial properties and good membrane selectivity [44]. Interestingly, the authors reported the first total synthesis strategy for xanthone based peptidomimetics. This versatile approach allowed the generation of a library by providing more modification options compared to semisynthetic methods using α-mangostin. Compounds were tested for their antibacterial and haemolytic properties in rabbit erythrocytes. SAR analysis revealed that the proper balance between charge and hydrophobicity is crucial to enhance the antibacterial activity and membrane selectivity of this class. Indeed, a positive charge drives selectivity towards zwitterionic mammalian cell membranes and promotes favourable electrostatic interactions with the negatively charged bacterial cells, while the hydrophobic portion helps to penetrate the bacterial membrane. Moreover, the small and conformationally rigid xanthone core facilitates penetration through the Gram-positive membrane. The fine tuning of charged and hydrophobic features led to the identification of two lead compounds (**15** and **16**), reported in Fig. **(24).**

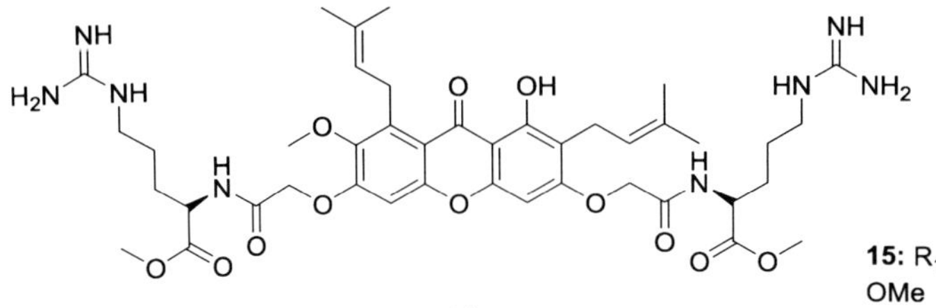

14

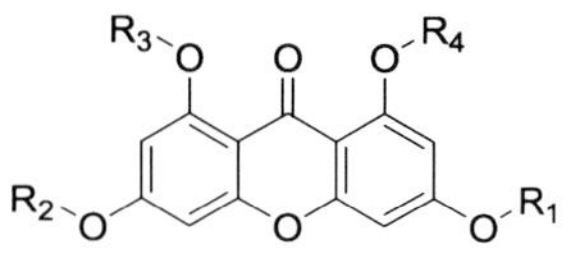

15: R_1=R_2= isoprenyl; R_3=R_4= CH_2-CO-Arg-OMe
16: R_1=R_2= isoprenyl; R_3=R_4= CH_2-CO-Arg-Arg-OMe

Fig. (24). Chemical structures of amphiphilic xanthones **14**, **15** and **16**.

Comprehensive biological studies highlighted the high therapeutic potential of this class. Compounds **15** and **16** were endowed with excellent bactericidal properties against Gram-positive bacteria and good membrane selectivity, as reported in Table **3**.

Table 3. ***In vitro*** **antibacterial activities against clinical isolates and hemolytic activities of compounds 15, 16, and vancomycin.**

Compound	MIC (µg/mL)				HC_{50}[a] (µg/mL)	Hemolysis (%)[b]
	S. aureus DM 4001R	*S. aureus* MRSA DM 9808R	*S. aureus* MRSA DM 21455	*Bacillus cereus* ATCC 11778		
15	0.78	0.78	1.56	3.13	750±18	42±2
16	1.53	3.13	3.13	3.13	>2000	9±1
Vancomycin	1.56	3.13	1.56	1.56	ND[c]	ND[c]

[a]The lowest concentration causing 50% hemolysis of red blood cells; [b]Percent hemolysis of red blood cells caused by **16** and **17** at 400 µg/mL; [c]Not determined.

Moreover, compound **15** was efficacious *in vivo* in a murine model of methicillin resistant *Staphylococcus aureus* (MRSA) corneal infection. Mode of action studies and molecular dynamics simulation confirmed the electronic discrimination over the mammalian cells and rapid penetration of the bacterial membrane, resulting in intracellular components leakage and cell death. As bacteria cannot achieve a rapid remodelling of their membrane, this class of antibacterials is not likely to develop resistance and can represent a valuable alternative for Gram-positive infections.

The same strategy was applied to identify novel agents against tuberculosis (TB). TB, caused by *Mycobacterium tuberculosis*, is the leading cause of death for infectious diseases. TB drug discovery is hampered by the emergence of drug resistance and a low success rate in clinical development. Therefore, there is a continuous need for novel chemical entities acting by innovative mechanisms of action [47 - 49]. The antimycobacterial activity of amphiphilic xanthones was investigated by Koh *et al.* in 2016 [50]. A fruitful combination of mechanistic studies and SAR analysis led to the development of potent and selective membrane targeting anti-TB agents. Interestingly, the structural criteria driving the antimycobacterial activities of these compounds were different from that of bacteria. More lipophilic and bulkier moieties enhanced anti-TB activities, suggesting that hydrophobic interactions are important to penetrate hydrophobic and waxier environment of the mycobacterial membranes. Amphiphilic xanthones included in this study rapidly killed mycobacteria by disrupting membrane integrity and inducing strong ATP leakage. This unprecedented and non-specific mechanism of action is different from that of the standard first-line anti-TB drugs and is less likely to generate resistance. Compound **17** (Fig. **25**) the hit of this series, displayed excellent properties also against multi-drug resistant (MDR) strains, was metabolically stable and showed low cytotoxicity Table **4.**

Table 4. *In vitro* antimycobacterial and hemolytic activities, cytotoxicity and metabolic stability in rat liver microsomes of compound 17.

Compound	cLog*P*	MIC[a]$_{90}$ (μM)		HC$_{50}$[b] (μM)	Citotoxicity[c] (CC$_{50}$, μM)	Metabolic Stability	
		M. Smegmatis	*M. Bovis*			% metabolized	$t_{1/2}$ (min)
17	10.18	3.2	3.2	>277.4	107.5	10.0	>30
Isoniazid	-0.67	15	6.25	ND[d]	ND[d]	ND[d]	ND[d]

[a]Minimal inhibitory concentration; [b] The lowest concentration causing 50% hemolysis of red blood cells; [c]Citotoxicity displayed in the ATP *via*bility assay; [d]not determined.

This compound was also able to kill persister mycobacteria in a suitable model of hypoxic nongrowing tubercle bacilli; as expected, its resistance mutation frequency in *M. bovis* was lower than 10^{-8} [51]. As its oral bioavailability was relatively low (14%), it was not suitable for establishing *in vivo* efficacy. Further hit-to-lead optimization efforts to improve PK parameters and *in vivo* proof-o--concept will disclose the therapeutic potential of this promising class of anti-TB candidates. Interestingly, the amphiphilic xanthone **AM-228** (Fig. **25**) was able to eradicate mycobacterial biofilms, which are the main obstacle to the treatment of non-tuberculosis mycobacterial (NTM) infections of the cornea [52].

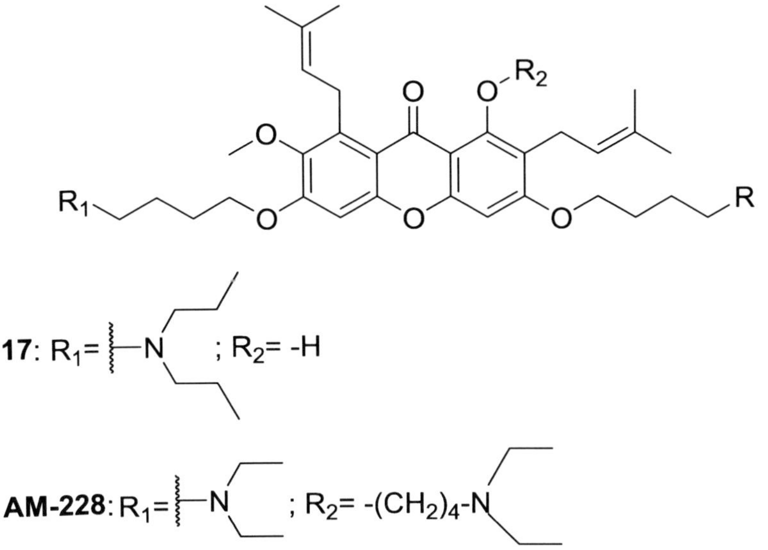

Fig. (25). Chemical structures of compound **17** and **AM-228**.

Amino Acid-Conjugated Xanthones

Despite their bactericidal activities, the potential of natural caged xanthones as antibacterial agents is hampered by their cytotoxicity [53]. In 2016, Chaiyakunvat *et al.* screened natural caged xanthones for their activities against the community-acquired MRSA USA300 strain SF8300 and explored their SARs to obtain less toxic antibacterial agents [54]. This study revealed that the carboxylic moiety at C30 is a key structural feature and suggested that replacing this substituent with less polar groups could be detrimental for the activity. Therefore, the scaffold of morellic acid (Fig. **26**) was conjugated with different amino acids *via* solid phase synthesis to obtain a new series of semisynthetic derivatives. Compound **18** (Fig. **26**) retained the antibacterial activity of the parent compound (MIC against MRSA strain SF8300 = 12.5 and 25 μM, respectively) but significantly decreased the cytotoxicity. Further experiments are needed to study how this semisynthetic caged xanthone could perturb intracellular invasion.

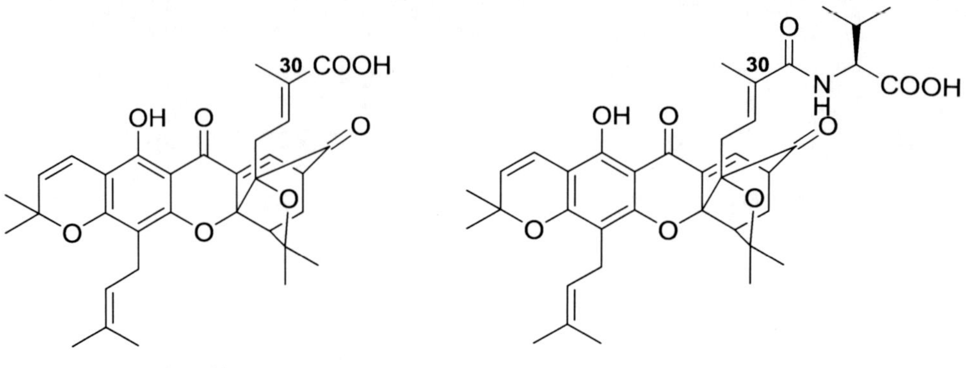

Fig. (26). Chemical structures of morellic acid and its semisynthetic derivative **18**.

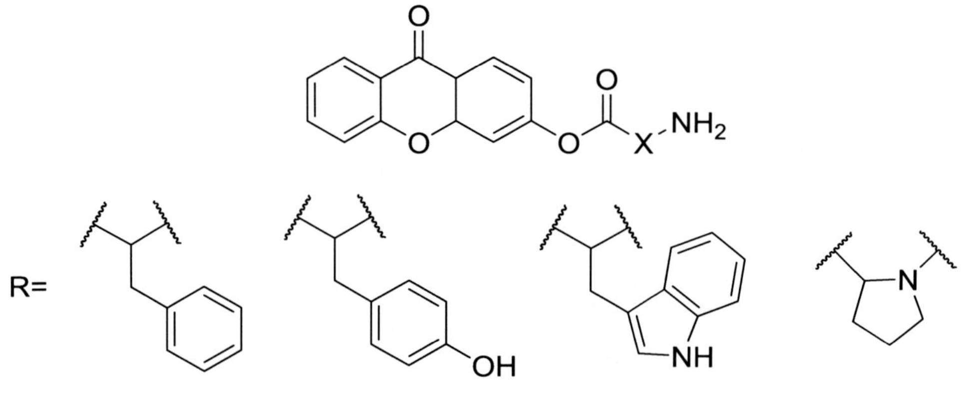

Fig. (27). General structures of 3-hydroxy amino acid-conjugate xanthones.

Chen *et al.* followed a similar approach and conjugated 3-hydroxyxanthones with different aminoacidic chains to obtain a series of potential membrane-disrupting agents (Fig. **27**) The conjugation with amino acids was crucial in determining the biological activity of these compounds, which showed promising antibacterial, antifungal and anti-inflammatory activities [55].

Miscellaneous Compounds

Very recently, an interesting study on halogenated derivatives of xanthones further expanded the SAR around this scaffold and highlighted important structural features for antibacterial and antifungal activities (Fig. **28**) Preliminary biological results revealed the potential for some of the synthesized derivatives, which might serve as a starting point for future optimization studies [56].

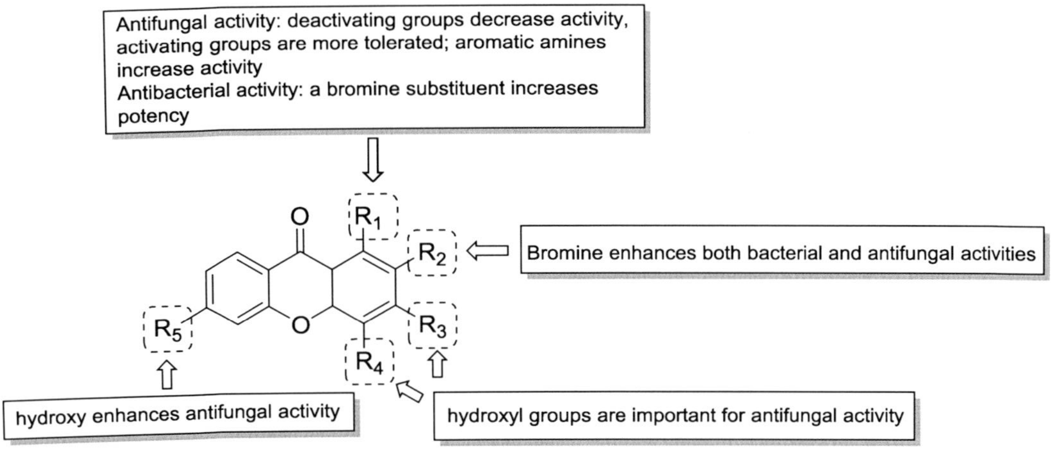

Fig. (28). SAR analysis of halogenated xanthone analogues.

O-carboxymethyl-*N,N,N*-trimethyl chitosan xanthones [57] (CTMC-Xan) are a class of putative membrane-disrupting agents (Fig. **29**) These compounds were designed to improve solubility and enhance the activity [58] of xanthones through the conjugation of *N,N,N*-trimethyl chitosan and showed an improved biological profile compared to the parent compounds. The scaffold of xanthones benefits from the insertion of the amino group both in terms of solubility and antibacterial properties. Indeed, the presence of a permanent positive charge increases water solubility and is likely to destabilize the negatively charged bacterial membrane, thereby increasing the permeation of CMTC-xanthones.

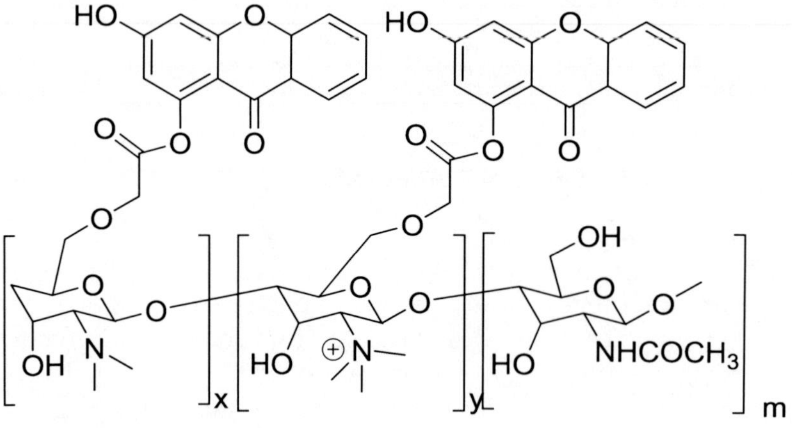

Fig. (29). General structure of CTMC-Xan.

Finally, Klesiewicz *et al.* designed a series of C3-substituted xanthone analogs to be evaluated against *H. pylori* [59] based on previous studies on *N*-substituted analogues of 2-oxo-2*H*-benzopyran-2-carboxamides [60]. The hit compound of this class of antibacterial agents was compound **19** (Fig. **30**), with a MIC of 5μg/mL against the *H. pylori* strain ATCC 43504. Interestingly, SAR analysis of these compounds suggested that the antibacterial activity of these compounds is determined by their structure and spherical conformation more than their hydrophilic character.

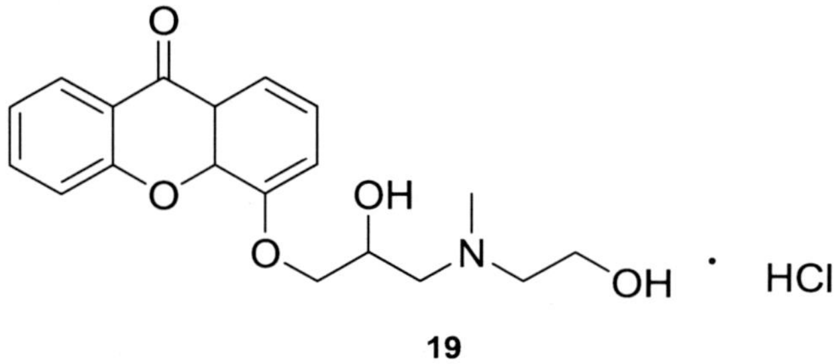

19

Fig. (30). Chemical structure of compound **19**.

ANTIFUNGAL XANTHONE SYNTHETIC DERIVATIVES

Inspired by the outstanding antibacterial properties of amphiphilic xanthones, the chemical scaffold of α-mangostin was modified to obtain a series of cationic amphiphilic xanthones as novel membrane-targeting antifungals [61]. A cationic moiety (arginine, guanidine, or amine) was incorporated in the scaffold to facilitate the electrostatic interaction with the negatively charged fungal membrane, while the hydrophobic isoprenyl groups and the xanthone core improved membrane permeabilization. Compounds **20** and **21** (Fig. **31**) were the most active ones and showed a unique biological profile. They displayed a broad spectrum of activity against a wide range of pathogen fungal, including resistant strains and showed negligible toxicities towards human cells, along with good electrostatic discrimination towards mammalian cells Table **5.** Their nonspecific mechanism of action is likely to prevent the development of drug resistance and was confirmed by a study that proved their ability to directly bind and disrupt fungal membranes. Compound **20** was highly efficacious in a murine model of fungal keratitis. It reduced 92.8% of the fungal burden at a concentration 25-fold lower than that of the standard dug natamycin, emerging as the lead compound of the class.

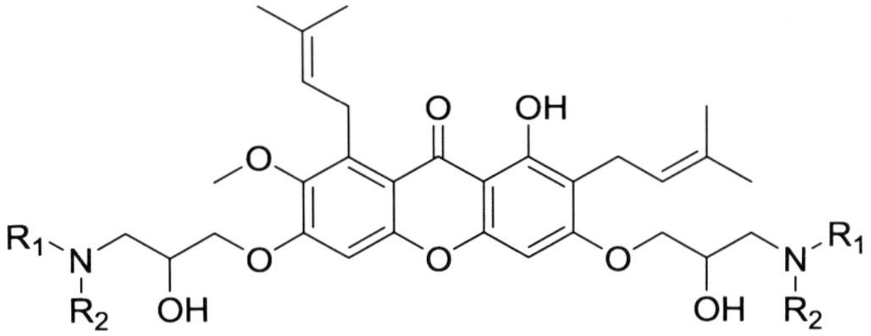

20: R_1=H; R_2= formamidyl
21: R_1= n-butyl; R_2= n-butyl

Fig. (31). Chemical structures of compounds **20** and **21**.

Table 5. *In vitro* antifungal and hemolytic activities of compounds 20 and 21 and α-mangostin.

Compound	cLog*P*	MIC against *C. albicans* ATCC 10231 (μg/mL)	MIC Against *C. albicans* DF2672R (μg/mL)	HC_{50} [a]	Selectivity (HC_{50}/MIC)
α-mangostin	5.07	>50	>50	9±2	<0.2
20	1.99	0.78	0.78	74.6±1.4	61
2	9.31	3.13	3.13	>400	>127.8
Natamycin	-	6.25	6.25	113.0±0.8	18.1

[a] The lowest concentration causing 50% hemolysis of red blood cells.

Chlorine-containing xanthones with different substitution patterns were also designed as potential antifungal agents. This class of synthetic xanthones showed moderate to good antifungal activities and requires further optimization but might serve as a scaffold to improve the activity profile and drug-like properties [2, 62].

ANTIMALARIAL XANTHONE SYNTHETIC DERIVATIVES

Novel antimalarial agents acting by innovative mechanisms of action are urgently needed to fight against the spread of parasite strains resistant to a majority of the drugs commonly employed in therapy [63, 64]. The mitochondrion of parasites is essential for survival and emerged as a validated target to develop novel antimalarial agents. Several studies demonstrated that GA is able to affect mitochondrial structure and function. In this context, Ke and co-workers designed a novel class of antimalarial agents by conjugating the caged xanthones scaffold with a triphenylphosphonium group [65] (Fig. **32**)

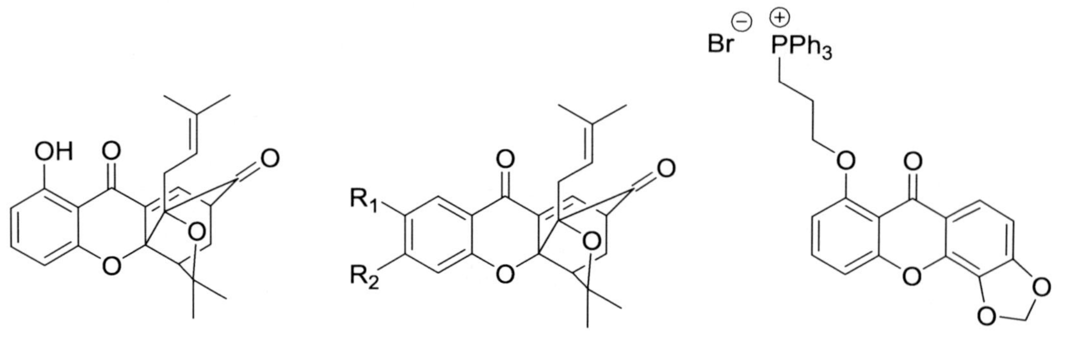

MAD28 **CR135**: R_1= -O-$(CH_2)_4PPh_3^+Br^-$; R_2= -H **SQ129**
CR142: R_1= -H; R_2=-O-$(CH_2)_4PPh_3^+Br^-$

Fig. (32). Chemical structures of the caged antimalarial xanthones **MAD28**, **CR135**, **CR142** and **SQ129**.

CR135 and **CR142** exhibited nanomolar potency against both drug sensitive and drug resistant *P. falciparum* strains. The insertion of a triphenylphosphonium group dramatically increased both the activity and the selectivity of human cells. The replacement of the CX structure with a planar xanthone caused a drop in potency, proving that the combination of a triphenylphosphonium group and a CX scaffold are the most profitable ones for optimal antimalarial activity. These compounds kill parasites at multiple asexual stages and induce distinct morphological changes. Biological data suggested that they are likely to target multiple pathways and act with different modes of action, which can be beneficial to prevent the insurgence of resistance. Further medicinal chemistry optimization of these hits could then increase the selectivity over human cells, leading to the development of optimal lead compounds for malaria treatment.

XANTHONE SYNTHETIC DERIVATIVES AS ANTI-INFLAMMATORY AGENTS

The aberrant inflammatory response plays a central role in various affections, such as cancer, metabolic disorders, autoimmune or neurodegenerative diseases, and it is related to grave tissue injury and dysfunction. Anti-inflammatory drugs commonly employed in therapy comprise mostly non-steroidal anti-inflammatory drugs and glucocorticoids, with related serious side effects and limited efficacy [17]. Prompted by the urgent need for new therapeutic approaches, several xanthone derivatives have been evaluated for their anti-inflammatory activities in the last few years.

Inspired by the anti-inflammatory effects exerted by the natural xanthone β-mangostin, Karunakaran *et al.* developed a series of monoacetate and *O*-alkylated β-mangostin semisynthetic derivatives [66] (Fig. **33**) Notwithstanding, the proposed compounds furnished worse anti-inflammatory profiles compared to the parent natural product. Hence, the IC_{50} values referred to the inhibitory activity against nitric oxide production were considerably higher (IC_{50} > 50 μM) than those provided by β-mangostin (IC_{50} 11.72 ± 1.16 μM), which remains the best candidate.

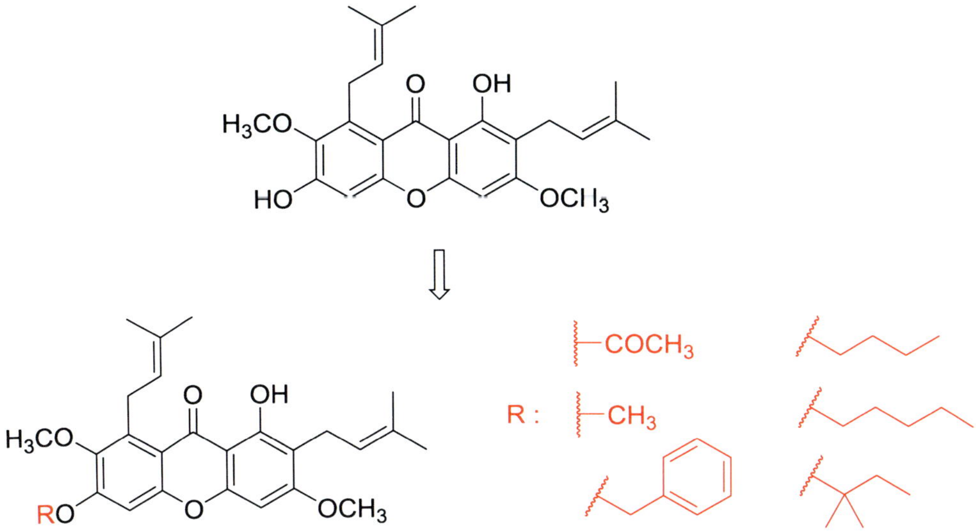

Fig. (33). Chemical structures of β-mangostin and the correspondant monoacetate and *O*-alkylated derivatives.

A different strategy to obtain novel anti-inflammatory agents explored by Chen *et al.* [55] in 2017 was to conjugate the xanthone scaffold with amino acids. The majority of the tested compounds exhibited greater *in vitro* anti-inflammatory activity than the standard drug indomethacin. Compounds containing aromatic (tryptophan, tyrosine, and phenylalanine) and sulphur (cysteine and methionine) amino acids were more active than those bearing aliphatic amino acids. *In silico* molecular docking studies were carried out to analyze the interaction of the most active candidates with secretory phospholipase A2 (sPLA2). As expected, xanthones conjugated with tryptophan and methionine had the highest docking scores. In particular, compound **22** inhibited the sPLA2 activity by establishing π–π stacking interaction with Gly29 and hydrogen bond with Asp48. These residues are located in the proximity of sPLA2's catalytic site and are crucial for the pro-inflammatory activity (Fig. **34**) These findings highlighted compound **23** as the hit for this series, but further investigation is needed to confirm the potential of this compound in *in vivo* inflammatory models.

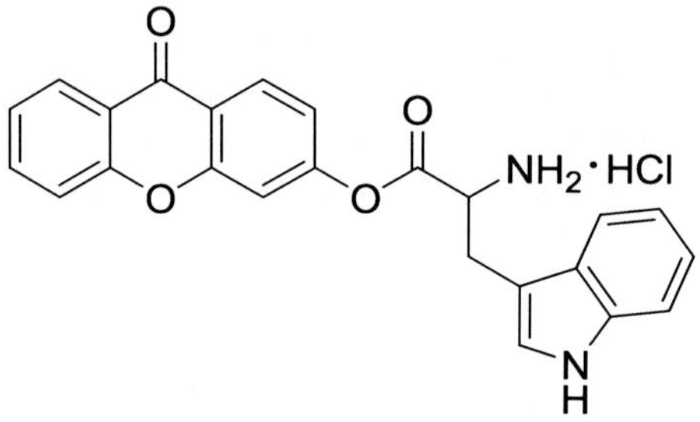

22

Fig. (34). Chemical structure of compound **22**.

ANTI-ALZHEIMER XANTHONE SYNTHETIC DERIVATIVES

Xanthones received considerable interest also as a valid therapeutic option for Alzheimer's disease (AD), a neurodegenerative disorder related to the progressive and irreversible cognitive detriment, regression in language and memory loss [67]. The current therapy for AD is based on acetylcholinesterase (AChE) inhibitors (AChEI) and only offers a symptomatic treatment. So far, no drugs have been discovered to prevent or arrest AD's progression. Thus, multiple strategies have been recently systematically evaluated. "Multi-target-directed ligands" (MTDLs), which can simultaneously interfere with the interconnected pathogenic factors involved in AD, represent a valuable strategy. In AD patients AChEI and cations, such as Cu^{2+} or Fe^{3+}/Fe^{2+}, facilitate the aggregation of A□ peptides [68]. Besides, the metal ions promote the release of ROS, thereby inducing oxidative stress, which also sustains AD's pathogenesis. In this field, xanthone derivatives have received significant attention as AChE inhibitors, metal chelators and antioxidant agents. SAR analysis of 1,3-dihydroxylated xanthones revealed that linking the xanthone core with tertiary or quaternary amino groups is crucial for an efficacious MTDLs strategy and to inhibit AChE both at the catalytic active (CAS) and the peripheral anionic sites (PAS) (Fig. **35**) Indeed, the tricyclic system interacts with PAS through π-π interactions with Tyr121 and Tyr334, π-anion interaction with Asp72, and hydrogen bond between the C1 hydroxyl group and Tyr334. On the other hand, the amino moiety establishes interaction with CAS, particularly forming π-alkyl interaction with Trp84. Moreover, the different length carbon chains act as linkers, bridging the right distance between the AChE active sites and thus accommodating the xanthone core and the amine moiety in the respective binding sites. The antioxidative property can be attributed to the phenolic hydroxyl groups and the electron-donating amines, which are well known to oxidize through lone pair donation. Ultimately, the hydroxyl and carbonyl groups of the xanthone core are effective chelating sites to metal ions.

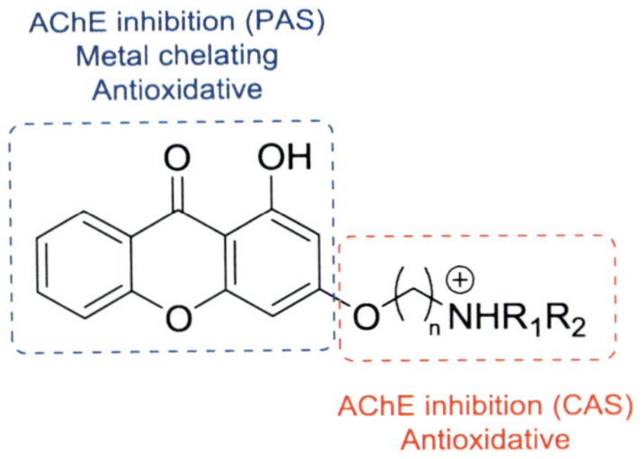

Fig. (35). SAR analysis of 3,4-dihydroxylated xanthones.

Based on these findings, Menéndez *et al.* reported a series of 1,3-dihydroxy xanthones linked to an amino group *via* different length carbon chains [69]. Molecular modeling studies showed that the *in vivo* positively charged amino moiety provides a new additional electrostatic interaction by establishing a salt bridge with Glu199 of AChE. Most of the derivatives were able to inhibit AChE in the micromolar range. Within the series, compound **23** (Fig. **36**) linked to piperidine *via* a five carbon chain linker was the most active one, with an IC_{50} value of 0.46 ± 0.02 μM, comparable to that of tacrine (IC_{50} = 0.029 ± 0.003 μM), an approved anti-AD drugs used as a standard.

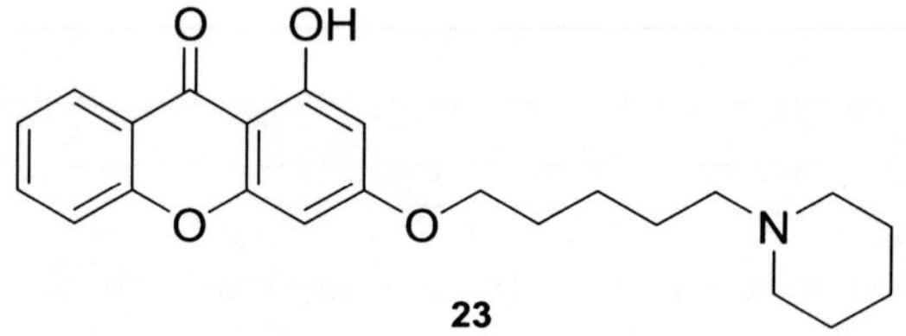

23

Fig. (36). Chemical structure of compound **23**.

In 2019, Kou *et al.* designed new 1,3-dihydroxyxanthones di-substituted with two tertiary amine-bearing carbon chain linkers [70]. The additional amino moiety provided multiple carbon-hydrogen interactions with Ser286, Arg289 and Ile 287 of AChE. Moreover, compounds with short linkers are expected to penetrate the blood-brain barrier more easily than those bearing longer carbon chains. The great Cu^{2+}chelating activity of each compound was confirmed by UV–vis spectrometry, and all the proposed derivatives emerged as greater antioxidant agents than vitamin C in the hydroxyl radicals scavenging assays performed with the Fenton reaction. Compound **24**, bearing pyrrolidine side chains (IC_{50} = 0.328 ± 0.001 µM), and its Cu(II) complex (IC_{50} = 0.193 ± 0.003 µM) were the best AChE inhibitors and exhibited the strongest antioxidant activity (Fig. **37**) The mono-substituted 1,3-dihydroxyxanthones exhibited great metal chelating and antioxidant properties as well [71]. In particular, xanthone derivative **256** (Fig. **37**) (IC_{50} = 2.403 ± 0.002 µM) and its Cu(II) complex (IC_{50} = 0.934 ± 0.002 µM) emerged as the best candidates of this series, yet less active than compound **245**.

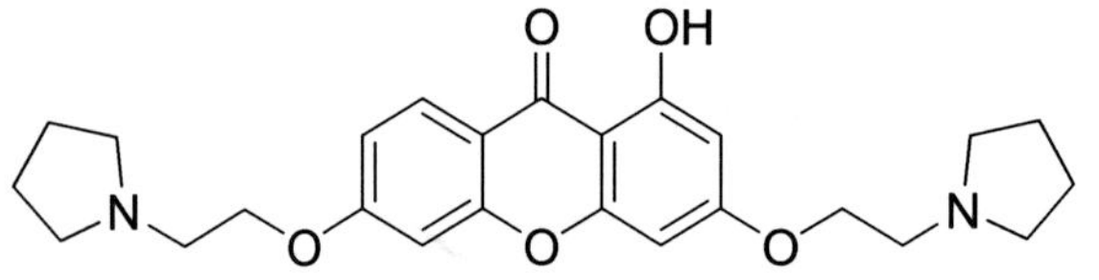

24

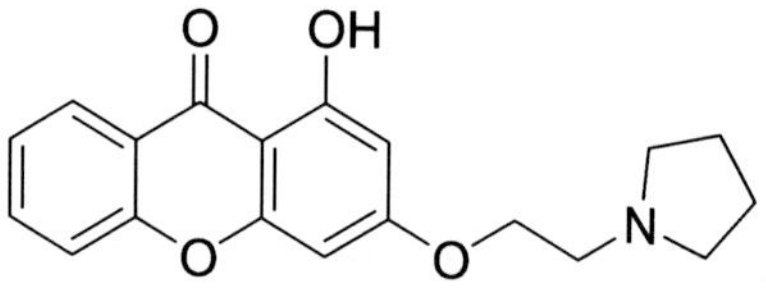

25

Fig. (37). Chemical structures of compounds **24** and **256**.

XANTHONE SYNTHETIC DERIVATIVES AS A-GLUCOSIDASE INHIBITORS

Type 2 diabetes (non-insulin-dependent diabetes mellitus) is the most widespread form of diabetes mellitus. Its treatment is based on the regulation and/or inhibition of the activity of carbohydrates hydrolytic enzymes. Accordingly, the inhibition of α-glucosidase, an enzyme promoting the hydrolysis of glycosidic bonds in carbohydrates, is a validated therapy to reduce postprandial blood glucose levels in diabetic patients. Previous studies successfully demonstrated the α-glucosidase inhibitory activity of xanthone derivatives [20]. Therefore, additional manipulations on the xanthone core have been investigated with the aim of designing novel anti-diabetic agents.

Wang's research group inserted various substitutions at C3–OH of 1,3-dihydroxyxanthones. The C3-substituted analogs emerged as non-competitive α-glucosidase inhibitors and acted by interacting with an allosteric binding site (Asp214, Glu276 and Asp349) of the enzyme. Hence, a series of 3-arylacyloxyxanthones were synthesized and evaluated as potential α-glucosidase inhibitors [72]. The enhanced activities of these compounds arose from the π-stacking or hydrophobic interactions established by the additional aromatic group introduced *via* the esterification of C3–OH. Furthermore, encouraging results were obtained through the insertion of polar hydroxyl, methoxy, methaminyl or alkylsilyloxyl groups on the aromatic moiety. Among the series, compound **26** (Fig. **4**) bearing the alkylsilyloxyl substituent, was more active (IC_{50} =10.6 μM) than the anti-diabetic drug 1-deoxynojirimycin (IC_{50} = 40 μM). However, the ester moiety significantly limits its potential effectiveness after oral administration. To address such stability issues, a series of novel analogs linked to triazole-bearing side chains *via* an ether bond were developed [73]. Several triazole-bearing derivatives were revealed to be good α-glucosidase inhibitors, more potent than 1-deoxynojirimycin. Notably, compound **27** provided the lowest IC_{50} value (2.06 ± 0.16 μM) (Fig. **38**) Moreover, the ability to increase the hepatic glucose was tested by exposing HepG2 cells to the most active candidates. Even though the presence of C1-OAc led to a less favorable α-glucosidase inhibitory profile, compound **28** (Fig. **38**) provided 61%, 90% and 163% glucose uptake in HepG2 cells at 0.625, 1.25 and 2.5 μM, respectively, better than the control rosiglitazone. Finally, to further explore the potential of this scaffold, novel oxazolylxanthones were obtained by including the C3-OH and C4 in the oxazole ring system [71]. Additional cyclohexyl or benzene rings decorated with electron-donating groups or halogens were introduced as oxazole substituents to establish new hydrophobic or π interactions. The best candidate of the series was compound **29** (Fig. **38**) with an IC_{50} = 6.3 ± 0.4 μM. Docking studies proposed that some derivatives can interact with distinct sites of α-glucosidase, raising the possibility of synergic inhibitory activities between the candidates.

Altogether, these findings confirmed that C3-OH substitutions of 1,3-dihydroxyxanthones with heterocycles are the most efficacious to design promising α-glucosidase inhibitors.

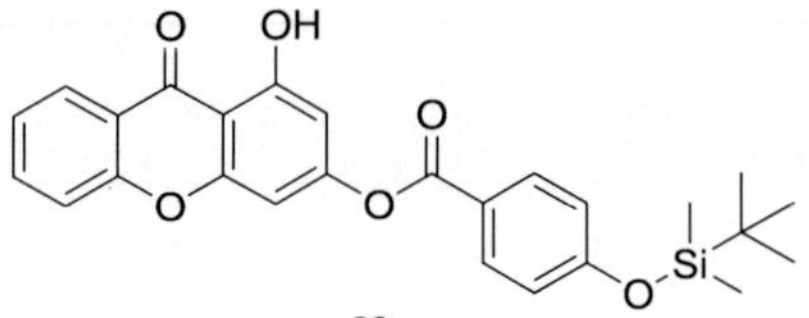

26

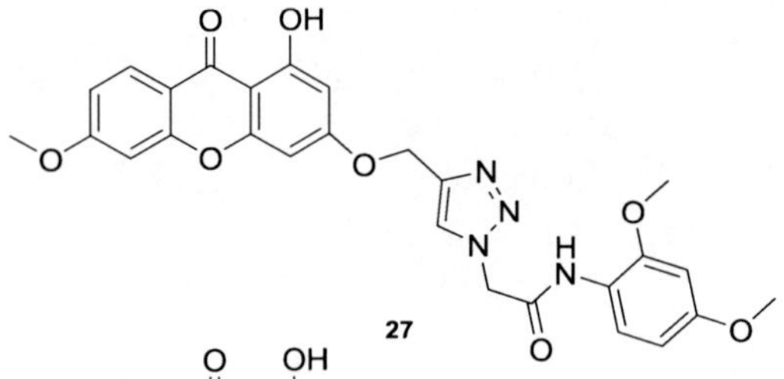

27

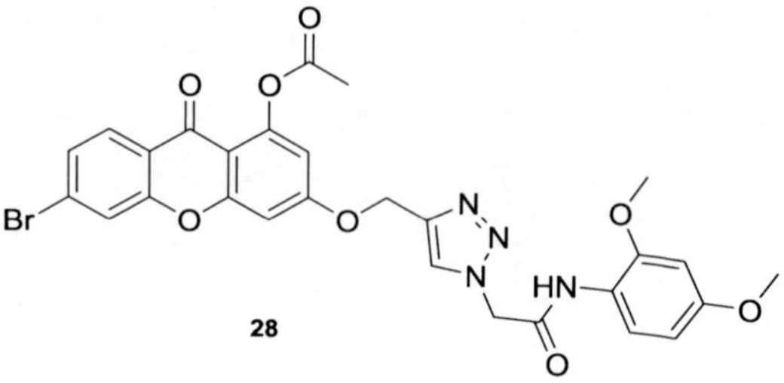

28

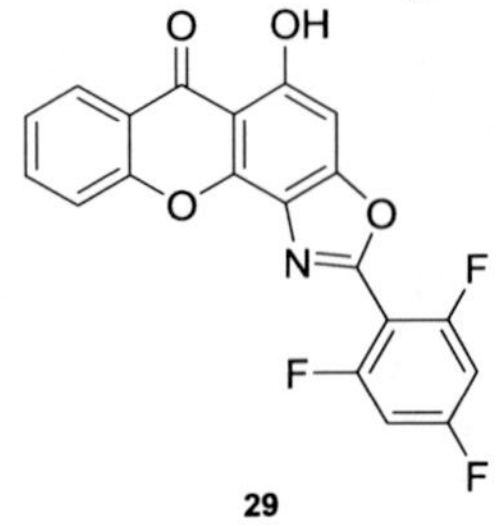

29

Fig. (38). Chemical structures of α-glucosidase inhibitors.

CONCLUDING REMARKS

Natural xanthones are a class of secondary metabolites occurring in a wide variety of natural sources and with a broad spectrum of biological activities. A combination of innovative synthetic methodologies and medicinal chemistry studies have provided several xanthone synthetic derivatives for different therapeutic purposes, including cancer, inflammation, AD, cardiovascular and infectious diseases. Some of them are endowed with outstanding antibacterial and antitumor activities and might be potential preclinical candidates. Notably, many of them, such as amphiphilic xanthones, act by innovative mechanisms of action and could significantly contribute to developing novel therapeutic agents. Xanthones have been an essential source to discover novel hits and leads over the last five years. Hopefully, continuous medicinal chemistry efforts to improve their drug-likeness and further exploration of the therapeutic potential of this promising scaffold will afford valuable clinical candidates.

CONSENT FOR PUBLICATION

Not applicable.

CONFLICT OF INTEREST

The authors declare no conflict of interest, financial or otherwise.

ACKNOWLEDGEMENT

Declared none.

REFERENCES

[1] Masters, K.S.; Bräse, S. Xanthones from fungi, lichens, and bacteria: the natural products and their synthesis. *Chem. Rev.,* **2012**, *112*(7), 3717-3776. [http://dx.doi.org/10.1021/cr100446h] [PMID: 22617028]

[2] Resende, D.; Pereira-Terra, P.; Inácio, Â.; Costa, P.; Pinto, E.; Sousa, E.; Pinto, M. Lichen xanthones as models for new antifungal agents. *Molecules,* **2018**, *23*(10), 2617. [http://dx.doi.org/10.3390/molecules23102617] [PMID: 30322037]

[3] Le Pogam, P.; Boustie, J. Xanthones of lichen source: a 2016 update. *Molecules,* **2016**, *21*(3), 294. [http://dx.doi.org/10.3390/molecules21030294] [PMID: 26950106]

[4] Ruan, J.; Zheng, C.; Liu, Y.; Qu, L.; Yu, H.; Han, L.; Zhang, Y.; Wang, T. Chemical and biological research on herbal medicines rich in xanthones. *Molecules,* **2017**, *22*(10), 1698. [http://dx.doi.org/10.3390/molecules22101698] [PMID: 29019929]

[5] Loureiro, D.R.P.; Soares, J.X.; Costa, J.C.; Magalhães, Á.F.; Azevedo, C.M.G.; Pinto, M.M.M.; Afonso, C.M.M. Structures, activities and drug-likeness of anti-infective xanthone derivatives isolated from the marine environment: a review. *Molecules,* **2019**, *24*(2), 243. [http://dx.doi.org/10.3390/molecules24020243] [PMID: 30634698]

[6] El-Seedi, H.; El-Barbary, M.; El-Ghorab, D.; Bohlin, L.; Borg-Karlson, A.K.; Göransson, U.; Verpoorte, R. Recent insights into the biosynthesis and biological activities of natural xanthones. *Curr. Med. Chem.,* **2010**, *17*(9), 854-901. [http://dx.doi.org/10.2174/092986710790712147] [PMID: 20156171]

[7] Banik, K.; Harsha, C.; Bordoloi, D.; Lalduhsaki Sailo, B.; Sethi, G.; Leong, H.C.; Arfuso, F.; Mishra, S.; Wang, L.; Kumar, A.P.; Kunnumakkara, A.B. Therapeutic potential of gambogic acid, a caged xanthone, to target cancer. *Cancer Lett.,* **2018**, *416*, 75-86. [http://dx.doi.org/10.1016/j.canlet.2017.12.014] [PMID: 29246645]

[8] Kashyap, D.; Mondal, R.; Tuli, H.S.; Kumar, G.; Sharma, A.K. Molecular targets of gambogic acid in cancer: recent trends and advancements. *Tumour Biol.,* **2016**, *37*(10), 12915-12925. [http://dx.doi.org/10.1007/s13277-016-5194-8] [PMID: 27448303]

[9] Ovalle-Magallanes, B.; Eugenio-Pérez, D.; Pedraza-Chaverri, J. Medicinal properties of mangosteen (Garcinia mangostana L.): A comprehensive update. *Food Chem. Toxicol.,* **2017**, *109*(Pt 1), 102-122. [http://dx.doi.org/10.1016/j.fct.2017.08.021] [PMID: 28842267]

[10] Chen, G.; Li, Y.; Wang, W.; Deng, L. Bioactivity and pharmacological properties of α-mangostin from the mangosteen fruit: a review. *Expert Opin. Ther. Pat.,* **2018**, *28*(5), 415-427. [http://dx.doi.org/10.1080/13543776.2018.1455829] [PMID: 29558225]

[11] Genovese, S.; Fiorito, S.; Taddeo, V.A.; Epifano, F. Recent developments in the pharmacology of prenylated xanthones. *Drug Discov. Today,* **2016**, *21*(11), 1814-1819. [http://dx.doi.org/10.1016/j.drudis.2016.06.033] [PMID: 27596926]

[12] Klein-Júnior, L.C.; Campos, A.; Niero, R.; Corrêa, R.; Vander Heyden, Y.; Filho, V.C. Xanthones and cancer: from natural sources to mechanisms of action. *Chem. Biodivers.,* **2020**, *17*(2), e1900499. [http://dx.doi.org/10.1002/cbdv.201900499] [PMID: 31794156]

[13] Araújo, J.; Fernandes, C.; Pinto, M.; Tiritan, M. Chiral derivatives of xanthones with antimicrobial activity. *Molecules,* **2019**, *24*(2), 314.
[http://dx.doi.org/10.3390/molecules24020314] [PMID: 30654546]

[14] Panda, S.S.; Chand, M.; Sakhuja, R.; Jain, S.C. Xanthones as potential antioxidants. *Curr. Med. Chem.,* **2013**, *20*(36), 4481-4507.
[http://dx.doi.org/10.2174/09298673113209990144] [PMID: 23834190]

[15] Jiang, D.J.; Dai, Z.; Li, Y.J. Pharmacological effects of xanthones as cardiovascular protective agents. *Cardiovasc. Drug Rev.,* **2004**, *22*(2), 91-102.
[http://dx.doi.org/10.1111/j.1527-3466.2004.tb00133.x] [PMID: 15179447]

[16] Bisi, A.; Micucci, M.; Gobbi, S.; Belluti, F.; Budriesi, R.; Rampa, A. Cardiovascular profile of xanthone-based 1,4 dihydropyridines bearing a lidoflazine pharmacophore fragment. *Molecules,* **2018**, *23*(12), 3088.
[http://dx.doi.org/10.3390/molecules23123088] [PMID: 30486354]

[17] Feng, Z.; Lu, X.; Gan, L.; Zhang, Q.; Lin, L. Xanthones, a promising anti-inflammatory scaffold: structure, activity, and drug likeness analysis. *Molecules,* **2020**, *25*(3), 598.
[http://dx.doi.org/10.3390/molecules25030598] [PMID: 32019180]

[18] Yang, H.; Bai, W.; Gao, L.; Jiang, J.; Tang, Y.; Niu, Y.; Lin, H.; Li, L. Mangiferin alleviates hypertension induced by hyperuricemia *via* increasing nitric oxide releases. *J. Pharmacol. Sci.,* **2018**, *137*(2), 154-161.
[http://dx.doi.org/10.1016/j.jphs.2018.05.008] [PMID: 29934052]

[19] Pinto, M.M.M.; Sousa, M.E.; Nascimento, M.S.J. Xanthone derivatives: new insights in biological activities. *Curr. Med. Chem.,* **2005**, *12*(21), 2517-2538.
[http://dx.doi.org/10.2174/092986705774370691] [PMID: 16250875]

[20] Shagufta, ; Ahmad, I. Recent insight into the biological activities of synthetic xanthone derivatives. *Eur. J. Med. Chem.,* **2016**, *116*, 267-280.
[http://dx.doi.org/10.1016/j.ejmech.2016.03.058] [PMID: 27111599]

[21] Chantarasriwong, O.; Althufairi, B.D.; Checchia, N.J.; Theodorakis, E. Caged Garcinia Xanthones: Synthetic Studies and Pharmacophore Evaluation In: Studies in Natural Products Chemistry; Atta-u--Rahman Elsevier Science B.: V: Amsterdam , **2018**; pp. 93-131.

[22] Wu, J.; Dai, J.; Zhang, Y.; Wang, J.; Huang, L.; Ding, H.; Li, T.; Zhang, Y.; Mao, J.; Yu, S. Synthesis of novel xanthone analogues and their growth inhibitory activity against human lung cancer A549 cells. *Drug Des. Devel. Ther.,* **2019**, *13*, 4239-4246.
[http://dx.doi.org/10.2147/DDDT.S217827] [PMID: 31853172]

[23] Zhang, X.; Li, X.; Sun, H.; Wang, X.; Zhao, L.; Gao, Y.; Liu, X.; Zhang, S.; Wang, Y.; Yang, Y.; Zeng, S.; Guo, Q.; You, Q. Garcinia xanthones as orally active antitumor agents. *J. Med. Chem.,* **2013**, *56*(1), 276-292.
[http://dx.doi.org/10.1021/jm301593r] [PMID: 23167526]

[24] Xu, X.; Wu, Y.; Hu, M.; Li, X.; Bao, Q.; Bian, J.; You, Q.; Zhang, X. Novel natural product-like caged xanthones bearing a carbamate moiety exhibit antitumor potency and anti-angiogenesis activity in vivo. *Sci. Rep.,* **2016**, *6*(1), 35771.
[http://dx.doi.org/10.1038/srep35771] [PMID: 27767192]

[25] Xu, X.; Wu, Y.; Hu, M.; Li, X.; Gu, C.; You, Q.; Zhang, X. Structure–activity relationship of Garcinia xanthones analogues: Potent Hsp90 inhibitors with cytotoxicity and antiangiogenesis activity. *Bioorg. Med. Chem.,* **2016**, *24*(19), 4626-4635.
[http://dx.doi.org/10.1016/j.bmc.2016.07.067] [PMID: 27527413]

[26] Li, X.; Wu, Y.; Wang, Y.; You, Q.; Zhang, X. 'Click Chemistry' synthesis of novel natural product-like caged xanthones bearing a 1,2,3-triazole moiety with improved druglike properties as orally active antitumor agents. *Molecules,* **2017**, *22*(11), 1834.

[http://dx.doi.org/10.3390/molecules22111834]

[27] Lee, C.H.; Ying, T.H.; Chiou, H.L.; Hsieh, S.C.; Wen, S.H.; Chou, R.H.; Hsieh, Y.H. Alpha-mangostin induces apoptosis through activation of reactive oxygen species and ASK1/p38 signaling pathway in cervical cancer cells. *Oncotarget,* **2017**, *8*(29), 47425-47439. [http://dx.doi.org/10.18632/oncotarget.17659] [PMID: 28537893]

[28] Chi, X.Q.; Zi, C.T.; Li, H.M.; Yang, L.; Lv, Y.F.; Li, J.Y.; Hou, B.; Ren, F.C.; Hu, J.M.; Zhou, J. Design, synthesis and structure–activity relationships of mangostin analogs as cytotoxic agents. *RSC Advances,* **2018**, *8*(72), 41377-41388. [http://dx.doi.org/10.1039/C8RA08409B] [PMID: 35559306]

[29] Shibata, M.A.; Hamaoka, H.; Morimoto, J.; Kanayama, T.; Maemura, K.; Ito, Y.; Iinuma, M.; Kondo, Y. Synthetic α□mangostin dilaurate strongly suppresses wide□spectrum organ metastasis in a mouse model of mammary cancer. *Cancer Sci.,* **2018**, *109*(5), 1660-1671. [http://dx.doi.org/10.1111/cas.13590] [PMID: 29601143]

[30] Ribeiro, J.; Veloso, C.; Fernandes, C.; Tiritan, M.E.; Pinto, M.M.M. Carboxyxanthones: bioactive agents and molecular scaffold for synthesis of analogues and derivatives. *Molecules,* **2019**, *24*(1), 180. [http://dx.doi.org/10.3390/molecules24010180] [PMID: 30621303]

[31] Daei Farshchi Adli, A.; Jahanban-Esfahlan, R.; Seidi, K.; Samandari-Rad, S.; Zarghami, N. An overview on Vadimezan (DMXAA): The vascular disrupting agent. *Chem. Biol. Drug Des.,* **2018**, *91*(5), 996-1006. [http://dx.doi.org/10.1111/cbdd.13166] [PMID: 29288534]

[32] Liu, J.; Zhou, F.; Zhang, L.; Wang, H.; Zhang, J.; Zhang, C.; Jiang, Z.; Li, Y.; Liu, Z.; Chen, H. DMXAA-pyranoxanthone hybrids enhance inhibition activities against human cancer cells with multi-target functions. *Eur. J. Med. Chem.,* **2018**, *143*, 1768-1778. [http://dx.doi.org/10.1016/j.ejmech.2017.10.074] [PMID: 29129511]

[33] Liu, J.; Zhang, J.; Wang, H.; Liu, Z.; Zhang, C.; Jiang, Z.; Chen, H. Synthesis of xanthone derivatives and studies on the inhibition against cancer cells growth and synergistic combinations of them. *Eur. J. Med. Chem.,* **2017**, *133*, 50-61. [http://dx.doi.org/10.1016/j.ejmech.2017.03.068] [PMID: 28376372]

[34] Zhou, B.D.; Zeng, L.L.; Tong, Y.G.; Fang, J.Y.; Ruan, Z.P.; Zeng, X.Y.; Fang, Y.Y.; Xu, G.F.; Hu, D.B. Synthesis and antitumor, antityrosinase, and antioxidant activities of xanthone. *J. Asian Nat. Prod. Res.,* **2018**, *20*(5), 467-476. [http://dx.doi.org/10.1080/10286020.2018.1454437] [PMID: 29597932]

[35] Liu, J., Bao, H.; Wang, H.; Luo, Q.; Zuo, J.; Liu, Z.; Qiu, S.; Sun, X.; Liu, X. Synthesis of xanthone derivatives and anti-hepatocellular carcinoma potency evaluation: induced apoptosis. *RSC Advances,* **2019**, *9*(70), 40781-40791. [http://dx.doi.org/10.1039/C9RA06408G] [PMID: 35540078]

[36] Martinez-Outschoorn, U.E.; Peiris-Pagés, M.; Pestell, R.G.; Sotgia, F.; Lisanti, M.P. Cancer metabolism: a therapeutic perspective. *Nat. Rev. Clin. Oncol.,* **2017**, *14*(1), 11-31. [http://dx.doi.org/10.1038/nrclinonc.2016.60] [PMID: 27141887]

[37] Wang, P.; Jiang, L.; Cao, Y.; Zhang, X.; Chen, B.; Zhang, S.; Huang, K.; Ye, D.; Zhou, L. Xanthone derivatives as phosphoglycerate mutase 1 inhibitors: Design, synthesis, and biological evaluation. *Bioorg. Med. Chem.,* **2018**, *26*(8), 1961-1970. [http://dx.doi.org/10.1016/j.bmc.2018.02.044] [PMID: 29530347]

[38] Wang, P.; Jiang, L.; Cao, Y.; Ye, D.; Zhou, L. the design and synthesis of N-xanthone benzenesulfonamides as novel Phosphoglycerate Mutase 1 (PGAM1) inhibitors. *Molecules,* **2018**, *23*(6), 1396. [http://dx.doi.org/10.3390/molecules23061396] [PMID: 29890679]

[39] Gomes, S.; Raimundo, L.; Soares, J.; Loureiro, J.B.; Leão, M.; Ramos, H.; Monteiro, M.N.; Lemos, A.; Moreira, J.; Pinto, M.; Chlapek, P.; Veselska, R.; Sousa, E.; Saraiva, L. New inhibitor of the

TAp73 interaction with MDM2 and mutant p53 with promising antitumor activity against neuroblastoma. *Cancer Lett.,* **2019**, *446*, 90-102.
[http://dx.doi.org/10.1016/j.canlet.2019.01.014] [PMID: 30664963]

[40] Lemos, A.; Gomes, A.S.; Loureiro, J.B.; Brandão, P.; Palmeira, A.; Pinto, M.M.M.; Saraiva, L.; Sousa, M.E. Synthesis, Biological evaluation, and in silico studies of novel aminated xanthones as potential P53-activating agents. *Molecules,* **2019**, *24*(10), 1975.
[http://dx.doi.org/10.3390/molecules24101975] [PMID: 31121972]

[41] Liu, C.; Zhang, M.; Zhang, Z.; Zhang, S.B.; Yang, S.; Zhang, A.; Yin, L.; Swarts, S.; Vidyasagar, S.; Zhang, L.; Okunieff, P. Synthesis and anticancer potential of novel xanthone derivatives with 3,6-substituted chains. *Bioorg. Med. Chem.,* **2016**, *24*(18), 4263-4271.
[http://dx.doi.org/10.1016/j.bmc.2016.07.020] [PMID: 27448774]

[42] Sypniewski, D.; Szkaradek, N.; Loch, T.; Waszkielewicz, A.M.; Gunia-Krzyżak, A.; Matczyńska, D.; Sołtysik, D.; Marona, H.; Bednarek, I. Contribution of reactive oxygen species to the anticancer activity of aminoalkanol derivatives of xanthone. *Invest. New Drugs,* **2018**, *36*(3), 355-369.
[http://dx.doi.org/10.1007/s10637-017-0537-x] [PMID: 29116476]

[43] Alves, A.; Correia-da-Silva, M.; Nunes, C.; Campos, J.; Sousa, E.; Silva, P.; Bousbaa, H.; Rodrigues, F.; Ferreira, D.; Costa, P.; Pinto, M. Discovery of a new xanthone against glioma: synthesis and development of (pro)liposome formulations. *Molecules,* **2019**, *24*(3), 409.
[http://dx.doi.org/10.3390/molecules24030409] [PMID: 30678085]

[44] Koh, J.J.; Zou, H.; Lin, S.; Lin, H.; Soh, R.T.; Lim, F.H.; Koh, W.L.; Li, J.; Lakshminarayanan, R.; Verma, C.; Tan, D.T.H.; Cao, D.; Beuerman, R.W.; Liu, S. Nonpeptidic amphiphilic xanthone derivatives: Structure-Activity Relationship and membrane-targeting properties. *J. Med. Chem.,* **2016**, *59*(1), 171-193.
[http://dx.doi.org/10.1021/acs.jmedchem.5b01500] [PMID: 26681070]

[45] Zou, H.; Koh, J.J.; Li, J.; Qiu, S.; Aung, T.T.; Lin, H.; Lakshminarayanan, R.; Dai, X.; Tang, C.; Lim, F.H.; Zhou, L.; Tan, A.L.; Verma, C.; Tan, D.T.H.; Chan, H.S.O.; Saraswathi, P.; Cao, D.; Liu, S.; Beuerman, R.W. Design and synthesis of amphiphilic xanthone-based, membrane-targeting antimicrobials with improved membrane selectivity. *J. Med. Chem.,* **2013**, *56*(6), 2359-2373.
[http://dx.doi.org/10.1021/jm301683j] [PMID: 23441632]

[46] Koh, J.J.; Lin, S.; Bai, Y.; Sin, W.W.L.; Aung, T.T.; Li, J.; Chandra, V.; Pervushin, K.; Beuerman, R.W.; Liu, S. Antimicrobial activity profiles of Amphiphilic Xanthone derivatives are a function of their molecular Oligomerization. *Biochim. Biophys. Acta Biomembr.,* **2018**, *1860*(11), 2281-2298.
[http://dx.doi.org/10.1016/j.bbamem.2018.05.006] [PMID: 29782818]

[47] Consalvi, S.; Scarpecci, C.; Biava, M.; Poce, G. Mycobacterial tryptophan biosynthesis: A promising target for tuberculosis drug development? *Bioorg. Med. Chem. Lett.,* **2019**, *29*(23), 126731.
[http://dx.doi.org/10.1016/j.bmcl.2019.126731] [PMID: 31627992]

[48] Appetecchia, F.; Consalvi, S.; Scarpecci, C.; Biava, M.; Poce, G. SAR analysis of small molecules interfering with energy-metabolism in Mycobacterium Tuberculosis. *Pharmaceuticals (Basel),* **2020**, *13*(9), 227.
[http://dx.doi.org/10.3390/ph13090227] [PMID: 32878317]

[49] Consalvi, S.; Poce, G.; Scarpecci, C.; Biava, M. Overcoming drug resistance in TB: an update. *Future Microbiol.,* **2020**, *15*(17), 1607-1609.
[http://dx.doi.org/10.2217/fmb-2020-0089] [PMID: 33215545]

[50] Koh, J.J.; Zou, H.; Mukherjee, D.; Lin, S.; Lim, F.; Tan, J.K.; Tan, D.Z.; Stocker, B.L.; Timmer, M.S.M.; Corkran, H.M.; Lakshminarayanan, R.; Tan, D.T.H.; Cao, D.; Beuerman, R.W.; Dick, T.; Liu, S. Amphiphilic xanthones as a potent chemical entity of anti-mycobacterial agents with membrane-targeting properties. *Eur. J. Med. Chem.,* **2016**, *123*, 684-703.
[http://dx.doi.org/10.1016/j.ejmech.2016.07.068] [PMID: 27517813]

[51] Mukherjee, D.; Zou, H.; Liu, S.; Beuerman, R.; Dick, T. Membrane-targeting AM-0016 kills

mycobacterial persisters and shows low propensity for resistance development. *Future Microbiol.*, **2016**, *11*(5), 643-650.
[http://dx.doi.org/10.2217/fmb-2015-0015] [PMID: 27158932]

[52] Aung, T.T.; Yam, J.K.H.; Lin, S.; Salleh, S.M.; Givskov, M.; Liu, S.; Lwin, N.C.; Yang, L.; Beuerman, R.W. Biofilms of pathogenic nontuberculous mycobacteria targeted by new therapeutic approaches. *Antimicrob. Agents Chemother.*, **2016**, *60*(1), 24-35.
[http://dx.doi.org/10.1128/AAC.01509-15] [PMID: 26459903]

[53] Anantachoke, N.; Tuchinda, P.; Kuhakarn, C.; Pohmakotr, M.; Reutrakul, V. Prenylated caged xanthones: Chemistry and biology. *Pharm. Biol.*, **2012**, *50*(1), 78-91.
[http://dx.doi.org/10.3109/13880209.2011.636176] [PMID: 22196584]

[54] Chaiyakunvat, P.; Anantachoke, N.; Reutrakul, V.; Jiarpinitnun, C. Caged xanthones: Potent inhibitors of global predominant MRSA USA300. *Bioorg. Med. Chem. Lett.*, **2016**, *26*(13), 2980-2983.
[http://dx.doi.org/10.1016/j.bmcl.2016.05.030] [PMID: 27216998]

[55] Chen, X.; Leng, J.; Rakesh, K.P.; Darshini, N.; Shubhavathi, T.; Vivek, H.K.; Mallesha, N.; Qin, H.L. Synthesis and molecular docking studies of xanthone attached amino acids as potential antimicrobial and anti-inflammatory agents. *MedChemComm*, **2017**, *8*(8), 1706-1719.
[http://dx.doi.org/10.1039/C7MD00209B] [PMID: 30108882]

[56] Resende, D.I.S.P.; Pereira-Terra, P.; Moreira, J.; Freitas-Silva, J.; Lemos, A.; Gales, L.; Pinto, E.; de Sousa, M.E.; da Costa, P.M.; Pinto, M.M.M. Synthesis of a small library of nature-inspired xanthones and study of their antimicrobial activity. *Molecules*, **2020**, *25*(10), 2405.
[http://dx.doi.org/10.3390/molecules25102405] [PMID: 32455828]

[57] Wang, H.; Zhang, Y.; Xue, W.; Zhang, X.; Jia, X.; Xue, T.; Guo, R.; Niu, B.; Yan, H. Preparation, characterization and antibacterial activity of a novel soluble polymer derived from xanthone and O-carboxymethyl-N, N, N-trimethyl chitosan. *Int. J. Biol. Macromol.*, **2020**, *164*, 836-844.
[http://dx.doi.org/10.1016/j.ijbiomac.2020.07.147] [PMID: 32693131]

[58] Amidi, M.; Romeijn, S.G.; Borchard, G.; Junginger, H.E.; Hennink, W.E.; Jiskoot, W. Preparation and characterization of protein-loaded N-trimethyl chitosan nanoparticles as nasal delivery system. *J. Control. Release*, **2006**, *111*(1-2), 107-116.
[http://dx.doi.org/10.1016/j.jconrel.2005.11.014] [PMID: 16380189]

[59] Klesiewicz, K.; Karczewska, E.; Budak, A.; Marona, H.; Szkaradek, N. Anti-Helicobacter pylori activity of some newly synthesized derivatives of xanthone. *J. Antibiot. (Tokyo)*, **2016**, *69*(11), 825-834.
[http://dx.doi.org/10.1038/ja.2016.36] [PMID: 27025351]

[60] Chimenti, F.; Bizzarri, B.; Bolasco, A.; Secci, D.; Chimenti, P.; Granese, A.; Carradori, S.; Rivanera, D.; Zicari, A.; Scaltrito, M.M.; Sisto, F. Synthesis, selective anti-Helicobacter pylori activity, and cytotoxicity of novel N-substituted-2-oxo-2H-1-benzopyran-3-carboxamides. *Bioorg. Med. Chem. Lett.*, **2010**, *20*(16), 4922-4926.
[http://dx.doi.org/10.1016/j.bmcl.2010.06.048] [PMID: 20630755]

[61] Lin, S.; Sin, W.L.W.; Koh, J.J.; Lim, F.; Wang, L.; Cao, D.; Beuerman, R.W.; Ren, L.; Liu, S. Semisynthesis and biological evaluation of xanthone amphiphilics as selective, highly potent antifungal agents to combat fungal resistance. *J. Med. Chem.*, **2017**, *60*(24), 10135-10150.
[http://dx.doi.org/10.1021/acs.jmedchem.7b01348] [PMID: 29155590]

[62] Klesiewicz, K.; Żelaszczyk, D.; Trojanowska, D.; Bogusz, B.; Małek, M.; Waszkielewicz, A.; Szkaradek, N.; Karczewska, E.; Marona, H.; Budak, A. Preliminary antifungal activity assay of selected chlorine-containing derivatives of xanthone and phenoxyethyl amines. *Chem. Biol. Drug Des.*, **2018**, *92*(5), 1867-1875.
[http://dx.doi.org/10.1111/cbdd.13356] [PMID: 29923674]

[63] Cowman, A.F.; Healer, J.; Marapana, D.; Marsh, K. Malaria: Biology and Disease. *Cell*, **2016**, *167*(3), 610-624.

[http://dx.doi.org/10.1016/j.cell.2016.07.055] [PMID: 27768886]

[64] Haldar, K.; Bhattacharjee, S.; Safeukui, I. Drug resistance in Plasmodium. *Nat. Rev. Microbiol.*, **2018**, *16*(3), 156-170.
[http://dx.doi.org/10.1038/nrmicro.2017.161] [PMID: 29355852]

[65] Ke, H.; Morrisey, J.M.; Qu, S.; Chantarasriwong, O.; Mather, M.W.; Theodorakis, E.A.; Vaidya, A.B. Caged Garcinia xanthones, a novel chemical scaffold with potent antimalarial activity. *Antimicrob. Agents Chemother.*, **2016**, *61*(1), e01220-e16.
[PMID: 27799215]

[66] Karunakaran, T.; Ee, G.C.L.; Ismail, I.S.; Mohd Nor, S.M.; Zamakshshari, N.H. Acetyl- and *O* -alkyl-derivatives of β-mangostin from *Garcinia mangostana* and their anti-inflammatory activities. *Nat. Prod. Res.*, **2018**, *32*(12), 1390-1394.
[http://dx.doi.org/10.1080/14786419.2017.1350666] [PMID: 28715912]

[67] Ballard, C.; Aarsland, D.; Cummings, J.; O'Brien, J.; Mills, R.; Molinuevo, J.L.; Fladby, T.; Williams, G.; Doherty, P.; Corbett, A.; Sultana, J. Drug repositioning and repurposing for Alzheimer disease. *Nat. Rev. Neurol.*, **2020**, *16*(12), 661-673.
[http://dx.doi.org/10.1038/s41582-020-0397-4] [PMID: 32939050]

[68] Cruz, M.I.; Cidade, H.; Pinto, M. Dual/multitargeted xanthone derivatives for Alzheimer's disease: where do we stand? *Future Med. Chem.*, **2017**, *9*(14), 1611-1630.
[http://dx.doi.org/10.4155/fmc-2017-0086] [PMID: 28832188]

[69] Menéndez, C.A.; Biscussi, B.; Accordino, S.; Paula Murray, A.; Gerbino, D.C.; Appignanesi, G.A. Design, synthesis and biological evaluation of 1,3-dihydroxyxanthone derivatives: Effective agents against acetylcholinesterase. *Bioorg. Chem.*, **2017**, *75*, 201-209.
[http://dx.doi.org/10.1016/j.bioorg.2017.09.012] [PMID: 28963904]

[70] Kou, X.; Song, L.; Wang, Y.; Yu, Q.; Ju, H.; Yang, A.; Shen, R. Design, synthesis and anti-Alzheimer's disease activity study of xanthone derivatives based on multi-target strategy. *Bioorg. Med. Chem. Lett.*, **2020**, *30*(4), 126927.
[http://dx.doi.org/10.1016/j.bmcl.2019.126927] [PMID: 31901382]

[71] Yang, A.; Yu, Q.; Ju, H.; Song, L.; Kou, X.; Shen, R. Design, synthesis and biological evaluation of xanthone derivatives for possible treatment of Alzheimer's disease based on multi-target strategy. *Chem. Biodivers.*, **2020**, *17*(10), e2000442.
[http://dx.doi.org/10.1002/cbdv.202000442] [PMID: 32692899]

[72] Li, G.L.; Cai, C.Y.; He, J.Y.; Rao, L.; Ma, L.; Liu, Y.; Wang, B. Synthesis of 3-acyloxyxanthone derivatives as α-glucosidase inhibitors: A further insight into the 3-substituents' effect. *Bioorg. Med. Chem.*, **2016**, *24*(7), 1431-1438.
[http://dx.doi.org/10.1016/j.bmc.2016.01.022] [PMID: 26917220]

[73] Ye, G.J.; Lan, T.; Huang, Z.X.; Cheng, X.N.; Cai, C.Y.; Ding, S.M.; Xie, M.L.; Wang, B. Design and synthesis of novel xanthone-triazole derivatives as potential antidiabetic agents: α-Glucosidase inhibition and glucose uptake promotion. *Eur. J. Med. Chem.*, **2019**, *177*, 362-373.
[http://dx.doi.org/10.1016/j.ejmech.2019.05.045] [PMID: 31158750]

Medicinal Chemistry Lessons From Nature, 2022, *Vol. 1*, 112-144

CHAPTER 4

Combretastatin Derivatives as Tubulin Inhibitors: A Fascinating Journey from Nature to Drug Discovery Strategies

Alessandra Ammazzalorso[1,*] and **Trond Vidar Hansen**[2]

[1] *Department of Pharmacy, Medicinal Chemistry Unit, G. d'Annunzio University of Chieti-Pescara, via dei Vestini, 66100 Chieti, Italy*

[2] *Department of Pharmacy, Section for Pharmaceutical Chemistry, University of Oslo, PO Box 1068 Blindern, N-0316 Oslo, Norway*

Abstract: The combretastatins are a family of stilbene phenolic natural products isolated from the bark of the South African bush willow tree *Combretum caffrum*. Since their isolation and structural elucidation, these molecules have attracted a lot of interest due to their potent cytotoxic activity against several human cancer cell lines. Combretastatin A-4, a *cis*-stilbene, is the most potent member of these natural products, has the ability to strongly inhibit tubulin polymerization, resulting in high cytotoxic activity. Indeed, it also displays an additional activity as a potent vascular disrupting agent. This interesting double bioactive profile accounts for the potent antiproliferative and antivascular action in tumors. However, combretastatin A-4, due to the sensitive *cis*-stilbene moiety, is prone to isomerization giving the less bioactive *trans*-isomer and exhibits diminished water solubility. Hence, a wide panel of synthetic derivatives were therefore developed with the aim of overcoming these limitations. The development of prodrugs such as fosbretabulin, ombrabulin and Oxi4503 isrepresentative of successful attempts to overcome pharmacokinetic disadvantages, whereas the most recent approaches aim to develop combretastatin prodrugs able to selectively target tumor site, possessing also theranostic properties. Herein, miscellaneous and the most potent synthetic analogues are presented. In addition, a general outlook on combretastatin derivatives and drug delivery approaches based on innovative nanoformulations is also presented.

Keywords: Anticancer, Combretastatin, Cytotoxic, Colchicine Binding Site, Drug Delivery System, Heterocyclic Derivatives, Natural Compounds, Nanoformulation, Prodrugs, Photoresponsive Hybrid, Stilbene, Structure-activity Relationships, Tubulin Polymerization, Vascular Disrupting Agent.

* **Corresponding author Alessandra Ammazzalorso:** Department of Pharmacy, G. d'Annunzio University, *via* dei Vestini 31, 66100 Chieti, Italy; E-mail: alessandra.ammazzalorso@unich.it

INTRODUCTION

Natural combretastatins were firstly isolated by Pettit in the 1980s from the bark of *Combretum caffrum* (Eckl. & Zeyh.) Kuntze, an African willow tree [1 - 3]. In the same years, their antimitotic activity was determined. Extracts from *Combretum caffrum* were traditionally used as a folk medicine for the treatment of scorpion stings, cardiovascular disorders and worm related diseases by the Xhosa tribe in South Africa. From a structural point of view, combretastatins are closely related to stilbenes, representing their *cis*-isomers. These bioactive compounds were classified into four families, namely combretastatin A (CA1 to CA6), combretastatin B (CB1 to CB4), combretastatin C-1 and combretastatin D (D1 to D4). The family A comprises stilbene-based compounds, whereas the family B dihydrostilbenes, phenanthrenes for C and macrocyclic lactones for D. In Fig. **1** the chemical structures of representative members for each family are presented. Overall, their general features are two phenyl rings (one trimethoxy substituted), linked by a *cis*-configure.d double bond. The mode of action of the combretastatins is closely related to colchicine, sharing with it the ability to bind tubulin and act as polymerization inhibitors. In fact, it was demonstrated that combretastatins bind at the colchicine binding site (CBS) on the β-tubulin in a similar orientation as colchicine. The most prominent representative of this group of compounds is combretastatin A-4 (CA4, 3'- hydroxy-3,4,4 ',5- tetramethoxy-*cis* -stilbene), whose principal structural features include a 3,4,5-trimethox--substituted phenyl ring (A), a B ring containing C3'-OH and C4'-OCH_3 substituents, and an ethylene bridge providing proper rigidity and spatial orientation of aromatic rings. These structural features were found essential to produce a potent interaction in CBS of tubulin and provide high levels of cytotoxicity [4]. CA4 displays potent antiproliferative effects as an inhibitor of tubulin polymerization, but it induces also marked anti-vascular and anti-angiogenic effects by acting as a vascular disrupting agent (VDA) [5]. The selective disruption of tumor microvessels determines the loss of nutrients, oxygen deprivation and irreversible vascular damage, leading to haemorrhagic necrosis and cell death.

It is interesting to underline that combretastatin A-1 (CA1) and its prodrugs can undergo activation to a cytotoxic *ortho*-quinone intermediate, which interacts with structural elements in proteins and nucleic acids producing oxidative stress through superoxide/hydrogen peroxide production. This chemical behaviour explains the superior antitumor effect played by CA1 compared to CA4, pointing out how little structure differences could affect different pathways into the organisms. Despite the potent cytotoxic, rather simple chemical structure and anti-angiogenic activity exerted by CA4 and CA1, these compounds suffer from some drawbacks, such as the low water solubility and the instability of the *cis* configuration. Many CA4 and CA1 derivatives were synthesized to overcome the solubility problems, including phosphate prodrugs: CA4 phosphate (fosbretabulin, Zybrestat®) represents a successful derivative, widely studied in many clinical studies alone or in combination with traditional chemotherapeutic agents or with radiotherapy. The isomerization of the *cis* configuration, occurring after *in vivo* administration or in the presence of light, heat, or acidic media, leads to the *trans*-stilbene isomer, significantly less potent at inhibiting tubulin polymerization and diminishing cancer cell growth [6].

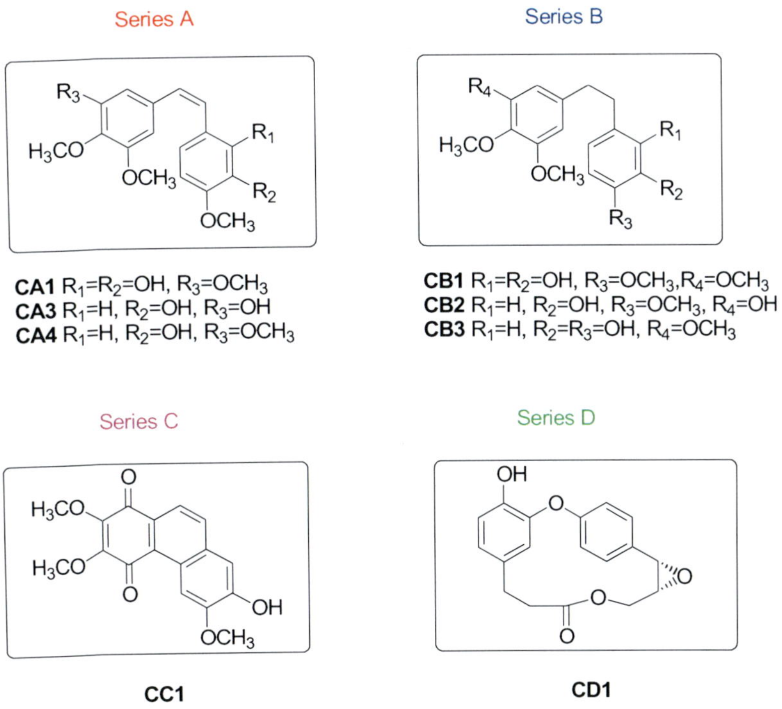

Fig. (1). Chemical structures of representative members of four families of combretastatins.

The potent anticancer profile of combretastatins attracted a lot of attention in medicinal chemistry research, stimulating the efforts of researchers to obtain derivatives with improved pharmacokinetic properties and tumor targeting selectivity [7, 8].

INSIGHTS ON MECHANISM OF ACTION OF COMBRETASTATINS

Combretastatins belong to the family of microtubule-binding agents, usually categorized in microtubule-stabilizing (taxanes, epothilones) and microtubule-destabilizing agents (colchicine, vinca alkaloids, combretastatins) when used in high concentration. The binding of combretastatins at the CBS, which is located at the interface between α- and β-tubulin, has been demonstrated, with action on microtubules similar to that of colchicine (Fig. **2**). Indeed, colchicine's clinical applications as anticancer agent are limited by its toxicity, narrow therapeutic index and development of resistance. Drugs able to bind to CBS and showing lesser undesired effects than colchicine might be of great interest as anticancer candidates. The ability to inhibit tubulin polymerization, together with the potent vascular disrupting activity, can make the combretastatins valuable targets in anticancer approaches. For these reasons, many research efforts have been focused to improve their anticancer activity, overcoming stability and solubility problems. These continuous efforts led some combretastatin derivatives to start clinical trials, as described in the next paragraph.

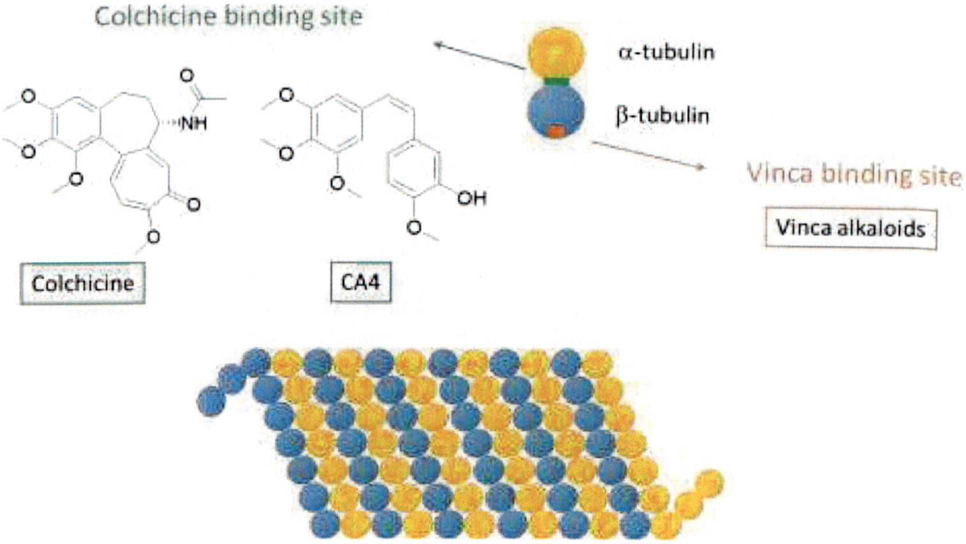

Fig. (2). Schematic representation of colchicine and vinca binding sites on microtubules.

Development of Combretastatin Prodrugs

With the aim to improve water solubility, several prodrugs have been developed both for CA4 and CA1. These prodrugs require chemical bioactivation by metabolic enzymatic processes into active forms. The first description of CA4 and CA1 prodrugs was realized by Pettit [9], who synthesized their phosphate prodrugs (Fig. **3**). The most successful prodrugs obtained to date are fosbretabulin (**1**) [10, 11] and Oxi4503 (**2**), the monophosphate and diphosphate salts of CA4 and CA1, respectively; they showed a faster conversion into active forms in tumor than in blood [12]. Their improved pharmacokinetic profile made them the preferred derivatives to progress into clinical trials. By adding a serinamide to the B ring of combretastatin, the prodrug AVE8062 (**3**) was synthesised, then marketed by Sanofi as ombrabulin; the action of aminopeptidases *in vivo* forms the active derivative.

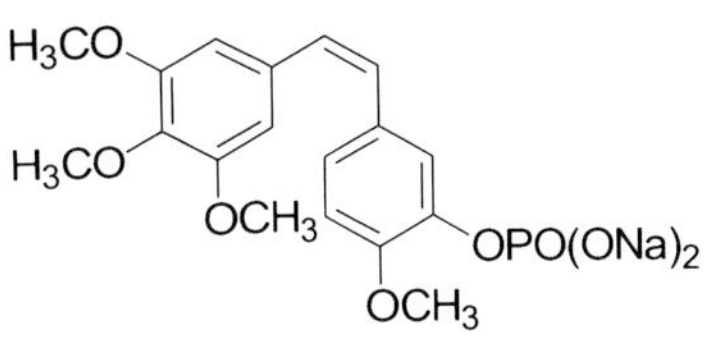

1 (CA4-P, fosbretabulin)

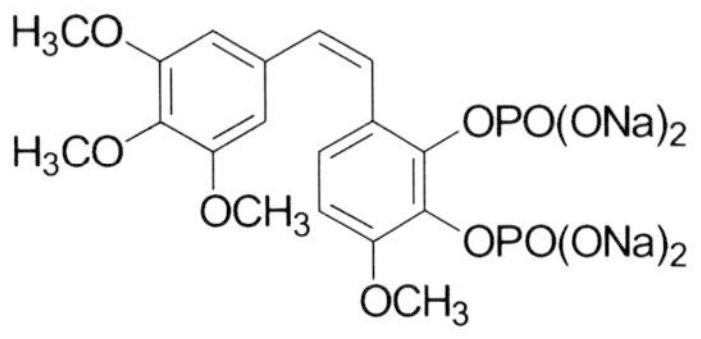

2 (Oxi4503)

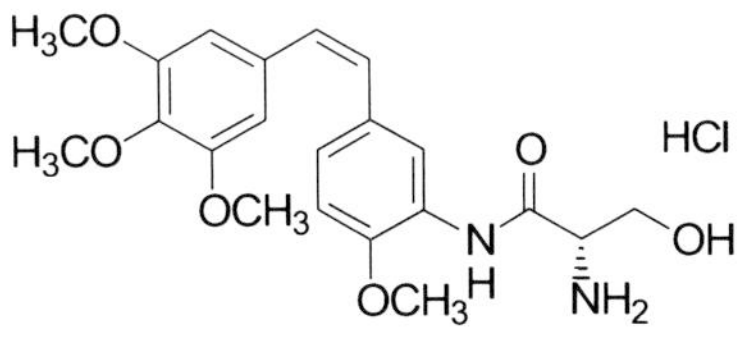

3 (AVE8062, ombrabulin)

Fig. (3). CA4 and CA1 prodrugs fosbretabulin, ombrabulin and Oxi4503.

Fosbretabulin, Ombrabulin and Oxi4503

Fosbretabulin is the most studied prodrug of CA4. As a VDA, it is able to destroy established tumor vasculature, in contrast to antiangiogenic compounds that prevent tumor neovascularization. The action of VDA is selective for tumor vasculature, giving its relative immaturity and instability compared to normal vasculature. However, preclinical studies evidenced that fosbretabulin has limited efficacy if used as a single agent, probably for the remaining *via*ble rim of cancerous cells. Combined approaches using combinations of fosbretabulin and antiangiogenic agents such as bevacizumab were studied for the treatment of ovarian cancer [13, 14]. Cardiovascular adverse events were described with the use of fosbretabulin, alone or in combination with other antiangiogenic agents: an acute but transient increase in blood pressure represents the most relevant toxicity associated with fosbretabulin [15].

Fosbretabulin completed multiple clinical trials for the treatment of patients with anaplastic thyroid carcinoma and other cancers in 2017 [16 - 18]. The combination of fosbretabulin with carboplatin and paclitaxel was well tolerated and displayed antitumor activity in treated patients with ovarian, oesophageal, small-cell lung cancer, and melanoma [19].

In clinical trial studies, the effects of fosbretabulin in combination with everolimus in neuroendocrine tumors have been evaluated [20, 21]. The combination of these two agents with distinct mechanisms of action may improve tumor control without additional toxicities and has the potential to reduce drug resistance. Tolerated doses and safety data were acquired from this study, displaying for fosbretabulin/everolimus combination a promising clinical efficacy in metastatic gastroenteropancreatic neuroendocrine tumor (GEPNET) patients.

Fosbretabulin completed phase II clinical trials for the therapy of advanced anaplastic thyroid cancer (ClinicalTrials.gov identifier: NCT00060242), pathologic myopia (ClinicalTrials.gov identifier: NCT01423149), and polypoidal choroidal vasculopathy (ClinicalTrials.gov identifier: NCT01023295). In addition, it is also undergoing phase III clinical trials for anaplastic thyroid cancer in combination with carboplatin/paclitaxel (ClinicalTrials.gov identifier: NCT00507429).

Ombrabulin (AVE8062, AC7700), the serine prodrug of 3′-amin--deoxycombretastatin CA4, was marketed by Sanofi Aventis as a derivative displaying superior solubility and oral bioavailability than its parent compound. It was widely studied in clinical trials in patients with advanced solid tumors, also in combination with standard chemotherapeutic drugs such as cisplatin and paclitaxel [22 - 24]. Ombrabulin was designed by EMA as an orphan drug in 2011 for the treatment of soft tissue sarcoma, but the orphan status and its clinical development were withdrawn in 2013 after the results of a phase 3 clinical trial. During this evaluation, the combination of ombrabulin and cisplatin significantly improved progression-free survival; however, no sufficient clinical benefit was observed in patients with advanced soft-tissue sarcomas to support its use as a therapeutic option [25].

Oxi4503, the diphosphate prodrug of CA1, received orphan drug approval by FDA in 2017 and it is in development for the treatment of acute myeloid leukaemia (AML) and myelodysplastic syndromes (MDS) by Mateon Therapeutics. Oxi4503 targets leukaemia by two different mechanisms of action: as VDA, it disrupts the shape of tumor bone marrow endothelial cells, and, in addition, it forms a cytotoxic *ortho*-quinone, acting as myeloperoxidase activator, able to directly kill tumor cells [26 - 28]. Clinical trials are undergoing for Oxi4503 in combination with cytarabine for the treatment of AML and MDS [29].

Combretastatin Prodrugs With Improved Drug Delivery Ability

In 2017, Kong *et al.* described the identification of a novel CA4 prodrug with additional theranostic ability to perform a specific drug delivery system with glutathione (GSH)-mediated prodrug activation [30]. The molecule YK-5-252 (**4**) was realized by a combination of three components: the CA4 scaffold, the dicyanomethylene-4*H*-pyran (DCM) as fluorophore, and a central disulfide linker subjected to cleavage by glutathione (Fig. **4**). While cancer cells present higher values of GSH than healthy cells, this system allows selective targeting of tumors. This novel prodrug was tested in a model of triple negative breast cancer (MDA-MB-231), affording selective toxicity against cancer cells. The authors, however, reported a reduced effect of the prodrug compared to the parent compound, rendering the need for further optimization studies to improve both the activity and selectivity of the prodrug.

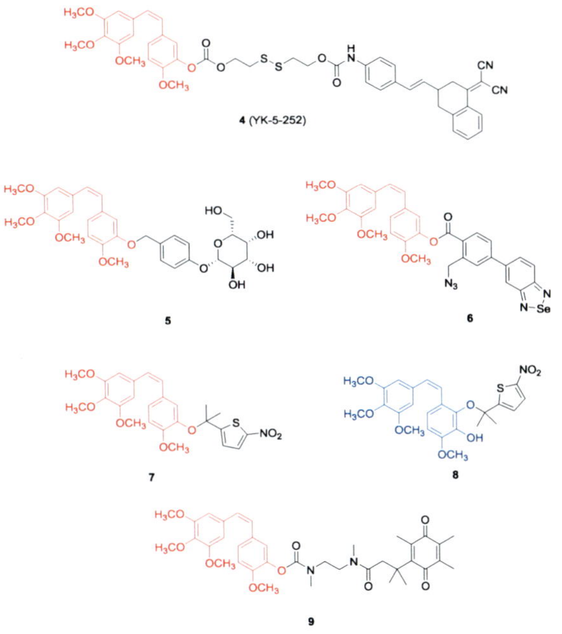

Fig. (4). Combretastatin prodrugs designed to obtain a tumor targeting delivery. CA4 skeleton is indicated in red, CA1 in blue.

β-Galactosidase activity has been found enhanced in some cancer cell lines, including ovarian, breast, colon cancers and gliomas. Doura *et al.* reported on a series of CA4 prodrugs, conjugated with β-galactose (CA4-βGals), developed as anticancer agents against ovarian cell lines [31]. A β-galactose moiety and a benzyl linker were connected to the 3-hydroxyl (ring B) of CA4, producing a novel prodrug (**5**) potentially useful for selective delivery to cancer cells (Fig. **4**). After the removal of β-galactose, the benzyl linker undergoes self-elimination, resulting in the liberation of bioactive CA4. The prodrug was completely inactive as a polymerization inhibitor, but it displayed strong cytotoxicity in ovarian cancer cell lines (OVCAR3 and OVK18). This study demonstrated that the cytotoxicity levels of CA4-βGals are dependent on intracellular β-galactosidase activity, and their cytotoxicity is ascribed to the bioactive compound CA4.

An intriguing methodology to obtain a controlled delivery of CA4 was recently described [32]. This approach takes advantage of the ability of triphenylphosphine (TPP) to induce a controlled drug release *via* the Staudinger reaction. To this aim, a prodrug combining CA4 and a seleno derivative was realized, given the excellent anticancer and radiosensitization effects of selenodiazoles, together with their high bioavailability and safety. The prodrug **6** (Fig. **4**). was synthesized by esterification of CA4 with the carboxylic group of an azide selenodiazole; the subsequent drug release in the presence of TPP was then studied. In *in vitro* experiments, **6** induced an improved antiproliferative effect against cervix cancer cells Caski compared to CA4. In addition, it displayed also excellent radiosensitization properties and greater inhibitory effects toward migration and invasiveness of cancer cells.

Bioreductive Prodrugs of Combretastatins

Hypoxia represents a common feature of many solid tumors that may offer specific prodrug strategies to obtain a selective delivery of anticancer drugs [33, 34]. Hypoxia-activated prodrugs undergo enzyme-mediated activation by one or two-electron reductase. The intriguing approach of hypoxia-targeted prodrugs has been applied also to combretastatins, producing both CA4 and CA1 bioreductive prodrugs. Thomson *et al.* developed a group of combreta-statin (CA4) nitrothiophene ether-linked conjugates, substituted on the α-carbon to modulate the rate of reductive elimination and the metabolic stability (Fig. **4**) [35]. Compound **7** emerged as the most promising derivative, displaying an effective and selective delivery of bioactive compounds into solid tumor environments. The same delivery strategy was applied to CA1 by using the nitrothiophene trigger to target NADPH-cytochrome P450 oxidoreductase (POR) [36]. Both nitrophenyl prodrugs of CA1 (**8**) and CA4 (**7**) were analyzed in this study, assessing the main chemical and biological features. Both *gem*-dimethyl combretastatin prodrugs were found inactive as tubulin polymerization inhibitors, demonstrating a hypoxia-selective activation in the A549 lung cancer cell line. *In vivo* dynamic bioluminescence imaging studies were performed using a 4T1 mouse breast tumor model, indicating **7** as a valuable prodrug candidate, able to induce the *in vivo* release of CA4 by POR and the subsequent vascular disruption.

NADPH quinone oxidoreductase 1 (NQO1), a two-electron reductase responsible for detoxification or bioactivation of some quinones, is overexpressed in different solid tumors, and for this reason, has been studied as a tumor-specific target in anticancer therapy [37, 38]. Prodrugs of CA4 based on NQO1-selective targeting have been developed, consisting of three structural moieties: the parent drug CA4, a NQO1-responsive trigger group, and a self-immolating linker containing carbonate or carbamate groups (Fig. **4**) [39]. Among synthesized prodrugs, **9** emerged as the most promising derivative: the trimethyl quinone propionic acid is the trigger group that undergoes an intramolecular cyclization after reductive activation of NQO1. Then, the *N*-methylcarbamate undergoes self-cyclization, enabling the release of CA4. **9** displayed a marked apoptotic effect on HepG2 cells and a reduction of tumor size in a xenograft liver tumor in mice. The interesting results obtained made this NQO1-responsive prodrug potentially useful for selective tumor-targeting treatment.

Photoresponsive Hybrid Prodrugs of Combretastatins

A photoresponsive hybrid prodrug (**10**) bearing both doxorubicin and CA4 was developed in a recent work with the aim to combine the beneficial effects against the tumor vasculature of two distinct bioactive compounds [40]. In this strategy, drugs could be liberated from parent prodrug by light irradiation, avoiding the use of carriers that could induce biocompatibility problems and off target interactions. The novel prodrug was obtained by a combination of two *ortho*-nitrobenzyl functional groups into an aromatic core, which was flanked by two hydrophilic side chains. CA4 was attached to this core by a carbonate group, whereas doxorubicin was linked by a carbamate linker (Fig. **5**). Studies performed on this novel hybrid prodrug showed a good stability profile and a satisfactory release of both active compounds by irradiation at proper wavelengths. The cytotoxicity of **10** was assessed in a breast cancer cell line (MDA-MB-231), where it exhibited significant cytotoxicity compared with doxorubicin and CA4 alone treated groups, suggesting a synergistic effect.

An innovative approach to combretastatin prodrugs was recently reported, where tissue-penetrable light (red and NIR) allows a selective release of the therapeutic agent [41]. A CA4 prodrug (**11**) was realized, using a core-modified porphyrin as a photosensitizer and an aminoacrylate linker responsible for the selective release of the active CA4. The irradiation with far-red light (690 nm) generates single oxygen (SO) that cleaves the electron-rich olefin, resulting in the subsequent release of the bioactive molecule (Fig. **5**). The synthesized prodrug **11** was evaluated in tissue culture, where it induced about a 6-fold increase in its IC_{50} value in MCF-7 after irradiation, most likely because of the released CA4. In a mouse tumor model (BALB/c mice), the prodrug had a valuable antitumor activity and did not show significant acute toxicity. This approach to tumor-targeted drug delivery appears intriguing and of great potentiality for chemotherapy, allowing selective targeting of bioactive compounds through a site-activated prodrug.

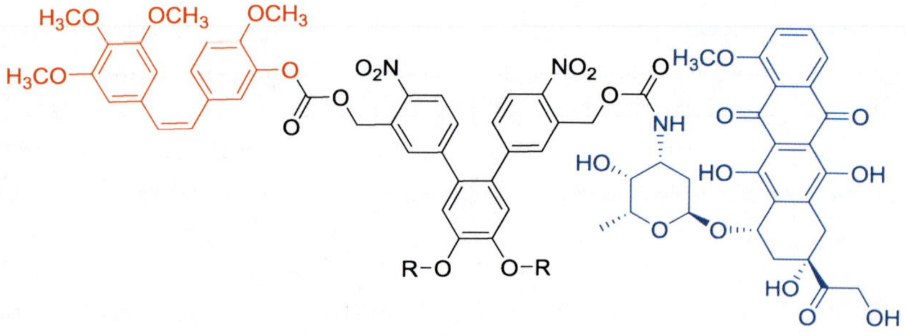

10

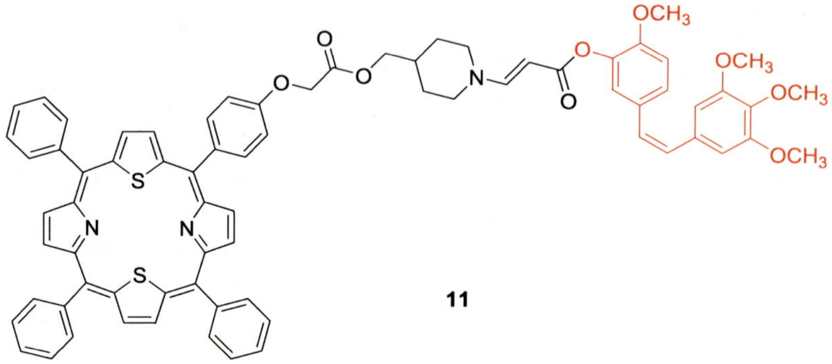

11

Fig. (5). Photoresponsive hybrid prodrugs of CA4. CA4 skeleton is indicated in red and doxorubicin in blue.

The same authors realized another CA4 prodrug based on a similar approach by generating the advanced multifunctioning prodrug **12** for fluorescence optical imaging and photodynamic therapy [42]. In this case, CA4 was combined with phthalocyanine as a fluorescent photosensitizer, linked through an SO-labile aminoacrylate portion (Fig. **6**). The cytotoxicity of this prodrug was lower than that of the parent drug CA4, but it showed enhanced cytotoxicity upon illumination when tested in a mice model.

By pursuing the same direction, the authors described an advanced light-activating prodrug strategy by adding a tumor-targeting group [43]. Folic acid was chosen as a vector for the selective delivery in cancer overexpressing the folate receptor in an attempt to minimize eventual side effects produced after broader illumination. Novel synthesized prodrug **13** comprises CA4 linked to an aminoacrylate linker, the fluorescent photosensitizer phthalocyanine (Pc), a polyethyleneglycol (PEG) spacer, connected to a folic acid portion (Fig. **6**). The choice to incorporate the hydrophilic and biocompatible PEG should improve the pharmacokinetic properties of prodrugs, avoiding aggregation and non-specific targeting into the organism. The PEG's length was varied to explore different linkers and determine the best requirements for efficient targeting. The prodrug with the longest PEG spacer gave the best results in terms of delivery to tumors when tested in mice; these positive results confirmed the good attractivity of this multifunctional prodrug strategy to obtain a selective and improved targeting of bioactive compounds to tumors. This strategy offers the advantage of being highly versatile and adaptable to many applications in selective targeting of chemotherapeutics.

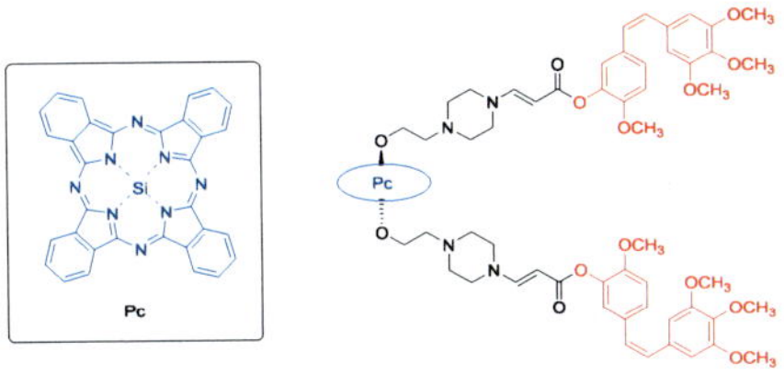

12

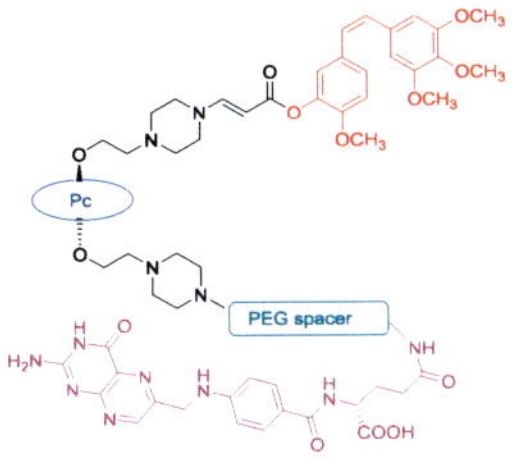

13

Fig. (6). Multifunctional CA4 prodrugs. CA4 skeleton is indicated in red, phthalocyanine (Pc) in blue, and folic acid in purple.

DEVELOPMENT OF COMBRETASTATIN DERIVATIVES

The potent anticancer profile of CA4 and its structural simplicity inspired medicinal chemistry researchers to manipulate its chemical structure to improve solubility, stability and therapeutic efficacy. A surprisingly high number of combretastatin derivatives have been synthesized, and many of them displayed potent anticancer effects. Overall, the pharmacophore of CA4 comprises three important features: ring A, with the trimethoxy substitution, the ethylene bridge, with a *cis* orientation, and ring B, which is more tolerant to modifications and substitutions. The detrimental effects on both tubulin inhibition and cytotoxic properties of changing the substitution pattern on ring A were reported by many studies. For these reasons, the main modifications performed on the combretastatin structure were on the ethylene bridge and on ring B, as summarized in Fig. (**7**).

In the next paragraphs, selected derivatives obtained by bridge modifications will be described, with a general outlook of the chemical structures and the activity profiles.

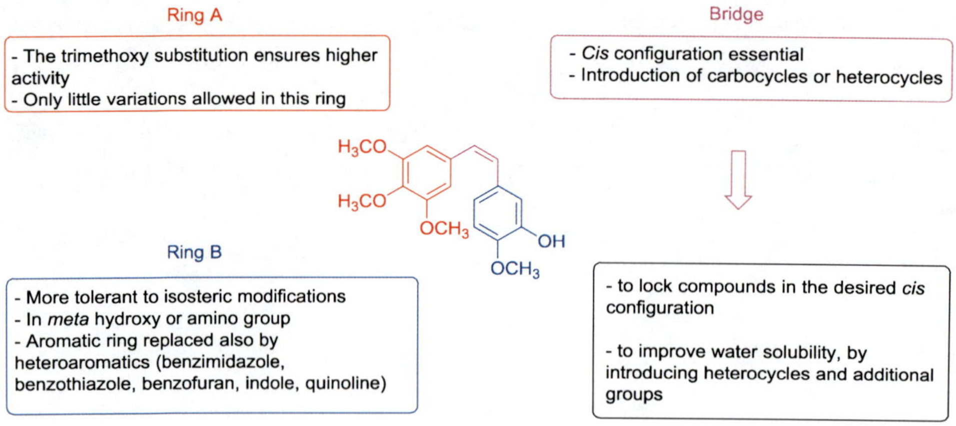

Fig. (7). Main modifications performed on three parts of the CA4 structure: ring A, bridge and ring B.

Combretastatin Derivatives Obtained by Bridge Modifications

A correlation between the bridge length (n) and the cytotoxicity was observed, with the order 2>1>3>4>0 for the structure of CA4. The two-atom bridge seems to be the optimal size, but there are many examples in the literature of active derivatives bearing a different length bridge. Among one-atom bridged analogues, benzophenone phenstatin (**14a**) and *iso*combretastatins (**15**) were reported as potent cytotoxic agents (Fig. **8**). The carbonyl derivative phenstatin, showing the same pattern of ring substitution of CA4, displays a comparable activity to CA4 but a minor ability to bind the colchicine binding site on tubulin [44]. Based on this evidence, the benzophenone analogue of CA1 was then synthesized, the hydroxyphenstatin (**14b**), a potent inhibitor of tubulin polymerization with activity comparable to that of combretastatin A1 [45]. *Iso*combretastatins A4 (**15a**) and A1 (**15b**) are olefin derivatives, displaying similar tubulin inhibitory activity and cytotoxicity to parent combretastatin. Among synthesized derivatives, *iso*CA4 **15a** displayed the best activity, with a 10-fold better cytotoxic activity than its carbonyl analogue phenstatin. Moreover, *iso*CA4 elicits its cytotoxicity in a similar fashion to CA4 by inhibiting tubulin polymerization, which leads to cell cycle arrest in G2/M [46]. Both classes of compounds, benzophenones and *iso*combretastatins, do not contain a *Z*-configure.d double bond, which is an advantage. A recent study summarizes the structure-activity relationships studies carried out on *iso*CA4, with a large panel of structural changes allowed on this molecule without significantly affecting its cytotoxic profile [47].

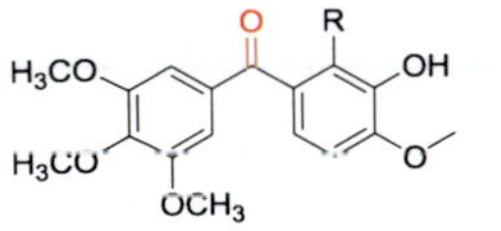

14

14a R = H **phenstatin**
14b R = OH **hydroxyphenstatin**

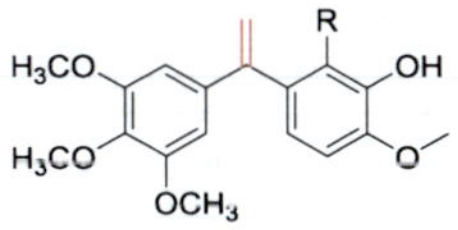

15

15a R = H ***iso*combretastatin A4**
15b R = OH ***iso*combretastatin A1**

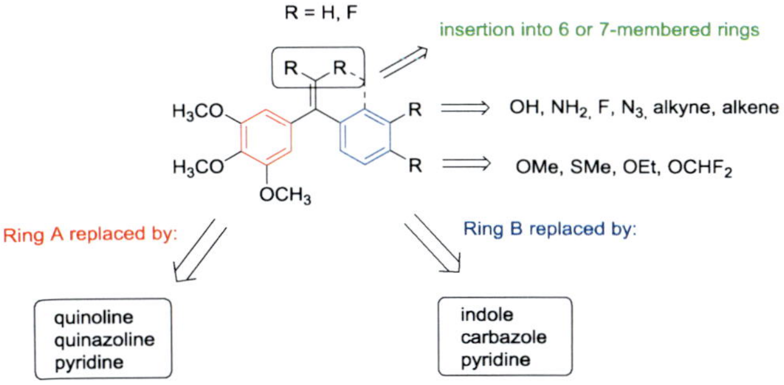

Fig. (8). Chemical structures of benzophenone and *iso*combretastatin derivatives. Main SAR studies for *iso*combretastatin A4 were adapted from [47].

Carbocyclic Derivatives

Different structural modifications of combretastatin were undertaken by replacing the double bond with carbo- and heterocyclic moieties, with the aim of locking compounds in the desired *cis* configuration. While the insertion of heteroaromatics could affect the polarity and, subsequently the binding to tubulin, the use of cycloalkane moieties is of great interest because it allows control of the geometry, keeping unaltered the overall polarity. Cyclopropane, as an alkene bioisostere, was used to obtain novel CA4 derivatives, in which antitumor activity and stereochemistry were studied. Furst *et al.* synthesized cyclopropyl analogues of CA4 (**16**) by varying the *meta* substituent on ring B: overall, all the derivatives, tested as racemates, were less active than corresponding stilbenes, but they retained a cytotoxic profile against cervical adenocarcinoma HeLa (IC_{50} 0.028-23.96 μM) and breast cancer cell line MCF7 (IC_{50} 0.063-14.01 μM) (Fig. **9**) [48]. The importance of stereochemistry was outlined by other studies, in which enantiomeric forms of CA4 cyclopropyl derivatives were synthesized [49]. The *meta*-hydroxy (**17a**) and *meta*-amino (**17b**) derivatives, both in racemic and enantiopure forms, were tested for their anti-tubulin activity and cytotoxicity against B16 melanoma cells. Contrary to what was observed in the anti-tubulin activity, with greater activity for the (-)-enantiomers, there was no significant difference in cytotoxic activity between racemates and enantiomers of tested compounds (**17a** IC_{50} 0.30-0.52 μM, **17b** IC_{50} 0.27-0.44 μM). The authors explained this discrepancy by supposing that tubulin as well as other molecular targets, could be involved in the cytotoxic effect observed in the cellular assays. Molecular docking studies confirmed the importance of stereochemistry for the interaction of the compounds with the colchicine binding site of tubulin.

Several 1,3-disubstituted cyclobutane derivatives (**18**) were synthesized and tested against human hepatocarcinoma (HepG2) and neuroblastoma (SK-N-DZ) cancer cell lines [50]. Both *cis***18a** and *trans***18b** derivatives exhibited weak cytotoxicity compared to CA4, with micromolar IC_{50}s. These results were attributed to a loss of specific tubulin inhibition, with a retained non-specific cytotoxicity. Results from molecular docking studies and molecular dynamic simulations within the colchicine binding site of tubulin were in agreement with experimental data, displaying a better interaction of isomer *cis* and less stable interactions compared to cyclopropylic derivatives, probably due to the higher conformational flexibility of cyclobutane derivatives.

Four to six membered carbocycles were incorporated into the CA4 skeleton, with the aim to explore in a deeper way the optimal geometry and ring size to retain the activity of the parent compound [51]. Cyclobutyl (**19**), cyclopentyl (**20**) and cyclohexyl (**21**) derivatives were synthesized and tested against a panel of haematological and solid tumors (acute T-lymphoblastic leukaemia CCRF-CEM, chronic myeloid leukaemia K562, lung A549 and colon HCT116, HCT116p53$^{-/-}$ adenocarcinomas, osteosarcoma U2OS). Overall, derivatives with larger carbocycles displayed lower cytotoxicity than analogues with smaller carbocycles: cyclobutene derivative **19** was identified as the most promising compound, with submicromolar activity against cancer cell lines but a low selectivity against healthy human fibroblasts. The cytotoxic behaviour shown by tested compounds was confirmed by an *in vitro* tubulin polymerization assay, in which novel compounds displayed activity comparable with nocodazole, a well-known inhibitor of tubulin polymerization.

Heterocyclic Derivatives

Several combretastatin derivatives were obtained by replacement of the olefinic bond with heterocyclic rings, such as pyridine, pyrimidine, quinoline, isoquinoline, oxazole, thiazole, triazole, pyrrole, pyrazole, imidazole, furan, thiophene and many others. In the next paragraphs, a general outlook of these derivatives will be presented and classified based on the size of the heterocyclic ring.

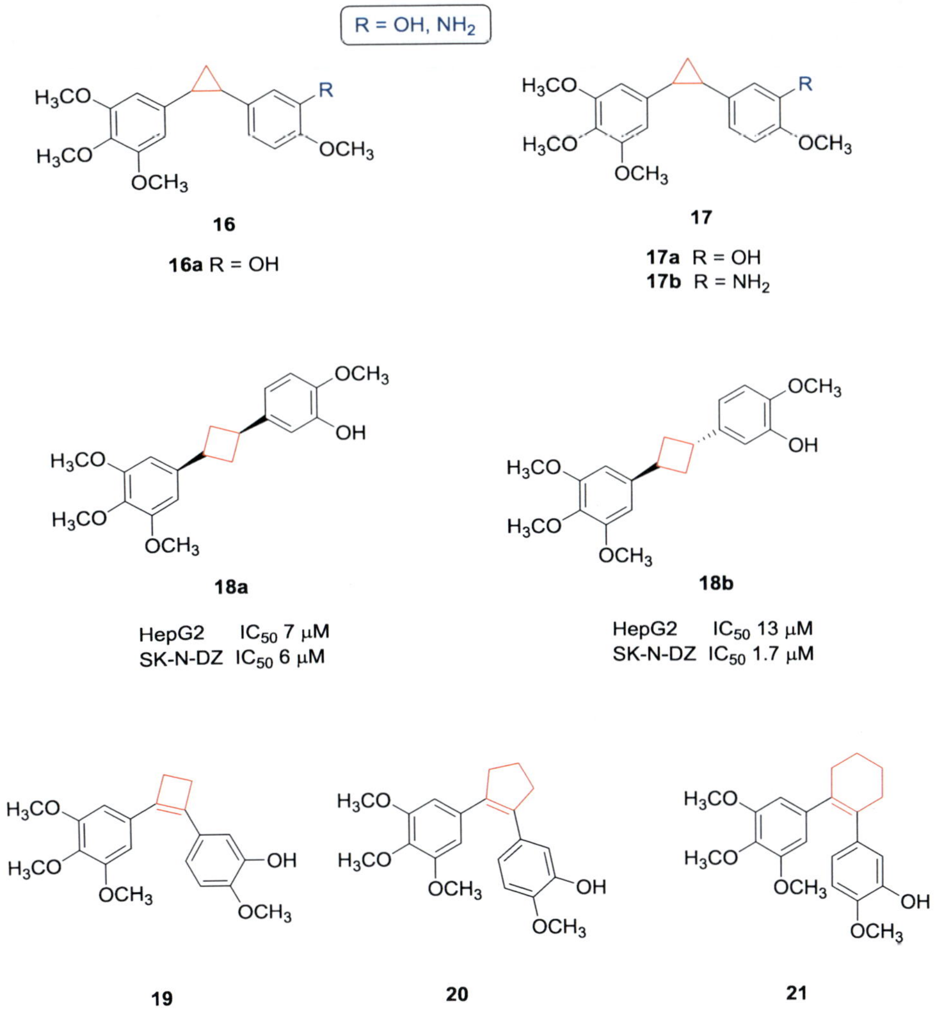

Fig. (9). Carbocyclic derivatives of CA4.

Three and Four-Membered Rings

A small number of combretastatin analogues bearing three or four-term heterocycles have been described as epoxides and β-lactams (**Fig. 10**). Hadfield *et al.* synthesized a small group of epoxide derivatives of CA4 [52]. Among these derivatives, the *trans* isomer **22** induced a potent cytotoxic effect against the human leukaemia K562 cell line (IC_{50} 90 nM); however, it failed to inhibit the assembly of tubulin.

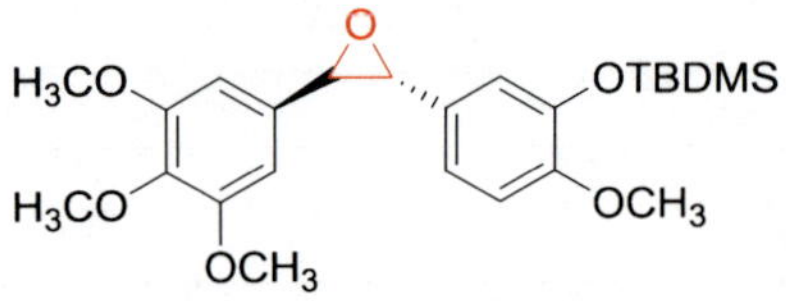

22

IC_{50} 90 nM

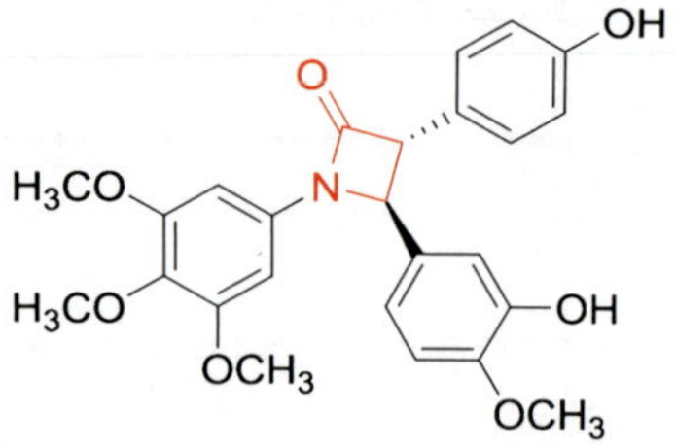

23

IC_{50} 0.34-50 nM

Fig. (10). Epoxide and β-lactam CA4 derivatives.

A wide series of 1,4-diaryl-2-azetidinones was synthesized as rigid analogues of CA4 (Fig. **10**) [53]. These compounds were also substituted at position 3 of the β-lactam ring with an aryl ring. The most potent compound **23** displayed subnanomolar activity in human breast cancer MCF-7 (IC_{50} 0.8 nM), in leukaemia cell lines HL-60 (IC_{50} 0.34 nM) and K562 (IC_{50} 0.89 nM). It was also found to inhibit tubulin polymerization with great efficacy. The cytotoxic profile of **23** was further studied in both *in vitro* and *in vivo* experiments: it was effective against CT-26 (IC_{50} 4.26 nM), Caco-2 (IC_{50} 15.3 nM), and HT-29 (IC_{50} 50 nM) adenocarcinoma cell lines and in a murine model of colon cancer [54].

Five-Membered Rings

Several studies have been dedicated to the discovery of heterocyclic analogues of combretastatins, incorporating five-term rings as rigidifying elements placed between two aromatic rings. Triazole, oxazole, isoxazole, imidazole and pyrazole derivatives of combretastatin are described in this paragraph as representative members of five-term heteroaryl derivatives.

Triazoles were widely used as mimetics of the olefinic bond of combretastatin. A group of 1,5-disubstituted 1,2,3-triazoles (**24**) was synthesized as CA4 analogues and tested for their cytotoxic activity against K562 leukaemia cell line, displaying IC_{50} values in the nanomolar range (Fig. **11**) [55]. The most potent compound, **24a,** showed antiproliferative activity at nanomolar concentration in a wide panel of cancer cell lines, including human melanoma (WM35 and WM239), ovarian (SKOV, OVCAR) and breast carcinoma (MDA-MB231, SK-BR 3). The ability of **24a** to inhibit tubulin polymerization was assessed, with an IC_{50} of 4.8 μM. Molecular modelling simulations predicted a good affinity for the colchicine binding site, with hydrogen bond interactions involving the triazole ring. The same authors reported a wider group of CA4 triazole derivatives, in which the effects of the position of nitrogen atoms in triazole and the linker length between two phenyls were studied [56]. Among several synthesized analogues, **25** and **26** (both amino derivatives in *meta* position of ring B) emerged as the most cytotoxic compounds when tested against the K562 leukaemia cell line (IC_{50} 0.73 and 0.38 μM, respectively). Indeed, they were not as active as parent triazole **24a** and were also lcss potent tubulin inhibitors, displaying IC_{50} values > 20 μM. A similar approach was pursued to obtain triazole analogues of CA1 (**27**), leading to novel derivatives acting as tubulin polymerization and angiogenesis inhibitors [57]. Most active compounds **27a-c** displayed cytotoxicity against selected cancer cell lines (MCF-7 human breast, H460 non-small-cell lung cancer and HT-29 colon cancer), a micromolar potency as angiogenesis inhibitors (0.3-3.2 μM) and tubulin inhibitors (5.2-15.6 μM).

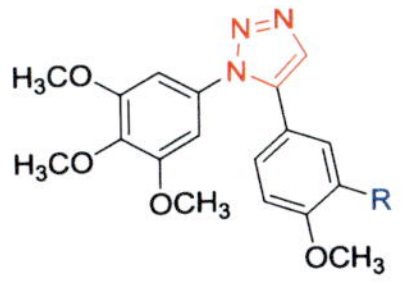

24

24a R = NH_2, IC_{50} 4-11 nM

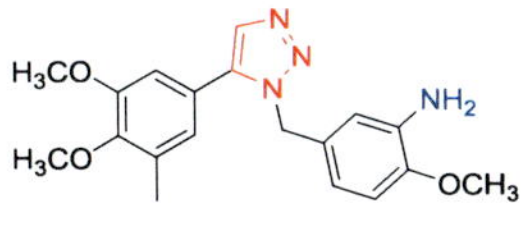

25 IC_{50} 0.73 μM

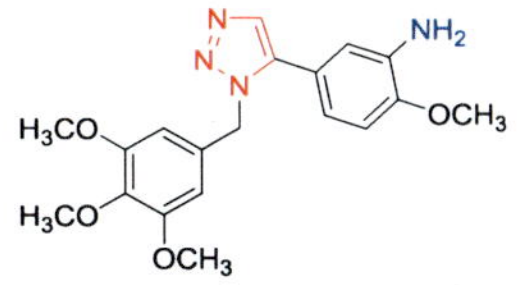

26 IC_{50} 0.38 μM

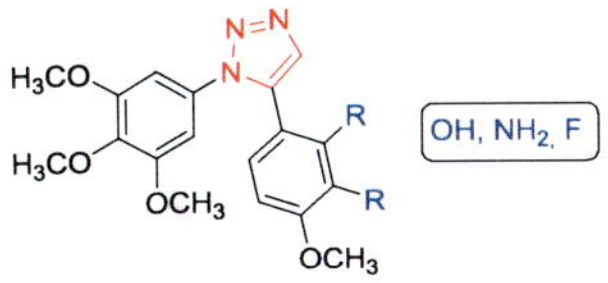

27

27a R = OH, IC_{50} 1.9-6.4 μM
27b R = NH_2, IC_{50} 17.2-38.8 μM
27c R = F, IC_{50} 1.9-26.7 μM

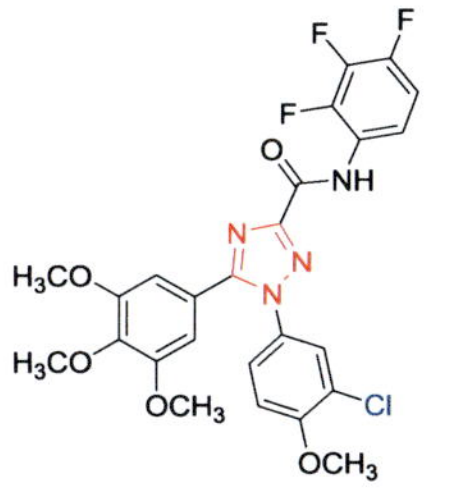

28 IC_{50} 0.04-2.66 μM

Fig. (11). 1,2,3- and 1,2,4-triazole derivatives of combretastatins.

1,2,4-Triazole derivatives of CA4 were reported as potent tubulin inhibitors [58]. In these compounds, the *meta* hydroxy group of B ring was successfully replaced by chlorine, and the *para* methoxy, in some derivatives, by fluorine. A further aromatic ring, spaced by an amide linker, was added in the attempt to target these compounds to both α- and β-subunits of colchicine. Among synthesized compounds, **28** displayed a submicromolar activity against HepG2, HL-60 and MCF-7 cancer cell lines (IC_{50} 0.04, 2.66, 2.10 μM, respectively), and a remarkable inhibition of tubulin polymerization (IC_{50} 0.76 μM).

Some interesting oxazole derivatives of CA4 were recently reported as potent antiproliferative agents [59]. By modulating the substitutions on both aromatic rings, a series of derivatives were synthesized and tested for their antiproliferative effects in selected cancer cell lines. The replacement of a methoxy group in ring A with a thiomethyl or bromine retained a good cytotoxic activity. The best cytotoxic effect was displayed by **29** and **30** against five cell lines (human epidermoid carcinoma A431, human cervical adenocarcinoma HeLa, human breast adenocarcinoma MCF-7 and MDA-MB-231, human ovarian adenocarcinoma SKOV-3), with IC_{50} in the low micromolar range (**29** IC_{50} 0.009-0.71 μM, **30** IC_{50} 0.43-2.78 μM) (Fig. **12**).

Some oxazole-bridged CA4 analogues with B-ring bearing additional -OH or -SMe groups were also reported [60]. Among synthesized compounds, the *para* thiomethyl derivative **31** displayed the best antiproliferative activity in human HL-60 leukaemia, 518A2 melanoma, and colon carcinomas HCT-116 and HT-29 cells (IC_{50} range 0.01-0.63 μM). Compound **31** was also found to inhibit the polymerization of tubulin *in vitro*.

Isoxazole analogues of combretastatin were also reported as antitubulin compounds [61]. Among synthesized compounds, the 4,5-diarylisoxazole **32** exhibited greater antitubulin activity than that of CA4 (0.75 *vs.* 1.2 μM) but modest antiproliferative activity against human colon adenocarcinoma cell line HT29 and transformed murine endothelial cell line SVEC 4-10 (IC_{50} 3.0 and 8.5 μM, respectively). In this study, minor variations in the chemical structure of the isoxazole and the position of two phenyl rings could strongly influence the antitubulin activity.

The isoxazole CA4 derivative **33** (XN05) was deeply studied for its cytotoxic activity exerted by disrupting the microtubule assembly [62]. It displayed antiproliferative activity when tested in a wide panel of cancer cell lines (leukaemia K562, breast cancer MCF-7, lung cancer A549, stomach cancer SGC-7901, oesophageal cancer ECA-109, prostate cancer PC3, hepatoma tumors BEL-7402 and SMMC-7721), with IC_{50} range 0.067-1.84 μM. Results from these investigations showed for **33** a great potential for therapeutic treatment of various malignancies.

A series of imidazole analogues of CA4 (Fig. **13**). that share a *meta* halogen substituted A-ring and a B-ring with *meta* halogen/amino and *para* ethoxy substitution were reported by Mahal and co-workers [63]. The most active compound **34** inhibited the growth of various cancer cell lines (melanoma 518A2, colon HT-29 and HCT-116, murine breast carcinoma cells MCF-7), with IC_{50} values in the low nanomolar range (5.1-72 nM). *In vitro* and *in vivo* experiments demonstrated that **34** effectively reduced the motility and invasiveness of cancer cells by initiating the formation of actin stress fibres and focal adhesions as a response to the extensive microtubule disruption.

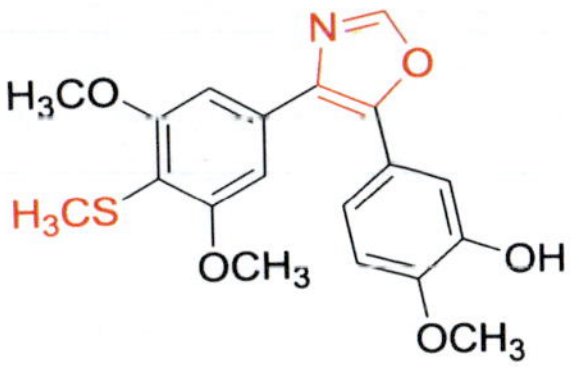

29

IC_{50} 0.009-0.71 μM

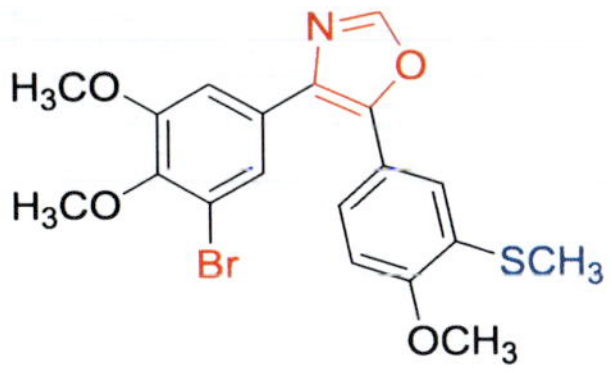

30

IC_{50} 0.43-2.78 μM

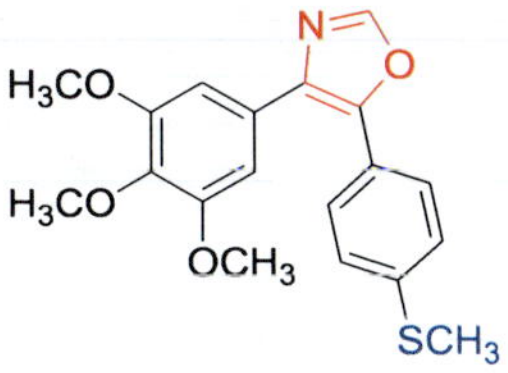

31

IC_{50} 0.01-0.63 μM

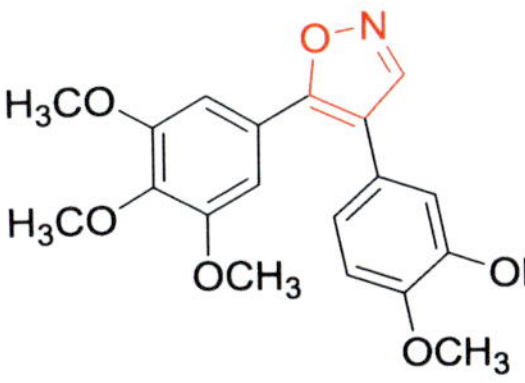

32

IC_{50} 3.0-8.5 μM

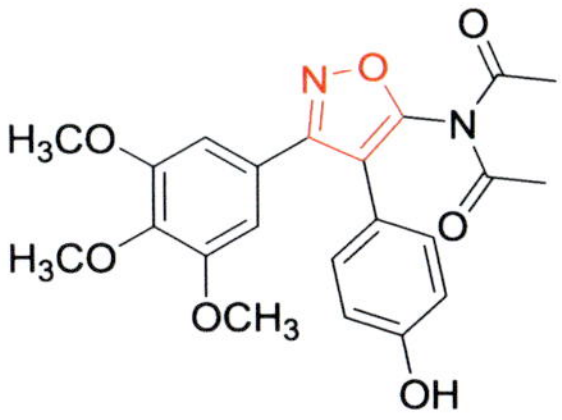

33 (XN05)

IC_{50} 0.067-1.84 μM

Fig. (12). Oxazole and isoxazole derivatives of combretastatins.

An intriguing approach for discovering CA4 related tubulin inhibitors was recently reported, with the assembly of 2-aminoimidazolecarbonyl as a bridging motif, trimethoxyphenyl as a ring, and different aryls and heteroaryls as the other ring [64]. The insertion of a carbonylic moiety was found to inhibit the tubulin assembly and enhance the antiproliferative effects. The most promising compound was the heteroaryl derivative **35**, presenting thiophene as ring B. The heterocycle **35** exerted potent cytotoxic effects on different cancer cell lines, including HeLa cervical cancer, MCF7 breast cancer, B16F10 skin melanoma, and A549 lung carcinoma, with IC_{50} in the range 36-1891 nM. The inhibition of tubulin assembly for this novel derivative was found to be similar to that of CA4 and colchicine.

The pyrazole ring was also used as a mimic of the *cis*-double bond of combretastatin, affording several derivatives with excellent cytotoxic properties. Romagnoli *et al.* reported on the synthesis of 1*H*-pyrazole analogues of CA4, in which some structure-activity relationships were also analyzed [65]. Among several analogues synthesized, compounds **36** and **37** gave excellent results when tested against six cancer cell lines (breast adenocarcinoma MCF7 and MDA-M--231, human cervix carcinoma HeLa, human colon adenocarcinoma HT-29, human promyelocytic leukaemia HL-60, human B-cell leukaemia SEM), with

IC_{50}s in the low nanomolar range (**36** IC_{50} 0.05-4.5 nM; **37** IC_{50} 0.06-0.7 nM) (Fig. **13**). The analogue **37** displayed a better activity than CA4 in tested cell lines, whereas the isomeric derivative **36** was less active than CA4 only against HL-60 cells. Both active compounds also strongly inhibited tubulin polymerization at submicromolar concentration. The antitumor effect *in vivo* of **37** was evaluated in an allograft tumor model developed in mice, where it significantly reduced tumor growth in a dose-dependent manner, even at the lower dose tested (5.0 mg/kg).

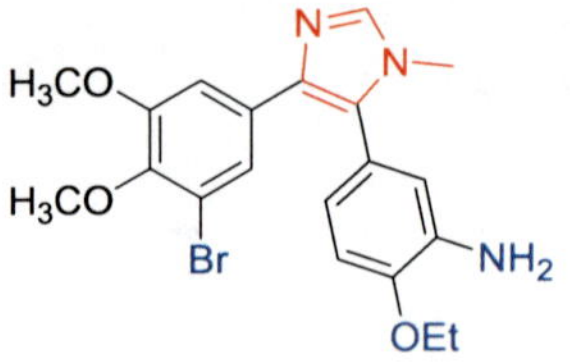

34

IC_{50} 5.1-72 nM

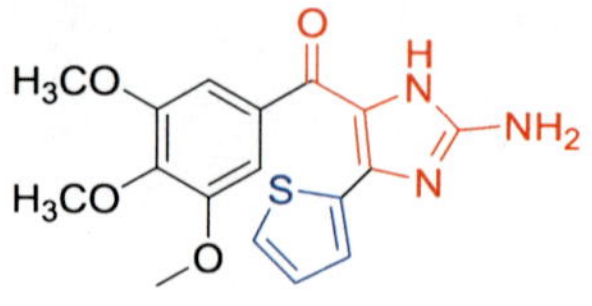

35

IC_{50} 36-1891 nM

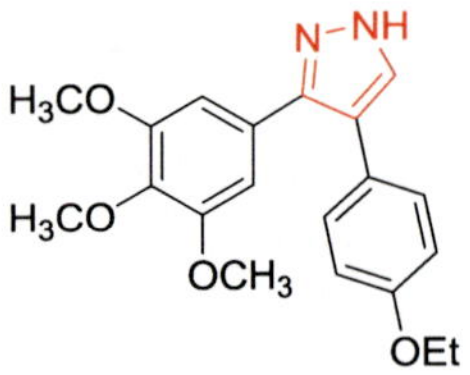

36

IC_{50} 0.05-4.5 nM

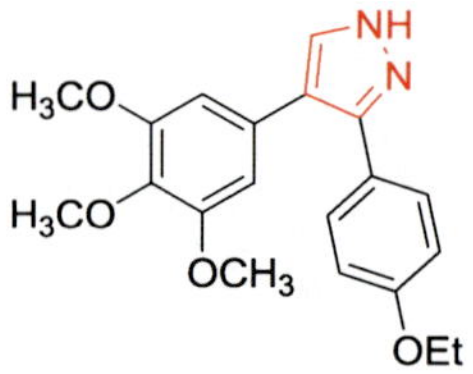

37

IC_5 0.06-0.7 nM

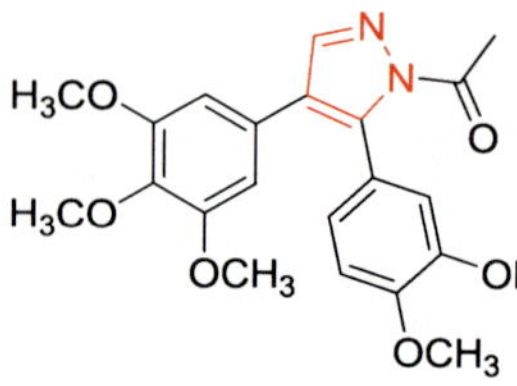

38

IC_{50} 9.3-22 nM

Fig. (13). Imidazole and pyrazole derivatives of combretastatins.

A large group of diarylpyrazoles was realized in which an extra acetyl group on the pyrazole and various substitutions with electron-donating and electron-withdrawing groups were introduced at different positions of the B ring [66]. Synthesized analogues were screened for their ability to inhibit cell proliferation in selected cancer cell lines (gastric adenocarcinoma SGC-7901 cells, mouth epidermal carcinoma KB cells and fibrosarcoma HT-1080 cells). Among target compounds, **38** showed the best antiproliferative activity against the three cell lines, with an IC_{50} range of 9.3-22 nM. Consistent with its antiproliferative activity, it also exhibited potent antitubulin activity (IC_{50} 7.73 μM).

Six-Membered Rings

Pyridine has been introduced to replace the *cis* double bond between the A and B rings of combretastatin (Fig. **14**) [67]. In these novel CA4 analogues the distance between the two phenyl rings is configure.d to be three or four atoms, including the nitrogen atom of pyridine. The cytotoxic profile and the antitubulin activity were found to be optimal for compounds with a linker length of three atoms and optimized substitutions in both aromatic rings. 2,6-Diphenylpyridines **39**, **40a** and **40b** displayed the best antiproliferative activity against three human cancer cell lines (MDA-MB-231, A549, and HeLa, IC_{50} range 0.0014-2.64 μM), arrested cell cycle, and blocked angiogenesis and vasculature formation *in vivo* in a similar way to CA4.

The pyridine ring was also inserted in *cis*-restricted benzimidazole and benzothiazole mimics of CA4, whose antiproliferative activity was studied in the cervix (HeLa), liver (HepG2), lung adenocarcinoma (A549) and prostate (DU-145) cancer cell lines [68]. Benzothiazole derivatives showed the greatest results, with nanomolar cytotoxic activity for trimethoxyphenyl derivative **41** (GI_{50} 0.06-0.26 μM) and trifluoromethyl-chlorophenyl analogue **42** (GI_{50} 0.04-0.091 μM). Tubulin polymerization assay confirmed for these derivatives a potent inhibition profile.

Pyrimidine bridged combretastatin (**43**) were recently described [69], in which the pyrimidine was placed as a three-carbon linker between the two aromatic rings, variously substituted with electron-withdrawing and electron-donating groups. These novel derivatives were tested against breast (MCF7) and lung (A549) cancer cell lines, displaying selective cancer cell toxicity at low micromolar concentration. Compound **43a** (IC_{50} 4.67 μM MCF7, 3.38 μM A549) was found to be a competitive inhibitor of colchicine in a tubulin binding assay; molecular modelling studies confirmed, for this derivative, a good fit in the colchicine binding pocket.

RECENT ADVANCES IN DRUG DELIVERY SYSTEMS OF COMBRETASTATIN

As for several bioactive compounds, also for combretastatin, drug delivery systems have been developed to overcome the limitations of the conventional drug delivery systems, including drug degradation and loss of activity, side-effects, low bioavailable concentrations in required tissues and pharmacokinetic instability. Delivery strategies, including nanoparticles, liposomes, micelles, nanospheres, nanogels and others, were applied both to combretastatin and to combinations of combretastatins with other chemotherapeutics in order to obtain synergistic effects (Fig. **15**). A brief overview of these strategies will be analyzed in this paragraph, pointing at the most representative studies.

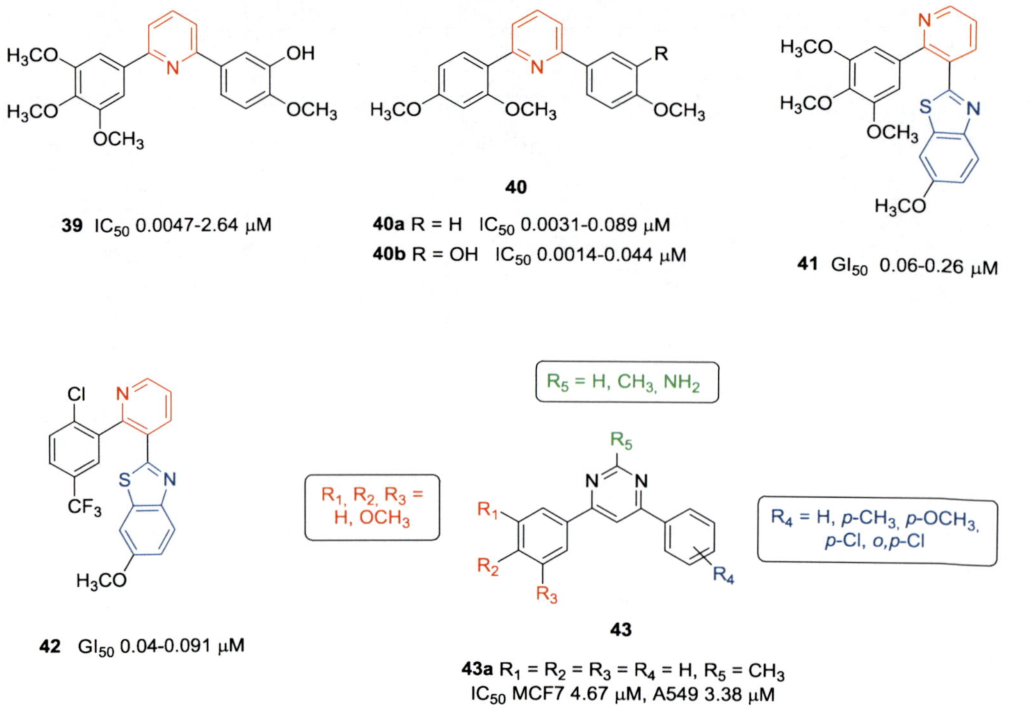

Fig. (14). Pyridine and pyrimidine derivatives of combretastatins.

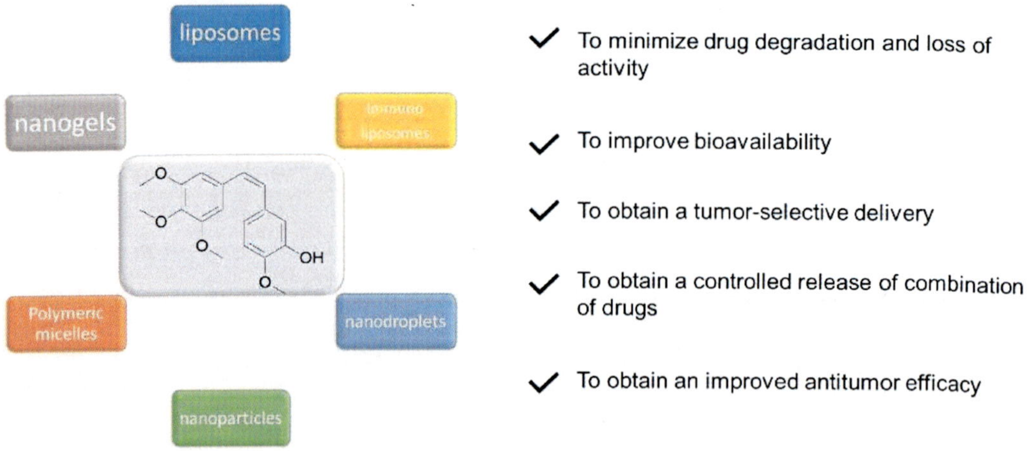

Fig. (15). Overview of drug delivery strategies successfully applied to combretastatins.

A liposome-based drug delivery system was applied to CA4 to obtain a specific delivery of drug to the solid tumor vasculature [70]. This approach started from the observation that cell adhesion molecules, such as $\alpha_v\beta_3$ integrins, were overexpressed on actively proliferating endothelium of the tumor vasculature. Liposomes composed of hydrogenated soybean phosphatidylcholine (HSPC), cholesterol, distearoyl phosphoethanolamine-polyethylene-glycol-2000 conjugate (DSPE-PEG), and DSPE-PEG-maleimide were prepared and coupled to cyclic RGD peptides, consisting of an Arg-Gly-Asp sequence, able to target $\alpha_v\beta_3$ integrin receptors. This system was effective in obtaining a selective targeting of CA4 to highly proliferating endothelium cells.

Pattillo *et al.* developed a drug delivery system for CA4 phosphate based on immunoliposomes [71]. In this approach, irradiation upregulated adhesion molecules on the surface of liposomes, preferentially targeting bioactive molecules to the irradiated tumor, so avoiding undesirable side effects of antivascular drugs on normal tissues. Anti-E-selectin was conjugated to liposomes containing CA4 phosphate, and this system resulted in a significant delay in tumor growth when administered in transplanted mammary tumors.

Lipid-stabilised oil nanodroplets (LONDs) containing CA4 were formulated and tested in SVR mouse pancreatic islet endothelial cells [72]. Different biocompatible oils were used to form LONDs with phospholipid coatings, and among these, tripropionin was chosen for the application in this study. CA4 was encapsulated in tripropionin LONDs and successfully released in cells, causing microtubule disruption.

The application of nanocarriers in drug delivery has received great attention to enhance the oral absorption of poorly bioavailable drugs. In the attempt to develop an oral formulation of CA4 phosphate, some authors established novel nanoparticles for oral administration by combining methoxy poly(ethylene glycol)-β-polylactide (PELA) and poly(D,L-lactic-co-glycolic acid) (PLGA) polymers [73]. Transport study was evaluated on Madin-Darby canine kidney cell models, widely used in oral permeability studies as it perfectly simulates the epithelial cells of the human intestinal tract. Antitumor efficacy was evaluated in subcutaneous xenotransplanted tumor models in mice. The nanoparticle formulation displayed better transcellular transport, enhanced the oral bioavailability and induced antitumor effects in *in vivo* model. This novel biodegradable polymer-based system deserves promising application in drug oral delivery.

Stimuli-responsive nanoparticles attracted much interest in tumor-selective drug delivery, given the possibility to direct drugs at unique features of the tumor microenvironment, such as pH, enzymes and ROS levels. Of these stimuli, higher concentrations of glutathione (GSH) were found in many tumors than in normal tissues; for these reasons, GSH-responsive nanodrugs could ensure selective targeting in tumor sites, avoiding undesired toxicity. PEGylated poly(alpha-lipoic acid) nanoparticles containing CA4 with GSH-responsive ability were proposed as novel tumor-selective drug delivery systems [74]. The realized nanoparticles were found stable under physiological conditions, whereas they underwent degradation in the presence of GSH. They achieved selective drug release at the tumor site, a long circulation time *in vivo* and significant antitumor effects in the 4T1 tumors of Balb/c nude mice.

In the last years, polymeric micelles have emerged as an attractive drug delivery platform for achieving passive targeting, along with the possibility of incorporating active targeting through appropriate surface functionalization. This attractive approach was realized by inserting CA4 in dendron-polymer conjugates, as reported by Sumer Bolu and co-workers [75]. A series of triblock dendron-polymer-dendron (DPD) conjugates were used as polymeric scaffolds, and CA4 was coupled to these through Huisgen type "click" chemistry. Minimal cytotoxicity was detected on human umbilical vein endothelial (HUVEC) cells by polymeric scaffold, whereas drug conjugated micelles induced a significant decrease in cell *via*bility, confirming these systems as suitable candidates as controlled drug delivery agents.

Innovative drug delivery systems were set up also for combinations of different chemotherapeutic agents, such as combretastatin and doxorubicin or methotrexate or paclitaxel, in order to obtain improved activity and selective targeting at tumor sites. A challenging delivery approach, based on a "nanocell", was proposed by Sengupta and co-workers, in which a nanoscale pegylated-phospholipid block-copolymer envelope coats a nuclear nanoparticle [76]. The nanocell is able to release, at different times, two drugs: the outer envelope first releases an anti-angiogenesis agent, causing vascular disruption, then the inner nanoparticle releases a chemotherapeutic agent directly into the tumor site. CA4 and doxorubicin were inserted in the nanocell, and the system was evaluated for its pharmacokinetic properties and activity in the tumor mice model of melanoma (B16/F10) and Lewis lung carcinoma. The observed reduced toxicity and enhanced antitumor effects outlined the success of this novel delivery strategy.

Arg-Gly-Asp (RGD)-modified liposomes loaded with both CA4 and doxorubicin were proposed for the delivery of combined chemotherapeutic agents [77]. The RGD peptide specifically binds to the $\alpha_V\beta_3$ integrins, whose increased expression has been observed in many tumors, such as melanoma. The selective targeting and release of drugs from liposomes was *in vitro* investigated on B16F10 melanoma cells and human umbilical vein endothelial cells (HUVECs). In *in vivo* experiments, liposomes effectively reduced the growth of subcutaneous B16F10 xenograft tumors in C57BL6 mice, showing a synergistic effect of combined drugs.

In a similar approach, the same combination of CA4-doxorubicin was encapsulated in liposomes based on cRGDyK-modified PEG-β-PLA co-polymers [78]. The cyclic peptide cRGDyK was used with the aim of obtaining a selective targeting of $\alpha_V\beta_3$ integrins. Liposomes were *in vitro* tested against three cell lines (melanoma B16-F10, breast cancer MCF-7, and HUVECs), which show a different integrin $\alpha_V\beta_3$ expression, and *in vivo* tested in C57BL/6 mice inoculated subcutaneously with B16-F10 cells. Results demonstrated a good release of both drugs and enhanced antitumor effect, supporting the active targeting and the combination therapy as a promising approach for cancer treatment.

A nanoparticulate delivery system based on poly(lactic-co-glycolic acid) (PLGA) and encapsulating paclitaxel and CA4 was also described [79]. The nanoparticles were decorated on the surface with a small peptide containing Arg-Gly-Asp (RGD) sequence in order to obtain a selective targeting of tumor overexpressing $\alpha_V\beta_3$ receptor. Subcutaneous B16F10 xenograft experiments in mice revealed tumor suppression by nanoparticles *via* vascular disruption, cellular proliferation inhibition, and apoptosis induction in the tumor microenvironment.

The combination of CA4 and methotrexate was studied in a pH-sensible target delivery system against hepatocellular carcinoma [80]. Pullulan, a ligand for hepatic asialoglycoprotein receptor (ASGPR), was modified with urocanic acid and then conjugated to methotrexate. The presence of the imidazole group in urocanic acid represents the element sensitive to pH: in fact, imidazole undergoes protonation in a mild acidic medium, as the tumor microenvironment, producing the swelling of nanoparticles and the release of drugs. After an intravenous injection to PLC/PRF/5-bearing nude mice, nanoparticles displayed enhanced antitumor and antiangiogenic effects, prolonged circulation time in blood, and selective delivery in the liver.

A dual-drug delivery system based on nanogel-incorporated injectable hydrogel was designed to locally deliver CA4 phosphate and doxorubicin for anti-angiogenesis and anticancer combination therapy [81]. Hydrogels exhibit great potential for local delivery of hydrophilic drugs, thanks to their ability to release high doses of drugs after simple injection, avoiding systematic side effects. pH and redox stimuli-responsive poly(acrylic acid-co-4-vinylphenylboronic acid) nanohydrogels were used as nanocarriers for doxorubicin delivery. These nanohydrogels were then incorporated into injectable hydrogels containing CA4 phosphate through reversible boronate ester bonds. The release of CA4 phosphate from hydrogel is quick, whereas subsequently, a slow release of doxorubicin occurs. The *in vivo* antitumor efficacy of the novel drug delivery system was carried out by a single peritumoral injection in xenograft tumor-bearing mice.

CONCLUDING REMARKS

In the field of natural compounds, combretastatins emerged as a fascinating scaffold to obtain novel anticancer drugs. The efforts by medicinal chemistry researchers led to an exceptional number of derivatives and prodrugs, endowed with improved anticancer efficacy and selective targeting of tumors. Nanoformulations and advanced drug delivery systems were developed for combretastatins, alone or in combination with other chemotherapeutic agents, leading to attractive and efficacious systems to selectively reach the tumor microenvironment. There are currently some combretastatin prodrugs under clinical evaluation for possible future application in chemotherapy.

ABBREVIATIONS

CBS	Colchicine binding site
CA4	Combretastatin A-4
VDA	Vascular disrupting agent
CA1	Combretastatin A-1
GEPNET	gastroenteropancreatic neuroendocrine tumor
AML	Acute myeloid leukaemia
MDS	Myelodysplastic syndromes
GSH	Glutathione
DCM	Dicyanomethylene-4*H*-pyran
CA4-βGal	Combretastatin A4-β-galactose
TPP	Triphenylphosphine
POR	NADPH-cytochrome P450 oxidoreductase
NQO1	NADPH quinone oxidoreductase 1
NIR	Near-infrared radiation
SO	Single oxygen
Pc	Phtalocyanine
PEG	Polyethylene glycol
HSPC	Hydrogenated soybean phosphatidylcholine
DSPE-PEG	Distearoyl phosphoethanolamine-polyethylene-glycol
RGD	Arg-Gly-Asp
LONDs	Lipid-stabilised oil nanodroplets

PELA	Poly(ethylene glycol)-β-polylactide
PLGA	Poly(D,L-lactic co glycolic acid
DPD	Dendron-polymer-dendron
ASGPR	Asialoglycoprotein receptor

CONSENT FOR PUBLICATION

Not applicable.

CONFLICT OF INTEREST

The authors declare no conflict of interest, financial or otherwise.

ACKNOWLEDGEMENT

Declared none.

REFERENCES

[1] Pettit, G.R.; Singh, S.B.; Niven, M.L.; Hamel, E.; Schmidt, J.M. Isolation, structure, and synthesis of combretastatins A-1 and B-1, potent new inhibitors of microtubule assembly, derived from *Combretum caffrum*. *J. Nat. Prod.,* **1987**, *50*(1), 119-131. [http://dx.doi.org/10.1021/np50049a016] [PMID: 3598594]

[2] Pettit, G.R.; Singh, S.B.; Schmidt, J.M.; Nixen, M.L.; Hamel, E.; Lin, C.M. Isolation, structure, synthesis, and antimitotic properties of combretastatins B-3 and B-4 from *Combretum caffrum*. *J. Nat. Prod.,* **1988**, *51*(3), 517-527. [http://dx.doi.org/10.1021/np50057a011] [PMID: 3404149]

[3] Pettit, G.R.; Singh, S.B.; Hamel, E.; Lin, C.M.; Alberts, D.S.; Garcia-Kendal, D. Isolation and structure of the strong cell growth and tubulin inhibitor combretastatin A-4. *Experientia,* **1989**, *45*(2), 209-211. [http://dx.doi.org/10.1007/BF01954881] [PMID: 2920809]

[4] Lin, C.M.; Singh, S.B.; Chu, P.S.; Dempcy, R.O.; Schmidt, J.M.; Pettit, G.R.; Hamel, E. Interactions of tubulin with potent natural and synthetic analogs of the antimitotic agent combretastatin: a structure-activity study. *Mol. Pharmacol.,* **1988**, *34*(2), 200-208. [PMID: 3412321]

[5] Dark, G.G.; Hill, S.A.; Prise, V.E.; Tozer, G.M.; Pettit, G.R.; Chaplin, D.J. Combretastatin A-4, an agent that displays potent and selective toxicity toward tumor vasculature. *Cancer Res.,* **1997**, *57*(10), 1829-1834. [PMID: 9157969]

[6] Pettit, G.R.; Rhodes, M.R.; Herald, D.L. Antineoplastic agents 393. Synthesis of the trans-isomer of combretastatin A-4 prodrug. *Anticancer Drug Des.,* **1998**, *13*(8), 981-993. [PMID: 10335271]

[7] Karatoprak, G.Ş.; Küpeli Akkol, E.; Genç, Y.; Bardakcı, H.; Yücel, Ç.; Sobarzo-Sánchez, E. Combretastatins: an overview of structure, probable mechanisms of action and potential applications. *Molecules,* **2020**, *25*(11), 2560. [http://dx.doi.org/10.3390/molecules25112560] [PMID: 32486408]

[8] McLoughlin, E.C.; O'Boyle, N.M. Colchicine-binding site inhibitors from chemistry to clinic: a

review. *Pharmaceuticals (Basel),* **2020**, *13*(1), 8.
[http://dx.doi.org/10.3390/ph13010008] [PMID: 31947889]

[9] Pettit, G.R.; Lippert, J.W., III Antineoplastic agents 429. Syntheses of the combretastatin A-1 and combretastatin B-1 prodrugs. *Anticancer Drug Des.,* **2000**, *15*(3), 203-216.
[PMID: 11049088]

[10] West, C.M.L.; Price, P. Combretastatin A4 phosphate. *Anticancer Drugs,* **2004**, *15*(3), 179-187.
[http://dx.doi.org/10.1097/00001813-200403000-00001] [PMID: 15014350]

[11] Siemann, D.W.; Chaplin, D.J.; Walicke, P.A. A review and update of the current status of the vasculature-disabling agent combretastatin-A4 phosphate (CA4P). *Expert Opin. Investig. Drugs,* **2009**, *18*(2), 189-197.
[http://dx.doi.org/10.1517/13543780802691068] [PMID: 19236265]

[12] Kirwan, I.G.; Loadman, P.M.; Swaine, D.J.; Shnyder, S.D.; Cooper, P.A.; Bibby, M.C. Comparative preclinical pharmacokinetic and metabolic studies of the combretastatin prodrugs combretastatin A4 phosphate and A1 phosphate. *Clin. Cancer Res.,* **2004**, *10*(4), 1446-1453.
[http://dx.doi.org/10.1158/1078-0432.CCR-0518-03] [PMID: 14977848]

[13] Monk, B.J.; Sill, M.W.; Walker, J.L. Randomized phase II evaluation of bevacizumab *versus* bevacizumab plus fosbretabulin in recurrent ovarian, tubal, or peritoneal carcinoma: an NRG oncology/gynecologic oncology group study. *J. Clin. Oncol.,* **2016**, *34*(19), 2279-2286.
[http://dx.doi.org/10.1200/JCO.2015.65.8153] [PMID: 27217446]

[14] Tewari, K.S.; Sill, M.W.; Coleman, R.L. Bevacizumab plus fosbretabulin in recurrent ovarian cancer: Overall survival and exploratory analyses of a randomized phase II NRG oncology/gynecologic oncology group study. *Gynecol. Oncol.,* **2020**, *159*(1), 79-87.
[http://dx.doi.org/10.1016/j.ygyno.2020.07.015] [PMID: 32723679]

[15] Grisham, R.; Ky, B.; Tewari, K.S.; Chaplin, D.J.; Walker, J. Clinical trial experience with CA4P anticancer therapy: focus on efficacy, cardiovascular adverse events, and hypertension management. *Gynecol. Oncol. Res. Pract.,* **2018**, *5*(1), 1.
[http://dx.doi.org/10.1186/s40661-017-0058-5] [PMID: 29318022]

[16] Mooney, C.J.; Nagaiah, G.; Fu, P. A phase II trial of fosbretabulin in advanced anaplastic thyroid carcinoma and correlation of baseline serum-soluble intracellular adhesion molecule-1 with outcome. *Thyroid,* **2009**, *19*(3), 233-240.
[http://dx.doi.org/10.1089/thy.2008.0321] [PMID: 19265494]

[17] Sosa, J.A.; Elisei, R.; Jarzab, B. Randomized safety and efficacy study of fosbretabulin with paclitaxel/carboplatin against anaplastic thyroid carcinoma. *Thyroid,* **2014**, *24*(2), 232-240.
[http://dx.doi.org/10.1089/thy.2013.0078] [PMID: 23721245]

[18] Granata, R.; Locati, L.D.; Licitra, L. Fosbretabulin for the treatment of anaplastic thyroid cancer. *Future Oncol.,* **2014**, *10*(13), 2015-2021.
[http://dx.doi.org/10.2217/fon.14.154] [PMID: 25396774]

[19] Rustin, G.J.; Shreeves, G.; Nathan, P.D. A Phase Ib trial of CA4P (combretastatin A-4 phosphate), carboplatin, and paclitaxel in patients with advanced cancer. *Br. J. Cancer,* **2010**, *102*(9), 1355-1360.
[http://dx.doi.org/10.1038/sj.bjc.6605650] [PMID: 20389300]

[20] Chauhan, A.; Arnold, S.; Slone, S.A.; Flynn, H.; Weiss, H.; Anthony, L.B. A phase I/II study of fosbretabulin in combination with everolimus in neuroendocrine tumors that have progressed after at least one prior regimen for metastatic disease. *J. Clin. Oncol.,* **2018**, *36*(15_suppl) Suppl., TPS4148-TPS4148.
[http://dx.doi.org/10.1200/JCO.2018.36.15_suppl.TPS4148]

[21] Chauhan, A.; Arnold, S.M.; Wu, J.; Nair, R.T.; Slone, S.A.; Van Meter Dressler, E.; Flynn, H.; Adams, V.R.; Weiss, H.; Evers, M.; Anthony, L.B. Clinical efficacy and toxicity data on phase I study of fosbretabulin in combination with everolimus in neuroendocrine tumors. *J. Clin. Oncol.,* **2019**.
[http://dx.doi.org/10.1200/JCO.2019.37.15_suppl.4114]

[22] Bahleda, R.; Sessa, C.; Del Conte, G. Phase I clinical and pharmacokinetic study of ombrabulin (AVE8062) combined with cisplatin/docetaxel or carboplatin/paclitaxel in patients with advanced solid tumors. *Invest. New Drugs,* **2014**, *32*(6), 1188-1196.
[http://dx.doi.org/10.1007/s10637-014-0119-0] [PMID: 24898305]

[23] Eskens, F A L.M.; Tresca, P.; Tosi, D. A phase I pharmacokinetic study of the vascular disrupting agent ombrabulin (AVE8062) and docetaxel in advanced solid tumours. *Br. J. Cancer,* **2014**, *110*(9), 2170-2177.
[http://dx.doi.org/10.1038/bjc.2014.137] [PMID: 24714750]

[24] Sessa, C.; Lorusso, P.; Tolcher, A. Phase I safety, pharmacokinetic and pharmacodynamic evaluation of the vascular disrupting agent ombrabulin (AVE8062) in patients with advanced solid tumors. *Clin. Cancer Res.,* **2013**, *19*(17), 4832-4842.
[http://dx.doi.org/10.1158/1078-0432.CCR-13-0427] [PMID: 23833302]

[25] Blay, J.Y.; Pápai, Z.; Tolcher, A.W. Ombrabulin plus cisplatin *versus* placebo plus cisplatin in patients with advanced soft-tissue sarcomas after failure of anthracycline and ifosfamide chemotherapy: a randomised, double-blind, placebo-controlled, phase 3 trial. *Lancet Oncol.,* **2015**, *16*(5), 531-540.
[http://dx.doi.org/10.1016/S1470-2045(15)70102-6] [PMID: 25864104]

[26] Cummings, J.; Zweifel, M.; Smith, N. Evaluation of cell death mechanisms induced by the vascular disrupting agent OXi4503 during a phase I clinical trial. *Br. J. Cancer,* **2012**, *106*(11), 1766-1771.
[http://dx.doi.org/10.1038/bjc.2012.165] [PMID: 22538971]

[27] Patterson, D.M.; Zweifel, M.; Middleton, M.R. Phase I clinical and pharmacokinetic evaluation of the vascular-disrupting agent OXi4503 in patients with advanced solid tumors. *Clin. Cancer Res.,* **2012**, *18*(5), 1415-1425.
[http://dx.doi.org/10.1158/1078-0432.CCR-11-2414] [PMID: 22235096]

[28] Rice, L.; Pampo, C.; Lepler, S.; Rojiani, A.M.; Siemann, D.W. Support of a free radical mechanism for enhanced antitumor efficacy of the microtubule disruptor OXi4503. *Microvasc. Res.,* **2011**, *81*(1), 44-51.
[http://dx.doi.org/10.1016/j.mvr.2010.10.003] [PMID: 20974154]

[29] Uckun, F.M.; Cogle, C.R.; Lin, T.L.; Qazi, S.; Trieu, V.N.; Schiller, G.; Watts, J.M. A phase 1B clinical study of combretastatin A1 diphosphate (OXi4503) and cytarabine (ARA-C) in combination (OXA) for patients with relapsed or refractory acute myeloid leukemia. *Cancers (Basel),* **2019**, *12*(1), 74.
[http://dx.doi.org/10.3390/cancers12010074] [PMID: 31888052]

[30] Kong, Y.; Smith, J.; Li, K.; Cui, J.; Han, J.; Hou, S.; Brown, M.L. Development of a novel near-infrared fluorescent theranostic combretastain A-4 analogue, YK-5-252, to target triple negative breast cancer. *Bioorg. Med. Chem.,* **2017**, *25*(7), 2226-2233.
[http://dx.doi.org/10.1016/j.bmc.2017.02.046] [PMID: 28284864]

[31] Doura, T.; Takahashi, K.; Ogra, Y.; Suzuki, N. Combretastatin A4-β-Galactosyl conjugates for ovarian cancer prodrug monotherapy. *ACS Med. Chem. Lett.,* **2017**, *8*(2), 211-214.
[http://dx.doi.org/10.1021/acsmedchemlett.6b00427] [PMID: 28197314]

[32] Hou, L.; Huang, W.; Cheng, J. The investigation and bioorthogonal anticancer activity enhancement of a triphenylphosphine-labile prodrug of seleno-combretastatin-4. *Chem. Commun. (Camb.),* **2020**, *56*(92), 14495-14498.
[http://dx.doi.org/10.1039/D0CC05498D] [PMID: 33150881]

[33] Wilson, W.R.; Hay, M.P. Targeting hypoxia in cancer therapy. *Nat. Rev. Cancer,* **2011**, *11*(6), 393-410.
[http://dx.doi.org/10.1038/nrc3064] [PMID: 21606941]

[34] Baran, N.; Konopleva, M. Molecular pathways: hypoxia-activated prodrugs in cancer therapy. *Clin. Cancer Res.,* **2017**, *23*(10), 2382-2390.
[http://dx.doi.org/10.1158/1078-0432.CCR-16-0895] [PMID: 28137923]

[35] Thomson, P.; Naylor, M.A.; Everett, S.A. Synthesis and biological properties of bioreductively targeted nitrothienyl prodrugs of combretastatin A-4. *Mol. Cancer Ther.*, **2006**, *5*(11), 2886-2894. [http://dx.doi.org/10.1158/1535-7163.MCT-06-0429] [PMID: 17121936]

[36] Winn, B.A.; Devkota, L.; Kuch, B. Bioreductively activatable prodrug conjugates of combretastatin A-1 and combretastatin A-4 as anticancer agents targeted toward tumor-associated hypoxia. *J. Nat. Prod.*, **2020**, *83*(4), 937-954. [http://dx.doi.org/10.1021/acs.jnatprod.9b00773] [PMID: 32196334]

[37] Zhang, K.; Chen, D.; Ma, K.; Wu, X.; Hao, H.; Jiang, S. NAD(P)H:Quinone Oxidoreductase 1 (NQO1) as a therapeutic and diagnostic target in cancer. *J. Med. Chem.*, **2018**, *61*(16), 6983-7003. [http://dx.doi.org/10.1021/acs.jmedchem.8b00124] [PMID: 29712428]

[38] Oh, E.T.; Park, H.J. Implications of NQO1 in cancer therapy. *BMB Rep.*, **2015**, *48*(11), 609-617. [http://dx.doi.org/10.5483/BMBRep.2015.48.11.190] [PMID: 26424559]

[39] Zhang, C.; Qu, Y.; Ma, X. NQO1-selective activated prodrugs of combretastatin A-4: Synthesis and biological evaluation. *Bioorg. Chem.*, **2020**, *103*, 104200. [http://dx.doi.org/10.1016/j.bioorg.2020.104200] [PMID: 32890998]

[40] Liu, W.; Liang, L.; Zhao, L. Synthesis and characterization of a photoresponsive doxorubicin/combretastatin A4 hybrid prodrug. *Bioorg. Med. Chem. Lett.*, **2019**, *29*(3), 487-490. [http://dx.doi.org/10.1016/j.bmcl.2018.12.017] [PMID: 30553736]

[41] Bio, M.; Rajaputra, P.; Nkepang, G.; Awuah, S.G.; Hossion, A.M.L.; You, Y. Site-specific and far-red-light-activatable prodrug of combretastatin A-4 using photo-unclick chemistry. *J. Med. Chem.*, **2013**, *56*(10), 3936-3942. [http://dx.doi.org/10.1021/jm400139w] [PMID: 23631389]

[42] Bio, M.; Rajaputra, P.; Nkepang, G.; You, Y. Far-red light activatable, multifunctional prodrug for fluorescence optical imaging and combinational treatment. *J. Med. Chem.*, **2014**, *57*(8), 3401-3409. [http://dx.doi.org/10.1021/jm5000722] [PMID: 24694092]

[43] Nkepang, G.; Bio, M.; Rajaputra, P.; Awuah, S.G.; You, Y. Folate receptor-mediated enhanced and specific delivery of far-red light-activatable prodrugs of combretastatin A-4 to FR-positive tumor. *Bioconjug. Chem.*, **2014**, *25*(12), 2175-2188. [http://dx.doi.org/10.1021/bc500376j] [PMID: 25351441]

[44] Pettit, G.R.; Toki, B.; Herald, D.L.; Verdier-Pinard, P.; Boyd, M.R.; Hamel, E.; Pettit, R.K. Antineoplastic agents. 379. Synthesis of phenstatin phosphate. *J. Med. Chem.*, **1998**, *41*(10), 1688-1695. [http://dx.doi.org/10.1021/jm970644q] [PMID: 9572894]

[45] Pettit, G.R.; Grealish, M.P.; Herald, D.L.; Boyd, M.R.; Hamel, E.; Pettit, R.K. Antineoplastic agents. 443. Synthesis of the cancer cell growth inhibitor hydroxyphenstatin and its sodium diphosphate prodrug. *J. Med. Chem.*, **2000**, *43*(14), 2731-2737. [http://dx.doi.org/10.1021/jm000045a] [PMID: 10893310]

[46] Messaoudi, S.; Tréguier, B.; Hamze, A. Isocombretastatins a *versus* combretastatins a: the forgotten isoCA-4 isomer as a highly promising cytotoxic and antitubulin agent. *J. Med. Chem.*, **2009**, *52*(14), 4538-4542. [http://dx.doi.org/10.1021/jm900321u] [PMID: 19530698]

[47] Hamze, A.; Alami, M.; Provot, O. Developments of isoCombretastatin A-4 derivatives as highly cytotoxic agents. *Eur. J. Med. Chem.*, **2020**, *190*, 112110. [http://dx.doi.org/10.1016/j.ejmech.2020.112110] [PMID: 32061961]

[48] Fürst, R.; Zupkó, I.; Berényi, Á.; Ecker, G.F.; Rinner, U. Synthesis and antitumor-evaluation of cyclopropyl-containing combretastatin analogs. *Bioorg. Med. Chem. Lett.*, **2009**, *19*(24), 6948-6951. [http://dx.doi.org/10.1016/j.bmcl.2009.10.064] [PMID: 19879758]

[49] Ty, N.; Pontikis, R.; Chabot, G.G.; Devillers, E.; Quentin, L.; Bourg, S.; Florent, J.C. Synthesis and

biological evaluation of enantiomerically pure cyclopropyl analogues of combretastatin A4. *Bioorg. Med. Chem.,* **2013**, *21*(5), 1357-1366.
[http://dx.doi.org/10.1016/j.bmc.2012.11.056] [PMID: 23369686]

[50] Malashchuk, A.; Chernykh, A.V.; Hurmach, V.V. Synthesis, biological evaluation, and modeling studies of 1,3-disubstituted cyclobutane-containing analogs of combretastatin A4. *J. Mol. Struct.,* **2020**, *1210*, 128025.
[http://dx.doi.org/10.1016/j.molstruc.2020.128025] [PMID: 32655187]

[51] Nowikow, C.; Fuerst, R.; Kauderer, M.; Dank, C. Synthesis and biological evaluation of cis-restrained carbocyclic combretastatin A-4 analogs: Influence of the ring size and saturation on cytotoxic properties. *Bioorg. Med. Chem.,* **2019**, *27*(19), 115032.
[http://dx.doi.org/10.1016/j.bmc.2019.07.048] [PMID: 31401010]

[52] Hadfield, J.A.; Gaukroger, K.; Hirst, N.; Weston, A.P.; Lawrence, N.J.; McGown, A.T. Synthesis and evaluation of double bond substituted combretastatins. *Eur. J. Med. Chem.,* **2005**, *40*(6), 529-541.
[http://dx.doi.org/10.1016/j.ejmech.2004.12.008] [PMID: 15922837]

[53] O'Boyle, N.M.; Carr, M.; Greene, L.M.; Bergin, O.; Nathwani, S.M.; McCabe, T.; Lloyd, D.G.; Zisterer, D.M.; Meegan, M.J. Synthesis and evaluation of azetidinone analogues of combretastatin A-4 as tubulin targeting agents. *J. Med. Chem.,* **2010**, *53*(24), 8569-8584.
[http://dx.doi.org/10.1021/jm101115u] [PMID: 21080725]

[54] Greene, L.M.; Wang, S.; O'Boyle, N.M.; Bright, S.A.; Reid, J.; Kelly, P.; Meegan, M.J.; Zisterer, D.M. Combretazet-3 a novel synthetic cis-stable combretastatin A-4- azetidinone hybrid with enhanced stability and therapeutic efficacy in colon cancer. *Oncol. Rep.,* **2013**, *29*(6), 2451-2458.
[http://dx.doi.org/10.3892/or.2013.2379] [PMID: 23564200]

[55] Odlo, K.; Hentzen, J.; dit Chabert, J.F.; Ducki, S.; Gani, O.A.B.S.M.; Sylte, I.; Skrede, M.; Flørenes, V.A.; Hansen, T.V. 1,5-Disubstituted 1,2,3-triazoles as cis-restricted analogues of combretastatin A-4: Synthesis, molecular modeling and evaluation as cytotoxic agents and inhibitors of tubulin. *Bioorg. Med. Chem.,* **2008**, *16*(9), 4829-4838.
[http://dx.doi.org/10.1016/j.bmc.2008.03.049] [PMID: 18396050]

[56] Odlo, K.; Fournier-Dit-Chabert, J.; Ducki, S.; Gani, O.A.B.S.M.; Sylte, I.; Hansen, T.V. 1,2,3-Triazole analogs of combretastatin A-4 as potential microtubule-binding agents. *Bioorg. Med. Chem.,* **2010**, *18*(18), 6874-6885.
[http://dx.doi.org/10.1016/j.bmc.2010.07.032] [PMID: 20708408]

[57] Akselsen, Ø.W.; Odlo, K.; Cheng, J.J.; Maccari, G.; Botta, M.; Hansen, T.V. Synthesis, biological evaluation and molecular modeling of 1,2,3-triazole analogs of combretastatin A-1. *Bioorg. Med. Chem.,* **2012**, *20*(1), 234-242.
[http://dx.doi.org/10.1016/j.bmc.2011.11.010] [PMID: 22137934]

[58] Mustafa, M.; Anwar, S.; Elgamal, F.; Ahmed, E.R.; Aly, O.M. Potent combretastatin A-4 analogs containing 1,2,4-triazole: Synthesis, antiproliferative, anti-tubulin activity, and docking study. *Eur. J. Med. Chem.,* **2019**, *183*, 111697.
[http://dx.doi.org/10.1016/j.ejmech.2019.111697] [PMID: 31536891]

[59] Stefański, T.; Mikstacka, R.; Kurczab, Design, synthesis, and biological evaluation of novel combretastatin A-4 thio derivatives as microtubule targeting agents. *Eur. J. Med. Chem.,* **2018**, *144*, 797-816.
[http://dx.doi.org/10.1016/j.ejmech.2017.11.050] [PMID: 29291446]

[60] Biersack, B.; Effenberger, K.; Schobert, R.; Ocker, M. Oxazole-bridged combretastatin A analogues with improved anticancer properties. *ChemMedChem,* **2010**, *5*(3), 420-427.
[http://dx.doi.org/10.1002/cmdc.200900477] [PMID: 20112324]

[61] Kaffy, J.; Pontikis, R.; Carrez, D.; Croisy, A.; Monneret, C.; Florent, J.C. Isoxazole-type derivatives related to combretastatin A-4, synthesis and biological evaluation. *Bioorg. Med. Chem.,* **2006**, *14*(12), 4067-4077.

[http://dx.doi.org/10.1016/j.bmc.2006.02.001] [PMID: 16510288]

[62] Wu, R.; Ding, W.; Liu, T.; Zhu, H.; Hu, Y.; Yang, B.; He, Q. XN05, a novel synthesized microtubule inhibitor, exhibits potent activity against human carcinoma cells *in vitro*. *Cancer Lett.,* **2009**, *285*(1), 13-22.
[http://dx.doi.org/10.1016/j.canlet.2009.04.042] [PMID: 19647933]

[63] Mahal, K.; Biersack, B.; Caysa, H.; Schobert, R.; Mueller, T. Combretastatin A-4 derived imidazoles show cytotoxic, antivascular, and antimetastatic effects based on cytoskeletal reorganisation. *Invest. New Drugs,* **2015**, *33*(3), 541-554.
[http://dx.doi.org/10.1007/s10637-015-0215-9] [PMID: 25678082]

[64] Hura, N.; Sawant, A.V.; Kumari, A.; Guchhait, S.K.; Panda, D. Combretastatin-inspired heterocycles as antitubulin anticancer agents. *ACS Omega,* **2018**, *3*(8), 9754-9769.
[http://dx.doi.org/10.1021/acsomega.8b00996] [PMID: 31459105]

[65] Romagnoli, R.; Oliva, P.; Salvador, M.K. Design, synthesis and biological evaluation of novel vicinal diaryl-substituted 1H-Pyrazole analogues of combretastatin A-4 as highly potent tubulin polymerization inhibitors. *Eur. J. Med. Chem.,* **2019**, *181*, 111577.
[http://dx.doi.org/10.1016/j.ejmech.2019.111577] [PMID: 31400707]

[66] Wang, C.; Yang, S.; Du, J.; Ni, J.; Wu, Y.; Wang, J.; Guan, Q.; Zuo, D.; Bao, K.; Wu, Y.; Zhang, W. Synthesis and bioevaluation of diarylpyrazoles as antiproliferative agents. *Eur. J. Med. Chem.,* **2019**, *171*, 1-10.
[http://dx.doi.org/10.1016/j.ejmech.2019.02.049] [PMID: 30901597]

[67] Zheng, S.; Zhong, Q.; Mottamal, M. Design, synthesis, and biological evaluation of novel pyridine-bridged analogues of combretastatin-A4 as anticancer agents. *J. Med. Chem.,* **2014**, *57*(8), 3369-3381.
[http://dx.doi.org/10.1021/jm500002k] [PMID: 24669888]

[68] Ashraf, M.; Shaik, T.B.; Malik, M.S. Design and synthesis of cis-restricted benzimidazole and benzothiazole mimics of combretastatin A-4 as antimitotic agents with apoptosis inducing ability. *Bioorg. Med. Chem. Lett.,* **2016**, *26*(18), 4527-4535.
[http://dx.doi.org/10.1016/j.bmcl.2016.06.044] [PMID: 27515320]

[69] Kumar, B.; Sharma, P.; Gupta, V.P.; Khullar, M.; Singh, S.; Dogra, N.; Kumar, V. Synthesis and biological evaluation of pyrimidine bridged combretastatin derivatives as potential anticancer agents and mechanistic studies. *Bioorg. Chem.,* **2018**, *78*, 130-140.
[http://dx.doi.org/10.1016/j.bioorg.2018.02.027] [PMID: 29554587]

[70] Nallamothu, R.; Wood, G.C.; Pattillo, C.B.; Scott, R.C.; Kiani, M.F.; Moore, B.M.; Thoma, L.A. A tumor vasculature targeted liposome delivery system for combretastatin A4: Design, characterization, and *in vitro* evaluation. *AAPS PharmSciTech,* **2006**, *7*(2), E7-E16.
[http://dx.doi.org/10.1208/pt070232] [PMID: 16796350]

[71] Pattillo, C.B.; Venegas, B.; Donelson, Radiation-guided targeting of combretastatin encapsulated immunoliposomes to mammary tumors. *Pharm. Res.,* **2009**, *26*(5), 1093-1100.
[http://dx.doi.org/10.1007/s11095-009-9826-1] [PMID: 19172383]

[72] Mico, V.; Charalambous, A.; Peyman, S.A.; Abou-Saleh, R.H.; Markham, A.F.; Coletta, P.L.; Evans, S.D. Evaluation of lipid-stabilised tripropionin nanodroplets as a delivery route for combretastatin A4. *Int. J. Pharm.,* **2017**, *526*(1-2), 547-555.
[http://dx.doi.org/10.1016/j.ijpharm.2017.05.009] [PMID: 28495582]

[73] Shen, Y.; Wu, L.; Qiu, L. Water-soluble combretastatin A4 phosphate orally delivered *via* composite nanoparticles with improved inhibition effect toward S180 tumors. *J. Pharm. Sci.,* **2017**, *106*(10), 3076-3083.
[http://dx.doi.org/10.1016/j.xphs.2017.05.031] [PMID: 28619603]

[74] Liu, Z.; Shen, N.; Tang, Z.; Zhang, D.; Ma, L.; Yang, C.; Chen, X. An eximious and affordable GSH stimulus-responsive poly(α-lipoic acid) nanocarrier bonding combretastatin A4 for tumor therapy. *Biomater. Sci.,* **2019**, *7*(7), 2803-2811.

[http://dx.doi.org/10.1039/C9BM00002J] [PMID: 31062006]

[75] Sumer Bolu, B.; Manavoglu Gecici, E.; Sanyal, R. Combretastatin A-4 conjugated antiangiogenic micellar drug delivery systems using dendron-polymer conjugates. *Mol. Pharm.,* **2016**, *13*(5), 1482-1490.
[http://dx.doi.org/10.1021/acs.molpharmaceut.5b00931] [PMID: 27019335]

[76] Sengupta, S.; Eavarone, D.; Capila, I.; Zhao, G.; Watson, N.; Kiziltepe, T.; Sasisekharan, R. Temporal targeting of tumour cells and neovasculature with a nanoscale delivery system. *Nature,* **2005**, *436*(7050), 568-572.
[http://dx.doi.org/10.1038/nature03794] [PMID: 16049491]

[77] Zhang, Y.; Wang, J.; Bian, D.; Zhang, X.; Zhang, Q. Targeted delivery of RGD-modified liposomes encapsulating both combretastatin A-4 and doxorubicin for tumor therapy: *In vitro* and *in vivo* studies. *Eur. J. Pharm. Biopharm.,* **2010**, *74*(3), 467-473.
[http://dx.doi.org/10.1016/j.ejpb.2010.01.002] [PMID: 20064608]

[78] Yang, T.; Wang, Y.; Li, Z. Targeted delivery of a combination therapy consisting of combretastatin A4 and low-dose doxorubicin against tumor neovasculature. *Nanomedicine,* **2012**, *8*(1), 81-92.
[http://dx.doi.org/10.1016/j.nano.2011.05.003] [PMID: 21664295]

[79] Wang, Z.; Chui, W.K.; Ho, P.C. Nanoparticulate delivery system targeted to tumor neovasculature for combined anticancer and antiangiogenesis therapy. *Pharm. Res.,* **2011**, *28*(3), 585-596.
[http://dx.doi.org/10.1007/s11095-010-0308-2] [PMID: 21057857]

[80] Wang, Y.; Chen, H.; Liu, Y. pH-sensitive pullulan-based nanoparticle carrier of methotrexate and combretastatin A4 for the combination therapy against hepatocellular carcinoma. *Biomaterials,* **2013**, *34*(29), 7181-7190.
[http://dx.doi.org/10.1016/j.biomaterials.2013.05.081] [PMID: 23791500]

[81] Yang, W.J.; Zhou, P.; Liang, L. Nanogel-incorporated injectable hydrogel for synergistic therapy based on sequential local delivery of combretastatin-A4 phosphate (CA4P) and doxorubicin (DOX). *ACS Appl. Mater. Interfaces,* **2018**, *10*(22), 18560-18573.
[http://dx.doi.org/10.1021/acsami.8b04394] [PMID: 29767951]

Medicinal Chemistry Lessons From Nature, 2022, *Vol. 1*, 145-172

CHAPTER 5

Natural Flavonoid and Chalcone Scaffolds as Leads for Synthetic Antitubercular Agents

Federico Appetecchia[1], **Mariangela Biava**[1] and **Giovanna Poce**[1,*]

[1] *Department of Chemistry and Technologies of Drug, Sapienza University of Rome, piazzale A. Moro 5, 00185 Rome, Italy*

Abstract: Tuberculosis is a leading cause of mortality and morbidity worldwide, claiming 1.2 million deaths (including 208 000 people with HIV) and 10 million new cases in 2019. Current treatment suffers from significant shortcomings such as length, dosage regimen, toxicity, and resistance development to currently used medicines. The emergence of multidrug-resistant tuberculosis and extensively drug-resistant tuberculosis is a major concern in controlling the disease. Therefore, there is an urgent need for new antitubercular drugs that are active against resistant strains, less toxic, and that act upon a different mechanism than the current drugs. Natural products can be a great source for the development of new anti-tubercular agents because of their rich chemical diversity with privileged antimicrobial activity. In this chapter, we focus our attention on flavonoids and chalcone scaffolds as leads for the development of new antitubercular agents.

Keywords: Antimicrobials, Antimycobacterials, Catechins, Chalcones, Coumarin, Epigallocatechin gallate, Flavanones, Flavonoids, Formononetin, Isoflavones, Liquiritigenin, Multi-drug resistant tuberculosis, *Mycobacterium tuberculosis*, Natural products, Quinolines, Secondary metabolites, Tuberculosis.

INTRODUCTION

Tuberculosis (TB) is a leading cause of mortality and morbidity worldwide, claiming 1.2 million deaths (including 208 000 people with HIV) and 10 million new cases in 2019. The annual number of TB deaths is falling globally (between 2015 and 2019 was 14%) less than halfway towards the 2020 milestone of a 35% reduction between 2015 and 2020 [1]. *Mycobacterium tuberculosis* (*Mtb*), the causative agent of TB, can survive within the host, switching between active and latent disease states and evading the immune system defenses. The current frontline TB therapy consists of a co-administration for 2 months of isoniazid

* **Corresponding Author Giovanna Poce:** Department of Chemistry and Technologies of Drug, Sapienza University of Rome, piazzale A. Moro 5, 00185 Rome, Italy; Tel.: +39 06 49913593; fax: +39 06 499133333; E-mail: giovanna.poce@uniroma1.it

(INH), rifampicin (RIF), ethambutol (EMB), and pyrazinamide (PZA) (Fig. **1**) followed by RIF and INH administration for 4 months. This treatment suffers from significant shortcomings such as length, dosage regimen, toxicity, and resistance development to currently used medicines. The emergence of multidrug-resistant TB (MDR-TB), defined as TB that is resistant to INH and RIF, and extensively drug-resistant TB (XDR-TB), classified as being resistant to INH and RIF in addition to any fluoroquinolone and injectable second-line drugs, is a major concern. The World Health Organization (WHO) estimates that in 2018 there were 484 000 new cases with resistance to rifampicin (RIF) (RR-TB), of which 78% had MDR-TB, and 8.5% of MDR-TB cases had XDR-TB [1].

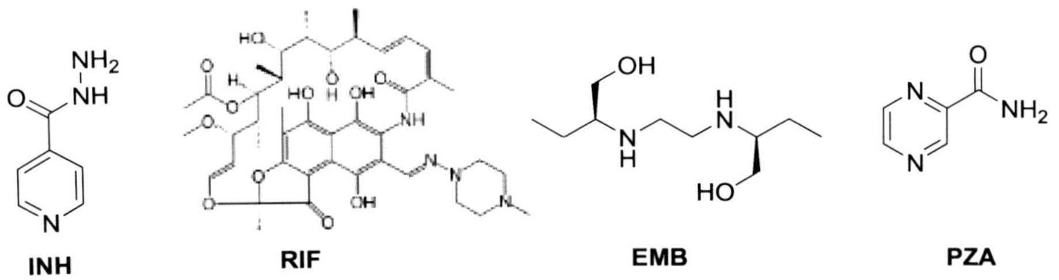

Fig. (1). Chemical structures of the frontline medicines isoniazid (INH), rifampicin (RIF), ethambutol (EMB), and pyrazinamide (PZA).

Therefore, there is an urgent need for new anti-TB drugs active against MDR and XDR strains, less toxic, and that act upon a different mechanism than the current drugs. Except for bedaquiline [2] and pretomanid [3] (Fig. **2**) approved by the Food and Drug Administration (FDA) in 2012 and 2019, respectively, and delamanid [4] (Fig. **2**)., approved by the European Medicines Agency (EMA) in 2014, very few molecules make it through the stringent bottlenecks of TB drug discovery.

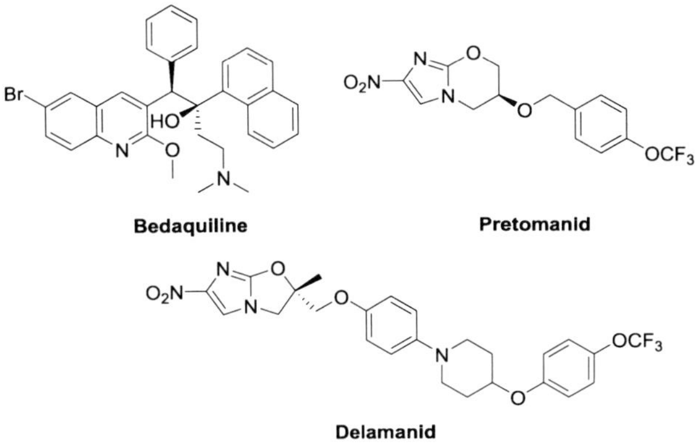

Fig. (2). Chemical structures of bedaquiline, pretomanid and delamanid.

Unfortunately, TB drug discovery was completely neglected for a long period of time, and only in the last two decades research all around the globe led to the discovery of new molecules with anti-TB potential [5, 6]. The majority of drugs that are currently being evaluated in clinical trials were identified using phenotypic screening. Indeed, most of the compounds identified by high-throughput screening campaigns and target-based drug design approaches failed to demonstrate activity against *Mtb* in a whole-cell screening assay. Natural products can be a great source for the development of new anti-tubercular agents because of their rich chemical diversity with privileged antimicrobial activity. In this chapter, we will focus our attention on flavonoids and chalcone scaffolds as leads for the development of new antitubercular agents.

FLAVONOIDS

Flavonoids are polyphenolic natural products commonly found in plants and fungi. A significant amount of literature is available that reports the antimycobacterial potential of naturally occurring flavonoids [7].

Epigallocatechin gallate (EGCG, (Fig. **3**) the main polyphenol found in green tea, showed several biological activities such as reducing inflammation and oxidative-stress [8] as well as anti-carcinogenic [9] and antimicrobial activity [10 - 12]. Unfortunately, EGCG showed low bioavailability and poor pharmacokinetics because of its rapid biotransformation and degradation after oral or parenteral administration in animal studies and the good *in vitro* results could not be translated into *in vivo* tests [13 - 15]. Banerjee *et al.* prepared triazolyl-flavonoids hybrids by combining the catechin/epicatechin fragment to a 1,4-triazole compounds **1**-**4**, (Fig. **3**) moiety as inhibitors of the FabG4 enzyme of *Mtb*. The role of the different fragments on the activity was evaluated building up structure-activity relationship (SAR) studies by substituting fragments linked to the 1- and 4-positions of the triazole ring with less interacting moieties.

Compounds **1** and **2** showed an inhibition constant (K*i*) of 3.97 and 0.88 μM, respectively, against FabG4 and a minimum inhibitory concentration (MIC) of 20 and 5 μg/ml against *M. smegmatis*, proving that both the catechin/epicatechin and the galloyl fragments play a crucial role in the inhibition potency [16].

Gaur *et al.* prepared a series of semi-synthetic derivatives of liquiritigenin LTG, (Fig. **4**) a flavanone found in a variety of plants, including *Glycyrrhiza glabra* that showed a MIC of 25 μg/ml against *Mtb* [17]. Plant extracted LTG was derivatized to four analogues: LTG-oxime (**5**), LTG-7,4'-diacetate (**6**), LTG-4'-acetate (**7**) and LTG-7,4'-dibenzoate (**8**) (Fig. **4**) Only the oxime **5** and the mono-acetate **7** showed some activity against *Mtb* with a MIC of 25 μg/ml, comparable to that of LTG, proving that the hydroxyl group at position 7 is essential for the activity.

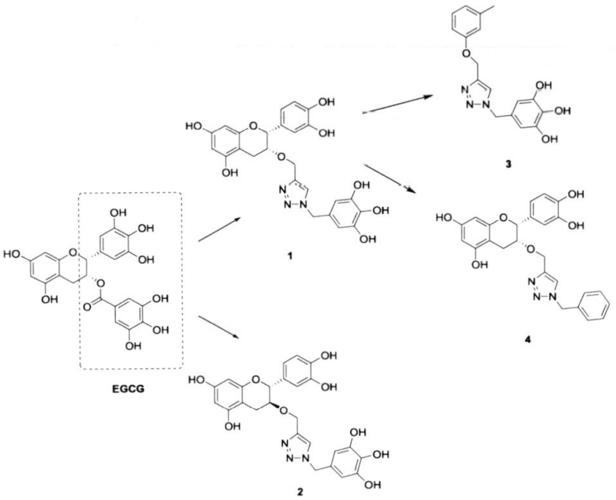

Fig. (3). Chemical structures of epigallocatechin gallate (EGCG) and compounds **1**-**4**.

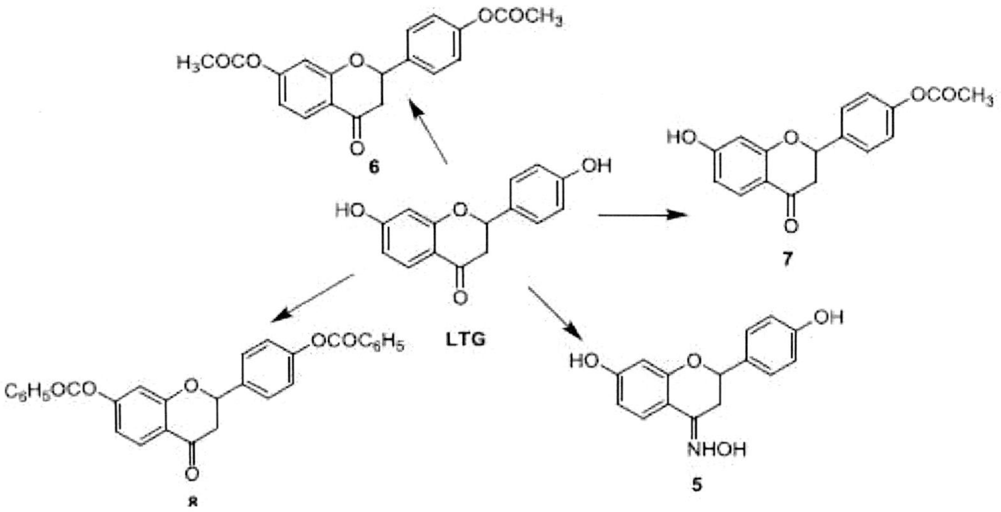

Fig. (4). Chemical structures of liquiritigenin (LTG), LTG-oxime (**5**), LTG-7,4'-diacetate (**6**), LTG-4-acetate (**7**) and LTG-7,4'-dibenzoate (**8**).

Formononetin, an *O*-methylated isoflavone that predominantly occurs in leguminous plants and Fabaceae, presented anti-infective activities as well as showed strong multi-drug resistance reversal effects by inhibiting the P-gp efflux pump [18, 19]. In 2015, Mutai *et al.* presented SARs studies on a series of formononetin derivatives built up by modifying both rings A and B as well as the benzopyranone linker. All modifications on formononetin led to a significant drop in activity, except for the introduction of a *tert*-butyl substituent on ring B, which improved the activity from 88% to 95% inhibition at 10 μM (Fig. **5**) [20].

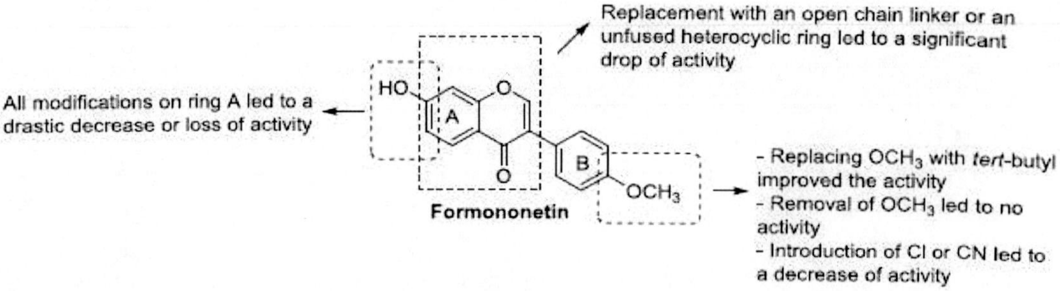

Fig. (5). Chemical structure of formononetin and SARs of its analogues.

Chalcones

Chalcone (1,3-diphenyl-2-propen-1-one) is a common and relatively simple scaffold found in many naturally occurring compounds. Chalcones exist in nature mainly as trans (*E*) isomers since cis (*Z*) isomers are thermodynamically less stable due to the strong steric effects between the carbonyl group and the A-ring (Fig. **6**) Chalcone scaffold is characterized by the presence of an α,β-unsaturated carbonyl system between two phenyl groups. As such, within cells, it can act as a Michael acceptor since the β carbon of the double bond is highly susceptible to the attack of nucleophiles, thus yielding toxic effects upon the formation of macromolecular adducts. On the other hand, this scaffold can afford a multiplicity of substitutions that can lead to analogs with reduced toxicity and certain therapeutic activities [21, 22]. Because of their relatively simple and small structure and because they are Michael acceptors, chalcones exhibit a broad spectrum of biological activities. Indeed, several chalcone-based compounds have been approved for clinical uses, such as metochalcone marketed as a choleretic drug and sofalcone, used as an antiulcer and mucoprotective drug [23].

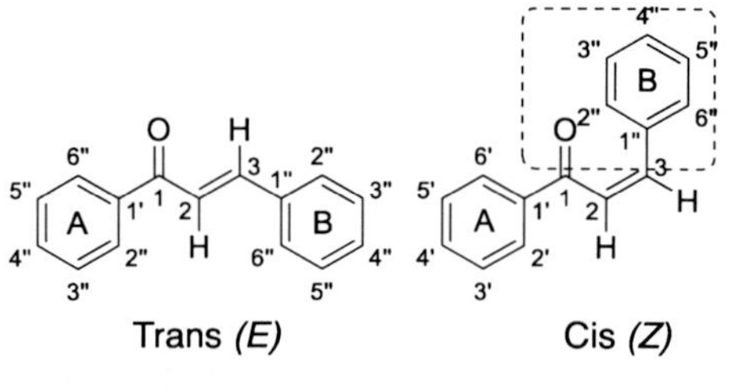

Fig. (6). Trans (*E*) and Cis (*Z*) chalcones.

Chalcones can be synthesized *via* diverse simple protocols. The general synthesis is represented by Claisen-Schmidt condensation in acid or basic condition, but other routes with different catalysts and conditions have also been used: photo-fires rearrangement, Meyer-Schuster rearrangement, Julia-Kocienski olefination, Mukaiyama-aldol reaction, one pot synthesis, Suzuki-coupling, Heck reaction,

Wittig reaction, Friedel-Crafts acylation with cinnamoyl chloride, deamination of aziridine, debromination of vicinal dibromides, oxidation of benzylic alcohols, dehydrogenation and deoxygenation [21, 24]. The high versatility of the chalcone scaffold has encouraged medicinal chemists to synthesize a large variety of biologically active compounds.

Simple-substituted Chalcones

Early studies on the effect of simple substitutions on the chalcone scaffold were performed by Lin *et al.*, who analyzed 25 chalcones to evaluate their inhibitory activity against *Mtb* H37Rv. Overall, chalcones devoided of halogens exhibited higher MICs compared to those with a halogen substitution, inferring that a series of halogenated derivatives could be designed in order to develop new antitubercular hits [25].

More recently, B-ring fluoro-substituted chalcones were designed and synthesized by Burmaoglu *et al.* using a base-catalyzed Claisen-Schmidt condensation and then screened against *Mtb* H37Rv. Chalcones presenting a fluorine atom at both positions 2 and 3 conjugated to a trimethoxy substitution on ring A showed increased anti-tubercular activity, with IC50 values <16.760 μM, which are comparable to the antitubercular drugs INH and EMB used as controls. When the B ring is 3-F or 2,5-difluoro substituted, the antitubercular activity becomes moderate Table **1** [26]. Molecular docking studies on these fluoro-substituted chalcones and others on DprE1, an essential mycobacterial enzyme involved in cell wall metabolism, marked the importance of the fluorine atom for such interaction and gave a good starting point to design novel DprE1 inhibitors [27].

Additional series of chalcones were synthesized to develop new drugs endowed with anti-inflammatory and antimycobacterial properties. Generally, all the studied chalcones met the pharmacokinetic parameters through *in silico* studies, and eight of them proved to be able to inhibit the growth of both *M. bovis* BCG and *Mtb* H37Rv strains in bacterial cultures and in infected macrophages. Among them, two halogenated chalcones, namely (*E*)-3-(4-chlorophenyl)-1-pheny-prop-2-en-1-one and (*E*)-1-(4-bromophenyl)-3-phenylprop-2-en-1-one, were found to have a MIC50 against *Mtb* H37Rv respectively of 13.0 ± 3.3 μM and 12.7 ± 1.9 μM. In addition, these two compounds showed activity against the hypervirulent *Mtb* strain M299 as well (MIC50 = 18.37 ± 3.9 μM and 11.7 ± 3.4 μM) Table **1** [28].

A series of 2-hydroxy chalcone analogs were also screened against *Mtb* H37Rv to prove the importance of the hydroxyl substitution on the specificity of the interaction with the two enzymes MtbPtpA and MtbPtpB, two mycobacterial tyrosine-phosphatases that mediate the extracellular signaling pathways leading to endorse the infection. The antitubercular results confirmed the improvement of the activity for the methoxy-substituted chalcones (at both rings) as well as for the halogenated ones at position 2 of the B ring [29].

InhA, an enzyme involved in the biosynthesis of mycolic acids that constitute a major component of mycobacterial cell walls, was also identified as a key target of some chalcones. This may indicate that different functional groups on chalcones play an important role in their mode of action. Recently, Anagani *et al.* evaluated the activity of 15 simple-substituted chalcones bearing both *meta*- and *para*- methoxyl groups on the A ring against *M. bovis* BCG and validated their direct inhibition against InhA. To do that, inhibition of mycolic acid biosynthesis was investigated using autoradiography thin layer chromatography (TLC) and confirmed by docking studies and activity assays against *M. bovis* BCG strains overexpressing InhA. Direct inhibition was further corroborated by using ligand binding tryptophan fluorescence assay. Interestingly, it was observed that chalcones, where all the R substituents on the B ring are hydrogens, were the most potent ones (MIC = 6.25 μg/ml) and with an acceptable safety profile. Such behavior indicated that more than electronic factors, the activity is dependent on the derived conformation of the molecule upon the halogen position [30].

A summary of the activities of the most active compounds prepared by introducing small substituents on both rings, A and B, is reported in Table **1**.

Table 1. Simple substitutions for favorable anti-TB activity.

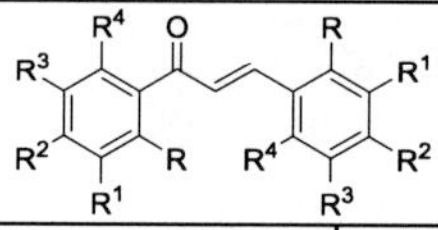

Ring A					Ring B					MIC[a] (μg/ml)
R	R^1	R^2	R^3	R^4	R	R^1	R^2	R^3	R^4	
OH								Cl		20.3
OH								I		31.5
OCH_3		OCH_3		OCH_3	F					ND
OCH_3		OCH_3		OCH_3		F				ND
		Br								43.9 ± 6.6[b]
							Cl			53.1 ± 13.5[b]
OCH_3	CH_3	OCH_3	CH_3	OH			OCH_3			1.6
OCH_3	CH_3	OCH_3	CH_3	OH	OCH_3	OCH_3	OCH_3			1.6
OCH_3	CH_3	OCH_3	CH_3	OH			$N(CH_3)_2$			1.6
OCH_3	CH_3	OCH_3	CH_3	OH		OEt	OCH_3			1.6
OCH_3	CH_3	OCH_3	CH_3	OH	F					6.25
OCH_3	CH_3	OCH_3	CH_3	OH	Cl					6.25
		SO_2CH_3								50

(Table 1) cont.....

Ring A					Ring B					MIC[a] (μg/ml)
R	R^1	R^2	R^3	R^4	R	R^1	R^2	R^3	R^4	
		SO_2CH_3					NO_2			50
		OCH_3	OCH_3							6.25[c]
		OCH_3	OCH_3				Br			12.5[c]
		OCH_3	OCH_3		Cl					12.5[c]

[a] MIC obtained against *Mtb* H37Rv strain; [b] MIC value has been converted from μM to μg/ml; [c] MIC obtained against *M. bovis* BCG; ND = Not determined.

In conclusion, while halogens at the *ortho*- and *meta*-positions of the A ring are not well tolerated, hydrophobic and/or hydrogen bond acceptor groups at the A ring are devoided of improved activity. Instead, the B ring tolerates polarizable groups. These results agree with the quantitative structure activity relationship (QSAR) studies conducted by Gomes *et al.*, although they speculated decreased activity upon any substitutions on the B ring [31].

Heteroaryl and Hybrid Chalcones

The antitubercular potential of chalcones has been widely explored using molecular modification strategies such as heteroaryl substitutions, bioisosterism and molecular hybridization. The replacement with cyclic functional moieties has involved both the double bond of the enone system and the two phenyl rings. On the whole, these approaches led to design compounds exhibiting improved potency, selectivity, and lower toxicity than the parent chalcones [21, 32].

Pyrazoline-based chalcones have been widely explored as antitubercular compounds [33 - 35]. The introduction of a five-membered heterocyclic ring between the two phenyl rings does not cause a significant change in the length of the molecule and may be ideal for drug effectiveness. Generally, the synthetic method for the preparation of pyrazoline-based chalcones goes *via* the cyclization of the double bond of the enone system with hydrazines (Fig. **7**).

Ahmad *et al.* synthesized pyrazoline derivatives by condensing either phenyl hydrazine or the antitubercular drug INH with chalcones prepared from paracetamol in an alkaline medium (Claisen-Schmidt reaction). Among the prepared compounds, the isoniazid-pyrazolines bearing either a 4-Cl, a 2,4-Cl or a 4-NO2 substituent on the phenyl ring compounds **9-11**, (Fig. **8**) showed good activities against *Mtb* with a MIC value of 3.12 μg/ml, which was even better than the standard drug streptomycin (MIC = 6.25 μg/ml) Table **2.** [36].

A series of *N*-phenyl-3-(4-fluorophenyl)-4-substituted pyrazoles were synthesized by Khunt *et al.* and tested *in vitro* against *Mtb* H37Rv. From this study emerged that the introduction of substituted pyrazole and pyrimidine rings at position 4 of the chalcone nucleus would lead to molecules with potent antitubercular activity compounds **12** and **13**, (Fig. **7**) with IC50 ranging from 0.47 to 118.0 μM Table **2**. A 3D-QSAR study was then performed using CoMFA and CoMSIA models to correlate the chemical structures with the biological activity to predict the activities of different analogues [37].

Table 2. Substitutions and activity against *Mtb* H37Rv of compounds 9-15.

Compound	R	MIC (μg/ml)	Assay
9	4-Cl	3.12	Agar dilution
10	2,4-Cl	3.12	Agar dilution
11	4-NO_2	3.12	Agar dilution
12	Ph-OH	0.37[a]	BACTEC 460 system
13	Ph	4.05[a]	BACTEC 460 system
14	4-F	12.5	Agar dilution
15	4-Br	12.5	Agar dilution

[a] MIC_{90}.

Other QSAR analyses using the SQ-MLR model were carried out by Gupta *et al.* on different nitro-chalcone derivatives, including pyrazoline-based chalcones. All derivatives bearing electron-withdrawing groups on ring B showed increased activity against *Mtb* H37Rv. Pyrazoline derivatives (compounds **14** and **15** showed MIC values of 12.5 μg/ml, Table **2**.) proved increased potency when compared to isoxazole and pyrimidine derivatives, however, it was not sufficient to overcome that of some simple-substituted chalcones [38].

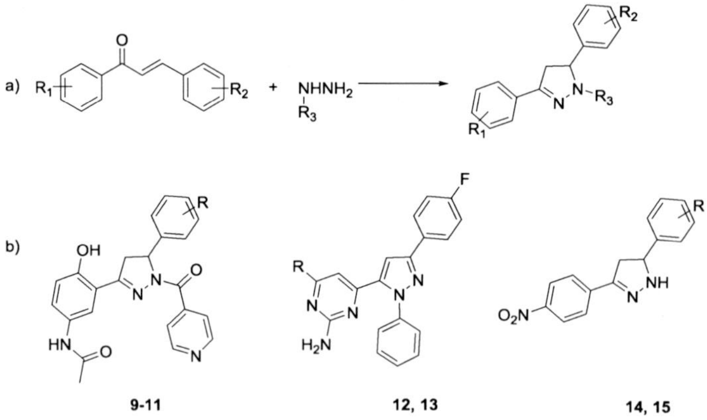

Fig. (7). a) Synthetic pathway for isoniazid-pyrazolines. **b)** chemical structures of compounds **9-15**.

In tuberculosis research, quinoline appears to be a promising moiety for drug development and novel chalcone-pyrazoline hybrids have been developed [5, 39]. In a study carried out by Rao *et al.*, among 42 quinoline-based compounds, pyrazoline analogs were obtained by conjugation with the quinoline nucleus. Quinoline-pyrazoline conjugates were synthesized by reacting the opportune hydrazine with the chalcone formed after condensation between the 4-substitute--2-methyl-3-acetylquinoline and substituted benzaldehydes. Overall, all the synthesized compounds displayed good ADME parameters and interesting activity with MIC ranging from 4 µg/ml (compound **16**, (Fig. **8**) to 64 µg/ml against both *Mtb* H37Rv and the rifampicin-resistant strains (rRif) Table **3**., meaning that also the quinoline plays an important role in *Mtb* infection control as suggested from previous studies. SAR studies indicated that the 4-methyl unit on the quinoline is favorable for the anti-tubercular activity and a fluorine atom is preferred at the *meta* position of the aromatic ring, while electron donating groups like -OCH_3 are more favorable at the *para* position. Furthermore, the most promising compounds were evaluated for their toxicity on MRC-5 lung fibroblast cells and positive results were obtained [40].

Recently, Kumar *et al.* [41] evaluated the antitubercular activity of 32 acrylic pyrazole-quinoline and acrylic pyrazole-coumarin chalcones synthesized by multiple-step reaction. Pyrazole intermediates were first synthesized and, prior to the Claisen-Schmidt condensation reaction with quinoline/coumarin derivatives, the Vilsmeier-Haack reaction was used to formylate position 4 of the pyrazole ring. Using the microplate Alamar Blue assay (MABA) method, Kumar's group identified two pyrazole-coumarin and one pyrazole-quinoline derivative (**17**-**19**, (Fig. **8**). showing MIC of 3.125 µg/ml and others with MICs ranging from 6.25 µg/ml to 12.5 µg/ml *versus Mtb* H37Rv strain. SAR analysis revealed that substituents like methyl and hydroxyl groups at the *para* position of the phenyl ring and substituents like –Cl and –Br at the sixth position of the coumarin ring were the most acceptable ones for antitubercular activity [41]. Molecular docking of the active compounds revealed good binding energy with the DprE1 enzyme, an interaction proposed by other authors in an antecedent paper during the analysis of the mode of action of some chalcones [27]. From this study, coumarin appears to play an important role in the interaction of these derivatives. Other coumarin derivatives were extensively studied for their interesting pharmacological properties in tuberculosis drug discovery. Several efforts have been made to synthesize coumarin-chalcone hybrids to be employed as antituberculars [42, 43]. For instance, Ahmad *et al.*, acknowledging the importance of lipophilicity in tuberculosis drugs and the influence of structural flexibility in protein interaction, investigated the antitubercular potential of a series of conformationally restricted chalcones hosting a coumarin nucleus. Compounds **20** and **21**, bearing amino alkyl groups at the *para* position of ring B

(Fig. **8**) showed MIC values of 3.5 μg/ml and 7.5 μg/ml, respectively, and were reported to be sufficiently selective towards *Mtb* being nontoxic *in vitro* Table **3**. [44].

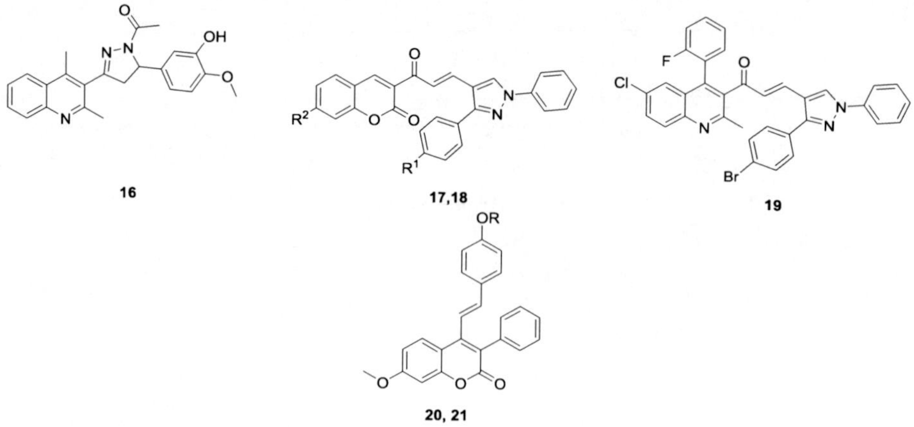

Fig. (8). Chemical structures of compounds **16-21**.

Table 3. Substitutions and activity against *Mtb* H37Rv of compounds 16-21.

Compound	**R**	**MIC[a] (μg/mL)**	**Assay**
16		4	Agar dilution
17	R^1= -CH_3; R^2 = -OCH_3	3.125	MABA
18	R^1 = -OH; R^2 = -H	3.125	MABA
19		3.125	MABA
20	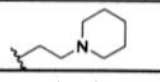	3.5	BACTEC 460
21	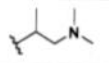	7.5	BACTEC 460

[a] MIC obtained against *Mtb* H37Rv strain.

Very potent compounds were obtained in a study carried out by Pallaepati *et al.* that evaluated a series of isoxazole appended 1-carboxamido-4,5-dihydro-1*H*-pyrazoles. Like pyrazole, isoxazole represents an important heterocyclic ring to develop anti-tubercular drugs, as seen for cycloserine and terizidone (both used in second line therapy). Therefore, Pallaepati *et al.* developed new molecules containing both isoxazole and pyrazoline moieties that could resemble INH and cycloserine by condensing isoxazolyl methoxy-substituted chalcones with semicarbazide. The majority of compounds showed enhanced activity than the respective chalcones and it was observed that the most potent derivatives **22**, **23** MIC= 0.1 μg/ml; INH MIC= 0.25 μg/ml, Table **4**. contained the concomitant presence of methoxyl groups and halogens (-Cl, -F) on the phenyl ring (Fig. **9**) Furthermore, both compounds resulted to be safe in normal human cell lines (IC_{50} > 40 μg/ml, Table **4.**), thus emerging as potential leads for antitubercular activity [45].

Table 4. Substitutions and activity against *Mtb* H37Rv of compounds 22-24.

Compound	R	MIC[a] (μg/mL)	Assay
22	R= -F; R^1 = $-OCH_3$; R^2= $-OCH_3$; R^3= -H; R^4= -H	0.1	MABA
23	R= -Cl; R^1 = -H; R^2= $-OCH_3$; R^3= -H; R^4= $-OCH_3$	0.1	MABA
24	R= $-OCH_3$; R^1= -H; R^2= $-OCH_3$; R^3= -H; R^4= $-OCH_3$	0.25	MABA

[a] MIC obtained against *Mtb* H37Rv strain.

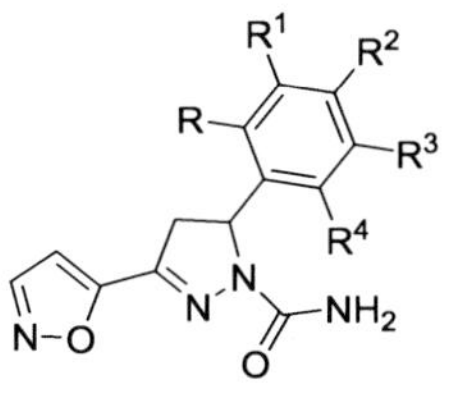

22-24

Fig. (9). Chemical structures of compounds **22-24**.

Recently, encouraging results came from the antimycobacterial evaluation of a new series of naphthyl chalcones and the corresponding pyrazoline derivatives, which showed MICs in the micromolar range. Particularly, compound **25** with 2-hydroxy-5-bromophenyl substitution (Fig. **10**) was the most potent one with a MIC of 6.25 μM (MIC_{INH} = 5.86 μM), and it was found to be nontoxic and mildly toxic to breast cancer and ovarian cells, respectively. Additionally, the predicted physicochemical values indicated that all the synthesized molecules fulfilled the criteria of Lipinski's rule of five, inferring that they possessed drug-likeness behavior [46]. Naphthyl chalcone-based hybrid molecules were already proposed as promising antitubercular agents by Chiaradia *et al.* that also explored the underlying mechanism of action. In their studies, naphthyl-chalcones proved to be competitive and selective inhibitors of PtpA and PtpB [47, 48], proteins belonging to the protein tyrosine-phosphatases (PTPs) family involved in the control of the phosphorylation state of tyrosines and important for *Mtb* pathogenesis [49].

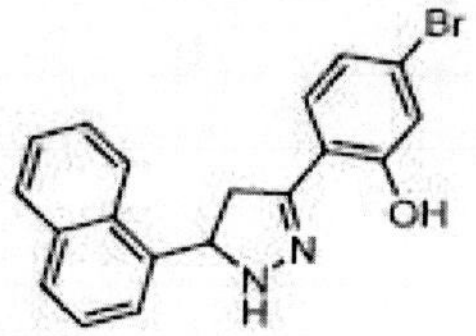

25

Fig. (10). Chemical structure of compound **25**.

Quinoxalines bearing a benzene ring fused with a pyrazine ring have been widely explored for their antitubercular potential [50 - 52]. Desai *et al.* were the first to synthesize quinoxalinyl chalcone hybrid scaffolds and to explore their mechanism of action against *Mtb*. Through molecular docking studies, they speculated an inhibitory action of this class of compounds against InhA [53]. However, Muradás *et al.* contended that the evidence of the mechanism of action was not conclusive since there was no inhibition of mycolic acid synthesis and further studies were needed. Particularly, Muradás *et al.* [54] performed a pre-clinical evaluation of 16 quinoxaline-derived chalcones differing in substituents on the phenyl ring. Six of them, mostly methoxylated on the phenyl ring, inhibited the growth of *Mtb* H37Rv with MIC values ranging from 3.13 µg/ml to 12.5 µg/ml Table **5.** Compound **26** (Fig. **11**) was the most potent one even against four drug-resistant clinical isolates (MICs between 1.56 µg/ml and 3.135 µg/ml, Table **5.**) and was subjected to deeper analysis [54]. Precisely, **26** demonstrated a synergistic effect in combination with moxifloxacin (FICI < 0.5) and to be not mutagenic or exhibiting genotoxic effects. However, significant inhibition of an important CYP450 enzyme isoform (CYP1A2) was observed through both *in silico* and *in vitro* studies [54].

Table 5. Substitutions and activity against *Mtb* H37Rv of compounds 26-29.

Compound	R	MIC[a] (µg/ml)	Assay
26	R= -OCH_3; R^1= -H; R^2= -H; R^3= -OCH_3; R^4= -H	3.13	REMA
27	R= -H; R^1= -OCH_3; R^2= -OCH_3; R^3= -OCH_3; R^4= -H	6.25	REMA
28	R= -H; R^1= - OCH_3; R^2= -H; R^3= -H; R^4= -H	5	REMA
29		2	Broth dilution

[a] MIC obtained against *Mtb* H37Rv strain.

Interesting data were also obtained by quinoxaline-1,4-di-*N*-oxide analogs. Particularly, it was observed that quinoxaline-1,4-di-*N*-oxide suffers from a bioreduction process under hypoxic conditions, ideal behavior in cases of tuberculous granulomas where the concentration of oxygen is very low [55, 56]. In an effort to develop new antitubercular drugs, Veliz *et al.* 51 found the quinoxaline-1,4-di-*N*-oxide–chalcone hybrid **29** (Fig. **11**) among 10 chalcone candidates to exhibit antibacterial activity at low concentrations. From a primary screening against *Mtb* H37Rv strain, it was observed that the *para* phenyl substitutions could significantly affect the results, with an electron withdrawing group to be preferred. **29** showed a MIC value of 2 µg/ml, which was 4- and 8-fold higher than derivatives with no substituent or electron donating group (-CH3) at the *para* position, respectively. Further analysis on INH-, RIF- and OFX-*Mtb* resistant strains and on *Mtb*-infected macrophages showed a significant inhibition rate, suggesting a different mechanism of action and confirming the great interest in this family of compounds [51]. (Fig. **11**) summarizes SARs of quinoxaline-derived chalcones.

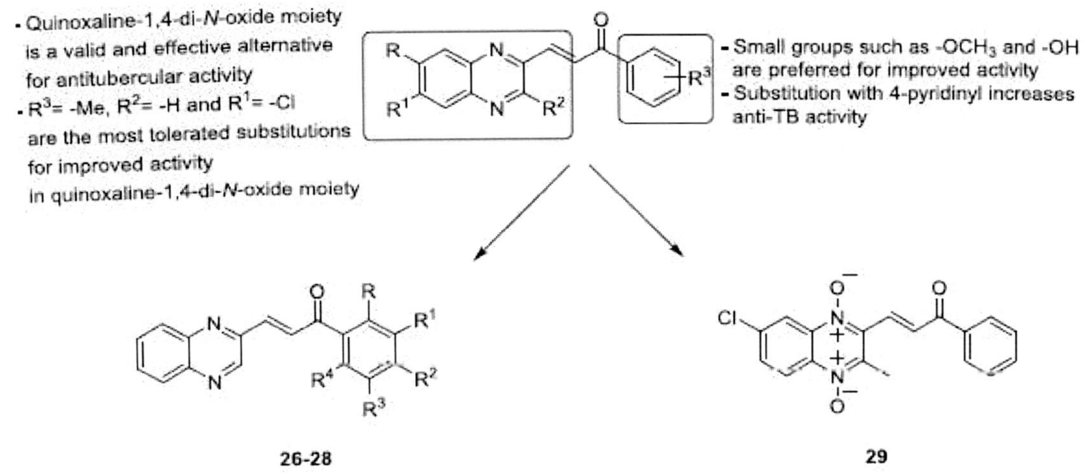

Fig. (11). SARs of quinoxaline-derived chalcones.

Several other nitrogen containing heterocycles fused to chalcones have been explored, such as a novel series of 2,4,6-trisubstituted-1,3,5-triazine-chalcone hybrid molecules synthesized and analyzed *in vitro* against *Mtb* H37Rv. Screening data revealed that the potency was modulated by substitutions on the phenyl ring, with considerable activity observed when halogens and some electron withdrawing or electron donating groups such as $-NO_2$ and $-OCH_3$ were present. Specially, the difluoro-substituted compound **30** (Fig. **12**). proved to be the most potent one with a MIC of 3.125 µg/ml Table **6**. [57].

Marrapu *et al.* [58] evaluated the anti-mycobacterial activity both *in vitro* and *in vivo* of aryloxy azolyl (imidazole or triazole) chalcones. From a series of 27 compounds bearing an imidazole/triazole moiety along with aryloxy/benzyloxy groups, 10 of them exhibited good MICs (in the range of 0.78-3.12 µg/ml, Table **6.**) and were further characterized. Cytotoxicity evaluation against mammalian cell line and mouse-bone marrow macrophages and *ex vivo* studies against intracellular bacilli identified two imidazolyl-based compounds (**31** and **32**, (Fig. **12**) showing the best profile. SAR evaluation suggested that chalcones with 4-imidazolyl moiety and benzyloxy group were more active than their triazolyl counterparts or than compounds with aryloxy groups. However, *in vivo* tests revealed that only compound **32** could be considered a lead candidate for optimization studies since it displayed an inhibition rate of 40% in infected mice [58].

A series of chalcone derivatives embedded with pyrido[1,2-*a*]imidazole, an extensively explored nucleus in this field, were found to be potent derivatives against *Mtb* H37Rv strain showing MIC values between 3.12 µg/ml and 25 µg/ml Table **6.** From screening and cytotoxicity data emerged that three butylamino-imidazo[1,2-*a*]pyridine chalcone derivatives **33-35**, (Fig. **12**) exhibited the best drug-profile since they displayed higher selectivity and safety values compared to cyclohexylamino-imidazo[1,2-*a*]pyridine chalcone derivatives with retained potency (3.12 µg/ml), hence could be promising antitubercular candidates to be further validated [59].

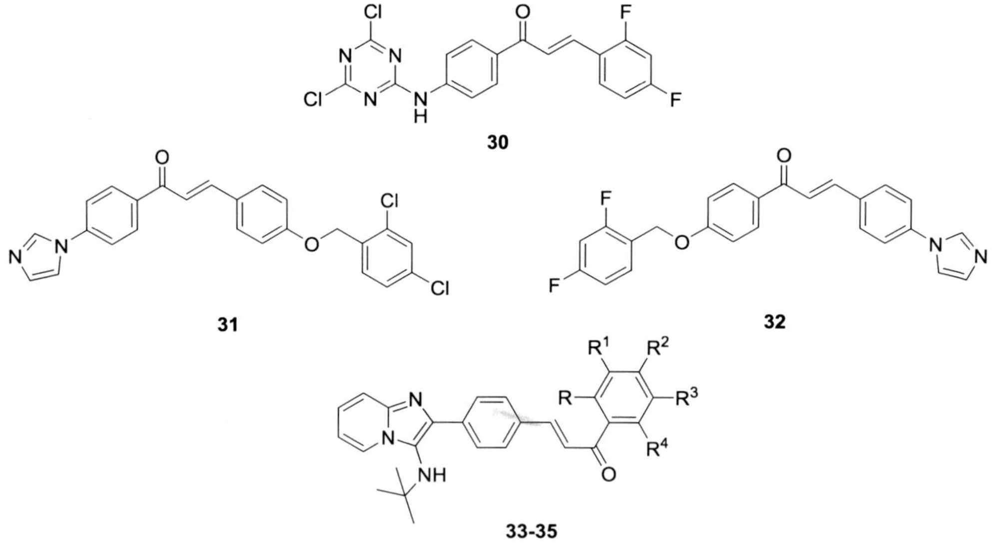

Fig. (12). Chemical structures of compounds **30-35**.

Table 6. Substitutions and activity against *Mtb* H37Rv of compounds 30-35.

Compound	R	MIC[a] (µg/mL)	Assay
30	-	3.125	MABA
31	-	3.12	Agar dilution
32	-	1.56	Agar dilution
33	R = -H; R^1 = -H; R^2 = -Br; R^3 = -H; R^4 = -H	3.12	Agar dilution
34	R= -H; R^1 = $-OCH_3$; R^2 = $-OCH_3$; R^3= $-OCH_3$; R^5 = -H	3.12	Agar dilution
35	R = -H; R^1= -H; R^2= -H; R^3= -H; R^4 = -H	3.12	Agar dilution

[a] MIC obtained against *Mtb* H37Rv strain.

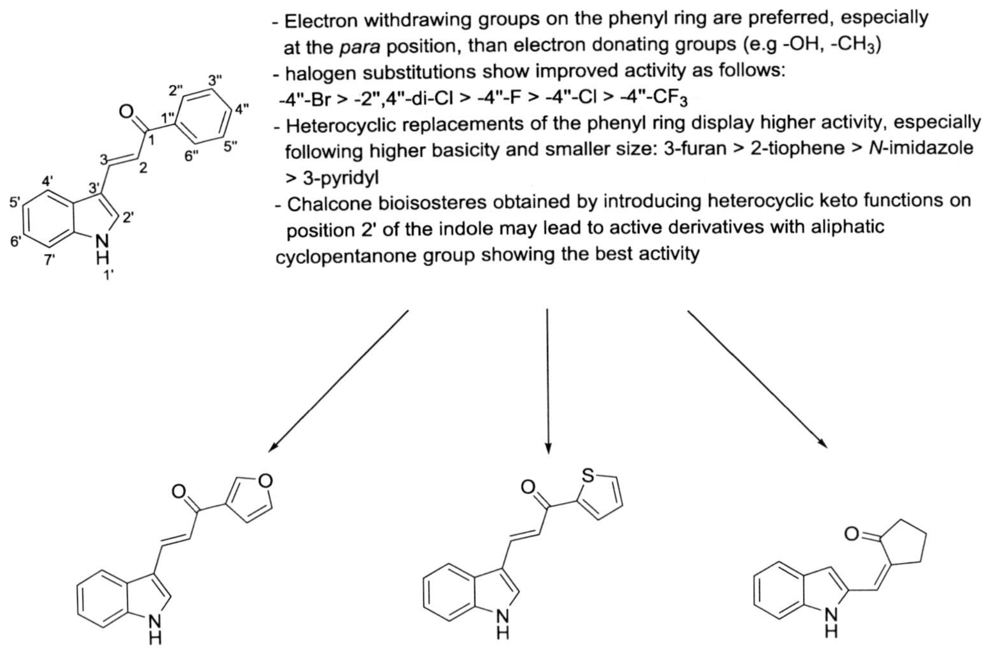

36 **37** **38**

Fig. (13). SARs of indole-based chalcones and chemical structures of compounds **36-38**.

Only recently, a novel class of indole-based chalcone derivatives has been studied. A series of 25 compounds differing on the phenyl ring substitutions were synthesized *via* Claisen-Schmidt condensation by Ramesh *et al.* All the derivatives showed a better ADME profile than INF and RIF; thus, they were screened against *Mtb* H37Rv strain using a Luciferase reporter mycobacteriophages (LRP) assay and structure-activity relationships were performed. Three derivatives **36-38**, (Fig. **13**) and Table **7.** with moderate anti-tubercular activity (MIC=197-236 μM) and displaying no toxicity to human megakaryocytes and murine B cells were identified as a potential starting point for the development of new anti-tubercular drugs. Docking studies showed a relevant binding affinity of **36** toward KasA protein similar to INH. SAR analysis is summarized in (Fig. **13**) [60].

Table 7. Activity against *Mtb* H37Rv of compounds 36-38.

Compound	MIC[a] (μg/mL)	Assay
36	49.82	LRP
37	49.90	LRP
38	49.86	LRP

[a] MIC obtained against *Mtb* H37Rv strain. Note: MIC value has been converted from μM to μg/mL.

PZA belongs to the first-line drugs for TB treatment and its derivatives have been intensely studied to endeavor to find novel anti-TB drugs. Therefore, also pyrazine analogs of chalcones were synthesized and their anti-mycobacterial activity was evaluated. In their research, Chlupakova *et al.* [61] identified pyrazine analogs of chalcones bearing an alkyl group at position 5 of the pyrazine ring as promising anti-TB compounds, particularly when the alkyl group is a *tert*-butyl one and the phenyl ring is bearing electron-withdrawing groups such as $-NO_2$ (compounds **39** and **40**, (Fig. **14**)., Table **8**.). However, the selectivity index (SI; the ratio between cytotoxicity and MIC) of the most promising compounds needs to be improved since result is lower than 10 [61, 62].

Recently, Hassan *et al.* [63] identified two chalcone derivatives among 31 pyrazine-based compounds with potent activity against *Mtb* and with SI largely higher than 10. Specifically, **41** showed the same potency as the reference compound PZA (MIC = 6.25 μg/ml) and compound **42** (Fig. (**14**)., Table **8**), a pyrazoline-1-carbothioamide derivative, showed double the activity (MIC = 3.12 μg/ml). *In silico* studies predicted a good ADME profile for the selected compounds, albeit **42** demonstrated a high risk of reproductive effect. Docking analysis of the active site of the pantothenate synthetase enzyme suggested this enzyme as a potential target [63].

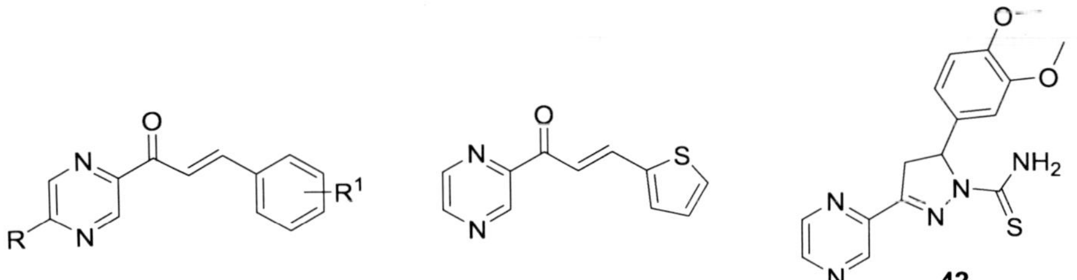

39,40 41 42

Fig. (14). Chemical structures of compounds **39-42**.

Table 8. Substitutions and activity against *Mtb* H37Rv of compounds 39-42.

Compound	R	MIC[a] (µg/mL)	Assay
39	R= -*i*Pr; R^1= 4-NO_2	6.25[b]	MABA
40	R= -*t*Bu; R^1= 4-NO_2	0.78	MABA
41	-	6.25	MABA
42	-	3.12	MABA

[a] MIC obtained against *Mtb* H37Rv strain; [b] MIC_{90}.

Given the wide range of biological activities of sulfonamides, Noreljaleel *et al.*[64] investigated the anti-tubercular activity of reduced chalcones condensed to different sulfonamide functionalities *via* the Mannich reaction. Nevertheless, only reduced chalcones **43** and **44** (Fig. **15**) showed potent growth inhibition at 10 µM (94-96%) and the most potent sulfanilamide-substituted reduced chalcone (**45**) only showed 14% of growth inhibition at that concentration despite high lipophilicity (Table **9**). Indeed, it was verified that high ClogP values (lipophilicity) correspond to high antitubercular activity since compounds are able to penetrate membrane barriers. Although reduced chalcones increase the lipophilicity of sulfanilamide, the poor activity might be attributed to the larger size of the derivate with respect to the reduced chalcone intermediate [64].

New chalcone-sulfonamide hybrids derived from 4-methoxyacetopenone were synthesized and submitted to biological assays against *Mtb* H37Rv strain by Castaño *et al.* [65]. The three most potent analogs (**46-48**, (Fig. **15**) exhibited MIC values in the range of 14-20 µM, albeit similar values of IC_{50} were obtained in toxicity tests against 3T3 mouse fibroblasts. Notwithstanding low selectivity, this novel class of hybrid chalcone-based compounds opened doors to optimization studies for the development of new potential leads in tuberculosis research [65].

Table 9. Substitutions and activity against *Mtb* H37Rv of compounds 43-48.

Compound	R	MIC[a] (μg/ml)	Assay
43	-3-OH	2.12[b]	BACTEC 460
44	-4-OH	2.12[b]	BACTEC 460
45	-	ND	BACTEC 460
46	-H	5.08	SPOTi
47	-Cl	4.93	SPOTi
48	-	10.14	SPOTi

[a] MIC obtained against *Mtb* H37Rv strain; [b] MIC value relative to >94% of growth inhibition of *Mtb* H37Rv strain using BACTEC 460 system; ND = Not determined; Note: MIC value has been converted from μM to μg/ml

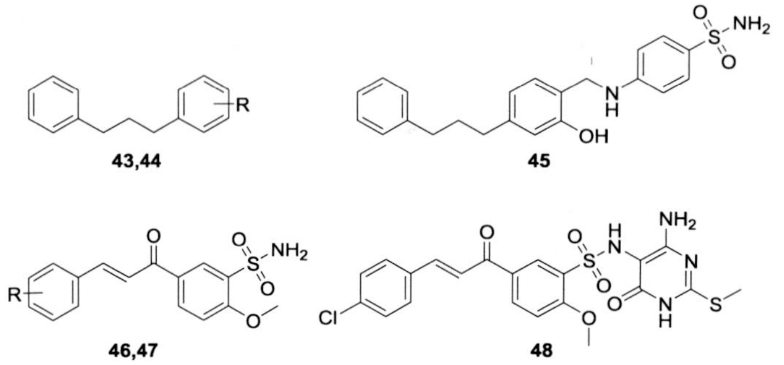

Fig. (15). Chemical structures of compounds **43-48**.

The past decade has witnessed a huge growth in the use of computer-aided drug design (CADD) for the development of new relevant drugs. Accordingly, QSAR modeling has been widely applied for the design of novel hits in tuberculosis research. Gomes *et al.* obtained remarkable results using QSAR models in the identification of new heteroaryl chalcone compounds with anti-TB activity. From 604 chalcones reported in the literature and selected over intriguing inhibition data, various QSAR models helped the researchers to choose 33 heteroaryl chalcones worth to be synthesized and evaluated *in vitro*. Therefore, the compounds were screened against *Mtb* H37Rv strain using LORA (hypoxic conditions) and MABA assays. Five designed compounds (**49-53**, (Fig. **16**) bearing either a nitrothiophene or nitrofuran ring showed exceptional activity in both assays (MABA MICs < 1 μM and LORA MICs < 10 μM, Table **10**). It was also observed that all compounds were modestly selective towards *Mtb* and surprisingly active against RMP and INH resistant strains, with compound **53** showing the lowest MIC values (MIC_{rRMP}= 0.14±0.01 μM; MIC_{rINH}=0.15±0.05 μM) [31].

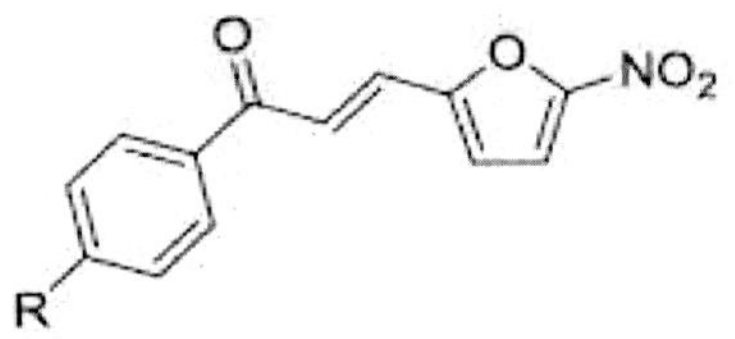

49-51

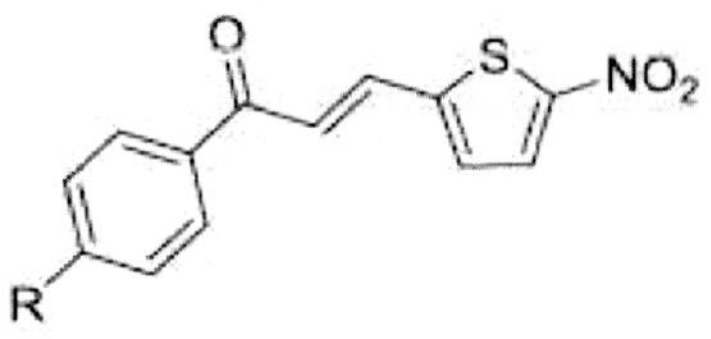

52,53

Fig. (16). Chemical structures of compounds **49-53**.

Table 10. Substitutions and activity against *Mtb* H37Rv of compounds 49-53.

Compound	R	MIC[a] (µg/ml)	Assay
49	-	0.26	MABA
50	$-CH_3$	0.15	MABA
51	-	1.12	MABA
52	-	0.05	MABA
53	-*t*Bu	0.07	MABA

[a] MIC obtained against *Mtb* H37Rv strain. Note: MIC value has been converted from µM to µg/ml.

A series of chalcone derivatives bearing a diphenyl ether system with variable substitution patterns were reported by Khade and colleagues [66]. The compounds were designed to possess a phenolic group at ring A as it was found to be essential for antitubercular activity, and a bioisosterism strategy was also applied by introducing a pyrroline nucleus *via* reaction of the enone system with nitromethane. As all the compounds were screened against *Mtb* H37Rv, derivative **54** (Fig. **17**) appeared to be the most promising one in the series with a MIC of 18 µM in MABA assay Table **11.**, probably due to the presence of the methyl group that induces higher lipophilicity to the molecule leading to a higher facility in crossing *Mtb*'s hydrophobic cell wall and phospholipid membrane. All the compounds were safe, showed good ADME properties *in silico* and strong interactions with InhA were detected through molecular docking analysis [66].

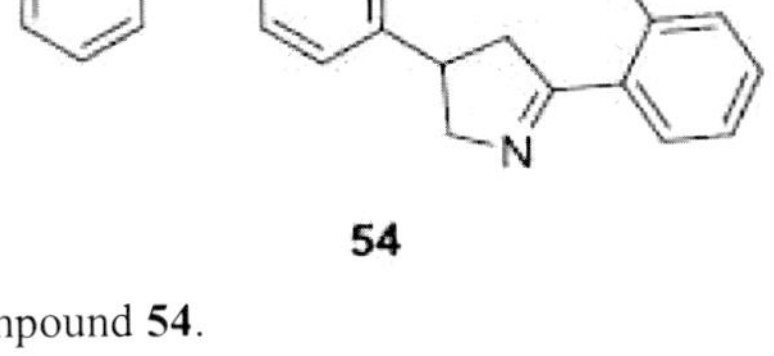

54

Fig. 17. Chemical structure of compound **54**.

Table 11. Activity against *Mtb* H37Rv of compound 54.

Compound	MIC[a] (μg/ml)	Assay
46	6.18	MABA

[a] MIC obtained against *Mtb* H37Rv strain. Note: MIC value has been converted from μM to μg/ml.

Ferrocenes, a class of derivatives consisting of two cyclopentadienyl groups complexed with iron, have achieved success in antimicrobial and antimalarial research and have offered an interesting alternative to the standard drugs against *Mtb* [67 - 70]. Therefore, Singh *et al.* [69] reported the synthesis and biological evaluation of new piperazyl-alkyl-ether linked 7-chloroquinolin--chalcone/ferrocenyl chalcone conjugates. The replacement of the phenyl ring with the ferrocene nucleus was realized by condensing ferrocene-carboxaldehydes with piperazine-linked 4-aminoquinoline-acetophenone conjugates. The ferrocene-based chalcones were then evaluated against the *Mtb* mc26230 strain and compared to the correspondent piperazine-linked 4-aminoquinoline-chalcone conjugates. It was observed that all compounds were safe *in vitro* towards the Vero cell lines and that the replacement with ferrocene nucleus improved the activity, with compound **55** (Fig. **18**) exhibiting the lowest MIC50 value Table **12.** [69].

Like chalcones, chromones are compounds linked to diverse biological functions that can serve as the backbone for developing new anti-TB chemotypes [71]. In this context, Mujahid *et al.* [72] reported the development and *in vitro* evaluation of novel spirochromone annulated chalcones conjugates. All the derivatives were then screened against *Mtb* H37Rv using the agar dilution method and five compounds out of 15 were identified as having good anti-TB properties with MIC values ranging between 3.13 μg/ml (**56**, (Fig. **18**), Table **12.** and 12.5 μg/ml. It was further observed that compounds bearing piperidinyl group instead of cycloalkyl group to form the spiro moiety were favored for anti-TB activity and halogen substitutions on the phenyl ring of the chalcone moiety are functional for improved activity. Finally, *in silico* analysis attributed a good ADME profile of the active compounds and validated the mechanism of action involving the PtpB enzyme as the putative target [72].

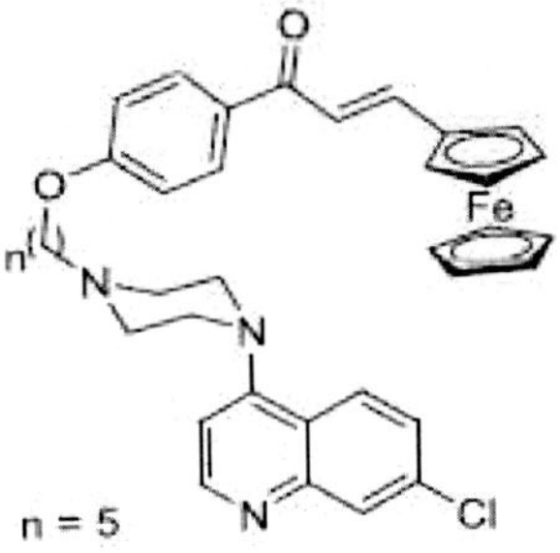

55

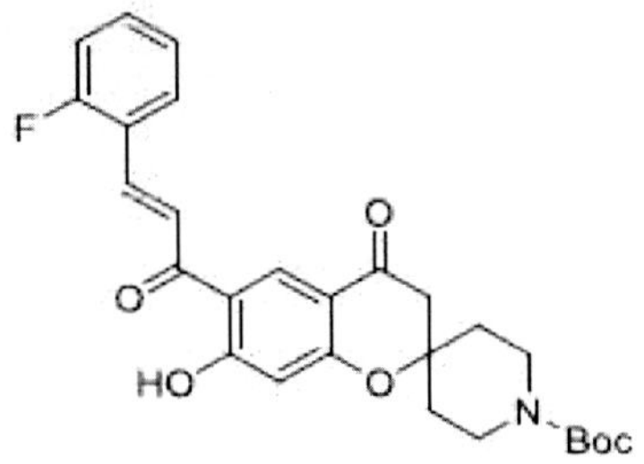

56

Fig. (18). Chemical structures of compounds **55** and **56**.

Table 12. Activity against *Mtb* H37Rv of compounds 55 and 56.

Compound	MIC (μg/ml)	Assay
55	14[a]	Broth dilution
56	3.13[b]	Agar dilution

[a] MIC_{50} value obtained against *Mtb* mc^{2}6230 strain [b] MIC value obtained against *Mtb* H37Rv strain.

CONCLUDING REMARKS

Nature is an unlimited source of biologically active substances; indeed, several drugs under clinical trial or in use are either of natural origin or were developed through planned chemical synthesis of natural products. Natural products can also be seen as novel original structural patterns that can represent a "molecular inspiration" for the design of new drugs.

In this book chapter we have examined several works on flavonoids and chalcones for developing new antitubercular entities. Several interesting leads have been found. As antitubercular compounds, flavonoids and chalcones showed optimal potential to be used as building blocks for novel semisynthetic compounds as a result of extensive SAR studies that provide much evidence to optimize their functionalities. Based on the wide range of studies, different substitutions could result in different targets and activity profiles, laying the ground for future development of hybrid compounds that display polypharmacology, a promising alternative to prevent resistance development. Particularly, the simple use of small electron withdrawing (*e.g.*, halogens) and electron donating (*e.g.*, para-methoxy group) substituents on chalcones change molecule conformation and thus the derived activity. Modifications with nitrogen-based heterocycles offer a variety of chemical strategies to significantly improve toxicity and selectivity profiles to resemble better novel anti-TB candidates.However, what is clear is that much has been done, but much more needs to be done in order to further develop these new antitubercular agents.

CONSENT OF PUBLICATION

Not applicable.

CONFLICT OF INTEREST

The author declares no conflict of interest, financial or otherwise.

ACKNOWLEDGMENT

This work has been supported by the Italian Ministry of Education, Universities and Research - Dipartimenti di Eccellenza - L. 232/2016.

REFERENCES

[1] WHO. **2020**.http://www.who.int/tb/publications/global_report/en/

[2] Deoghare, S. Bedaquiline: A new drug approved for treatment of multidrug-resistant tuberculosis. *Indian J. Pharmacol.,* **2013**, *45*(5), 536-537. [http://dx.doi.org/10.4103/0253-7613.117765] [PMID: 24130398]

[3] Keam, S.J. Pretomanid: First Approval. *Drugs,* **2019**, *79*(16), 1797-1803. [http://dx.doi.org/10.1007/s40265-019-01207-9] [PMID: 31583606]

[4] Xavier, A.S.; Lakshmanan, M. Delamanid: A new armor in combating drug-resistant tuberculosis. *J. Pharmacol. Pharmacother.,* **2014**, *5*(3), 222-224. [http://dx.doi.org/10.4103/0976-500X.136121] [PMID: 25210407]

[5] Appetecchia, F.; Consalvi, S.; Scarpecci, C.; Biava, M.; Poce, G. SAR analysis of small molecules interfering with energy-metabolism in Mycobacterium tuberculosis. *Pharmaceuticals (Basel),* **2020**, *13*(9), 227. [http://dx.doi.org/10.3390/ph13090227] [PMID: 32878317]

[6] Consalvi, S.; Scarpecci, C.; Biava, M.; Poce, G. Mycobacterial tryptophan biosynthesis: A promising target for tuberculosis drug development? *Bioorg. Med. Chem. Lett.,* **2019**, *29*(23), 126731. [http://dx.doi.org/10.1016/j.bmcl.2019.126731] [PMID: 31627992]

[7] Boniface, P.K.; Ferreira, E.I. Opportunities and Challenges for flavonoids as potential leads for the treatment of tuberculosis. *Studies in Natural Products Chemistry; Atta-ur-Rahman.,* **2020**, *Vol. 65*, 85-124. [http://dx.doi.org/10.1016/B978-0-12-817905-5.00003-2]

[8] Yang, C.S.; Ho, C.T.; Zhang, J.; Wan, X.; Zhang, K.; Lim, J. Antioxidants: differing meanings in food science and health science. *J. Agric. Food Chem.,* **2018**, *66*(12), 3063-3068. [http://dx.doi.org/10.1021/acs.jafc.7b05830] [PMID: 29526101]

[9] Yang, C.S.; Wang, X.; Lu, G.; Picinich, S.C. Cancer prevention by tea: animal studies, molecular mechanisms and human relevance. *Nat. Rev. Cancer,* **2009**, *9*(6), 429-439. [http://dx.doi.org/10.1038/nrc2641] [PMID: 19472429]

[10] Chakrawarti, L.; Agrawal, R.; Dang, S.; Gupta, S.; Gabrani, R. Therapeutic effects of EGCG: a patent review. *Expert Opin. Ther. Pat.,* **2016**, *26*(8), 907-916. [http://dx.doi.org/10.1080/13543776.2016.1203419] [PMID: 27338088]

[11] Reygaert, W.C. The antimicrobial possibilities of green tea. *Front. Microbiol.*, **2014**, *5*, 434. [http://dx.doi.org/10.3389/fmicb.2014.00434] [PMID: 25191312]

[12] Maiolini, M.; Gause, S.; Taylor, J.; Steakin, T.; Shipp, G.; Lamichhane, P.; Deshmukh, B.; Shinde, V.; Bishayee, A.; Deshmukh, R.R. The war against tuberculosis: a review of natural compounds and their derivatives. *Molecules,* **2020**, *25*(13), 3011. [http://dx.doi.org/10.3390/molecules25133011] [PMID: 32630150]

[13] Lambert, J.D.; Lee, M.J.; Lu, H. Epigallocatechin-3-gallate is absorbed but extensively glucuronidated following oral administration to mice. *J. Nutr.*, **2003**, *133*(12), 4172-4177. [http://dx.doi.org/10.1093/jn/133.12.4172] [PMID: 14652367]

[14] Mereles, D.; Hunstein, W. Epigallocatechin-3-gallate (EGCG) for clinical trials: more pitfalls than promises? *Int. J. Mol. Sci.*, **2011**, *12*(9), 5592-5603. [http://dx.doi.org/10.3390/ijms12095592] [PMID: 22016611]

[15] Ramachandran, B.; Jayavelu, S.; Murhekar, K.; Rajkumar, T. Repeated dose studies with pure Epigallocatechin-3-gallate demonstrated dose and route dependant hepatotoxicity with associated dyslipidemia. *Toxicol. Rep.*, **2016**, *3*, 336-345. [http://dx.doi.org/10.1016/j.toxrep.2016.03.001] [PMID: 28959554]

[16] Banerjee, D.R.; Dutta, D.; Saha, B.; Bhattacharyya, S.; Senapati, K.; Das, A.K.; Basak, A. Design, synthesis and characterization of novel inhibitors against mycobacterial β-ketoacyl CoA reductase FabG4. *Org. Biomol. Chem.*, **2014**, *12*(1), 73-85. [http://dx.doi.org/10.1039/C3OB41676C] [PMID: 24129589]

[17] Chokchaisiri, R.; Suaisom, C.; Sriphota, S.; Chindaduang, A.; Chuprajob, T.; Suksamrarn, A. Bioactive flavonoids of the flowers of Butea monosperma. *Chem. Pharm. Bull. (Tokyo),* **2009**, *57*(4), 428-432. [http://dx.doi.org/10.1248/cpb.57.428] [PMID: 19336944]

[18] Khan, I.A.; Avery, M.A.; Burandt, C.L.; Goins, D.K.; Mikell, J.R.; Nash, T.E.; Azadegan, A.; Walker, L.A. Antigiardial activity of isoflavones from Dalbergia frutescens bark. *J. Nat. Prod.,* **2000**, *63*(10), 1414-1416. [http://dx.doi.org/10.1021/np000010d] [PMID: 11076565]

[19] Gyémánt, N.; Tanaka, M.; Antus, S.; Hohmann, J.; Csuka, O.; Mándoky, L.; Molnár, J. In vitro search for synergy between flavonoids and epirubicin on multidrug-resistant cancer cells. *In Vivo,* **2005**, *19*(2), 367-374. [PMID: 15796199]

[20] Mutai, P.; Pavadai, E.; Wiid, I.; Ngwane, A.; Baker, B.; Chibale, K. Synthesis, antimycobacterial evaluation and pharmacophore modeling of analogues of the natural product formononetin. *Bioorg. Med. Chem. Lett.*, **2015**, *25*(12), 2510-2513. [http://dx.doi.org/10.1016/j.bmcl.2015.04.064] [PMID: 25977095]

[21] Gomes, M.; Muratov, E.; Pereira, M. Chalcone derivatives: promising starting points for drug design. *Molecules,* **2017**, *22*(8), 1210. [http://dx.doi.org/10.3390/molecules22081210] [PMID: 28757583]

[22] Rozmer, Z.; Perjési, P. Naturally occurring chalcones and their biological activities. *Phytochem. Rev.*, **2016**, *15*(1), 87-120. [http://dx.doi.org/10.1007/s11101-014-9387-8]

[23] Zhou, B.; Xing, C. Diverse Molecular targets for chalcones with varied bioactivities. *Med. Chem. (Los Angeles),* **2015**, *5*(8), 388-404. [http://dx.doi.org/10.4172/2161-0444.1000291] [PMID: 26798565]

[24] Zhuang, C.; Zhang, W.; Sheng, C.; Zhang, W.; Xing, C.; Miao, Z. Chalcone: a privileged structure in medicinal chemistry. *Chem. Rev.*, **2017**, *117*(12), 7762-7810. [http://dx.doi.org/10.1021/acs.chemrev.7b00020] [PMID: 28488435]

[25] Lin, Y.M.; Zhou, Y.; Flavin, M.T.; Zhou, L.M.; Nie, W.; Chen, F.C. Chalcones and flavonoids as anti-Tuberculosis agents. *Bioorg. Med. Chem.*, **2002**, *10*(8), 2795-2802.
[http://dx.doi.org/10.1016/S0968-0896(02)00094-9] [PMID: 12057669]

[26] Burmaoglu, S.; Algul, O.; Gobek, A.; Aktas Anil, D.; Ulger, M.; Erturk, B.G.; Kaplan, E.; Dogen, A.; Aslan, G. Design of potent fluoro-substituted chalcones as antimicrobial agents. *J. Enzyme Inhib. Med. Chem.*, **2017**, *32*(1), 490-495.
[http://dx.doi.org/10.1080/14756366.2016.1265517] [PMID: 28118738]

[27] Yalcin, G.; Burmaoglu, S.; Yildiz, I.; Algul, O. Molecular docking studies on fluoro-substituted chalcones as potential DprE1 enzyme inhibitors. *J. Mol. Struct.*, **2018**, *1164*, 50-56.
[http://dx.doi.org/10.1016/j.molstruc.2018.02.087]

[28] Ventura, T.; Calixto, S.; Abrahim-Vieira, B. Antimycobacterial and anti-inflammatory activities of substituted chalcones focusing on an anti-tuberculosis dual treatment approach. *Molecules*, **2015**, *20*(5), 8072-8093.
[http://dx.doi.org/10.3390/molecules20058072] [PMID: 25951004]

[29] Anandam, R.; Jadav, S.S.; Ala, V.B.; Ahsan, M.J.; Bollikolla, H.B. Synthesis of new C-dimethylated chalcones as potent antitubercular agents. *Med. Chem. Res.*, **2018**, *27*(6), 1690-1704.
[http://dx.doi.org/10.1007/s00044-018-2183-z]

[30] Anagani, B.; Singh, J.; Bassin, J.P. Identification and validation of the mode of action of the chalcone anti-mycobacterial compounds. *Cell Surf.*, **2020**, *6*, 100041.
[http://dx.doi.org/10.1016/j.tcsw.2020.100041] [PMID: 32743153]

[31] Gomes, M.N.; Braga, R.C.; Grzelak, E.M.; Neves, B.J.; Muratov, E.; Ma, R.; Klein, L.L.; Cho, S.; Oliveira, G.R.; Franzblau, S.G.; Andrade, C.H. QSAR-driven design, synthesis and discovery of potent chalcone derivatives with antitubercular activity. *Eur. J. Med. Chem.*, **2017**, *137*, 126-138.
[http://dx.doi.org/10.1016/j.ejmech.2017.05.026] [PMID: 28582669]

[32] Zampieri, D.; Mamolo, M.G. Hybridization approach to drug discovery inhibiting Mycobacterium tuberculosis. An overview. *Curr. Top. Med. Chem.*, **2021**, *21*(9), 777-788.
[http://dx.doi.org/10.2174/1568026620666200819151342] [PMID: 32814528]

[33] Harikrishna, N.; Isloor, A.M.; Ananda, K.; Obaid, A.; Fun, H.K. Synthesis, and antitubercular and antimicrobial activity of 1′-(4-chlorophenyl)pyrazole containing 3,5-disubstituted pyrazoline derivatives. *New J. Chem.*, **2016**, *40*(1), 73-76.
[http://dx.doi.org/10.1039/C5NJ02237A]

[34] Xu, Z.; Gao, C.; Ren, Q.C.; Song, X.F.; Feng, L.S.; Lv, Z.S. Recent advances of pyrazole-containing derivatives as anti-tubercular agents. *Eur. J. Med. Chem.*, **2017**, *139*, 429-440.
[http://dx.doi.org/10.1016/j.ejmech.2017.07.059] [PMID: 28818767]

[35] Poce, G.; Consalvi, S.; Venditti, G. Novel pyrazole-containing compounds active against Mycobacterium tuberculosis. *ACS Med. Chem. Lett.*, **2019**, *10*(10), 1423-1429.
[http://dx.doi.org/10.1021/acsmedchemlett.9b00204] [PMID: 31620228]

[36] Ahmad, A.; Husain, A.; Khan, S.A.; Mujeeb, M.; Bhandari, A. Synthesis, antimicrobial and antitubercular activities of some novel pyrazoline derivatives. *J. Saudi Chem. Soc.*, **2016**, *20*(5), 577-584.
[http://dx.doi.org/10.1016/j.jscs.2014.12.004]

[37] Khunt, R.C.; Khedkar, V.M.; Chawda, R.S.; Chauhan, N.A.; Parikh, A.R.; Coutinho, E.C. Synthesis, antitubercular evaluation and 3D-QSAR study of N-phenyl-3-(4-fluorophenyl)-4-substituted pyrazole derivatives. *Bioorg. Med. Chem. Lett.*, **2012**, *22*(1), 666-678.
[http://dx.doi.org/10.1016/j.bmcl.2011.10.059] [PMID: 22104148]

[38] Gupta, R.A.; Kaskhedikar, S.G. Synthesis, antitubercular activity, and QSAR analysis of substituted nitroaryl analogs: chalcone, pyrazole, isoxazole, and pyrimidines. *Med. Chem. Res.*, **2013**, *22*(8), 3863-3880.

[http://dx.doi.org/10.1007/s00044-012-0385-3]

[39] Liu, B.; Li, F.; Zhou, T.; Tang, X.Q.; Hu, G.W. Quinoline derivatives with potential activity against multidrug-resistant tuberculosis. *J. Heterocycl. Chem.*, **2018**, *55*(8), 1863-1873. [http://dx.doi.org/10.1002/jhet.3241]

[40] Rao, N.S.; Shaik, A.B.; Routhu, S.R. New quinoline linked chalcone and pyrazoline conjugates: molecular properties prediction, antimicrobial and antitubercular activities. *ChemistrySelect,* **2017**, *2*(10), 2989-2996. [http://dx.doi.org/10.1002/slct.201602022]

[41] Kumar, G.; Siva Krishna, V.; Sriram, D.; Jachak, S.M. Pyrazole–coumarin and pyrazole–quinoline chalcones as potential antitubercular agents. *Arch. Pharm. (Weinheim),* **2020**, *353*(8), 2000077. [http://dx.doi.org/10.1002/ardp.202000077] [PMID: 32484273]

[42] Pires, C.T.A.; Scodro, R.B.L.; Cortez, D.A.G.; Brenzan, M.A.; Siqueira, V.L.D.; Caleffi-Ferracioli, K.R.; Vieira, L.C.C.; Monteiro, J.L.; Corrêa, A.G.; Cardoso, R.F. Structure–activity relationship of natural and synthetic coumarin derivatives against *Mycobacterium tuberculosis. Future Med. Chem.,* **2020**, *12*(17), 1533-1546. [http://dx.doi.org/10.4155/fmc-2018-0281] [PMID: 32820960]

[43] Mali, H.M.; Sabale, S.S.; Degani, M.S.; Borkute, R.; Choudhari, A.S.; Sarkar, D.; Krishna, V.S.; Sriram, D. Rational design of coumarin derivatives as antituberculosis agents. *Future Med. Chem.,* **2018**, *10*(20), 2431-2444. [http://dx.doi.org/10.4155/fmc-2018-0015] [PMID: 30325198]

[44] Ahmad, I.; Thakur, J.P.; Chanda, D. Syntheses of lipophilic chalcones and their conformationally restricted analogues as antitubercular agents. *Bioorg. Med. Chem. Lett.,* **2013**, *23*(5), 1322-1325. [http://dx.doi.org/10.1016/j.bmcl.2012.12.096] [PMID: 23369537]

[45] Palleapati, K.; Kancharlapalli, V.R.; Shaik, A.B. Synthesis, characterization and antitubercular evaluation of some new isoxazole appended 1-carboxamido-4,5-dihydro-1H-pyrazoles. *Journal of Research in Pharmacy,* **2019**, *23*(2), 156-163. [http://dx.doi.org/10.12991/jrp.2019.120]

[46] Pola, S.; Banoth, K.K.; Sankaranarayanan, M.; Ummani, R.; Garlapati, A. Design, synthesis, in silico studies, and evaluation of novel chalcones and their pyrazoline derivatives for antibacterial and antitubercular activities. *Med. Chem. Res.,* **2020**, *29*(10), 1819-1835. [http://dx.doi.org/10.1007/s00044-020-02602-8]

[47] Chiaradia, L.D.; Martins, P.G.A.; Cordeiro, M.N.S. Synthesis, biological evaluation, and molecular modeling of chalcone derivatives as potent inhibitors of Mycobacterium tuberculosis protein tyrosine phosphatases (PtpA and PtpB). *J. Med. Chem.,* **2012**, *55*(1), 390-402. [http://dx.doi.org/10.1021/jm2012062] [PMID: 22136336]

[48] Chiaradia, L.D.; Mascarello, A.; Purificação, M. Synthetic chalcones as efficient inhibitors of Mycobacterium tuberculosis protein tyrosine phosphatase PtpA. *Bioorg. Med. Chem. Lett.,* **2008**, *18*(23), 6227-6230. [http://dx.doi.org/10.1016/j.bmcl.2008.09.105] [PMID: 18930396]

[49] Wong, D.; Chao, J.D.; Av-Gay, Y. Mycobacterium tuberculosis-secreted phosphatases: from pathogenesis to targets for TB drug development. *Trends Microbiol.,* **2013**, *21*(2), 100-109. [http://dx.doi.org/10.1016/j.tim.2012.09.002] [PMID: 23084287]

[50] Wang, T.; Tang, Y.; Yang, Y. Discovery of novel anti-tuberculosis agents with pyrrolo[1,2- a]quinoxaline-based scaffold. *Bioorg. Med. Chem. Lett.,* **2018**, *28*(11), 2084-2090. [http://dx.doi.org/10.1016/j.bmcl.2018.04.043] [PMID: 29748048]

[51] Santivañez-Veliz, M.; Pérez-Silanes, S.; Torres, E.; Moreno-Viguri, E. Design and synthesis of novel quinoxaline derivatives as potential candidates for treatment of multidrug-resistant and latent tuberculosis. *Bioorg. Med. Chem. Lett.,* **2016**, *26*(9), 2188-2193. [http://dx.doi.org/10.1016/j.bmcl.2016.03.066] [PMID: 27025343]

[52] Vicente, E.; Pérez-Silanes, S.; Lima, L.M. Selective activity against Mycobacterium tuberculosis of new quinoxaline 1,4-di-N-oxides. *Bioorg. Med. Chem.*, **2009**, *17*(1), 385-389. [http://dx.doi.org/10.1016/j.bmc.2008.10.086] [PMID: 19058970]

[53] Desai, V.; Desai, S.; Gaonkar, S.N.; Palyekar, U.; Joshi, S.D.; Dixit, S.K. Novel quinoxalinyl chalcone hybrid scaffolds as enoyl ACP reductase inhibitors: Synthesis, molecular docking and biological evaluation. *Bioorg. Med. Chem. Lett.*, **2017**, *27*(10), 2174-2180. [http://dx.doi.org/10.1016/j.bmcl.2017.03.059] [PMID: 28372908]

[54] Muradás, T.C.; Abbadi, B.L.; Villela, A.D. Pre-clinical evaluation of quinoxaline-derived chalcones in tuberculosis. *PLoS One*, **2018**, *13*(8), e0202568. [http://dx.doi.org/10.1371/journal.pone.0202568] [PMID: 30114296]

[55] Azqueta, A.; Arbillaga, L.; Pachón, G.; Cascante, M.; Creppy, E.E.; Cerain, A.L. A quinoxaline 1,4-di-N-oxide derivative induces DNA oxidative damage not attenuated by vitamin C and E treatment. *Chem. Biol. Interact.*, **2007**, *168*(2), 95-105. [http://dx.doi.org/10.1016/j.cbi.2007.02.013] [PMID: 17420013]

[56] Cheng, G.; Sa, W.; Cao, C.; Guo, L.; Hao, H.; Liu, Z.; Wang, X.; Yuan, Z. Quinoxaline 1,4-di-N-oxides: biological activities and mechanisms of actions. *Front. Pharmacol.*, **2016**, *7*, 64. [http://dx.doi.org/10.3389/fphar.2016.00064] [PMID: 27047380]

[57] Dwarampudi, S.R.; Dannana, G.S.; Avupati, V.R.; Bendi, V.S.M. Synthesis, characterization and in vitro biological evaluation of some new 1,3,5-triazine-chalcone hybrid molecules as Mycobacterium tuberculosis H37Rv inhibitors. *Eur. J. Chem.*, **2014**, *5*(4), 570-576. [http://dx.doi.org/10.5155/eurjchem.5.4.570-576.1098]

[58] Marrapu, V.K.; Chaturvedi, V.; Singh, S.; Singh, S.; Sinha, S.; Bhandari, K. Novel aryloxy azolyl chalcones with potent activity against Mycobacterium tuberculosis H37Rv. *Eur. J. Med. Chem.*, **2011**, *46*(9), 4302-4310. [http://dx.doi.org/10.1016/j.ejmech.2011.06.037] [PMID: 21764184]

[59] Pandey, A.K.; Sharma, R.; Purohit, P.; Dwivedi, R.; Chaturvedi, V.; Chauhan, P.M.S. Synthesis of pyrido[1,2-a]imidazo-chalcone *via* 3-component Groebke- Blackburn-Bienayme reaction and their bioevaluation as potent antituberculosis agents. *J. Chem. Biol. Interfaces,* **2016**, *6*, 10.

[60] Ramesh, D.; Joji, A.; Vijayakumar, B.G.; Sethumadhavan, A.; Mani, M.; Kannan, T. Indole chalcones: Design, synthesis, *in vitro* and in silico evaluation against Mycobacterium tuberculosis. *Eur. J. Med. Chem.*, **2020**, *198*, 112358. [http://dx.doi.org/10.1016/j.ejmech.2020.112358] [PMID: 32361610]

[61] Kucerova-Chlupacova, M.; Kunes, J.; Buchta, V.; Vejsova, M.; Opletalova, V. Novel pyrazine analogs of chalcones: synthesis and evaluation of their antifungal and antimycobacterial activity. *Molecules,* **2015**, *20*(1), 1104-1117. [http://dx.doi.org/10.3390/molecules20011104] [PMID: 25587786]

[62] Bousquet, A.; Bugier, S.; Larréché, S.; Bigaillon, C.; Weber, P.; Delacour, H.; Valade, E.; De Briel, D.; Mérens, A. Clinical isolates of Escherichia coli solely resistant to mecillinam: prevalence and epidemiology. *Int. J. Antimicrob. Agents,* **2018**, *51*(3), 493-497. [http://dx.doi.org/10.1016/j.ijantimicag.2017.11.001] [PMID: 29154843]

[63] Hassan, N.W.; Saudi, M.N.; Abdel-Ghany, Y.S.; Ismail, A.; Elzahhar, P.A.; Sriram, D.; Nassra, R.; Abdel-Aziz, M.M.; El-Hawash, S.A. Novel pyrazine based anti-tubercular agents: Design, synthesis, biological evaluation and in silico studies. *Bioorg. Chem.*, **2020**, *96*, 103610. [http://dx.doi.org/10.1016/j.bioorg.2020.103610] [PMID: 32028062]

[64] Noreljaleel, A.E.M.; Wilhelm, A.; Bonnet, S.L.; van der Westhuizen, J.H. Synthesis and bioactivity of reduced chalcones containing sulfonamide side chains. *J. Nat. Prod.*, **2018**, *81*(1), 41-48. [http://dx.doi.org/10.1021/acs.jnatprod.7b00570] [PMID: 29309141]

[65] Castaño, L.F.; Cuartas, V.; Bernal, A. New chalcone-sulfonamide hybrids exhibiting anticancer and

antituberculosis activity. *Eur. J. Med. Chem.*, **2019**, *176*, 50-60. [http://dx.doi.org/10.1016/j.ejmech.2019.05.013] [PMID: 31096118]

[66] Khade, A.B.; Boshoff, H.I.M.; Arora, K.; Vandana, K.E.; Verma, R.; Shenoy, G.G. Design, synthesis, evaluation, and molecular dynamic simulation of triclosan mimic diphenyl ether derivatives as antitubercular and antibacterial agents. *Struct. Chem.*, **2020**, *31*(3), 983-998. [http://dx.doi.org/10.1007/s11224-019-01478-8]

[67] Xiao, J.; Sun, Z.; Kong, F.; Gao, F. Current scenario of ferrocene-containing hybrids for antimalarial activity. *Eur. J. Med. Chem.*, **2020**, *185*, 111791. [http://dx.doi.org/10.1016/j.ejmech.2019.111791] [PMID: 31669852]

[68] Zampino, D.; Pedotti, S.; Ussia, M.; Dattilo, S.; Mancuso, M.; Zaccone, R.; Patti, A. Preparation, characterization, and antimicrobial activity of ferrocene-containing polymeric materials. *J. Appl. Polym. Sci.*, **2021**, *138*(7), 49852. [http://dx.doi.org/10.1002/app.49852]

[69] Singh, A.; Viljoen, A.; Kremer, L.; Kumar, V. Synthesis and antimycobacterial evaluation of piperazyl-alkyl-ether linked 7-chloroquinoline-chalcone/ferrocenyl chalcone conjugates. *ChemistrySelect,* **2018**, *3*(29), 8511-8513. [http://dx.doi.org/10.1002/slct.201801453]

[70] Ludwig, B.S.; Correia, J.D.G.; Kühn, F.E. Ferrocene derivatives as anti-infective agents. *Coord. Chem. Rev.*, **2019**, *396*, 22-48. [http://dx.doi.org/10.1016/j.ccr.2019.06.004]

[71] Singh, A.; Fong, G.; Liu, J. Synthesis and preliminary antimicrobial analysis of isatin-ferrocene and isatin-ferrocenyl chalcone conjugates. *ACS Omega,* **2018**, *3*(5), 5808-5813. [http://dx.doi.org/10.1021/acsomega.8b00553] [PMID: 30023926]

[72] Mujahid, M.; Yogeeswari, P.; Sriram, D.; Basavanag, U.M.V.; Díaz-Cervantes, E.; Córdoba-Bahena, L.; Robles, J.; Gonnade, R.G.; Karthikeyan, M.; Vyas, R.; Muthukrishnan, M. Spirochromone-chalcone conjugates as antitubercular agents: synthesis, bio evaluation and molecular modeling studies. *RSC Advances,* **2015**, *5*(129), 106448-106460. [http://dx.doi.org/10.1039/C5RA21737G]

CHAPTER 6

In Silico Approaches to Naturally Existing Chalcones and Flavonoids on Mao Inhibitory Action: A Boon to CNS Drug Discovery

Arafa Musa[1,2], Della Grace Thomas Parambi[3], Mutairah Shaker Alshammari[4], Rania Bakr[3], Mohammed A. Abdelgawad[3,5], Dibya Sundar Panda[6], Manoj Kumar Sachidanandan[7], Vaishnav Bhaskar[8], Leena K. Pappachen[8] and **Bijo Mathew[8,*]**

[1] *Department of Pharmacognosy, College of Pharmacy, Jouf University, Sakaka, Al Jouf, 72341, Saudi Arabia*

[2] *Department of Pharmacognosy, Faculty of Pharmacy, Al-Azhar University, Cairo-11371, Egypt*

[3] *Department of Pharmaceutical Chemistry, College of Pharmacy, Jouf University, Sakaka, Al Jouf, 72341, Saudi Arabia*

[4] *Department of Pharmaceutical Analytical Chemistry, Jouf University, Sakaka, Al Jouf, 72341, Saudi Arabia*

[5] *Department of Pharmaceutical Organic Chemistry, Beni-Suef University, Beni-Suef, 62514Egypt*

[6] *Department of Pharmaceutics, College of Pharmacy, Jouf University, Sakaka, Al Jouf, 72341, Saudi Arabia*

[7] *Department of Oral and maxillofacial surgery and diagnostics, College of Dentistry, Hail University, Hail Province,2440, Saudi Arabia*

[8] *Department of Pharmaceutical Chemistry, Amrita School of Pharmacy, Amrita Vishwa Vidyapeetham, Amrita Health Science Campus, Kochi-682 041, India*

Abstract: *In silico* studies or computer-aided drug design (CADD) have led to advancement in drug discovery and development of neurodegenerative disorders (NDDs) and neuropsychiatric disorders. CADD is being increasingly used by universities and industries and provides a clear understanding of molecular interactions. Predicting molecular interactions provides relevant information to extract the potential of bioactive compounds. At present, more interest is on natural entities as therapeutic agents with different heterocyclic categories. Various heterocyclic structures are suggested to show MAO (monoamine oxidase) inhibitory activity by CADD and preclinical studies. Among these, chalcones and flavonoids play a major role in MAO inhibitory action because of the phenolic ring. In this chapter, we discuss *in silico* studies of natural chalcones and flavonoids with MAO inhibitory by considering the

* **Corresponding author Bijo Mathew, Associate Professor:** Department of Pharmaceutical Chemistry, Amrita School of Pharmacy, Amrita Vishwa Vidyapeetham, Amrita Health Science Campus, Kochi-682 041, India; E-mails: bijomathew@aims.amrita.edu, bijovilaventgu@gmail.com

Simone Carradori (Ed.)

complexity of the brain and the multifactorial nature of neurodegenerative disorders. These *in silico* studies prove that phytoconstituents from herbal medicine with therapeutic properties can serve as lead drug molecules for the treatment of NDDs.

Keywords: Apigenin, Chalcone, Flavonoids, *In silico*, Isoflavonoids, Kaempferol, Luteolin, MAO-inhibitor, Neurodegenerative Disorders, Quercetin, Xanthones.

INTRODUCTION

Neurodegenerative disorders are remarked as disorders of the central nervous system often resulting in selective loss of neurons. The research illustrated that deposition of amyloid proteins causes neuronal degeneration. As information pile up to date, no treatments are available for NDDs and are increasing the mortality and morbidity rates in developed countries and the same in developing countries. The reports say that abnormalities in MAOs (monoamine oxidases) lead to various neurological disorders and they have a major role in CNS and peripheral organs. Recent reports also indicate that abnormalities in mitochondria and the enzymes present in the mitochondria, like monoamine oxidases (MAOs), catechol-*O*-methyl transferases, and dopa decarboxylase [1 - 3], lead to NDDs. At this moment, the focus is on the flavin-containing enzyme called monoamine oxidase B (MAO-B), which is present in the outer membrane of mitochondria. MAO-B acts by catalyzing the oxidative deamination of neurotransmitters (dopamine, noradrenaline, and serotonin) and exogenous amines, which are targets for the diseases like Alzheimer's disease (AD), Parkinson's disease (PD), cardiovascular diseases, and also depression [4, 5]. MAO-B is directly involved in damaging neuronal cells by creating reactive oxygen species (ROS), which is the key reason for cell oxidative injury [5]. Identifying the MAO enzymes was a breakthrough in the history of drug discovery.

It is a long-standing tradition to use herbal drugs to treat and cure many diseases, mainly as medicines or sources of unique lead molecules for drug discovery and development of novel medicines [6 - 8]. Reports indicate that half of the top best-selling medicines are natural products, and their sales account for US 16 billion dollars, indicating that herbal medicines can be pre-optimized to be potentially bioactive compounds. Several chemoinformatics analyses also reveal that natural products can act as" drug-like" or "lead-like" and their physicochemical and structural properties can make them leads or drugs. Numerous reports suggest that natural products can act as therapeutic and lead compounds in neurodegenerative diseases [9]. The rational treatment of CNS disorders by natural products is still in its infancy due to the multifactorial nature and complexity of CNS and the complex chemistry and pharmacology of natural compounds.

Several human MAO inhibitors are now used as antianxiety anti-depression agents, whereas human MAO-B inhibitors can be used alone or in combination therapy for Alzheimer's and Parkinson's disease. Phytochemicals have the capacity to alternate the line of treatment in neurodegenerative disease. Herbal compounds have antioxidant properties and the capability to interact with several targets especially signaling pathways, neuroinflammation, and protein folding [10 - 13]. For example, several reports depict that natural compounds containing chalcones and flavonoids exert antioxidant properties directly interacting in Nrf2 pathways by scavenging reactive oxygen species (ROS). It is reported that many antioxidant properties of echinatin, licochalcone, and chalcones are due to proton transfer and electron transfer mechanisms [14], and natural and synthetic analogues like morpholine, naphthoquinone, amphetamine, coumarins, piperine, β-carboline, and caffeine have shown to exhibit appreciable MAO and neuroprotection [15 - 17]. Several synthetic compounds were developed incorporating the basic structure of chalcone and flavonoids as the basic moiety [18 - 23]. This book chapter mainly emphasizes the chalcones and flavonoids containing natural products related to their MAO-B action.

CHALCONES

The name" chalcone" was coined by the scientists Stanislaw Kostanneki and Josef Tambor. Chalcones are open-chain and chemically a three α, β-carbon unsaturated carbonyl system joined to two aromatic rings [24, 25] (Fig. **1**) They are also known to be the major precursor in the biosynthesis of some heterocyclic compounds like pyrazolines, benzothiazepine, flavones, and 1,4-diketones.

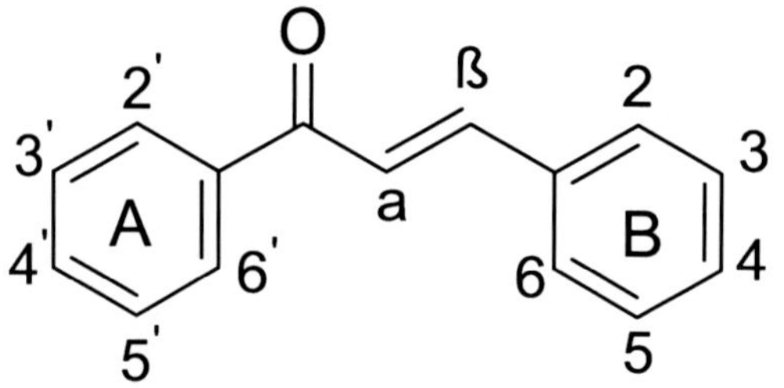

Fig. (1). Chemical structure of chalcone.

Chalcones are known as a biogenetic precursor of most flavonoids found in fruits (apple, citrus, and tomato), vegetables (potatoes, bean sprouts, and shallots), edible plants like licorice, but do not accumulate much in plants and are abundantly found in Leguminosae, Moraceae, and Asteraceae families. Chalcones are studied for their broad-spectrum activities like antimicrobial, antimicrobials, antioxidant, antifungal, cytotoxic, chemopreventive, and proapoptotic. They have long been used in traditional medicine and many of the chalcones isolated from the plants are now under clinical trials for their treatment in viral, cancer, cardiovascular diseases, and CNS disorders and cosmetic preparations [26].

Prenylated Chalcone: Xanthoangelol and 4-Hydroxyderricin

Two prenylated chalcones found in *Angelica keiskei* are xanthoangelol (**1**) and 4-hydroxyderricin (**2**) (Fig. **2**). They were extracted by activity-guided fractionation and evaluated for their MAO inhibitory activity. Xanthoangelol is found to be a nonselective MAO inhibitor with IC_{50} values of 43.4 μM and 43.9 μM for MAO-A and MAO-B inhibition, respectively [27].

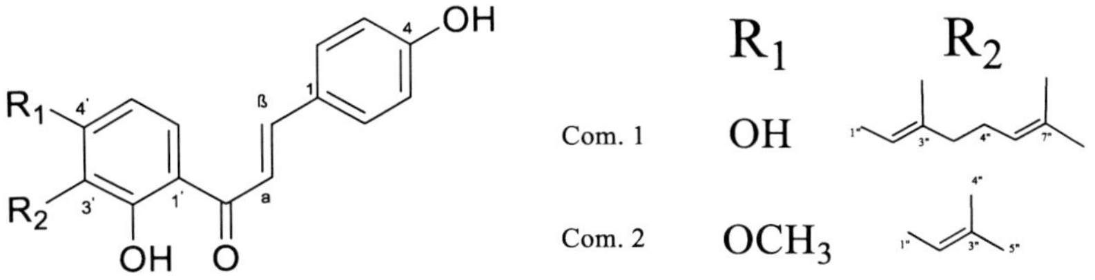

Fig. (2). Prenylated chalcones: xanthoangelol (**1**) and 4-hydroxyderrin (**2**).

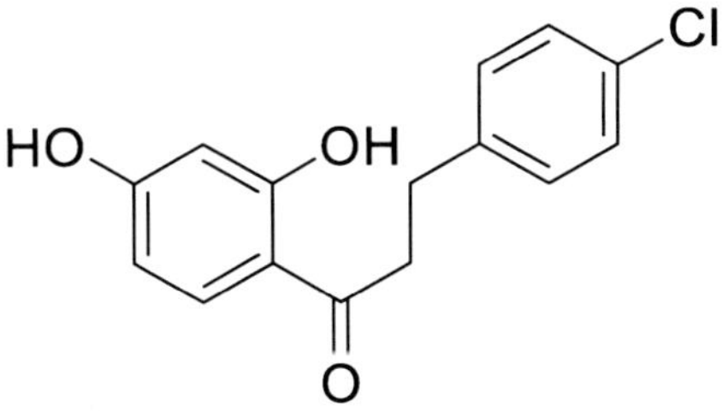

Fig. (3). 3-(4-chlorophenyl)-1-(2,4-dihydroxyphenyl)-propan-1-one.

Synthetic derivatives of the same were prepared and tested for human monoamine oxidases A and B (hMAO-A and hMAO-B) inhibition. It is ascertained that compounds that contain chlorine, methoxyl or hydroxyl substituents on the 4th position of the chalcone demonstrated selective hMAO-B inhibition in the concentration of nano- and micromolar ranges. The *in-silico* studies were conducted to analyze the enzyme-inhibitor interaction and to justify the selectivity of the lead compound for hMAO-B inhibitory action. In all docking poses, H-bonds stabilize the identification of ligands and the hydroxyl-phenyl ring was located near the cofactor. The most active compound among them was 3-(--chlorophenyl)-1-2,4-dihydroxy phenyl)-propan-1-one (Fig. **3**). exhibiting hydrogen-pi interactions with chlorophenyl ring and two hydrogen bonds with FAD and Tyr435, respectively [28].

Resveratrol

Resveratrol is chemically a 3,5,4-trihydroxystilbene known as "red phenol" with a stilbene backbone. Resveratrol exists in two isomeric forms, namely *cis* and *trans-resveratrol* (Fig. **4**). among which *trans*-resveratrol is biologically the most active form.

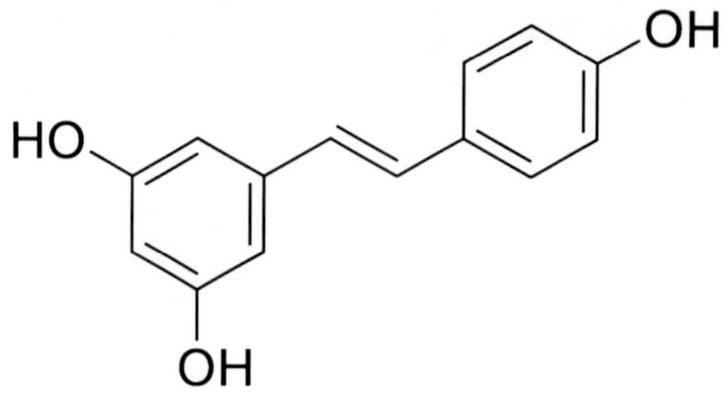

Fig. (4). Chemical structure of Resveratrol.

Resveratrol is a fat-soluble compound found in over 100 edible plants synthesized by fungal or bacterial infection [29 - 31]. It is also richly found in the skin of peanuts, berries, and grapes [32]. Resveratrol is found to have multiple functions on CNS by modulating different pathways in AD pathology. It is known to be a neuroprotector by acting as a calorie restriction mimetic *via* the sirtuin pathway, thereby preventing apoptosis. It also protects blood vessels and nerves against Aβ insults [33, 34]. Rodacka and coworkers reported the neuroprotective effects of resveratrol through the superoxide anion radical-induced inactivation of glyceraldehyde-3-phosphate dehydrogenase (GADPH). This effect is confirmed by docking studies with an enzyme that proves that resveratrol radical ion is more efficient in GADPH inactivation than the superoxide anion alone [35].

In a docking and molecular simulation study by Carpene *et al.*, resveratrol was taken as a ligand along with other natural chalcone-containing herbs for a comparison of different herbal components, and docking scores were calculated for MAO-A and B by Schrodinger's software. Docking studies paved some important outcomes and explained that resveratrol interacted non-covalently within the MAO-A and MAO-B interaction sites. All the natural ligands interacted with in substrate pockets near flavin moiety. The H-acceptor for resveratrol is found to be the Pro102 containing a back bone oxygen atom. The oxidation of tyramine moiety, as MAO-dependent oxidation, was blocked by resveratrol [36].

Dihydrochalcones

A study by Haraguchi and coworkers suggests that the traditional medicine *Gentiana lutea* is a potent inhibitor of rat MAOs. The study explains that the methanolic extract of *Gentiana* is fractionated using ethyl acetate and water. Ethyl acetate fraction was subjected to column chromatography and 4 compounds were isolated. The compounds (Fig. **5**) 3-3” linked-(2’-hydroxy-4”-*O*-isoprenylchalcone)-2’’’-hydroxy-4”-*O*-isoprenylchalcone) (**3**), 2-methoxy-3-(1,10 -dimethylallyl)-6a,10a-dihydrobenzo[1,2-*c*] chroman-6-one (**4**) were the potential lead MAO inhibitors isolated from *G. lutea.* A hydrolysis product (**5**) also inhibited MAOs. The hydrolysis product (**5**) from dimeric chalcone derivative (**3**) exhibited high potent MAO-B inhibition than MAO-A [37].

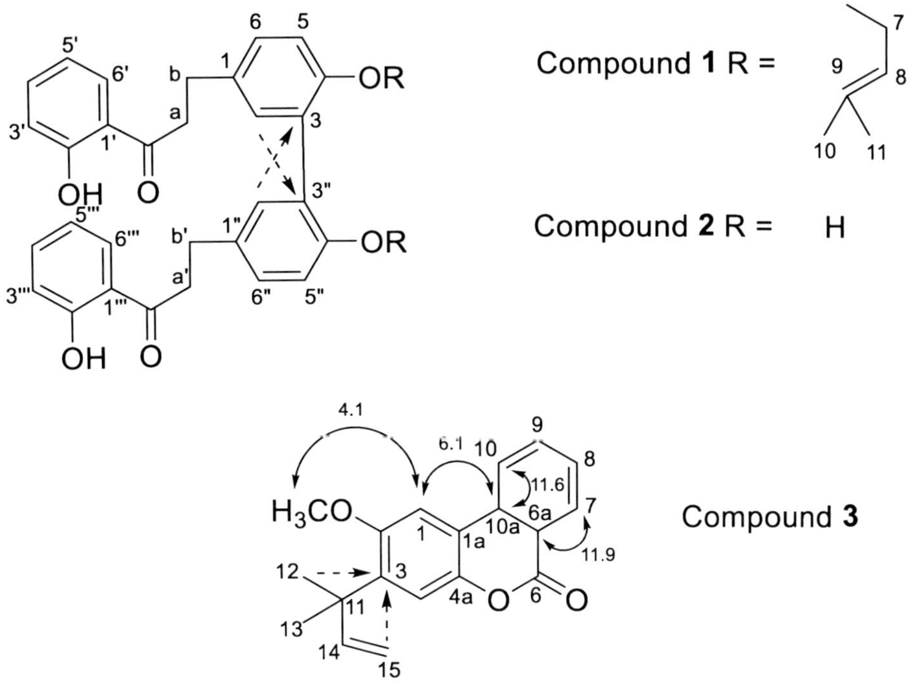

Fig. (5). structure of MAOIs isolated from *Gentiana lutea*..

Flavonoids

Flavonoids are important plant polyphenolic metabolites reported for their potential activity against MAO enzymes. Epidemiological proof suggests that consuming flavonoids can promote human health by modulating physiological functions that depend upon the physical-chemical properties and substitution pattern on the molecule [38 - 40]. Flavonoids are characterized by an extremely reactive hydroxyl group(s) that can scavenge free radicals to less reactive compounds by oxidation, which in turn, reduces oxidative stress. Emerging research suggests that these compounds can induce necessary mitochondrial enzymes involved in respiration and chelate divalent metal ions. The latest information gathered by different surveys depicts that lifetime utilization of various herbs rich in flavonoids can reduce the rate of depression in the elderly. Comparative research has been put forward by different scientists to assess the impacts of flavonoid-rich intercessions on mood [41].

Quercetin

Quercetin is chemically 3,3',4',5,7-pentahydroxyflavone, a subclass of flavonoids that has overwhelming existence in food and herbs (Fig. **6**). It consists of a fused ring system with phenyl substituents having benzopyran as the aromatic ring. Apples, citrus fruits, berries, and cherries, and also vegetables like broccoli, onions, and beverages such as red wine and tea are rich sources of quercetin [42, 43].

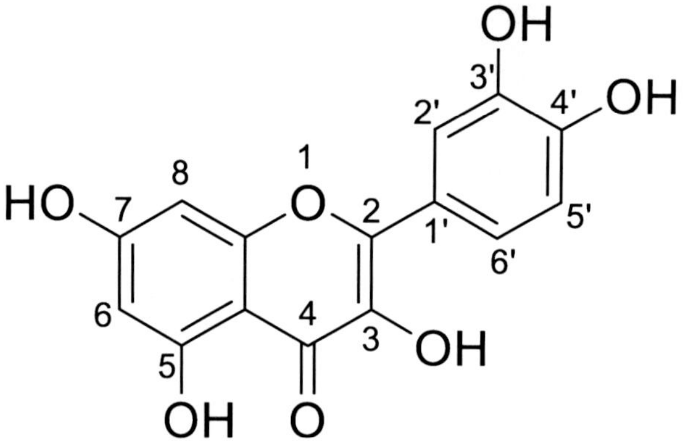

Fig. (6). Chemical structure of quercetin.

A plant that is rich in quercetin, *Hypericum hircinum* was evaluated for MAO-A and B by *in vitro* tests. *In silico* analysis was done by applying the graphical user interface using Schrödinger. Molecular interactions during the experiments emphasized a great relationship with trial restraint information and affirmed the MAO action. The quercetin fits better hMAO-A over in the restricting pocket of hMAO-B due to the foundation of most extreme pi-pi interactions and intermolecular hydrogen bonding [44].

Xanthones

Xanthones hold a unique 9*H*-xanthen-9-one scaffold, which mainly occurs in the plant families like Hypericaceae and Gentianaceae as well as in lichens and fungi (Fig. 7) [45]. Varieties of types of xanthones are identified, like xanthone glycosides, oxygenated xanthones, prenylated xanthones, xanthonolignoids, and miscellaneous types, too [46].

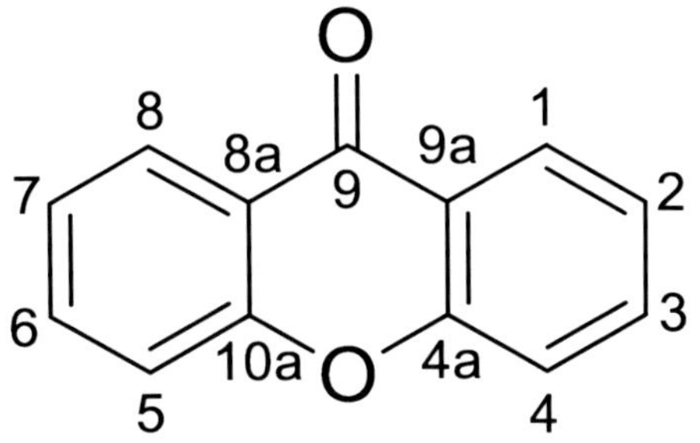

Fig. (7). Chemical structure of xanthone.

In an *in-silico* approach performed by Zang and coworkers, a comparison is done to know the effects produced by xanthones and quercetin on MAO enzymes. The OH groups of xanthones in positions 1 and 3 reacted with OH at other positions. As discussed in the previous studies, quercetin, simulated against hMAO-B, has maximum interaction on the 5th or 7th positions with a score of 61.5. In the case of quercetin, the significant contributor to binding and increasing enzyme inhibition is ring B of catechol, whereas xanthone does not require this ring for binding interaction. Ring B of flavonoids can rotate through the C2-C10 bond, which allows altering their orientation to fit inside the potential pockets of various proteins [47].

Homoisoflavonoids

Homoisoflavonoids are natural products commonly found in the rhizomes, roots, and bulbs of the Hyacinthaceae and Caesalpinioideae families. They have structural similarities to flavonoids and they are classified into 3 groups: 3-benzylidenechroman-4-ones, 3-benzylchroman-4-ones, and 3-benzyl-4*H*-chromen-4-ones (Fig. **8**) [48, 49].

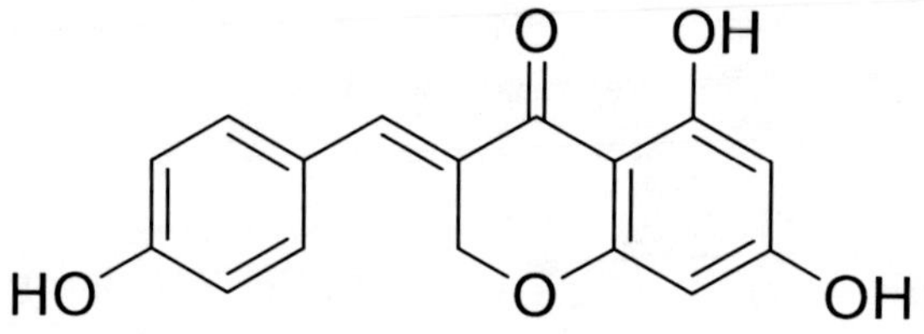

(E)-5,7-dihydroxy-3-(4-hydroxybenzylidene)chroman-4-one

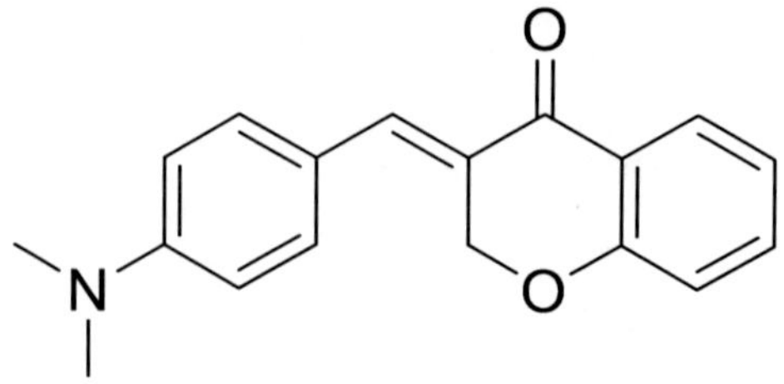

(E)-3-(4-(Dimethylamino)benzylidene)chroman-4-one

Fig. (8). Chemical structure of homoisoflavonoids.

Desideri and coworkers experimented on homoisoflavonoids and synthesized compounds to test the *in vitro* inhibitory activity of hMAO isoforms of A and B. *In silico* studies paved the way for the inhibitory action of homoisoflavonoids and the best poses of (*E*)-3-(4-(dimethylamino)benzylidene)chroman-4-one and (*E*)-5,7-dihydroxy-3-(4-hydroxybenzylidene)chroman-4-one suggested that chromone rings were located very near to the FAD in human monoamine oxidase-A. The closeness of the phenolic hydroxyl group due to an H-bond with an N_5 atom of FAD is the distinction in the hMAO-A coupling association. (*E*)-3--4-(dimethylamino) benzylidene) chroman-4-one was found to involve hydrophobic interactions with TYR444 and ASN181, whereas (*E*)-5,7-dihydro-y-3-(4-hydroxybenzylidene)chroman-4-one with TYR69 [50].

Thioflavones

Studies done on the potential class of thioflavones revealed their hMAO inhibitory action and subjected to *in silico* studies by Glide to examine both (*R*) and (*S*) enantiomers of 2-(4-fluorophenyl)-7-methyl-2,3-dihydrochromen-4-one and to assess the capacity to bind with hMAO isoforms. It was found that both enantiomers fit inside both hMAO isomeric forms and possess the best inhibitory action (Fig. **9**) [51].

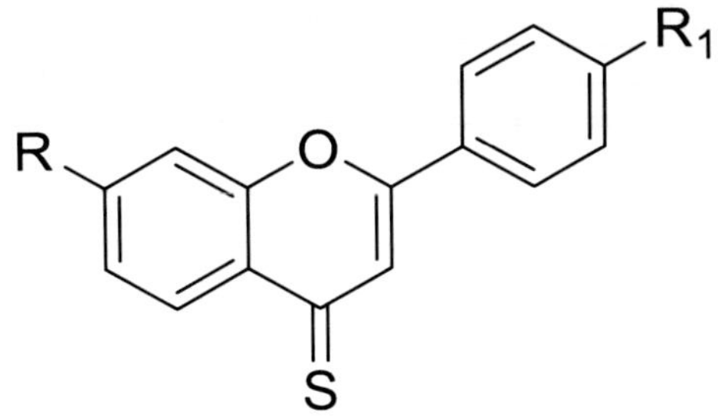

Fig. (9). Chemical structure of thioflavone.

Sideritis Flavonoids

The genus *Sideritis* belongs to the Lamiaceae family and is known to contain essential oils, diterpenes, and flavonoids [52 - 55]. It has over 500 species spread over the Mediterranean-Macaronesian region. These species have been used in traditional medicine as infusions for the treatment of gastrointestinal disorders, common colds, anticonvulsants, analgesics, tonics, sedatives, and diuretics. It is also used for improving cognitive functions and memory.

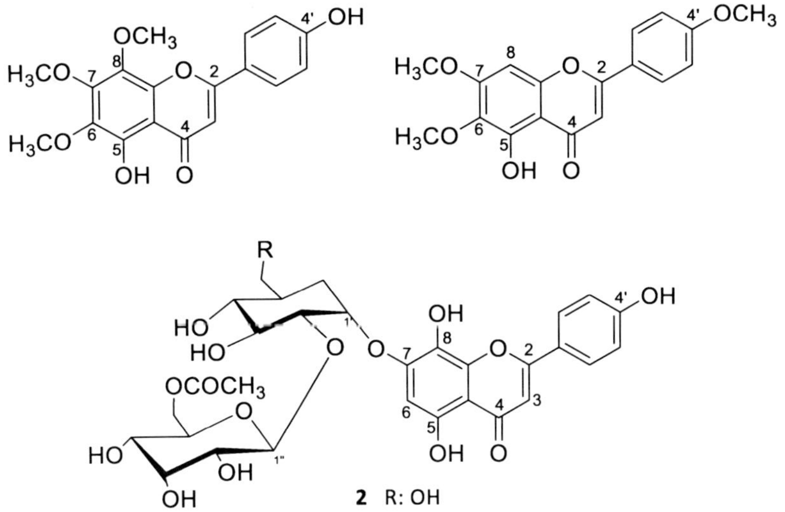

2 R: OH

3 R: $OCOCH_3$

Fig. (10). Structures of the four studied flavonoids: xanthomicrol (1), isoscutellarein 7-*O*-[6”’-*O*-acetyl--‐D-allopyranosyl]-ß-D-glucopyranoside (2), isoscutellarein 7-*O*-[6”’-*O*-acetyl-ß-D-allopyranosyl]-6”-*O*-acetyl-ß-D-gluco-pyranoside (3) and salvigenine (4).

Recently Turkmenoglu and his team studied the hMAO inhibitory capability of *Sideritis* flavonoids like xanthomicrol, isoscutellarein 7-*O*-[6”’-*O*-acetyl--‐D-allopyranosyl-1→2)]-6”-*O*-acetyl-β-D-glucopyranoside, isoscutellarein 7-*O*-

[6'''-*O*-acetyl-β-D-allopyranosyl-(1→2)]-6''-*O*-acetyl-β-D-gluco-pyranoside, salvigenin (Fig. **10**). using recombinant hMAO isoenzymes. *In-silico* tests revealed that strong electrostatic and van der Waals connections exist with the active site of hMAO-A. Also, the benzene ring of coumarin moiety of salvigenin formed two pi-pi interactions with TYR444 and TYR407, making salvigenin a powerful MAO-A inhibitor. Xanthomicrol established five hydrogen bonds with the side chains of the A isoform, which is also the reason for a promising effect on hMAO-A. The coumarin ring of xanthomicrol was found to be sandwiched between the TYR407 and TYR444 and established a pi-pi interaction with TYR407, which is known to be placed in the hydrophobic region of the active site [56].

Studies on Apigenin, Kaempferol, Quercetin and Luteolin

Phytoconstituents like apigenin, kaempferol, quercetin, and luteolin (Fig. **11**) have attained remarkable attention on their clinical efficiency in traditional medicine for the treatment of neurodegenerative disorders. Apigenin [57], kaempferol [58], and quercetin [59] are established as antiepileptic agents, whereas luteolin [60, 61] and quercetin [62] also act as neuroprotective agents against multiple sclerosis.

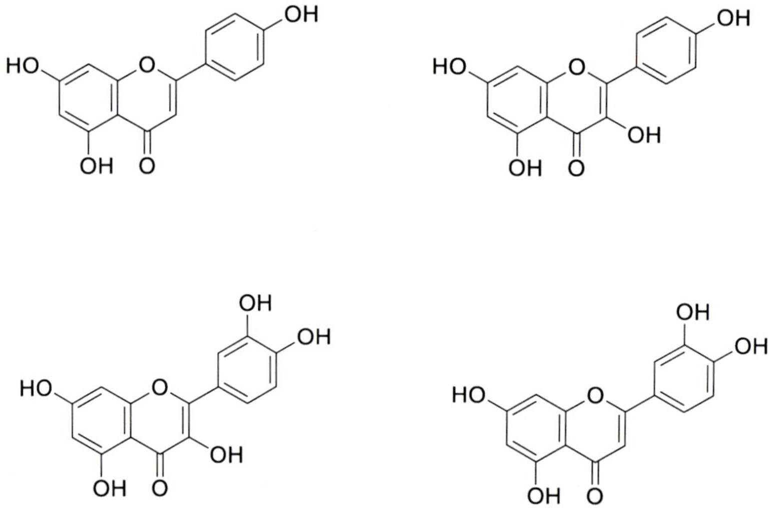

Fig. (11). Apigenin (1), Kaempferol (2), Quercetin (3) and Luteolin (4).

MAO inhibitory affinity of apigenin, kaempferol, quercetin, and luteolin were assessed by *in silico* docking study using Auto Dock tools. Lamarckian Genetic

Algorithm (LGA) is used to compute the binding free energy and inhibition constants. Interactions with various residues are given in Fig. **(12).**

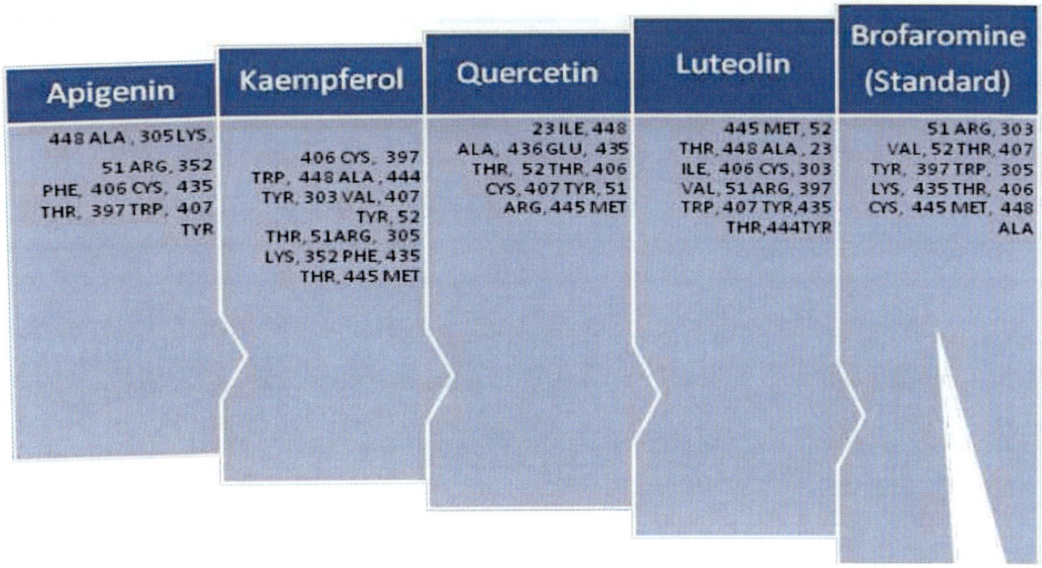

Fig. (12). In silico docking studies about flavonoids like apigenin, kaempferol, quercetin, and luteolin and their site of interaction with amino acids.

The Figure indicates that the four flavonoids interacted in a similar way except for some distinct bonds. Apigenin, kaempferol, quercetin, and luteolin have similar interactions with ALA448, CYS406, THR435, and TYR407 amino acid residues. Furthermore, luteolin formed interactions similar to the standard brofaromine, and amino acid residues involved were ARG51, VAL303, THR407, MET445, CYS406, ALA448, TRP397, and THR435 [63].

PRENYLAPIGENIN

Belula *et al.* isolated 6-prenylapigenin (5,7-dihydroxy-2-(4-hydroxyphenyl--6-(3-methyl-but-2-en-1-yl)-4H-chromen-4-one) as a major flavanone (Fig. **13**) containing an isoprenyl sidechain, from *Achyranthes aspera*, family Amaranthaceae.

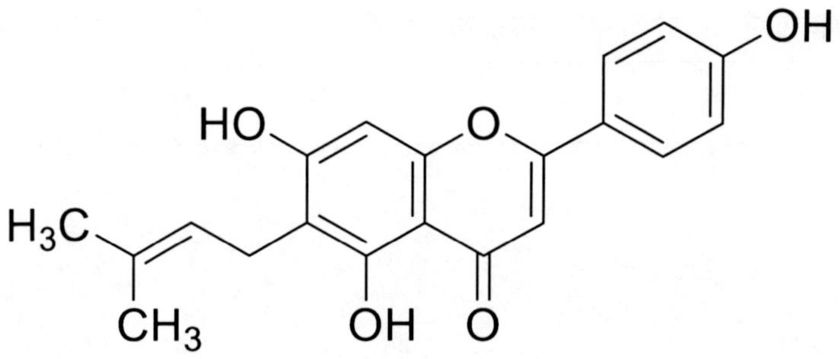

Fig. (13). 6-prenylapigenin.

His team also performed molecular docking to assess the binding modes towards monoamine oxidase-A enzyme by AutoDock experiments. It explicates that 6-prenylapigenin is a potential MAO-A inhibitor having a score of -8.06 kcal/mol and an inhibition constant of 1.23 μM. To understand the structural role, the structure was into three different fragments of the flavone skeleton, and the phenolic group was placed on the second position of the nucleus and the distal side chain on the 6th position. An interesting fact is that the π electrons of the phenolic side chain are placed in between the side chain of amino acid residues like TYR407 and TYR444, which form a hydrophobic portion of the enzyme. Another site for π-π stacking interaction is flavone and TRP441 amino acid residue on the surface of the hMAO-A binding site.

Bavachinin and Bavachin

Zarmouh and associates [64] identified two new MAO-B inhibitors, bavachinin (BNN) and bavachin (BVN), from the ethanolic extract of *Psoralea corylifolia* seeds. They are chemically prenyl flavanones and are known for their neuroprotective [65] and antioxidant properties (Fig. **14**) [66].

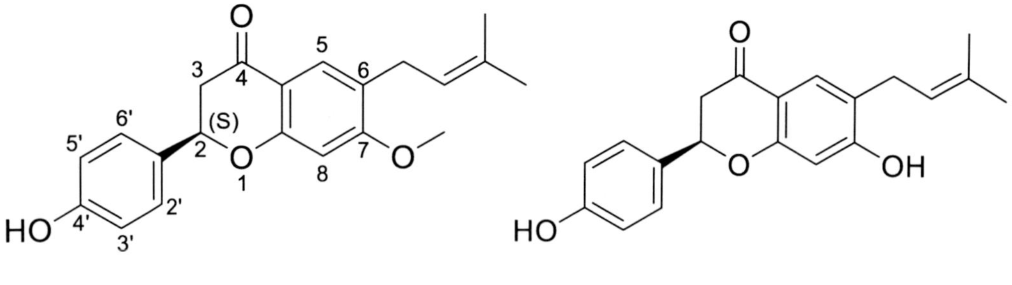

Fig. (14). Chemical structures of bavachinin (BNN) and bavachin (BVN).

Both ethanolic extract of *Psoralea corylifolia* and BNN inhibited stronger hMAO-B than hMAO-A. BNN exhibited selective hMAO-B inhibition with IC_{50} of 8.82 µM to hMAO-A with IC_{50} of 189.28 µM. Molecular docking examination of BNN suggested that the C-7-methoxy group allows selectivity, reversibility, and affinity to MAO-B Table **1.** [64].

Table 1. Summary of the docking scores, H-bonds formed, and isoform selectivity data.

Compound	MAO-A active site		MAO-B active site		General bonds		Selectivity to MAO isoform
	Docking score	H-Bond formed	Docking score	H-bond formed	H-bond formed	Amino acid residues	
Bavachin (BVN)	-8.69	H_2O-726	-3.95	0	-	-	-
Bavachinin (BNN)	-1.54	0	-6.82	2	OH....HN OH....O	Thr:201:A Thr:201:A	B
Safinamide	-0.25	0	-6.12	3	NH....O NH....O NH....O	Thr:201:A GLU:84:A PRO:102:A	B

Genistein

Genistein (GST) is an isoflavone traditionally found in medicinal herbs such as bakuchi [67], soybean [68], and red clover (Fig. **15**) [69].

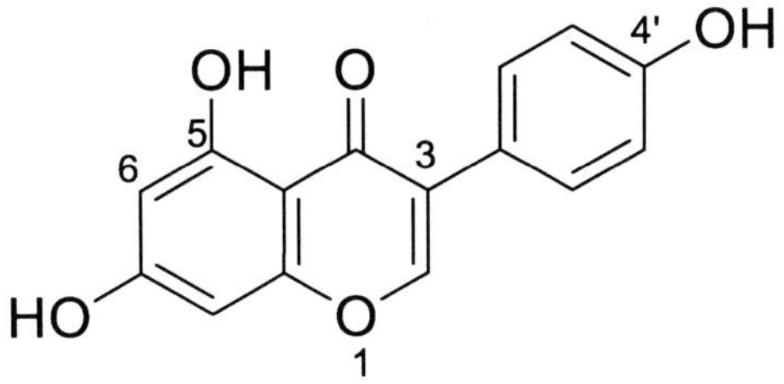

Fig. (15). Chemical structure of Genistein.

Zarmouh and coworkers [70] reported on the isoflavone genistein (GST) and its analogue daidzein (DZ) for MAO inhibition. GST demonstrated hMAO–B inhibition with an IC_{50} value of 6.81 µM, and its hMAO-A inhibition was higher than the reference deprenyl. It is also shown to be a time-dependent reversible and competitive hMAO–A and hMAO–B inhibitor with a lower K_i for hMAO–B. Docking studies illustrated that reversibility and selectivity inhibition is due to the C5-OH effects on its spatial arrangement and its interactions with THR201 of the active site. It is assumed that GST can interact with MAO-B better than MAO-A depending upon their strength to retard tyramine and luciferin derivative substrate from interacting and thereby reduce the production of H_2O_2 as a byproduct in the brain Table **2**.

Table 2. Summary of the docking scores, H-bonds formed and amino acids involved.

Name of the Lead	MAO-A		MAO-B		Bond Length Distance Å	Amino Acid
	Docking Score	Predicted H-Bond	Docking Score	Predicted H-Bond		
Genistein (GST)	-7.3	0	-12.8	2 (OH..... N)	2.27	THR:201:A
Daidzein (DZ)	-6.8	0	-12.8	1 (O.....HN)	2.32	THR:201:A

Phytochemicals from *Clitoria Ternatea*

Clitoria ternatea is a popular herbal drug used in "*Medhya Rasayana*" as a brain and nervine medicine traditionally practiced in traditional medicine in treating neurological diseases and revitalizing neurons [71, 72]. Margret and coworkers suggested the MAO inhibitory activity of 26 isolated phytoconstituents from the methanolic extract of *Clitoria ternatea*. Docking experiments was carried out on phytocomponents such as myricetin-3-glucoside, myricetin-3-neohesperidoside, myricetin-3-rutinoside, delphinidin 3,3,5-triglucoside, kaempferol derivatives (kaempferol 3-rutinoside, kaempferol 3-glucoside, kaempferol 3-neohesperidoside), quercetin derivatives (quercetin 3-2G-rhamnosyl rutinoside, quercetin 3-rutinoside, quercetin 3-neohesperidoside and quercetin 3-glucoside) on target proteins. The important interaction between n-hexadecanoic acid and MAO-A was contributed by the amino acids MET445 and ALA68. The interaction between (*Z*)-9,17-octadecadienal and MAO-A was contributed by the amino acids ALA68 and TYR69. Among the docked compounds, kaempferol---monoglucoside showed the least score of -13.90/-12.95 kcal/mol. The competitive binding was displayed among the four isolated compounds and (*Z*)-9,17-octadecadienal was established with low, restricting binding affinity -6.50--7.71 kcal/mol with both MAO forms and n-hexadecanoic acid with a minimum docking score of -10.5001 kcal/mol against MAO-B Table **3.** [73].

O-Methylated Flavonoids

O-Methylated flavonoids were isolated from plants like *Senecio roseiflorus* (1), *Polygonum senegalense* (2 and 3), *Bhaphia macrocalyx* (4), *Gardenia ternifolia* (5), and *Psiadia punctualata* (Fig. **16**). *In vitro* studies proved that the interaction with MAO-A characterized these plant species. Compounds 1, 2, and 5 exhibited selective inhibition of MAO-A, while 4 and 6 showed selective inhibition of

MAO-B. The *in silico* studies proved that compound 1 binds with the active site of human MAO-A near N5 of FAD (Fig. **17**) The binding free energy calculation reveals that the *O*-methylated flavonoids (1 and 4–6) and chalcones (2 and 3) to MAO-A matched closely with the trend in the experimental IC_{50}'s. Binding-free analysis proved the better interaction of 4 and 6 with MAO-B than with MAO-A [74].

Table 3. ***In silico*** **data of isolated compounds from** ***Clitoria ternatea*****.**

Compound	Binding Score Energy Value	No. of Hydrogen Bonds	Interacting Amino Acid Residue
kaempferol-mono glucoside	-14.9178 (MAO-A) -13.9653 (MAO-B)	7 (MAO-A) 3 (MAO-B)	ASN181, GLN443, GLN66, GLN443, MET445, TYR69, ALA68 (MAO-A) LYS296, TYR60, GLY434 (MAO-B)
malvidin-3-*O*-glucoside	-7.86773 (MAO-A) 0 (MAO-B)	3 (MAO-A) 0 (MAO-B)	TYR69, GLN215, ALA68 (MAO-A)
n-hexadecanoic acid	-5.4457 (MAO-A) -10.5192 (MAO-B)	3 (MAO-A) 1 (MAO-B)	ALA68, MET445, ALA68 (MAO-A) TYR60 (MAO-B)
Quercetin	-11.4556 (MAO-A) -10.9755 (MAO-B)	2 (MAO-A) 1 (MAO-B)	ASN181, PHE208 (MAO-A) GLY434 (MAO-B)

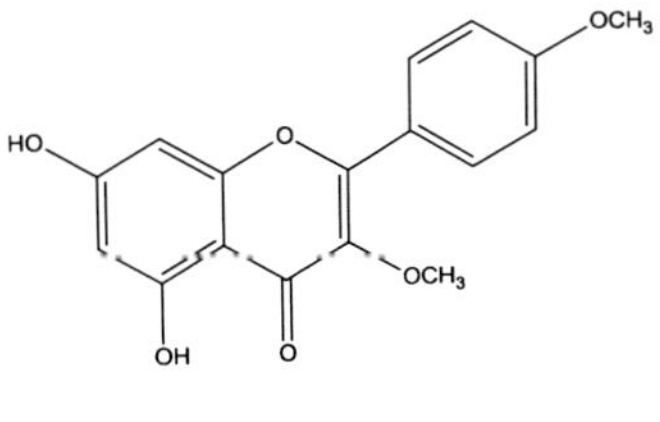

1

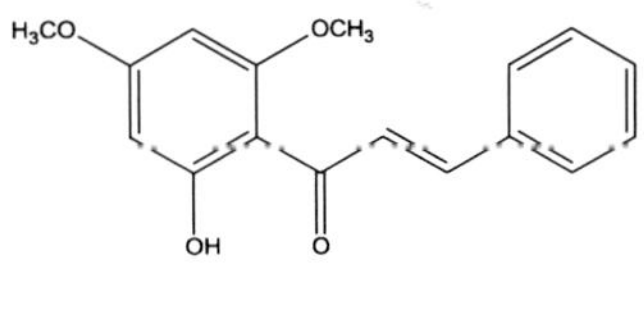

2

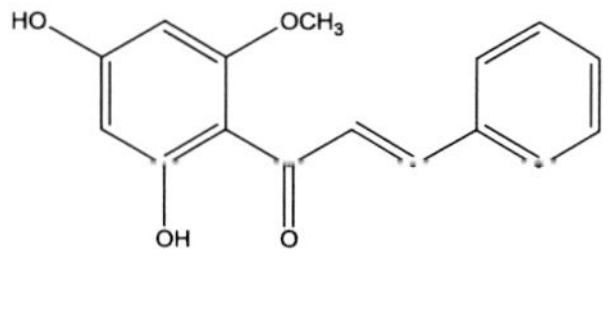

3

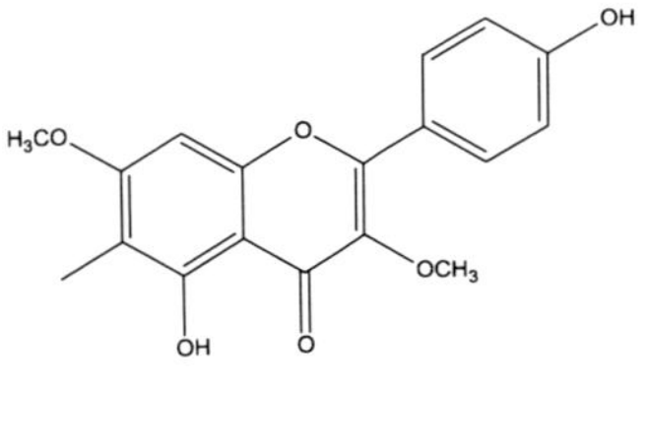

4

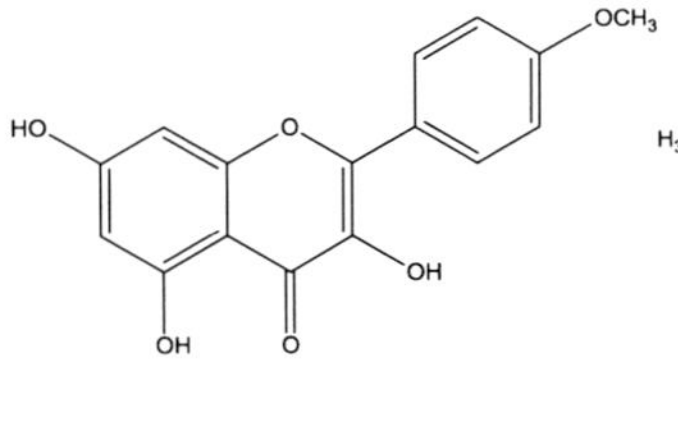

5

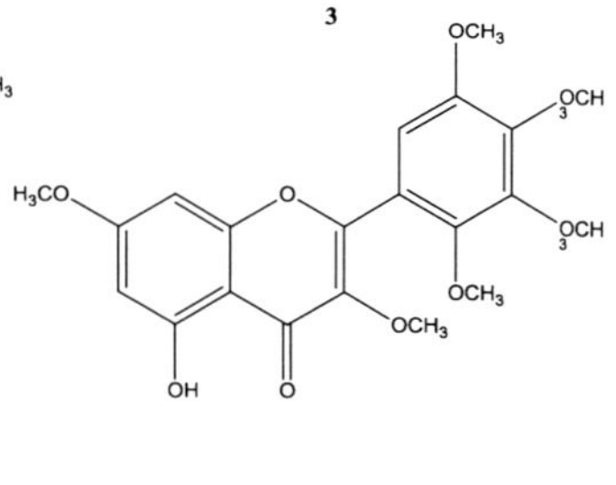

6

Fig. (16). Chemical structures of *O*-methylated flavonoids (**1-6**).

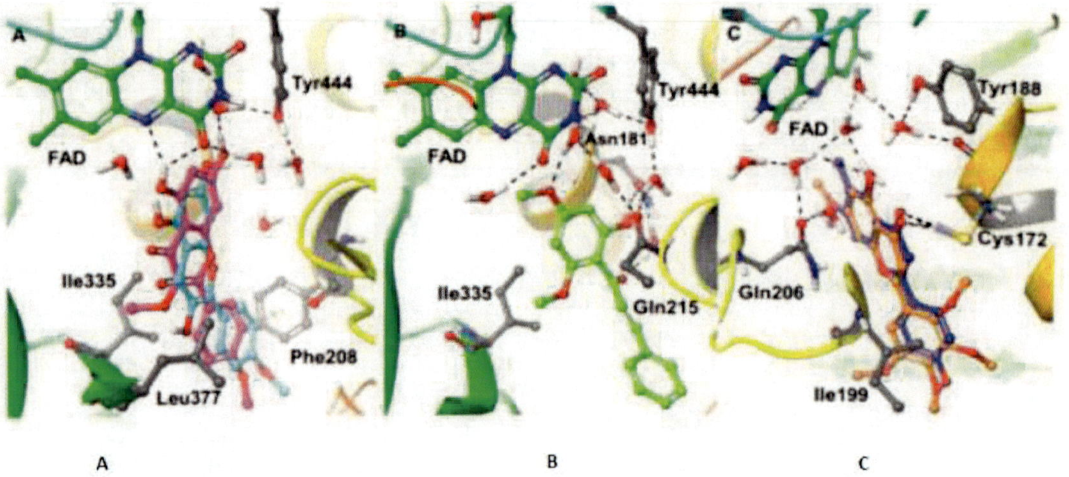

Fig. (17). 3D representation of protein-ligand interaction of compounds **1-6** with X-ray crystal structures of MAO-A and B. **(A)1** (C magenta, stick model) and **5** (C cyan, stick model) with MAO-A, **(B)2** (C light green, stick model) with MAO-A, **(C)4** (C blue, stick model), and **6** (C orange, stick model) with MAO-B. Some crystallographic water molecules (O red, H white, stick model), FAD (C dark green), and the important residues of MAO-A and MAO-B (C gray) are also shown. The black dashed lines represent H-bonding.

CONCLUDING REMARKS

Plant metabolites are known to be efficient scaffolds for the critical design of unique and potential drugs against neurodegenerative diseases evolved by the increased activity of biological amines within the areas of CNS. Computational modeling in human mono oxidase has led to advancement in drug design and the treatment of various neurodegenerative diseases. Exploration of bioactive components that can exert MAO inhibitory action and prevent the progression of neurodegenerative diseases may provide important insight into developing novel and highly effective treatments for CNS disorders such as Alzheimer's disease, Parkinson's disease, depression, and anxiety. Chalcones and flavonoids were consistently associated with a variety of reassuring MAO inhibitory actions, giving a template for pharmaceutical industries to design and synthesize moieties helpful in treating nervous disorders. The free radical scavenging properties of phenolic groups present in most chalcones and flavonoids make them a favorite candidate. Many medicinal chemists work on computational design with new potent and specific MAO inhibitors endowed with a better safety profile.

Along with docking, the crystallographic structures of MAO, lead hybridization, and COMFA analyses pave the way to discover new and effective solutions for NDDs. Based on the structural requirements and essential modifications, there are numerous ongoing research activities to design novel molecules. Chalcones and flavonoids remain the most crucial and stimulating field of research and future chemical changes for preclinical and clinical studies. In the future, based on the simulation results of the reported chalcones and flavonoids, the active and improved derivatives can be tested in-vitro for evaluation of their inhibitory activity against the MAO-B enzyme. Thus, it can provide safer and more potent MAO inhibitors to treat neurodegenerative diseases.

CONSENT FOR PUBLICATION

Not applicable.

CONFLICT OF INTEREST

The author declares no conflict of interest, financial or otherwise.

ACKNOWLEDGEMENTS

Declared none.

REFERENCES

[1] von Campenhausen, S.; Bornschein, B.; Wick, R.; Bötzel, K.; Sampaio, C.; Poewe, W.; Oertel, W.; Siebert, U.; Berger, K.; Dodel, R. Prevalence and incidence of Parkinson's disease in Europe. *Eur. Neuropsychopharmacol.*, **2005**, *15*(4), 473-490. [http://dx.doi.org/10.1016/j.euroneuro.2005.04.007] [PMID: 15963700]

[2] Gershanik, O.S. Improving L -dopa therapy: The development of enzyme inhibitors. *Mov. Disord.*, **2015**, *30*(1), 103-113. [http://dx.doi.org/10.1002/mds.26050] [PMID: 25335824]

[3] Dar, A.; Khan, K.M.; Ateeq, H.S.; Khan, S.; Rahat, S.; Perveen, S.; Supuran, C.T. Inhibition of monoamine oxidase–A activity in rat brain by synthetic hydrazines: Structure-activity relationship (SAR). *J. Enzyme Inhib. Med. Chem.*, **2005**, *20*(3), 269-274. [http://dx.doi.org/10.1080/14756360400026212] [PMID: 16119198]

[4] Bayazit, V.; Khan, K.M. Evaluation of carbonic anhydrase (CA) and monoamine oxidase (MAO) enzyme activations in organs and blood of goat (*Capra aegagrus hircus*). *J. Chem. Soc. Pak.*, **2005**, *27*, 306-313.

[5] Yu, P.H. Pharmacological and clinical implications of MAO-B inhibitors. *Gen. Pharmacol.*, **1994**, *25*(8), 1527-1539. [http://dx.doi.org/10.1016/0306-3623(94)90352-2] [PMID: 7721026]

[6] Ambure, P.; Bhat, J.; Puzyn, T.; Roy, K. Identifying natural compounds as multi-target-directed ligands against Alzheimer's disease: an *in silico* approach. *J. Biomol. Struct. Dyn.*, **2019**, *37*(5), 1282-1306. [http://dx.doi.org/10.1080/07391102.2018.1456975] [PMID: 29578387]

[7] Newman, D.J.; Cragg, G.M. Natural products as sources of new drugs over the last 25 years. *J. Nat. Prod.*, **2007**, *70*(3), 461-477. [http://dx.doi.org/10.1021/np068054v] [PMID: 17309302]

[8] Paterson, I.; Anderson, E.A. Chemistry. The renaissance of natural products as drug candidates. *Science*, **2005**, *310*(5747), 451-453. [http://dx.doi.org/10.1126/science.1116364] [PMID: 16239465]

[9] Chen, X.; Decker, M. Multi-target compounds acting in the central nervous system designed from natural products. *Curr. Med. Chem.*, **2013**, *20*(13), 1673-1685.

[http://dx.doi.org/10.2174/0929867311320130007] [PMID: 23410166]

[10] Essa, M.M.; Vijayan, R.K.; Castellano-Gonzalez, G.; Memon, M.A.; Braidy, N.; Guillemin, G.J. Neuroprotective effect of natural products against Alzheimer's disease. *Neurochem. Res.*, **2012**, *37*(9), 1829-1842.
[http://dx.doi.org/10.1007/s11064-012-0799-9] [PMID: 22614926]

[11] Mazzio, E.; Harris, N.; Soliman, K. Food constituents attenuate monoamine oxidase activity and peroxide levels in C6 astrocyte cells. *Planta Med.*, **1998**, *64*(7), 603-606.
[http://dx.doi.org/10.1055/s-2006-957530] [PMID: 9810264]

[12] Zhou, C.; Huang, Y.; Przedborski, S. Oxidative stress in Parkinson's disease: a mechanism of pathogenic and therapeutic significance. *Ann. N. Y. Acad. Sci.*, **2008**, *1147*(1), 93-104.
[http://dx.doi.org/10.1196/annals.1427.023] [PMID: 19076434]

[13] Wang, J.; Huang, L.; Cheng, C.; Li, G.; Xie, J.; Shen, M.; Chen, Q.; Li, W.; He, W.; Qiu, P.; Wu, J. Design, synthesis and biological evaluation of chalcone analogues with novel dual antioxidant mechanisms as potential anti-ischemic stroke agents. *Acta Pharm. Sin. B,* **2019**, *9*(2), 335-350.
[http://dx.doi.org/10.1016/j.apsb.2019.01.003] [PMID: 30972281]

[14] Liang, M.; Li, X.; Ouyang, X.; Xie, H.; Chen, D. Antioxidant mechanisms of echinatin and licochalcone A. *Molecules,* **2018**, *24*(1), 3.
[http://dx.doi.org/10.3390/molecules24010003] [PMID: 30577443]

[15] Ferino, G.; Vilar, S.; Matos, M.J.; Uriarte, E.; Cadoni, E. Monoamine oxidase inhibitors: ten years of docking studies. *Curr. Top. Med. Chem.*, **2012**, *12*(20), 2145-2162.
[http://dx.doi.org/10.2174/156802612805220048] [PMID: 23231393]

[16] Viña, D.; Serra, S.; Lamela, M.; Delogu, G. Herbal natural products as a source of monoamine oxidase inhibitors: a review. *Curr. Top. Med. Chem.*, **2012**, *12*(20), 2131-2144.
[http://dx.doi.org/10.2174/156802612805219996] [PMID: 23231392]

[17] Helguera, A.M.; Perez-Machado, G.; Cordeiro, M.N.; Borges, F. Discovery of MAO-B inhibitors - present status and future directions part I: oxygen heterocycles and analogs. *Mini Rev. Med. Chem.*, **2012**, *12*(10), 907-919.
[http://dx.doi.org/10.2174/138955712802762301] [PMID: 22420569]

[18] Mathew, B.; Ucar, G.; Yabanogclu-Ciftci, S.; Baysal, I.; Suresh, J.; Mathew, G.; Vilapurathu, J.; Nadeena, A.M.; Nabeela, P.; Lakshmi, V.; Haridas, A.; Fathima, F. Development of fluorinated thienylchalcones as monoamine oxidase-b inhibitors: Design, synthesis, biological evaluation, and molecular docking studies. *Lett. Org. Chem.*, **2015**, *12*(9), 605-613.
[http://dx.doi.org/10.2174/1570178612666150903213416]

[19] Mathew, B.; Suresh, J.; Mathew, G.E.; Haridas, A.; Suresh, G.; Sabreena, P. Synthesis, ADME studies, toxicity estimation, and exploration of molecular recognition of thiophene based chalcones towards monoamine oxidase-A and B. Beni-Seuf Univ. *J. Appl. Sci. (Faisalabad),* **2016**, *5*, 396-401.

[20] Carradori, S.; Gidaro, M.C.; Petzer, A.; Costa, G.; Guglielmi, P.; Chimenti, P.; Alcaro, S.; Petzer, J.P. Inhibition of human monoamine oxidase: Biological and molecular modeling studies on selected natural flavonoids. *J. Agric. Food Chem.*, **2016**, *64*(47), 9004-9011.
[http://dx.doi.org/10.1021/acs.jafc.6b03529] [PMID: 27933876]

[21] Suresh, J.; Baek, S.C.; Ramakrishnan, S.P.; Kim, H.; Mathew, B. Discovery of potent and reversible MAO-B inhibitors as furanochalcones. *Int. J. Biol. Macromol.*, **2018**, *108*, 660-664.
[http://dx.doi.org/10.1016/j.ijbiomac.2017.11.159] [PMID: 29195801]

[22] Parambi, D.G.T.; Oh, J.M.; Baek, S.C.; Lee, J.P.; Tondo, A.R.; Nicolotti, O.; Kim, H.; Mathew, B. Design, synthesis and biological evaluation of oxygenated chalcones as potent and selective MAO-B inhibitors. *Bioorg. Chem.*, **2019**, *93*, 103335.
[http://dx.doi.org/10.1016/j.bioorg.2019.103335] [PMID: 31606547]

[23] Mathew, B. Unraveling the Structural Requirements of Chalcone Chemistry Towards Monoamine

Oxidase Inhibition. *Cent. Nerv. Syst. Agents Med. Chem.*, **2019**, *19*(1), 6-7. [http://dx.doi.org/10.2174/1871524919666190131160122] [PMID: 30706795]

[24] Kumar, D.; Kumar, M.; Kumar, A.; Singh, S. Chalcone and curcumin derivatives: a way ahead for malarial treatment. *Mini Rev. Med. Chem.*, **2013**, *13*(14), 2116-2133. [http://dx.doi.org/10.2174/13895575113136660101] [PMID: 24160709]

[25] Schmidt, T.J.; Khalid, S.A.; Romanha, A.J.; Alves, T.M.; Biavatti, M.W.; Brun, R.; Da Costa, F.B.; de Castro, S.L.; Ferreira, V.F.; de Lacerda, M.V.; Lago, J.H.; Leon, L.L.; Lopes, N.P.; das Neves Amorim, R.C.; Niehues, M.; Ogungbe, I.V.; Pohlit, A.M.; Scotti, M.T.; Setzer, W.N.; de N C Soeiro, M.; Steindel, M.; Tempone, A.G. The potential of secondary metabolites from plants as drugs or leads against protozoan neglected diseases - part II. *Curr. Med. Chem.*, **2012**, *19*(14), 2176-2228. [http://dx.doi.org/10.2174/092986712800229087] [PMID: 22414104]

[26] Ni, L.; Meng, C.Q.; Sikorski, J.A. Recent advances in therapeutic chalcones. Expert Opin Ther Patents **2004**, *14*, 1669-1691.

[27] Kim, J.H.; Son, Y.K.; Kim, G.H.; Hwang, K.H. Xanthoangelol and 4-hydroxyderricin are the major active principles of the inhibitory activities against monoamine oxidases on Angelica keiskei K. *Biomol. Ther. (Seoul)*, **2013**, *21*(3), 234-240. [http://dx.doi.org/10.4062/biomolther.2012.100] [PMID: 24265870]

[28] Chimenti, F.; Fioravanti, R.; Bolasco, A.; Chimenti, P.; Secci, D.; Rossi, F.; Yáñez, M.; Orallo, F.; Ortuso, F.; Alcaro, S. Chalcones: a valid scaffold for monoamine oxidases inhibitors. *J. Med. Chem.*, **2009**, *52*(9), 2818-2824. [http://dx.doi.org/10.1021/jm801590u] [PMID: 19378991]

[29] Malhotra, A.; Bath, S.; Elbarbry, F. An Organ System Approach to Explore the Antioxidative, Anti-Inflammatory, and Cytoprotective Actions of Resveratrol. *Oxid. Med. Cell. Longev.*, **2015**, *2015*, 1-15. [http://dx.doi.org/10.1155/2015/803971] [PMID: 26180596]

[30] Vallianou, N.G.; Evangelopoulos, A.; Kazazis, C. Resveratrol and Diabetes. *Rev. Diabet. Stud.*, **2013**, *10*(4), 236-242. [http://dx.doi.org/10.1900/RDS.2013.10.236] [PMID: 24841877]

[31] Walle, T. Bioavailability of resveratrol. *Ann. N. Y. Acad. Sci.*, **2011**, *1215*(1), 9-15. [http://dx.doi.org/10.1111/j.1749-6632.2010.05842.x] [PMID: 21261636]

[32] Liu, K.; Zhou, R.; Wang, B.; Mi, M.T. Effect of resveratrol on glucose control and insulin sensitivity: a meta-analysis of 11 randomized controlled trials. *Am. J. Clin. Nutr.*, **2014**, *99*(6), 1510-1519. [http://dx.doi.org/10.3945/ajcn.113.082024] [PMID: 24695890]

[33] Villaflores, O.B.; Chen, Y.J.; Chen, C.P.; Yeh, J.M.; Wu, T.Y. Curcuminoids and resveratrol as anti-Alzheimer agents. *Taiwan. J. Obstet. Gynecol.*, **2012**, *51*(4), 515-525. [http://dx.doi.org/10.1016/j.tjog.2012.09.005] [PMID: 23276553]

[34] Anekonda, T.S. Resveratrol—A boon for treating Alzheimer's disease? *Brain Res. Brain Res. Rev.*, **2006**, *52*(2), 316-326. [http://dx.doi.org/10.1016/j.brainresrev.2006.04.004] [PMID: 16766037]

[35] Rodacka, A.; Strumillo, J.; Serafin, E.; Puchala, M. Effect of resveratrol and tiron on the inactivation of glyceraldehyde-3- phosphate dehydrogenase induced by superoxide anion radical. *Curr. Med. Chem.*, **2014**, *21*(8), 1061-1069. [http://dx.doi.org/10.2174/0929867311320666027 4] [PMID: 24059224]

[36] Carpéné, C.; Hasnaoui, M.; Balogh, B.; Matyus, P.; Fernández-Quintela, A.; Rodríguez, V.; Mercader, J.; Portillo, M.P. FernándezQuintela, A.; Rodríguez, V.; Mercader, J.; Portillo, M.P. Dietary phenolic compounds interfere with the fate of hydrogen peroxide in human adipose tissue but do not directly inhibit primary amine oxidase activity. *Oxid. Med. Cell. Longev.*, **2016**, *2016*, 1-15. [http://dx.doi.org/10.1155/2016/2427618] [PMID: 26881018]

[37] Haraguchi, H.; Tanaka, Y.; Kabbash, A.; Fujioka, T.; Ishizu, T.; Yagi, A. Monoamine oxidase

inhibitors from. *Phytochemistry,* **2004**, *65*(15), 2255-2260.
[http://dx.doi.org/10.1016/j.phytochem.2004.06.025] [PMID: 15587710]

[38] Hwang, S.L.; Shih, P.H.; Yen, G.C. Neuroprotective effects of citrus flavonoids. *J. Agric. Food Chem.,* **2012**, *60*(4), 877-885.
[http://dx.doi.org/10.1021/jf204452y] [PMID: 22224368]

[39] Matos, M.J.; Vazquez-Rodriguez, S.; Uriarte, E.; Santana, L. Potential pharmacological uses of chalcones: a patent review (from June 2011−2014). Expert Opin. Ther. Pat. **2015**, *25*, 351-366.

[40] Kumar, S.; Pandey, A.K. Chemistry and biological activities of flavonoids: an overview. *ScientificWorldJournal,* **2013**, *2013*, 1-16.
[http://dx.doi.org/10.1155/2013/162750] [PMID: 24470791]

[41] Gong, J.; Huang, J.; Ge, Q.; Chen, F.; Zhang, Y. Advanced research on the antidepressant effect of flavonoids. *Curr. Opin. Complement. Altern. Med.,* **2014**, *1*, e00011.

[42] Erlund, I. Review of the flavonoids quercetin, hesperetin, and naringenin. Dietary sources, bioactivities, bioavailability, and epidemiology. *Nutr. Res.,* **2004**, *24*(10), 851-874.
[http://dx.doi.org/10.1016/j.nutres.2004.07.005]

[43] Nijveldt, R.J.; van Nood, E.; van Hoorn, D.E.C.; Boelens, P.G.; van Norren, K.; van Leeuwen, P.A.M. Flavonoids: a review of probable mechanisms of action and potential applications. *Am. J. Clin. Nutr.,* **2001**, *74*(4), 418-425.
[http://dx.doi.org/10.1093/ajcn/74.4.418] [PMID: 11566638]

[44] Chimenti, F.; Cottiglia, F.; Bonsignore, L.; Casu, L.; Casu, M.; Floris, C.; Secci, D.; Bolasco, A.; Chimenti, P.; Granese, A.; Befani, O.; Turini, P.; Alcaro, S.; Ortuso, F.; Trombetta, G.; Loizzo, A.; Guarino, I. Quercetin as the active principle of Hypericum hircinum exerts a selective inhibitory activity against MAO-A: extraction, biological analysis, and computational study. *J. Nat. Prod.,* **2006**, *69*(6), 945-949.
[http://dx.doi.org/10.1021/np060015w] [PMID: 16792415]

[45] Cardona, M.L.; Fernández, I.; Pedro, J.R.; Serrano, A. Xanthones from *Hypericum reflexum. Phytochemistry,* **1990**, *29*(9), 3003-3006.
[http://dx.doi.org/10.1016/0031-9422(90)87123-C]

[46] Peres, V.; Nagem, T.J. Trioxygenated naturally occurring xanthones. *Phytochemistry,* **1997**, *44*(2), 191-214.
[http://dx.doi.org/10.1016/S0031-9422(96)00421-9]

[47] Ji, H.F.; Zhang, H.Y. Theoretical evaluation of flavonoids as multipotent agents to combat Alzheimer's disease. *J. Mol. Struct. THEOCHEM,* **2006**, *767*(1-3), 3-9.
[http://dx.doi.org/10.1016/j.theochem.2006.04.041]

[48] Al Nakib, T.; Bezjak, V.; Meegan, M.J.; Chandy, R. Synthesis and antifungal activity of some 3-benzylidenechroman-4-ones, 3-benzylidenethiochroman-4-ones and 2-benzylidene-1-tetralones. *Eur. J. Med. Chem.,* **1990**, *25*(5), 455-462.
[http://dx.doi.org/10.1016/0223-5234(90)90010-Z]

[49] Desideri, N.; Olivieri, S.; Stein, M.; Sgro, R.; Orsi, N.; Conti, C. Synthesis and anti-picornavirus activity of homo-isoflavonoids. *Antivir. Chem. Chemother.,* **1997**, *8*(6), 545-555.
[http://dx.doi.org/10.1177/095632029700800609]

[50] Desideri, N.; Bolasco, A.; Fioravanti, R.; Proietti Monaco, L.; Orallo, F.; Yáñez, M.; Ortuso, F.; Alcaro, S. Homoisoflavonoids: natural scaffolds with potent and selective monoamine oxidase-B inhibition properties. *J. Med. Chem.,* **2011**, *54*(7), 2155-2164.
[http://dx.doi.org/10.1021/jm1013709] [PMID: 21405131]

[51] Chimenti, F.; Fioravanti, R.; Bolasco, A.; Chimenti, P.; Secci, D.; Rossi, F.; Yáñez, M.; Orallo, F.; Ortuso, F.; Alcaro, S.; Cirilli, R.; Ferretti, R.; Sanna, M.L. A new series of flavones, thioflavones, and flavanones as selective monoamine oxidase-B inhibitors. *Bioorg. Med. Chem.,* **2010**, *18*(3), 1273-

1279.
[http://dx.doi.org/10.1016/j.bmc.2009.12.029] [PMID: 20045650]

[52] Obon de Castro, C.; Rivera-Nunez, D. Phanerogamarum Monographiae Tomus XXI: A Taxonomic Revision of the Section Sideritis (genus Sideritis) (Labiatae). **1994**,

[53] Ezer, N.; Akcoş, Y. Flavonoids from *Sideritis lycia. J. Hacettepe Univ. Fac. Pharm.*, **1995**, *15*, 81-87.

[54] Knörle, R. Extracts of Sideritis scardica as triple monoamine reuptake inhibitors. J. Neural Transm. 2012, 119, 1477–1482. *Molecules*, **2015**, *20*, 7471.

[55] González-Burgos, E.; Carretero, M.E.; Gómez-Serranillos, M.P. *Sideritis* spp.: Uses, chemical composition and pharmacological activities—A review. *J. Ethnopharmacol.*, **2011**, *135*(2), 209-225. [http://dx.doi.org/10.1016/j.jep.2011.03.014] [PMID: 21420484]

[56] Turkmenoglu, F.; Baysal, İ.; Ciftci-Yabanoglu, S.; Yelekci, K.; Temel, H.; Paşa, S.; Ezer, N.; Çalış, İ.; Ucar, G. Flavonoids from Sideritis species: human monoamine oxidase (hMAO) inhibitory activities, molecular docking studies and crystal structure of xanthomicrol. *Molecules*, **2015**, *20*(5), 7454-7473. [http://dx.doi.org/10.3390/molecules20057454] [PMID: 25915461]

[57] Song, J.; Parker, L.; Hormozi, L.; Tanouye, M.A. DNA topoisomerase I inhibitors ameliorate seizure-like behaviors and paralysis in a Drosophila model of epilepsy. *Neuroscience*, **2008**, *156*(3), 722-728. [http://dx.doi.org/10.1016/j.neuroscience.2008.07.024] [PMID: 18703119]

[58] Jäger, A.K.; Krydsfeldt, K.; Rasmussen, H.B. Bioassay-guided isolation of apigenin with GABA-benzodiazepine activity from *Tanacetum parthenium. Phytother. Res.*, **2009**, *23*(11), 1642-1644. [http://dx.doi.org/10.1002/ptr.2816] [PMID: 19441011]

[59] Dib, B.; Falchi, M. Convulsions and death induced in rats by Tween 80 are prevented by capsaicin. *Int. J. Tissue React.*, **1996**, *18*(1), 27-31.
[PMID: 8880377]

[60] Theoharides, T.C. Luteolin as a therapeutic option for multiple sclerosis. *J. Neuroinflammation*, **2009**, *6*(1), 29.
[http://dx.doi.org/10.1186/1742-2094-6-29] [PMID: 19825165]

[61] Sternberg, Z.; Chadha, K.; Lieberman, A.; Drake, A.; Hojnacki, D.; Weinstock-Guttman, B.; Munschauer, F. Immunomodulatory responses of peripheral blood mononuclear cells from multiple sclerosis patients upon *in vitro* incubation with the flavonoid luteolin: additive effects of IFN-β. *J. Neuroinflammation*, **2009**, *6*(1), 28.
[http://dx.doi.org/10.1186/1742-2094-6-28] [PMID: 19825164]

[62] Theoharides, T.C., Asadi, S.; Panagiotidou, S. A case series of a luteolin formulation (NeuroProtek®) in children with autism spectrum disorders. *Int. J. Immunopathol. Pharmacol.*, **2012**, *25*(2), 317-323. [http://dx.doi.org/10.1177/039463201202500201] [PMID: 22697063]

[63] Beula, S.J.; Raj, V.B.A.; Mathew, B. Isolation and molecular recognization of 6-prenyl apigenin towards MAO-A as the active principle of seeds of *Achyranthes aspera. Biomedicine & Preventive Nutrition*, **2014**, *4*(3), 379-382.
[http://dx.doi.org/10.1016/j.bionut.2014.03.003]

[64] Zarmouh, N.; Eyunni, S.; Mazzio, E.; Messeha, S.; Elshami, F.; Soliman, K. Bavachinin and genistein, two novel human monoamine Oxidase-B (MAO-B) inhibitors in the *Psoralea corylifolia* seeds. *FASEB J.*, **2015**, *29*(S1), 771-772.
[http://dx.doi.org/10.1096/fasebj.29.1_supplement.771.2]

[65] Im, A.R.; Chae, S.W.; Zhang, G.; Lee, M.Y. Neuroprotective effects of *Psoralea corylifolia* Linn seed extracts on mitochondrial dysfunction induced by 3-nitropropionic acid. *BMC Complement. Altern. Med.*, **2014**, *14*(1), 370.
[http://dx.doi.org/10.1186/1472-6882-14-370] [PMID: 25277760]

[66] Xiao, G.; Li, G.; Chen, L.; Zhang, Z.; Yin, J.J.; Wu, T.; Cheng, Z.; Wei, X.; Wang, Z. Isolation of antioxidants from *Psoralea corylifolia* fruits using high-speed counter-current chromatography guided

by thin layer chromatography-antioxidant autographic assay. *J. Chromatogr. A,* **2010**, *1217*(34), 5470-5476.
[http://dx.doi.org/10.1016/j.chroma.2010.06.041] [PMID: 20663508]

[67] Kong, L.D.; Tan, R.X.; Woo, A.Y.H.; Cheng, C.H.K., II Inhibition of rat brain monoamine oxidase activities by psoralen and isopsoralen: implications for the treatment of affective disorders. *Pharmacol. Toxicol.,* **2001**, *88*(2), 75-80.
[http://dx.doi.org/10.1034/j.1600-0773.2001.d01-86.x] [PMID: 11169165]

[68] Xu, L.; Du, B.; Xu, B. A systematic, comparative study on the beneficial health components and antioxidant activities of commercially fermented soy products marketed in China. *Food Chem.,* **2015**, *174*, 202-213.
[http://dx.doi.org/10.1016/j.foodchem.2014.11.014] [PMID: 25529671]

[69] Booth, N.L.; Overk, C.R.; Yao, P.; Burdette, J.E.; Nikolic, D.; Chen, S.N.; Bolton, J.L.; Breemen, R.B.; Pauli, G.F.; Farnsworth, N.R. The chemical and biologic profile of a red clover (*Trifolium pratense* L.) phase II clinical extract. *J. Altern. Complement. Med.,* **2006**, *12*(2), 133-139.
[http://dx.doi.org/10.1089/acm.2006.12.133] [PMID: 16566672]

[70] Zarmouh, N.O.; Messeha, S.S.; Elshami, F.M.; Soliman, K.F.A. Evaluation of the Isoflavone Genistein as Reversible Human Monoamine Oxidase-A and -B Inhibitor. *Evid. Based Complement. Alternat. Med.,* **2016**, *2016*, 1-12.
[http://dx.doi.org/10.1155/2016/1423052] [PMID: 27118978]

[71] Chuneker, K.C. Bhavaprakasa Nighantu. **1982**, , 202-203.

[72] Nadkarni, K.M. Indian Materia Medica. **1976**, *Vol. 1*, 9-10.

[73] Margret, A.A.; Begum, T.N.; Parthasarathy, S.; Suvaithenamudhan, S. A strategy to Employ Clitoria ternatea as a prospective brain drug confronting monoamine oxidase (MAO) against neurodegenerative diseases and depression. *Nat. Prod. Bioprospect.,* **2015**, *5*(6), 293-306.
[http://dx.doi.org/10.1007/s13659-015-0079-x] [PMID: 26667936]

[74] Chaurasiya, N.D.; Midiwo, J.; Pandey, P.; Bwire, R.N.; Doerksen, R.J.; Muhammad, I.; Tekwani, B.L. Selective Interactions of O-Methylated Flavonoid Natural Products with Human Monoamine Oxidase-A and -B. *Molecules,* **2020**, *25*(22), 5358.
[http://dx.doi.org/10.3390/molecules25225358] [PMID: 33207635]

CHAPTER 7

Lignins and Lignans – Recent Developments and Trends Regarding their Pharmaceutical Properties

Luc Zongo[1] and **Heiko Lange**[2,*]

[1] *Department of Pharmacy, University of Saint Dominic of West Africa (USDAO), Doulougou, Burkina Faso*

[2] *Department of Environmental and Earth Sciences, University of Milano-Bicocca, Milan, Italy*

Abstract: Lignins and lignans as natural polyphenols exhibit a rather broad variety of common physico-chemical features that can be of interest with respect to their use in the pharmaceutical sector. While polyphenol types have antioxidant, antiinflammatory, antibacterial and eventually antiviral activities in common, structural features beyond the polyphenol aspect differ enormously: isolated lignins are oligomers and/or polymers of monolignol C9-building blocks, while lignans are based on dimers thereof. The structural differences caused lignin to be exploited in the pharmaceutical sector mainly as material for the generation of matrices and carrier for drug delivery, while lignans are tested for the suitability as APIs. The chapter gives an overview of this situation, including the biological backgrounds of the two interesting natural polyphenols, isolation and methods for their characterisation.

Keywords: Antioxidant, Anti-Inflammatory, Antibacterial, Antivirus, Antitumor, Carrier, Delivery, Film, Lignin, Lignan, Microcapsules, Nanoparticles, Nanocapsules, Polyphenols, Renewable Resources.

INTRODUCTION

From all the renewable components present in land-based and aqueous biomass, natural polyphenols, namely lignin, lignans and tannins, are respectively important structural materials in the support tissues of vascular plants and valuable products of secondary plant metabolism that have a fundamental role in different stages of plant life, participating mostly in ecological mechanisms of interaction with other organisms and with the surrounding environment, and allowing plants to cope with the adversities. The natural polyphenols offer a wide range of heterogeneous intrinsic reactivities and activities that render them ideal starting oligomeric and polymeric materials for the preparation of functional

* **Corresponding author Heiko Lange:** Department of Environmental and Earth Sciences, University of Milano-Bicocca, Piazza della Scienza 1, 20126 Milan, Italy; E-mail: heiko.lange@unimib.it

macromolecules and the development of highly value-added materials. Nevertheless, due to the complexity and heterogeneity of their structures, especially in case of lignin and its isolated forms, and a type of historical lack in suitable, *i.e.*, useful detailed structural characterisation and the slow adaption of new structural insights by the wider community, their potential remains somewhat underexploited. Benefitting, however, more than ever simply from sheer necessity to actually find *via*ble substitutes for fossil-based materials, valorisation of natural polyphenols in the form of lignin, lignans and tannins is a booming research area, as the development of publications related to the field is indicating.

LIGNIN

Lignin interacts chemically and physically with the other two major components of the plant biomass, *i.e.*, cellulose and hemicelluloses [1]. The tight interplay between these three major plant biopolymers renders the plant cell wall impermeable, confers mechanical strength and rigidity, and overall serves to provide stability to the plants and confers resistance to microbial attacks.

The different functions of lignin in the plant cause its distribution to vary significantly within the different parts of the plant, *i.e.*, among stem, branching points, branches and leaves, and between the different walls of the plant cells themselves [2, 3]. The concentrations of lignin in the middle lamella and the primary cell wall are higher than the lignin concentration in the secondary cell wall. Nonetheless, the majority of the total amount of lignin present in the plant, 75–85%, is located in the secondary wall, due to its considerably large volume. Lignin abundancy is different for every plant species, ranging from ca. 20% in hardwoods, ca. 28% in softwoods and herbaceous angiosperms, to ca. 15% in monocots, accounting overall for 15–35% in average in dry wood [2, 4 - 6]. Unlike the structurally very regular and well-understood cellulose and hemicelluloses, lignin seems to exhibit only random sequences of various interunit bonding motifs [7].

Biosynthesis and Structural Features of Lignins

Lignin formation in cells has been proposed to be a *post-mortem* process in plant cells [8, 9]. The three monolignol building blocks for lignin, *i.e.*, *p*-coumaryl alcohol, coniferyl alcohol, and sinapyl alcohol (Fig. **1**) are produced presumably from *l*-tyrosine [10 - 13] or phenylalanine [14, 15] in adjacent living cells and transported into dead cells for lignification of the dead cell in a radical polymerisation process. While being induced by enzymatic activation of the monomers, the polymerisation proceeds most probably without any influence of the dirigent protein.

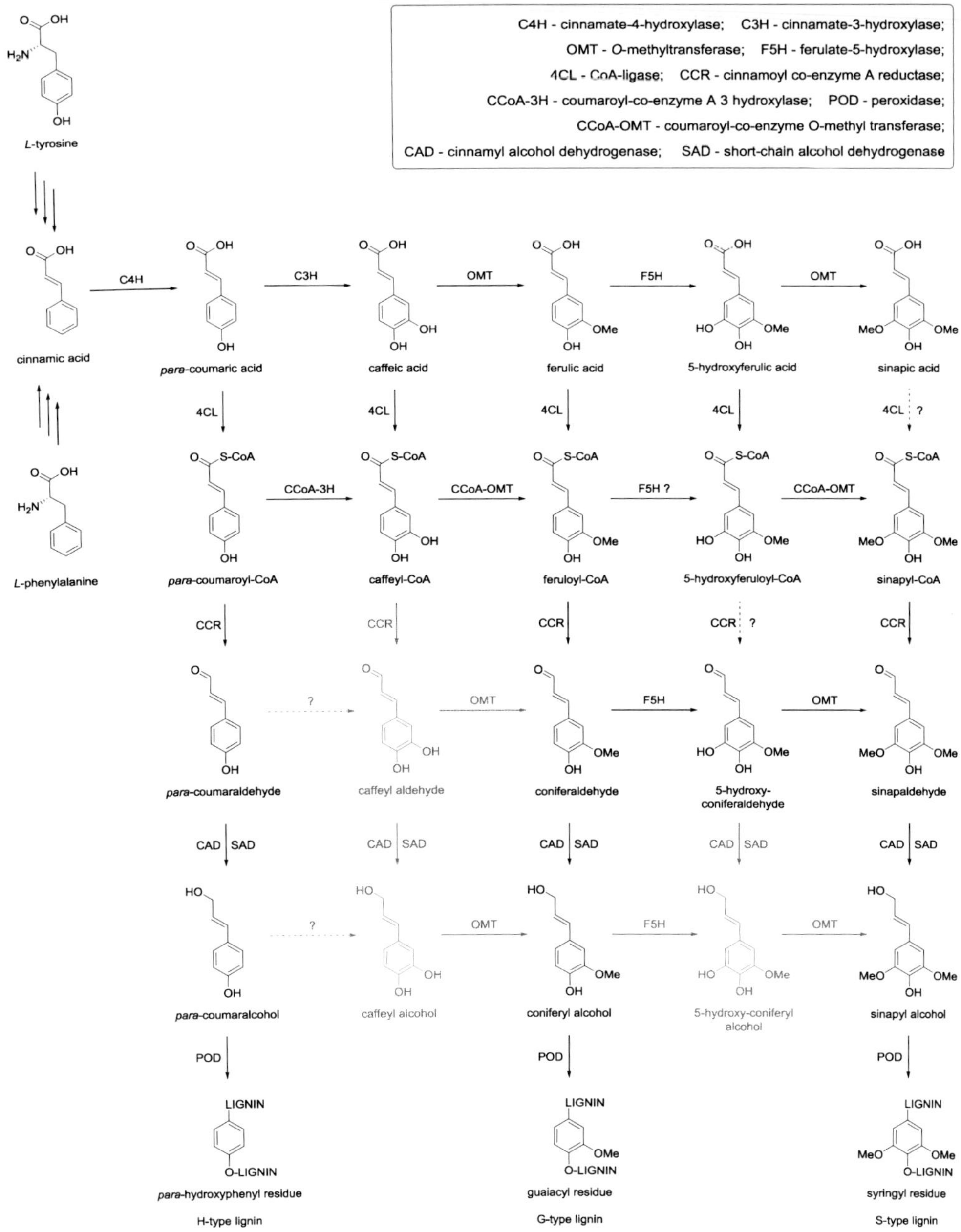

Fig. (1). Elements of the biosynthesis of lignins. For references, refer to the main text.

This assumption would explain the observed lack of a defined primary structure, and the fact that lignins have yet been found only in racemic form [16 - 18]. Bond motifs in lignin formation might be governed, however, by the microenvironments surrounding the polymerisation site, including mechanical stress, *etc* [19, 20]. Linking motifs leading to oligomeric and polymeric lignin molecules are comprised of ether and carbon-carbon bonds between the H-, G-, and S-type monolignols (Fig. **1**) [4, 10, 11, 13, 21]. Relative abundances of the different lignin types vary especially as the function of the type of plant the lignin is isolated from: lignin of gymnosperms consists almost entirely of G-type lignin (G-lignin); dicotyledonous angiosperms produce a mixture of G- and S-type lignins (GS-lignin). All three types of lignin can be found in different quantities in monocotyledonous lignin (GSH-lignin).

The structural complexity of lignins manifests itself in the form of variability in a couple of bonding motifs generally found in isolated lignins (Fig. **2**) [4, 13, 17]: enzyme-generated monolignol radicals couple to form an initial dehydro-dimer (Fig. **2**). The coupling itself is favoured at monolignol β-positions, resulting in arylglycerol- β-aryl ether (β-*O*-4'), pinoresinol (β-β'), phenylcoumaran (β-5'), spirodienone (SD), and diphenylethane (β-1') dimeric motifs. Dilignol coupling could also take place at positions 4 and 5, yielding diphenyl (5-5') and dimers diaryl ether (4-*O*-5') (not shown). In a subsequent step, after intermediate dehydrogenation and recurrent oxidative enzyme activation, coupling with another monomer radical in an end-wise coupling mode can occur [1, 22]. Coupling of two lignin oligomers yields 4-*O*-5' and 5-5' coupling motifs. In turn, 5-5' subunits undergo α-β-*O*-4-4' coupling to dibenzodioxocin units (DBDO) [11]. The phenylpropane (C9) units are thus attached to one another by a series of characteristic linkages (β-*O*-4', β-5', β-β', β-1',). Lignin cross linking bonds are accepted to be generated by post polymerisation chain coupling (5-5', DBDO, and 4-*O*-5') [6, 23]. It is currently still controversially discussed whether lignin is a branched, three-dimensional polymer *in planta*, or whether it consists of linear chains that are primarily oligomeric, as found for some isolated lignins that are believed to best resemble native lignins (Fig. **3**) [24].

Difficulties in answering these questions do not only arise due to the fact that analysis tools for investigating plant polymers and oligomers in their natural environment, *i.e.*, in the plant cells, are still in their infancy, but also due to the fact that any form of biomass isolation induces structural changes in the isolated biopolymer. Thus any analysis of "isolated" lignins inevitably carries the burden of not dealing with the "real", *i.e.*, natural lignin. While the analysis of lignins *in planta*, as discussed below, is suitable to get a good, but still only initial idea regarding the features of the lignin present in the plant under analysis, a detailed structural characterisation of lignin is, however, only possible using an isolated lignin, and applying a combination of different types of analyses techniques - independent of the lignin type.

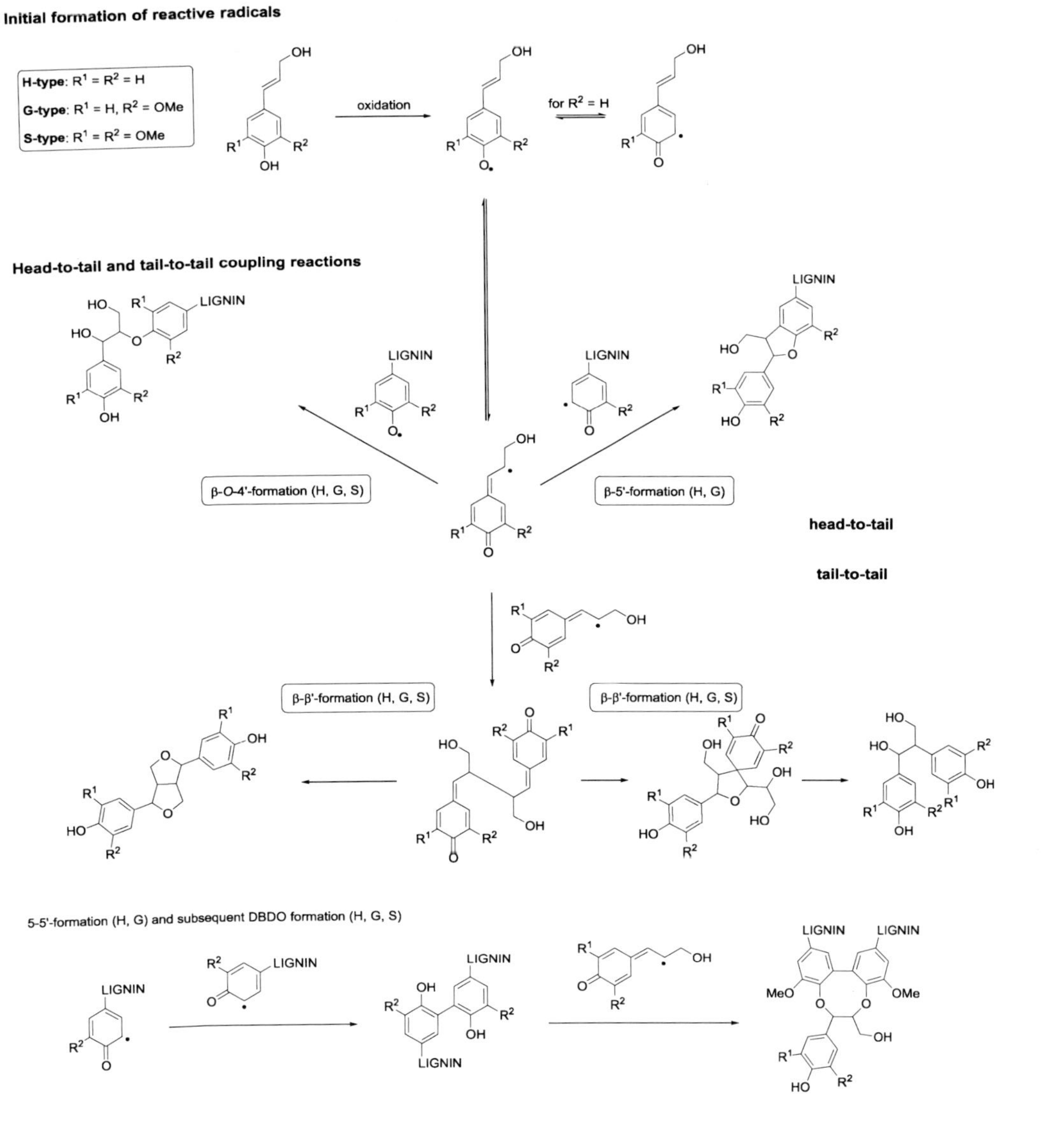

Fig. (2). Formation of typical bonding motifs found in lignins.

As mentioned before, any research on and with lignin will require analytical insight into its characteristics, especially structural features. A standard repertoire of analysis techniques was established for this purpose [24 - 27]. Any of the main techniques discussed in the dedicated paragraph (*vide infra*) unfolds its true potential, however, only in combination with the others.

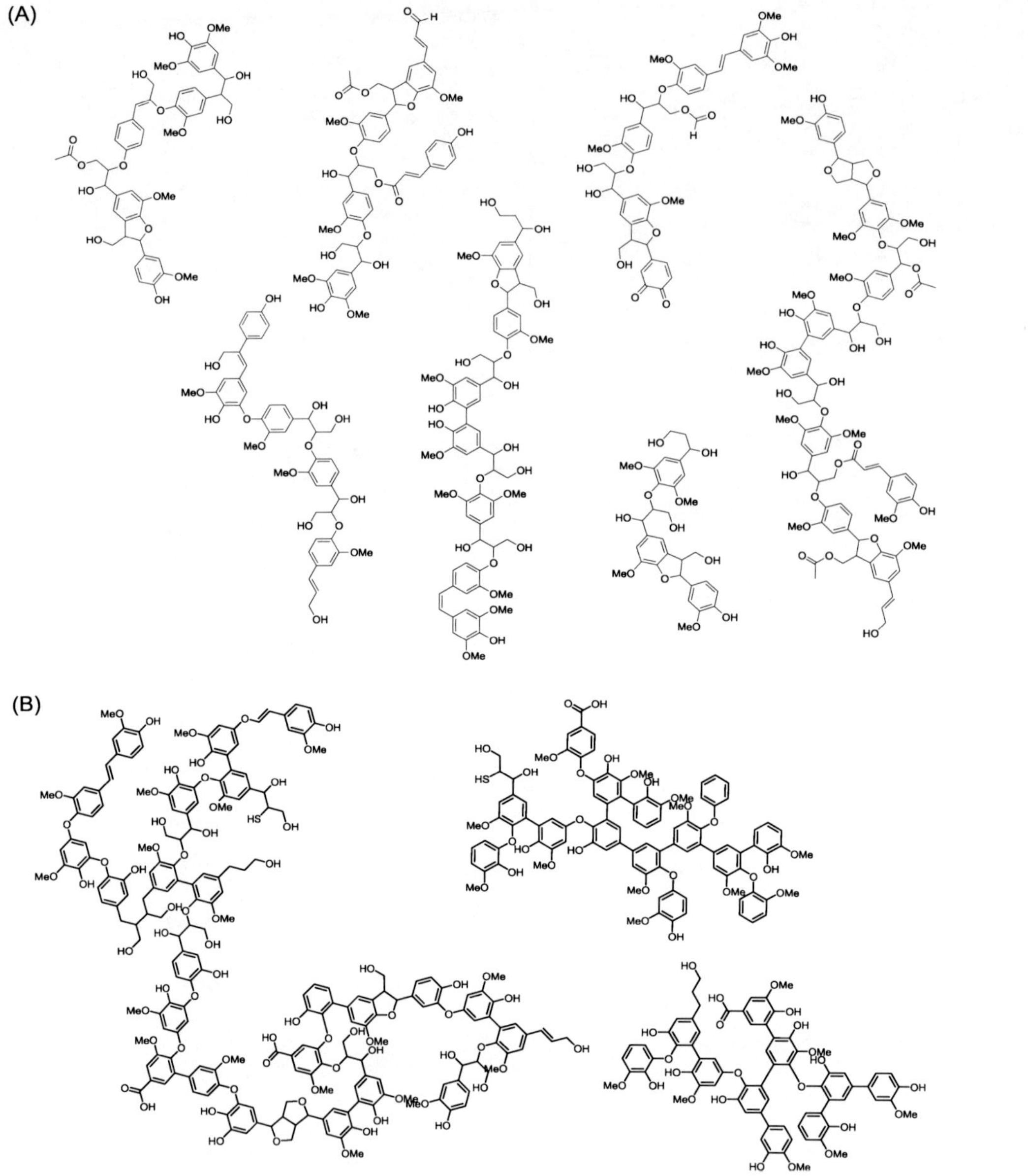

Fig. (3). Lignin structures (A) linear chains of oligomeric organosolv wheat straw lignin (**OSL**) [28]; (C) polymeric and oligomeric fraction of Lignoboost softwood kraft lignin (**SKL**) [29].

Isolation of Lignins

Novel biorefinery technologies co-exist together with established, classical pulp-and-paper processes as fundamental sources of isolated lignins. Obviously, various processes are suitable for furnishing different quantities of lignins, with the latter differing also substantially in their physico-chemical characteristics. Among the most important types of isolated lignins are: i) milled wood lignin (**MWL**), used mainly as laboratory reference in basic studies [30], iii) organosolv lignin (**OSL**) [31 - 33], iv) kraft lignin (**KL**) [34 - 36], and v) lignosulfonates (**LS**) [37]. Any of the procedures is suitable to modify the natural structure of lignin either by physical means, chemical means or combinations thereof; the isolation methods can introduce new functional groups and/or cause partial lignin degradation. The introduction of 'alien' functional groups, i.e., thiol groups in KL and sulfonate groups in LS, do obviously affect chemical and biological properties of these technical lignins with respect to 'more natural' lignins as obtained in the form of **MWL** and **OSL**.

Dehydrogenation polymers (**DHP**) have been proposed as 'synthetic lignins' by reacting monolignols in the presence of oxidative enzymes [38 - 40]. In terms of circular economy and sustainability aspects, this approach has to be seen critically though.

Using genetically modified plants with the aim to better control lignin formation such as to reduce structural variety and to eventually ease delignification during the biorefinery processes to reduce introduction of additional functional groups would render eventually the use of lignin more easy and the bioethanol and biofuel production industrially streamlined [41 - 48]. This approach is, however, scientifically very challenging, and bears other socio-economic challenges.

Lignin Fractionation

The main drawback for lignin valorisation is its wide structural diversity and heterogeneity. The impossibility to get reproducible lignin batches from sequential biomass treatments results in a scarcely defined material that can be hardly value added. Several studies are in course in order to develop lignin fractionation and purification processes with the aim to get reproducible lignin streams possessing defined molecular weight ranges and solubility characteristics. Fractionation of lignins has been identified as a promising technique for refining technical lignins in terms of structural and/or molecular size features since the early 1950s [49, 50]. Common fractionation strategies comprise: i) sequential precipitation out of alkaline solutions [51], ii) fractional precipitation of re-dissolved kraft lignin and a wheat straw lignin in a gradually changed binary solvent system [28, 52], iii) (sequential) extractions using different solvents [51,

53 - 61], and iv) fractionation by ultrafiltration of black liquor using ceramic membranes [62 - 64]. Some very recent reviews give more extensive overviews and discuss also the challenges that would still eventually need to be overcome [65, 66]. Importantly and interestingly, form a regulatory point of view, fractionation of isolated lignins offers the possibility to arrive at repeatable structural features that can be seen as a prerequisite for use in biomedical and pharmaceutical fields.

LIGNANS

Biosynthesis and Structural Features of Lignans

Lignans can be found in many plant species as dimers of phenylpropanoid units which are linked *via* their β-carbon atoms (Fig. **4**); neolignans, on the other hand, refers to dimeric phenylpropanoid structures linked by other motifs [1, 67, 68]. General similarities to lignin structural units are obvious (Fig. **1**).

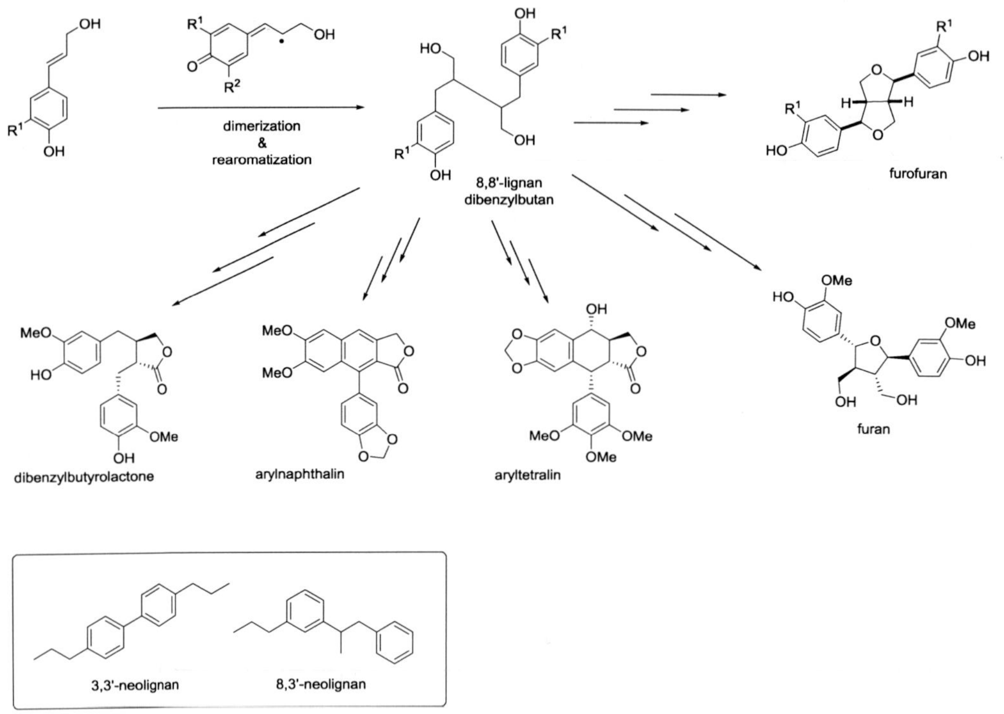

Fig. (4). Structural features of lignans and neolignans.

The structural repertoire is additionally enriched by chemical derivatisations leads to a broad variety of derivatives (Fig. **4**) Lignins are stereochemically generally considered to exist in racemic form with respect to all possible chiral centres, and also lignans are present in both forms, albeit different stereoisomers are found across different plant species or even organs of the same species (*vide infra*) [68]. This represents an eventually very interesting aspect with respect to potential applications.

Lignans and lignins share common features with respect to biosynthesis. The monolignol precursors for lignan biosynthesis are presumably formed in the general phenylpropanoid and the monolignol pathways (compare also (Fig. **1**) [11, 21]. Just as in case of lignin, not everything is known regarding the specific steps leading to the biosynthesis of complex lignan structures [67, 69 - 74].

It is controversially postulated that the presence of dirigent protein leads to the exclusive formation of (+)-pinoresinol in *Forsythia intermedia* in the dimerization of coniferyl alcohol as an initial step [75]. Dirigent proteins or genes encoding them were also detected in other plant species, allowing for hypothesising that the enantiomeric purity of lignans is determined at the oxidative coupling step [76]. Yet opposite enantiomers of the same lignin are found in different plants also of the same family [68], excluding eventually a very uniform pathway. The participation of such dirigent proteins and the enantioselective formation of chiral centers represent eventually (*vide infra*) an interesting and significant, sharp difference in the biosynthetic pathway leading to lignin, taking into account what is currently known (*vide supra*) with respect to lignin formation. (+)-Pinoresinol is reduced *via* (+)-lariciresinol to (−)-secoisolariciresinol by pinoresinol-lariciresinol reductase and subsequently oxidised to (−)-matairesinol [69, 77 - 81]. Despite remaining gaps in terms of knowledge of the biosynthetic pathway, matairesinol is believed to be a central intermediate leading to all diverse lignan structures (Fig. **5**).

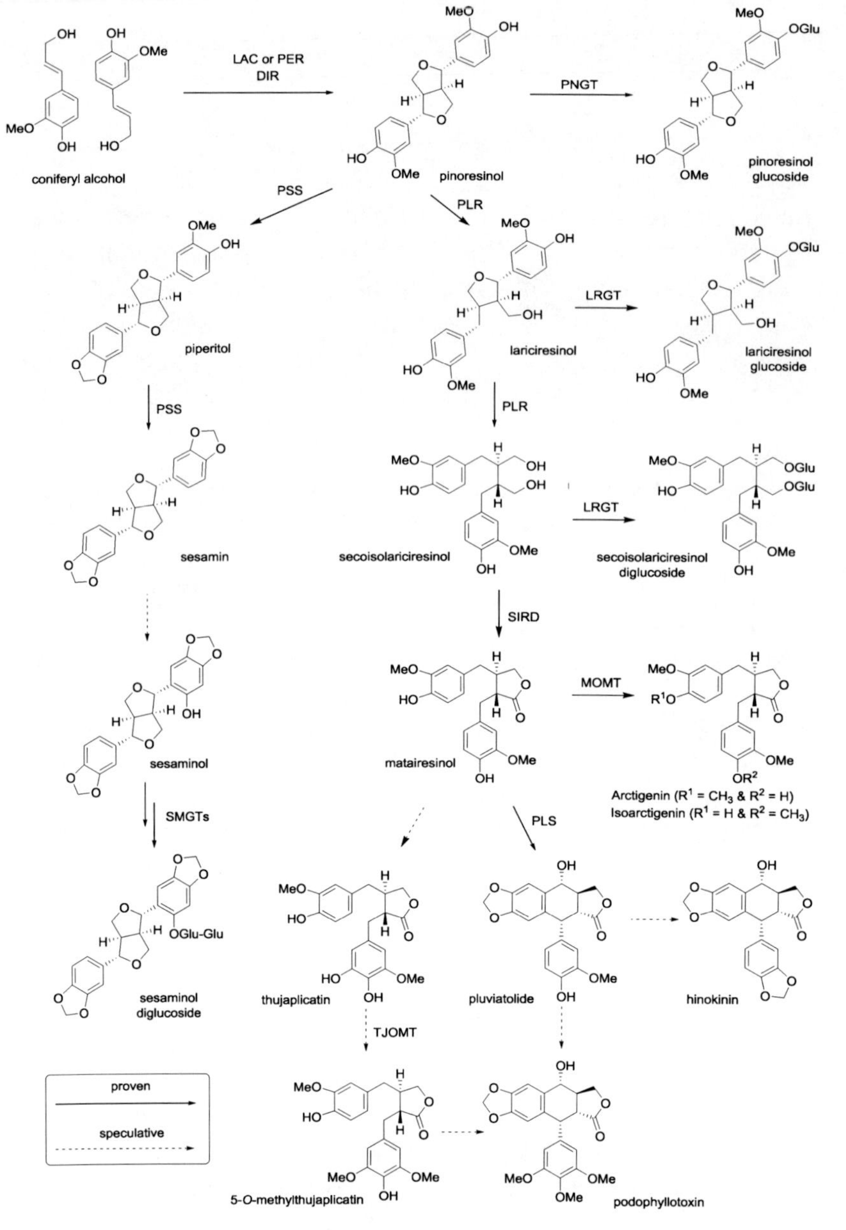

LAC - laccase; PER - peroxygenase; DIR - dirigent protein; PNGT - putative pinoresinol glycosyltransferase; PSS - epiperitol-sesamin synthase; PLR - pinoresinol-lariciresinol reductases; LRGT - lariciresinol glycosyltransferase; SIRD - secoisolariciresinol dehydrogenase; MOMT - matairesinol *O*-methytransferase; SMGT - sesaminol 2-*O*-glucosyltransferase.

Fig. (5). Proven and hypothesised steps in the biosynthesis of lignans (refer to main text for references).

ANALYTICAL TOOLS FOR ANALYSES OF LIGNINS AND LIGNANS

Several methods exist for the structural and physico-chemical characterisation of isolated lignins. Classical wet-chemical and spectroscopic techniques can provide qualitative and quantitative information on functional groups and linkages of constituents in lignin as well as the degradation products. While wet-chemical analyses are often destructive with respect to the lignin backbone, especially modern nuclear magnetic resonance (NMR)-based techniques allow an analysis of isolated lignins without touching the oligo- or polymeric structure. In the following, some traditional as well as modern techniques shall be discussed, given the importance of structural understanding with respect to insights into observed/intended physiological actions. The interested reader is encouraged to refer to dedicated overviews for more information [25, 82 - 86]. Principally, the presented analytical techniques are suitable for the structural and physical-chemical characterisation of both lignans and lignins [67, 87].

Fourier-Transform Infrared Spectroscopy and Raman Spectroscopy

The continued use of FT-IR for structural characterisation also in the field of natural products like lignins and lignans is due to its facile applicability, either in the traditional form of potassium bromide (KBr) pellets or newer ATR technique. Careful application of band deconvolution [88, 89], band fitting [90], and combinations thereof [91] allow for more detailed insights.

In 1984, the first reports were published regarding the use of Raman Spectroscopy to characterise lignin model compounds [92, 93]. In combination with *in silico* studies on lignin model compounds, a sound database could be generated that facilitates the application of Raman spectroscopy to lignin analysis [94]. Since then, numerous efforts have been made to overcome initial low sensitivity stemming from the interfering natural fluorescence of lignin, and from the visible light absorption by lignin, which made it necessary to develop tailor-made irradiation sources [95].

NMR Spectroscopy-Based Analysis Methods

Overall superior structural information can be obtained using NMR spectroscopy-based analysis methods, since NMR spectroscopy allows obtaining both detailed qualitative structural information and robust quantitative data using external, internal or intrinsic standards [85, 96 - 100]. The main difficulty in the NMR analyses is the low solubility of lignins in the typical NMR solvents like deuterated chloroform ($CDCl_3$) or deuterated dimethyl sulfoxide (DMSO-d_6). Derivatisation of the hydroxyl groups along the backbone, for example in the form of acetylation, can improve the situation.

QQ-HSQC is a potential method for the acquisition of quantitative HSQC spectra, but often the available NMR equipment dictates the method that should be employed. In case a high-field (400 MHz or more) NMR machine equipped with a cryo-probe is available, either a QQ-HSQC pulse sequence [101], or an approach consisting of a series of HSQC-measurements with incremented repetition times and mathematical backward-extrapolation, called $HSQC_0$ [102], can be adopted for the acquisition of lignin spectra [28, 103 - 105]. In both QQ-HSQC and $HSQC_0$, quantification is achieved based on the intrinsic standard represented by the distinct shifts of the aromatic hydrogen atoms in 2-position, which can be easily detected, summed up, and used as a reference. As a third option, the quantification of a high-quality standard ^1H-^{13}C HSQC spectrum can be achieved on the basis of a quantitative ^{13}C NMR analysis of the very same sample used for acquisition of the HSQC, given the sample exhibits the necessary structural stability in the solvent of choice in the time frames needed for the separate measurements [106].

Both the number and the nature of free hydroxyl groups can be determined using ^{31}P NMR spectroscopy on phosphitylated lignins in the presence of an internal standard like cholesterol [85, 96, 107, 108]. Quantitative ^{31}P NMR can be seen as one of the standard analytical tools in lignin chemistry. Advantages in the use of ^{31}P NMR lie in the low amount of sample needed, reduced analysis time, ease in sample preparation, and reproducibility. Cholesterol is used as an internal standard using a suitable pulse sequence for obtaining quantitative results after a phosphitylation reaction with 2-chloro-3,3,4,4-tetramethyl-1,3,2-dioxophospholane [96, 109]. The different electromagnetic environments around the phosphorus atoms lead to characteristic shifts, which in turn allows for differentiation and quantification.

Although not specifically applied to lignans yet, ^{31}P NMR could be used to confirm a hydroxyl group-mapping that was achieved using ^1H and ^{13}C NMR analysis, and could, in analogy to what is possible in terms of tannins analysis *via* quantitative ^{31}P NMR [110, 111], be used for determining sample purities and sample fingerprinting.

Size Exclusion and Gel Permeation Chromatographic Methods

A more promising way of determining molecular weight key features of lignins, such as mean average molecular weight (M_n), weight average molecular weight (M_w) and polydispersity (PD) is the use of size exclusion chromatography (SEC) or gel permeation chromatography (GPC) [112 - 118]. The structural differences between different lignins theoretically require a set of tailor-made standards for achieving a calibration of the SEC setup that fits the characteristics of the lignin analyte. It has been shown, however, that universal calibrations do not lead to better results than a much more feasible calibration based on commercially available polystyrene standards. Different detector types are known to lead to different results: commonly used UV-based detectors and refractive index detectors have been shown to perform poorly compared to molecular weight sensitive detectors based on viscosimetry [119] or laser light scattering detectors [120 - 124].

Mass Spectrometry Methods

Structural insights can be obtained in the area of lignins using an MS-based sequencing strategy for lignin oligomers [125]. MALDI-ToF-based mass analysis eventually allows additional structural insights especially due to the fact that analysis is independent of solubility issues and structural aspects, and results can be claimed to be more accurate [126]. Especially newer MALDI-ToF MS/MS methods, that are principally capable of determining molecular mass and structural aspects simultaneously, showed promising performance as an effective substitute for the combined NMR and SEC analysis, even for *in situ* lignin [127, 128]. The major challenge in this area lies, however, obviously in a careful evaluation of the most suitable matrix for a given lignin. Also quadrupole (Qp) ToF-MS analysis in combination with atmospheric pressure photoionization (APPI) MS has been applied to the analysis of lignins [129, 130].

With respect to lignans, given their reduced molecular size with respect to lignin, especially HPLC-MS-based methods are applicable, also in combination with NMR and UV-spectroscopy [131 - 136]. Exploiting available or custom-made databases in combination with modern MS-analysers allows for reliable lignan characterisation.

Anti-Oxidant Activity Assays

Antioxidant activity is one of the most important properties of natural polyphenols such as lignins and lignans. Various methods allow for quantifying this activity: TRAP (Total Radical-Trapping Antioxidant Parameter) [137], ORAC (Oxygen-Radical Absorbance Capacity) [138], superoxide radicals scavenging [139], peroxyl radical scavenging [140], 2,2-diphenyl-1-picrylhydrazyl (DPPH) method [141] and the 2,2'-azino-bis(3-ethylbenzothiazoline-6-sulphonic acid) (ABTS) radical cation assay [142, 143].

Most of methods express the activity of the sample as µm standard antioxidant equivalents per gram of freshly weighted samples. Gallic acid (GAE), tannic acid (TAE), trolox, ascorbic acid (AAE) equivalents and others can be used as standard antioxidants. Solubility issues are eventually encountered especially when analysing lignins, so that occasionally emulsifiers might be used to ensure full sample dissolution.

LIGNINS FOR USE IN PHARMACEUTICAL AREA

Lignin shows very interesting properties from a material's point of view in a broad range of areas [3, 144, 145], but with respect to its use in the pharmaceutical and/or biomedical field, especially as a leading ingredient, the situation is very different [146, 147]. Despite years of research in the field, this situation is still changing only very slowly, a fact that is indicative of a series of challenges that are commonly faced and that are intrinsic to the biopolymer lignin. One of the main reasons lies in the, in comparison to other biopolymers, complex and irregular structure (*vide supra*), which comes with a rather complex and changing reactivity profile. Nevertheless, structural analysis of lignins is becoming mature, and fractionation protocols applied to isolated lignins (*vide supra*) are about to allow for a narrowing down of structural diversities in generated fractions. Additionally, both chemical and biotechnological routes to tailored lignins are subject to current research efforts that are basically suitable for rendering lignins more, or more easily suitable for pharmaceutical applications [148].

Lignin as Source of Pharmaceutical Activity

Comparably few studies exist that see lignin, or derivatives thereof, as the main pharmaceutically active ingredient; its role consists here principally in furnishing simple beneficial actions such as antioxidant, anti-inflammatory [149] or as UV-shielding activities [150]. Structure-activity relationship studies in the classical sense are difficult, some initial trials exist and have been recently discussed [146]; the challenges in this context can be understood in light of the difficulties that would be encountered in correctly describing the regularly irregular poly- and oligomeric lignin structure *in silico*.

In light of its anti-inflammatory and anti-oxidant activities, lignin seems predisposed as an active, or at least a source of actives that exhibit anti-tumour actions [151]: in several studies involving i) polyphenols with structural motifs found in lignin, ii) mixtures of monomers lignin is composed of, and/or iii) small aromatic molecules that could be the enzymatic degradation products of lignin, it was elucidated if and to which extend these lignin derivatives affect tumour development and growth, and how the underlying and connected signalling pathways are disturbed [152, 153]. It is speculated that cytotoxic activity of lignin and lignin derivatives emerges from interactions of lignin with other biologically relevant substances like ascorbic acid [154].

Despite the structural challenges with respect to regulatory aspects, the suitability of lignin as an excipient for the production of conventional tablets has been reported [155 - 157]. Incorporating standard actives such as acetylsalicylic acid or paracetamol, the presence of lignin or chemically derived carboxylated lignin led to altered release profiles for the active ingredient; generally, the presence of lignin increased the release efficiency compared to controls [156].

Reports exist on research activities focusing on potential anti-viral activities of lignin derivatives, also against HIV [158, 159].

Lignin-carbohydrate complexes (LCCs, Fig. **6**) [160 - 163], controversially discussed in detail still in terms of structure and general natural occurrence, have been tested in various more or less isolated forms with respect to a series of pharmacological activities, including antiviral, antibacterial and anti-inflammatory effects [164 - 171].

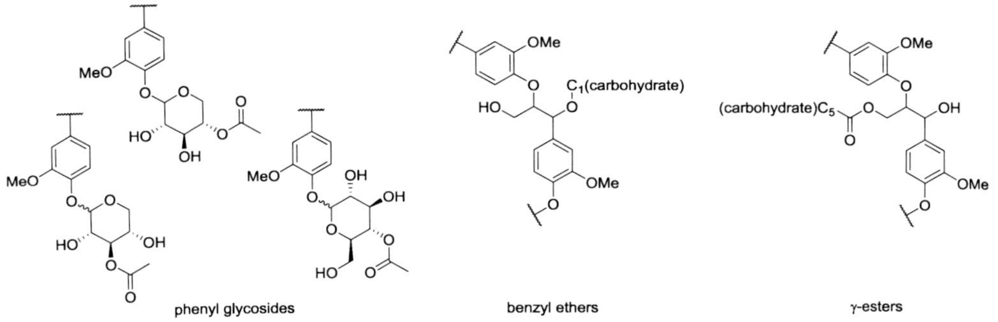

Fig. (6). General structural motifs attributed to lignin-carbohydrate complexes (LCCs), linking carbohydrate and lignin moieties.

The effects are hence the same as those found for some lignins. Since LCC motifs are commonly found in isolated lignins as function of feedstock and biorefinery method, it is difficult to judge whether the observed activities stem from the polyphenol part alone or from the connection between lignin and carbohydrates. Since the described activity profiles are normally not attributable to carbohydrates, it seems most likely that a polyphenolic moiety plays a major role. More research is necessary, however, using a very pure isolated sample of LCCs, obtainable, *e.g.*, *via* fractionation of isolated lignins [172 - 174], in comparison to LCC-free polyphenol preparations in order to arrive at general structure-activity relationships.

LIGNIN AS MATERIAL FOR MICRO- AND NANOSTRUCTURES FOR PHARMACEUTICAL USE

Given the interesting and well-investigated properties of lignin in the fields of material science, in combinations with especially the aforementioned UV-shielding and anti-oxidant properties, the use of lignins for the fabrication of materials and matrices within the pharmaceutical context is attractive. Fabrication of lignin particles, capsules and films in nano- and microscales has been achieved. Being currently a very active field of research, several recent reviews exist that highlight the various recent developments [147, 175 - 181]. Some main research lines will be discussed below.

Lignin-Containing Film Preparations for Pharmaceutical Applications

Lignin has been used as an ingredient in various film preparations, exploiting its anti-oxidant and anti-inflammatory activities. Films have been developed for applications in wound healing and tissue engineering. Table 1 lists selected works with the respective references. An incorporation of actives has not been reported.

Table 1. Selection of lignin-containing film preparations for pharmaceutical and biomedical applications.

Composition (Lignin Source, Technique)[a]	Field of Application	Year/ [Ref.]
PLA-lignin fibres (alkali lignin, electrospinning)	tissue engineering	2016/ [182]
PEO-chitin nanofibrils-lignin fibres (organosolv lignin, electrospinning)	wound healing	2016/ [183]
PVA-lignin fibres (lignin as decoration for multi-walled nanotubes, electrospinning)	wound healing/tissue engineering	2018/ [184]
PVA-PGS-lignin fibres (kraft lignin in form of commercialised nanoparticles, electrospinning)	tissue engineering/ regeneration	2019/ [185]
PCL-lignin fibres (kraft lignin in form of commercialised nanoparticles, electrospinning)	tissue engineering/ regeneration	2020/ [186]

a: PLA – poly(lactic acid); PVA – poly(vinyl alcohol); PGS – poly(glycerol sebacate); PCL – poly(caprolactone); PEO – poly(ethylene oxide).

Challenges in the area of lignin-containing films exist in the form of compatibility of lignin with the main matrix polymer, lignin solubility, and often affected mechanical stabilities and/or homogeneities of films when lignin concentrations exceed a certain concentration. While thermal stability often found to benefit from lignin presence, controlling mechanical stability becomes more challenging due to the varying plasticizer characteristics of different lignins. Some reported applications do actually not use lignin as integral part of the fibres, but as nanoparticulate additive during the fibre generation. Most of the publications used kraft or alkali lignins, which in crude form might expose higher risks in terms of cytotoxicity compared to lignins stemming from other biorefinery approaches like organosolv processes.

NANOPARTICLES

Three main routes have emerged for generating lignin nanoparticles. The most common method for the preparation of lignin NPs involves solvent exchange by adding an anti-solvent to a solution of lignin, or *vice versa*, resulting in the formation of solid spheres (Fig. **7**) A-C [187]. Aqueous and non-aqueous tetrahydrofuran [188, 189], dioxane [190], dimethyl sulfoxide [191, 192], acetone [192 - 194], and ethanol [195, 196] have been used for solubilising the starting lignins. Pure water served as anti-solvent in most cases.

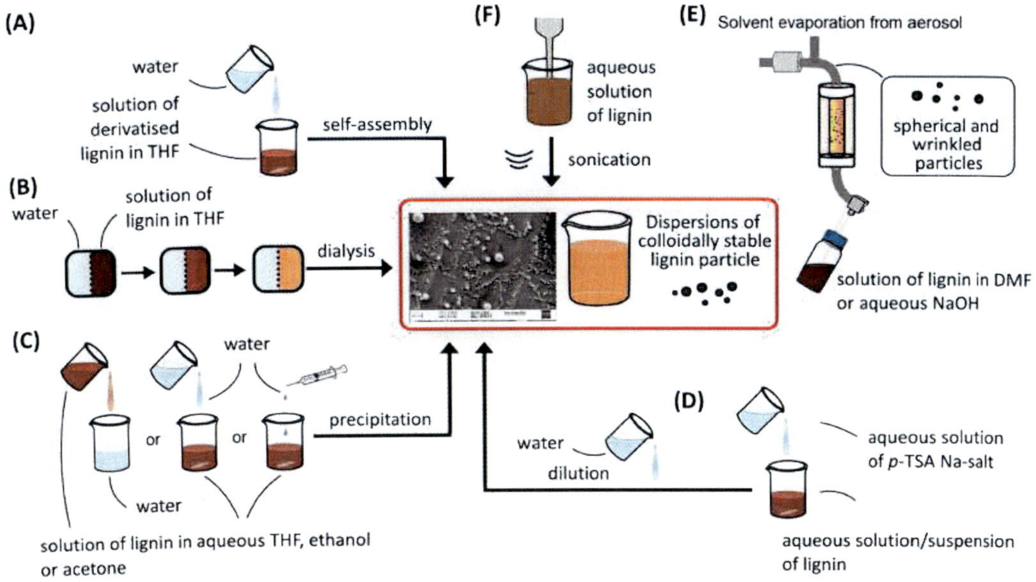

Fig. (7). Fabrication modes for generating of nano- and microscale lignin particles: **(A)** adding water into THF solution of suitable or suitably modified lignin; **(B)** dialysing a solution of suitable lignin in THF against deionised water; **(C)** nanoprecipitation by adding water into a solution of a suitable lignin; **(D)** formation of lignin nanoparticles using a hydrotropic system; **(E)** formation of micro- and nanoparticles in an aerosol flow reactor; **(F)** formation of non-spherical lignin nanoparticles upon ultrasonication of aqueous lignin solutions. Refer to the main text and Table **3.** for references. Figure realised on the basis of ref [177].

Sodium *para*-toluene sulfonate (**Na-PTSA**) was used in an autotrophic approach to generate lignin nanoparticles (Fig. **7D**) [197]. These precipitated upon rapid dilution of an acidic aqueous solution containing kraft lignin and **Na-PTSA** with water.

Aerosol technology is another approach to prepare lignin nano- and microparticles (Fig. **7E**) [198]. In this process, solvent is vaporised from a solution of lignin, forming particles at the hydrophobic solvent-air interface; the particles formed do not necessarily exhibit a spherical shape in this case.

Non-spherical particles were obtained also in a ultrasonication-based formation of lignin nanoparticles (Fig. **7F**), starting from an aqueous solution of lignin [199].

It is then commonly found that lignin nanoparticles show the antioxidant and UV-protective properties that are typical for the starting lignins [200]. This finding goes together with elucidations that confirm that the lignins remain chemically, *i.e.*, structurally unaltered [197, 201]. The latter aspect is especially important with respect to regulatory issues and an eventually guaranteed biodegradability of the lignin part of any pharmaceutical product on the basis of lignins.

Micro- and Nanoscaled Core-shell Structures

With respect to applications in the pharmaceutical sector, usage of lignin particles as delivery vehicle is most obvious; such actives would have to be co-precipitated upon particle formation, requiring a comparable solubility profile (*vide infra*). Restrictions that emerge from this aspect can eventually be circumvented using core-shell structures, *i.e.*, capsules rather than solid particles.

Oil-in-water emulsions have been used as templates for the preparation of lignin microcapsules (0.3–1.4 μm) by ultrasonication (Fig. **8**) [202 - 206]. Applying the same approach, the generation of lignin-metal frameworks as shell material was demonstrated as well [207]. Ultrastirring of lignin-containing emulsions has been demonstrated to be applicable to lignin micro- and nanoparticle formation [208].

Synthesis of lignin nanotubes has been conducted using aluminium with interpenetrating holes as sacrificial templates [209]. The length (11–19 μm) and diameter (about 200 nm) of the nanotubes were influenced only slightly by the different types of lignin raw materials used.

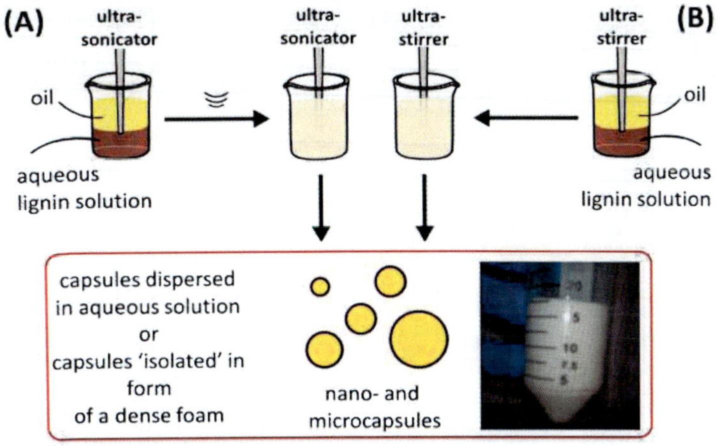

Fig. (8). Modes for generating of nano- and microscale lignin capsules: (A) ultrasonication of emulsions of an oil and an aqueous solution of a suitable lignin; (B) ultrastirring of an emulsion of an oil and an aqueous solution of a suitable lignin. Refer to main text and Table **3**. for references.

As in the case of most of the discussed lignin-based formation of particles, no chemical derivatisation of the lignins is necessary to achieve capsule strictures with decent stabilities and eventually tuneable decomposition characteristics, allowing once more for generating materials that exhibit unaltered biodegradation. A slightly different situation is encountered in this respect, of course, when emulsion-phase polymerisation and cross-linking are applied for the generation of nanoparticles, nanocapsules and/or porous microparticles [203, 210].

Incorporation of Actives in Lignin Particle and Lignin Capsule Structures

The typical characteristics of lignins in terms of UV-shielding and anti-oxidant properties can be exploited in the use of the above-described lignin particles and capsules as green delivery vehicles in various fields of application. Such carrier systems are capable of trigger-related slow or fast release of entrapped or encapsulated actives, which are protected from external, eventually degrading factors such as UV-radiation or molecules. *Vice versa*, biological and or environmental matrices in which particles and capsules will be eventually immersed are protected from the active ingredients unless matrix characteristics change to trigger slow or fast particle and capsule decomposition. Due to the slow rate of biodegradation of lignin, it can contribute to maintaining the soil carbon balance [211].

Entrapment, encapsulation, adsorption, and covalent binding are common methods for loading actives into lignin materials (Fig. **9**). The loading of the cargo may take place during or after the formation of nanoparticles, nanocapsules, by entrapment or encapsulation. The main hurdle being in both cases is a sufficient, compatible solubility of the active, which in case of generations from biphasic systems can become challenging given the ultimately necessary hydrophilicity of most actives.

Entrapment *Vs.* Encapsulation *Vs.* Adsorption

Entrapment is the most common method for incorporating small active molecules into solid lignin particles. The current view is that lignin NPs form by supramolecular assembly of poorly water-soluble molecules *via* electric interactions with aromatic rings [188, 201, 212]. As could be expected from this mechanism, most of the substances currently successfully entrapped in lignin NPs are poorly water-soluble lower molecular weight compounds. A couple or pioneering reports describe the loading of pharmaceutically relevant small molecules and biological macromolecules such as antibodies and enzymes; the works are discussed in form of Table **1**.

Encapsulation can be used to dissolve lipophilic drugs in the water-immiscible cores of capsules dispersed in aqueous media, and *vice versa*. The ratio of sphere volume to surface area equals diameter/6, and therefore microcapsules appear more efficient than nanocapsules if compared solely based on the volume available for loading of the active. However, nanocapsules with diameters of around 200 nm have exhibited benefits over microcapsules in drug delivery to cancer cells (Fig. **9**) [59, 84, 85].

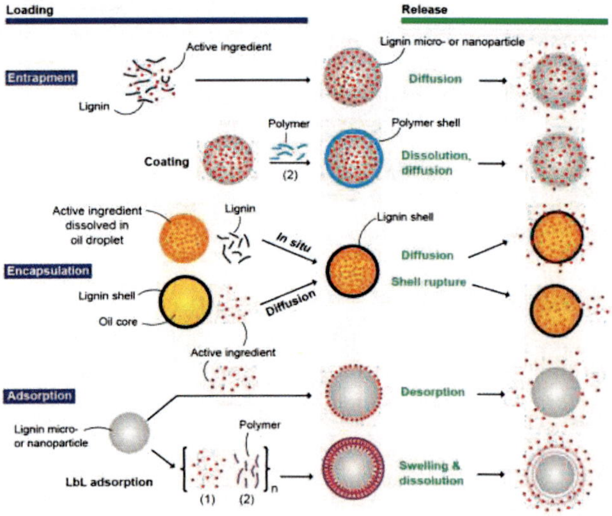

Fig. (9). General methods for loading and releasing actives from a variety of different carriers. Used with permission from Ref [177]. Copyright (2019) Wiley VCH.

As a means of measuring the success of any entrapment of encapsulation efforts, entrapment/encapsulation efficiencies (EE-%) are commonly determined. Reported values are found to range from 4% to >95%, depending on type and formation process of the lignin-based carrier and the type of active Table **1**. Whether the reported numerical differences do actually reflect real differences in terms of hosting capability of the carrier system is currently questionable, since a type of gold standard' for determining loading capacity and EE-% does not exist.

Immobilisation of macromolecules, including oligopeptides and enzymes is normally achieved *via* covalent surface-linking or simple electrostatic adsorption. Yet this method of incorporation of actives in the context of lignin-based particulate and capsule systems represents a smaller fraction in the context of lignin-based carrier systems, and has been used only for enzymes in pharmaceutically relevant applications: in order to increase enzyme stability, lipase was adsorbed on composite material consisting of chitin and oxidised kraft lignin [213], and cutinases and porcine pancreatic α-amylase were adsorbed on acetic acid lignin [214].

Table **2** lists a selection of recent works in which lignin-based particulate or capsule systems have been employed for supporting actives relevant to the pharmaceutical sector. Listed are systems that were used entrapping, encapsulating and adsorbing actives. Systems used for hosting substances relevant to the agricultural sector, such as pesticides, herbicides and insecticides have not been considered here, but should of course, be taken into account for the valuable insights they deliver on a general technical ground. The relatively small number of entries compared to the overall relatively high number of publications, as well as patents detailing synthesis and potential use of lignin microcapsules is once more indicative of the misbalance in terms of envisaged fields of application.

Table 2. Micro- and nanoscaled particle and capsule systems based on lignin for use as carrier systems. Selected examples report incorporation of drugs or drug-like substances.

Nanoscaled System (Lignin Source)[a]	**Active[b]**	**Active Incorporation[c]**	**Entrapment/ Encapsulation/ Adsorption Efficiency (%)[d]**	**Loading Capacity (wt%)[d]**	**Year/[Ref.]**
LNPs (**SKL**)	Methylene blue	ET	18 (hydrotropic) 35 (precipitation)	n.a.	2020/ [197]
LNPs (**WS** soda lignin)	Budesonide	ET	35	3.5	2018/ [201]
LNPs (**KL**, Sigma-Aldrich)	DOX, GFLX	ET	43 DOX 5–37 GFLX	n.a.	2018/ [215]

(Table 2) cont.....

Nanoscaled System (Lignin Source)[a]	Active[b]	Active Incorporation[c]	Entrapment/ Encapsulation/ Adsorption Efficiency (%)[d]	Loading Capacity (wt%)[d]	Year/[Ref.]
LNPs (**OSL**)	Tyrosinase	ET	69	12	2018/ [216]
LNPs (**SKL**)	BZL, SFN	ET	77 BZL, 68 SFN	8 BZL, 7 SFN	2017/ [217]
LNPs (alkali lignin from HT-pretreated corn cobs)	Resveratrol	ET	71–95	19–26	2017/ [218]
LNPs (succinylated **SKL**)	Benzazulene	ET	50–57	9–11	2017/ [219]
Lignin-based complex micelles (alkali lignin)	Ibuprofen	ET	74	46	2017/ [220]
Chitosan-LNPs (calcium-**LS**)	RNase A	ET	61–40	6.6–43	2013/ [221]
lignin microcapsules (alkali lignin)	Avermectin	ET	76-85	4.4-4.7	2020/ [208]
LNCs (**SLS**)	Thymol derivatives	EC	10-76	n.a.	2020/ [222]
Chitosan-coated LNPs (**SKL**)	Ciprofloxacin	EC	n.a.	n.a.	2019/ [223]
hollow LNPs (enzymatically hydrolyzable lignin (**EHL**))	Doxorubicin	EC	45-65	6-14	2019/ [224]
LNC (**EHL**)	Avobenzone, Octinoxate	EC	98	53	2018/ [225]
Cationic LNPs (**SKL**)	Lipase, cutinase	AD	96	5.5	2018/ [226]
Lignin NPs (**OSL**)	Tyrosinase	AD	71–90	12–15	2018/ [216]
Silica-lignin composite (alkali lignin)[a]	Lipase	AD	1.7	42	2017/ [227]
LNPs (acetic acid lignin from bamboo shoot shells)	α-Amylase	AD	n.a.	1.9	2017/ [214]

(Table 2) cont.....

Nanoscaled System (Lignin Source)[a]	Active[b]	Active Incorporation[c]	Entrapment/ Encapsulation/ Adsorption Efficiency (%)[d]	Loading Capacity (wt%)[d]	Year/[Ref.]
LNPs and LNCs (**KL**)	2-Propyl-pyridine	EC	n.a.	n.a.	2017/ [203]
Complex micelles (**SKL**)	Ibuprofen	EC	74	46	2017/ [220]
SLS-CTAB microspheres	Avermectin	EC	63	71	2017/ [228]
Lignin microcapsules (poplar alkali lignin)	Avermectin	ET	61	17	2016/ [229]
LNCs (alkali lignin)[a]	Coumarin 6	EC	70–90	n.a.	2016/ [207]
LNCs (**SLS**)	Coumarin 6	EC	n.a.	n.a.	2016/ [204]
Chitin-**KL** composite	Lipase	AD	1.0–2.0	33–11	2015/ [213]
LNCs (**SLS**)	Sulfo-rhodamine	EC	n.a.	n.a.	2014/ [230]
LMC (alkali lignin)[a]	Coumarin 6	EC	n.a.	n.a.	2014/ [202]

a: LNPs, lignin nanoparticles; **WS**, wheat straw, **KL**, kraft lignin. **SKL**, softwood kraft lignin. **HT**, hydrothermal. **OSL**, organosolv lignin. **LS**; lignosulfonate, **SLS**, sodium lignosulfonate. **ALS**, ammonium lignosulfonate, **EHL**, enzymatically hydrolyzable lignin; b: BZL, benzazulene; SFN, sorafenib; DOX, doxorubicin; GFLX, gatifloxacin; c: entrapment (ET); encapsulation (EC); adsorption (AD); d: n.a., not available.

Covalent and Electrostatic Surface Functionalisation

Chemical modifications of base material used for carriers and grafting of biologically relevant functional motifs are common methods to render micro- and nanoscaled structures more suitable for an intended application. Compared to the abundant literature on the preparation of lignin-based nano- and microstructures as such, reports regarding their surface modification is relatively scarce. Caicedo *et al.* [209] functionalised lignin nanotubes (LNTs) with avidin for specific immobilisation onto desthiobiotin-grafted glass surfaces. Figueiredo *et al.* [219] succinylated softwood kraft lignin and used the product to generate carboxylated lignin particles (CLNPs) that were further modified by chemically attaching a block copolymer comprising poly(ethylene glycol) (PEG), poly(histidine) and a cell-penetrating peptide.

Anionic LNPs have been modified by adopting a layer-by-layer (LbL) technique generating a layer of cationic polymers such as poly(diallyldimethylammonium chloride) on their surfaces [188, 231]. This simple possibility allowed for amplifying the potential application range of the particles. Using a variation of the LbL-approach, adsorption of chitosan on LNPs was shown to form colloidally stable cationic particles that fully stabilised olive oil-in-water emulsions [223].

Instead of cationic polymers, LNPs coated with proteins [232] are expected to improve biocompatibility and reduce clearance rate; however, these important aspects need yet to be demonstrated under physiological conditions.

Zhong *et al.* [233] reported antibacterial silver nanoparticle composites in a matrix of poly(vinyl alcohol) and lignin isolated from spent pulping liquor to arrive at nanomaterials that exhibit a boosted antibacterial activity. Silica/lignin hybrid particles comprising silver NPs have been reported for the same purpose [234]. Commercial silica material was modified with *N*-(2-aminoethyl--3-aminopropyltrimethoxysilane to increase affinity to kraft lignin oxidised with sodium periodate. Silver NPs grafted onto the resulting silica/lignin hybrids were stable and active against *Pseudomonas aeruginosa.* Silver-ion-containing lignin nanoparticles have been realised as an eco-friendly alternative to silver nanoparticles in antimicrobial applications [235].

PHARMACEUTICAL PROPERTIES OF LIGNANS

While the polymeric lignins are not present in large quantities in human diets, and therefore do not seem to play a major role in the context of health-promoting diets, lignans as low molecular weight secondary plant metabolites present in human diets do exhibit properties relevant for human health, mainly as antioxidants, anti-allergic, anti-inflammatory, anticancer, antihypertensive, and antimicrobial agents [236 - 240]. In this respect, a particular attention should be paid to lignans, which are polyphenols found in plants, part of the phytoestrogen family, with well-known health properties. Lignans have been studied also more specifically for specific effects on various pathologies. Representing essentially dimeric structures, more classical structure-activity relationship considerations can be tested in the various fields in which activity was observed.

Extensive overviews were presented roughly a decade ago [241], and several reviews in the last ten years described further advances in the use of lignans and neolignans as plant-derived actives in various fields [87, 236, 242 - 245]. This chapter will thus highlight selected findings that emerged during the last decade in which lignans showed interesting properties from a pharmaceutical point of view. The discussed selection of newer findings is additionally summarised, including structural features of the various lignans, in form of Table **3**. at the end of this paragraph.

Dietary Value of Lignans in Health Promotion

The health benefits of natural food products have been considered for different goals since ancient times. More than 2000 years ago Hippocrates expressed his famous statement: "Let food be thy medicine and medicine be thy food". [246] Choosing a balanced diet has become an essential part of a healthy lifestyle and many studies have shown that people who follow a specific diet (especially polyphenol-rich diets) have a low risk for a range of chronic diseases, such as obesity, diabetes, cancer, heart disease, *etc* [239, 246 - 250].

Monomeric and oligomeric plant polyphenols such as lignans and tannins are generally considered to have anticancer, anti-inflammatory, antiviral, antimicrobial, and immunomodulatory effects, which explain their promotion for human health [239, 251 - 253]. Lignans, in line with other natural compounds, have been shown to contribute significantly to disease prevention and health promotion [249]; Several studies have shown the potential of lignan-rich diets in preventing the development of various diseases, particularly hormone-dependent cancer, cardiovascular diseases, and diabetes [247, 249 - 251, 254 - 257].

Plant-based foods confer considerable health benefits, partly attributable to their abundant micronutrient, *e.g.*, lower molecular weight polyphenol content. Interest in the activity of (low) oligomeric polyphenols is largely focused on the contribution of their antioxidant activity to the prevention of various disorders [258]. For these properties, lignans are considered an important aspect in nutraceuticals and functional foods.

Among plant polyphenols, lignans have recently been studied as potential modulators of the gut-brain axis. In particular, gut bacterial metabolism is able to convert dietary lignans into therapeutically relevant polyphenols, *i.e.*, enterolignans, such as enterolactone and enterodiol [244]. Enterolignans are characterised by various biologic activities, including tissue-specific estrogen receptor activation, together with anti-inflammatory and apoptotic effects [244].

Mechanisms of the anticancer effects of oligomeric polyphenols such as lignans. It was found that they can block the initiation of carcinogenesis by inactivating, on the basis of their antioxidant activity, reactive oxygen species (ROS) as important representative of exogenous or endogenous genotoxic molecules [259].

Antiaging Potential of Lignans

Among the bioactivities of lignin has to be listed presumably also an antiaging potential; however, this antiaging potential has not been well elucidated yet. Su *et al.* [260] isolated from *Arctium lappa*, a well-known traditional medicinal plant in

China and Europe, six lignans, namely arctigenin, matairesinol, arctiin, (iso)lappaol A, lappaol C, and lappaol F, to study their antioxidant and antiaging properties using *Caenorhabditis elegans* as a relevant animal model. All lignans had the potential to significantly extended the mean life span of *C. elegans* at noteworthy concentrations of 10 and 100 μM. In case of matairesinol, when applied at a concentration of 100 μM, the life span of the worms could be extended by 25% [260]. Fittingly, it was observed that five lignans, once more on the basis of their strong free radical-scavenging activity *in vitro* and *in vivo* could improve survival rates of *C. elegans* under oxidative stress conditions. More interestingly, the study demonstrated that lignans can induce the nuclear translocation of the transcription factor DAF-16 and up-regulate its expression, suggesting that a possible underlying mechanism of the observed longevity-promoting activity of lignans depends on DAF-16 mediated signalling pathway. All lignans studied up-regulated the expression of jnk-1, indicating that lignans may promote the *C. elegans* longevity and stress resistance through a JNK--DAF-16 cascade [260].

Anti-Inflammatory Properties of Lignans

The anti-inflammatory properties of lignans have been investigated by Szopa *et al.* using *Schisandra rubriflora* and *Schisandra Chinensis* extracts [261]. *Schisandra rubriflora* is a dioecious plant of increasing importance due to its lignan composition and the possible therapeutic properties emerging thereof. In this context, the anti-inflammatory activity of extracts of fruits, leaves and shoots of the pharmacopoeial species *S. chinensis*, as well as extracts of *S. rubriflora* and individual lignans were tested *in vitro* for the inhibition of 15-lipooxygenase (15-LOX), phospholipases A2 (sPLA2) as well as cyclooxygenase 1 and 2 (COX-1; COX-2) enzyme activities. The results of anti-inflammatory assays revealed higher activity of *S. rubriflora* extracts. Individual lignans showed significant inhibitory activity against 15-LOX, COX-1 and COX-2 enzymes.

Table 3. Selected lignans and their pharmacological properties.

Lignan	Chemical Structure	Activity	Ref.
Arctigenin		- antiaging - antioxidant - free radical scavenger	[260]
Arctiin		- antiaging - antioxidant - free radical scavenger	[260]
Bicyclol		- anticancer - antiviral (venereal wart and chronic hepatitis B)	[245]

(Table 3) cont.....

Lignan	Chemical Structure	Activity	Ref.
Carbohydrate-lignan conjugates (CLCs)		- drug design (assessment of their ADMET profile and their lead-like / drug-like establishment)	[262]
Enterolignans (Enterodiol)		- antioxidant - neuroprotective effects - anticancer (*e.g.*, breast cancer) - cardiovascular disease	[256, 263, 264]
Enterolignans (Enterolactone)		- antioxidant - anti-inflammatory - apoptotic effects - lowered risk of heart disease, menopausal symptoms, osteoporosis and breast cancer	[265 - 268]
Hinokinin		- cytotoxic activities - anti-inflammatory - antimicrobial activities (*e.g.*, anti-trypanosomal activity)	[253]
Honokiol		- anti-inflammatory - antiapoptotic - antifibrotic activities	[252, 269, 270]
Macelignan		- antibacterial - anti-inflammatory - anticancer - antidiabetes - hepatoprotective activities - neuroprotective activities	[265]
Magnolol		- anti-inflammatory - antiapoptotic - antifibrotic activities	[252, 269, 270]
Matairesinol		- antiaging - antioxidant	[260]
Podophyllotoxin		- anticancer (cytotoxicity) - antiviral (venereal wart and chronic hepatitis B) - immunoregulatory activities - drug design (for the synthesis of etoposide and teniposide)	[236, 245, 263, 271, 272]
Schisandrin		- anti-inflammatory - antiapoptotic - antifibrotic activities	[239]
Sesamin		- antihypertensive - anticancer - hypocholesterolemic activities - protection against several hormone related diseases (*via* enterolignans its metabolite)	[239]

(Table 3) cont.....

Lignan	Chemical Structure	Activity	Ref.
Sesaminol		- antihypertensive - anticancer - hypocholesterolemic activities	[239]
Sesamol		- antihypertensive - anticancer - hypocholesterolemic activities	[239]
Sesamolin		- antihypertensive - anticancer - hypocholesterolemic activities	[239]

Anticancer Properties of Lignans

Cancer is a major problem of public health and one of the main causes of death around the globe [271]. Indeed, malignant diseases are the second mortality cause within the human population. Despite the serious progress in establishing and introduction of novel specifically targeted drugs, the therapy of these diseases remains severe medical and social problem. Several phenolic and alkaloid compounds have been demonstrated to have anticancer effects on various types of cancers. Anti-cancer activity exhibited by secondary metabolites medicinal plants such as phenolic acids, flavonoids, tannins, stilbenes, curcuminoids, xanthones, coumarins and especially lignans involves removing free radicals and thus lowering oxidative stress, leading to anticarcinogenic, antimutagenic, and anti-estrogenic effects, as well as induction of apoptosis, cell cycle arrest and inhibition of angiogenesis [242, 264, 273, 274].

Some of the most effective cancer treatments to date are based on natural products or compounds derived from plant products [242, 247, 250, 256, 257, 262]. Among the anticancer drugs, about 50% come from natural products as isolated or semisynthetic or related synthetic compounds: Taxol, vinca alkaloids, camptothecin, and podophyllotoxins, as well as their semisynthetic or synthetic derivatives, are the most important plant-derived anticancer drugs [271].

Traditionally, health benefits attributed to lignans have included a reduced risk of heart disease, menopausal symptoms, osteoporosis and breast cancer [258]. In addition, it was observed that several members of lignans and neolignans group, namely enterolactone and its biochemical precursors also known as phytoestrogens, possess important protective properties.

The fact that structural motives present in lignans also serve as an important starting point in the development of anticancer drugs can be described using the most famous products within this class of compounds, etoposide and teniposide, synthetic derivatives of podophyllotoxin, are used in the clinical treatment of lymphocytic leukemia as well as certain brain tumour and lung tumours since 20 years [236].

In addition to the cancer-preventing activities of lignans that can be traced back to their antioxidant activities, it was found that another mechanism underlying the anticancer effects of polyphenols consists in the inhibition of activity and synthesis of carcinogen-metabolising enzymes [275]. Lignans could also, on the other hand, induce the expression of genes encoding for antioxidant and detoxification enzymes, important factors in preventing the initiation of carcinogenesis [275].

Antibiotic Properties of Lignans

Lignans have attracted attention as plant derived biologically active compounds also due to their anti-biotic properties. In particular, genus *Bursera,* which belongs to the family of Burseraceae, has been used in traditional Mexican medicine for treating some pathophysiological disorders *via* their antioxidant, apoptotic, anti-cancer, anti-inflammatory, anti-bacterial, anti-viral, anti-fungal, and anti-protozoal properties [276]. Some lignans *Bursera* spp., such as dibenzyl butyrolactone lignans, dibenzyl butane diol lignans and aryltetraline lignans, have been developed to approved therapeutics, and others are considered as lead structures for new antibiotics [87].

Given the increasing microbial resistance as a pressing problem in antibiotic therapy, identification and investigation of potential synergistic effect of plant-derived polyphenols like lignans in combination with conventional antimicrobial agents against clinical multidrug-resistant microorganisms is representing another important active research line [238]. In particular, macelignan found in the nutmeg mace of *Myristica fragrans* gained attention as a new antibacterial active, that would additionally display activities anti-inflammatory, anti-cancer, anti-diabetes, as well as hepatoprotective and neuroprotective activities [265].

Hinokinin is another lignan, isolable from several plant species, that has been recently demonstrated to exhibit antimicrobial activity. As in many other lignan cases, this activity comes together with proven cytotoxic and anti-inflammatory toxicity; particularly interesting is its notable anti-trypanosomal activity [253].

Antiviral Properties of Lignans

Among their diverse pharmacological properties, lignans were also discussed to exhibit antiviral activities [245, 272, 277, 278]. Two types of antiviral lignans, podophyllotoxin and bicyclol, are used to treat venereal warts and chronic hepatitis B (CHB) in clinical trials.

In other respects, the antiviral and immunostimulant activities of *Andrographis paniculate* have been investigated [263]. *Andrographis paniculata* is a medicinal plant which was reported before to have anti-HIV, anti-pathogenic bacteria and immunoregulatory activities [279]. The research purpose was to investigate the activity of *Andrographis paniculata* ethanol extracts, presumably rich in lignans, as antiviral compound and immunostimulant. The result indicated that the *A. paniculata* ethanol extract inhibited the multiplication of Simian Retro Virus (SRV) virus in A549 cells, while not being toxic to the A459 cell line itself. Furthermore, the low concentration (1 μg/mL) of *A. paniculata* extracts was found to stimulate lymphocyte cell proliferation about 38% [263].

Hepatoprotective Effects of Lignans

Parenchymal hepatic cell survival, hepatic stellate cell (HSC) deactivation, and extracellular matrix (ECM) degradation by interfering with multiple targets and signaling pathways are discussed in antifibrotic effects of lignans [252], especially schisandrin B, honokiol, magnolol and sauchinone. Schisandrin B is an important bioactive lignan derived from a well-known herbal medicine named *Schisandra chinensis* that has been used for liver protection in recent years. Schisandrin B significantly attenuated liver damage and liver fibrosis progression in rat models, and also significantly suppressed HSC-T6 activation. Schisandrin B could further exert antifibrotic effects by increasing the Nrf2-ARE signaling pathway and decreasing the TGF-β/Smad signaling pathway [280]. This lignan also attenuated lipopolysaccharide- (LPS-) induced HSCs activation by upregulating Nrf2 expression [281]. Additionally performed transcriptomic analyses suggest that metabolic pathways, CYP450 enzymes, and the PPAR signaling pathway are the major targets of schisandrin B action [282].

In recent years, studies focused on the hepatoprotective effect of honokiol and magnolol; honokiol and magnolol are the main bioactive lignans isolated from *Magnolia officinalis* [269]. Treatment with honokiol alle*via*ted ConA-induced liver fibrosis by downregulating hydroxyproline, α-SMA, and collagen fiber deposition, which was associated with restoring antioxidant defense, regulating inflammatory cascades, and inhibiting the TGF-β/Smad/MAPK signaling pathway [283]. *In vitro* experiments further indicated that honokiol can induce apoptotic cell death in activated rat HSCs through the release of mitochondrial cytochrome C. Magnolol also attenuated ConA-induced liver fibrosis and suppressed human LX2 HSC activation, which was closely related to inhibiting Th17 cell differentiation by suppressing IL-17A generation [284]. In addition, other honokiol derivatives, such as 4′-*O*-ethylhonokiol, also prevented from HSC activation and induced apoptosis *via* regulation of Bak1 and Bcl-2 expression [270].

Sauchinone is a bioactive lignan that is mainly extracted from *Saururus chinensis* and has been widely used for treating fever, edema, jaundice, and several inflammatory diseases [285]. With respect to the effect of sauchinone on liver fibrosis, experimental results indicate that sauchinone at 10 and 20 mg/kg alleviated CCl_4-induced liver fibrosis and inhibited TGF-β1-induced HSC activation, which might be associated with suppressing autophagy and oxidative stress in HSCs [286]. Sauchinone also has liver protection effect to resist liver fibrosis. For instance, sauchinone protected the liver from toxicity induced by iron accumulation [287].

The Neuroprotective Effects of Lignans

Some studies assessed the neuroprotective properties of lignans [265, 266, 288]. In this respect, Reddy *et al.* [288] investigated the transformation of lignans into physiologically active and neuroprotector compounds through gut bacterial metabolism. These gut bacterial metabolites exert their neuroprotective effects in various neurodegenerative diseases, such as Alzheimer's disease (AD) and Parkinson's disease (PD), and also have protective effects against other diseases including cardiovascular diseases, cancer, and diabetes. For example, enterolactone and enterodiol, therapeutically relevant polyphenols, are formed as secondary gut bacterial metabolites of lignans. These compounds are also acetylcholinesterase inhibitors, and thereby have potential applications as therapeutics in AD and other neurological diseases. Polyphenols are also advanced glycation end product (AGE) inhibitors (antiglycating agents), and thereby exert neuroprotective effects in cases of AD. It is hypothesised that gut bacterial metabolism-derived polyphenols, when combined with the nanoparticle-based blood–brain barrier (BBB)-targeted drug delivery, may prove to be effective therapeutics for various neurological disorders, including traumatic brain injury (TBI), AD, and PD.

The Physicochemical Properties of Lignans in Drug Design

Classical lignans, neolignans, flavonolignans and carbohydrate-lignan conjugates (CLCs) were analysed by Pilkington [262], to assess their ADMET profiles and establish if these compounds are lead-like/drug-like and thus have potential to be or act as leads in the development of future therapeutics. It was found that while no studied compounds were lead-like, a very large proportion (< 75%) fulfilled all the requirements to be deemed as present in drug-like space and almost all compounds studied were in the known drug space. Principal component analysis was an effective technique that enabled the investigation of the relationship between the studied molecular descriptors and was able to separate the lignans from their sugar derivatives and flavonolignans, primarily according to the parameters that are considered when defining chemical space (i.e., number of hydrogen bond donors, acceptors, rotatable bonds, polar surface area and molecular weight). These results indicate that while CLCs and flavonolignans are less drug-like, lignans show a particularly high level of drug-likeness, an observation that coupled with their potent biological activities, demands future pursuit into their potential for use as therapeutics.

CONCLUDING REMARKS AND FUTURE PERSPECTIVES

The overview indicates, in terms of research regarding the use of lignin in pharmaceutical contexts, that the field has essentially matured from a technical point of view, agreeing on the fact that most benefits can be obtained when using lignin as a material for carrier systems. The practically exponentially growing number of articles detailing the formation of such carrier systems from essentially all types of currently available lignins can be interpreted as that a technological plateau has been reached, and the methods for generation of particles and capsules have become mainstream. Various actives are incorporated, and tuning is possible to achieve stability profiles that would suit specific applications. The main drawback, however, is only scarcely touched at the moment. The research in this field is still lacking final proofs regarding the real-life applicability of the developed systems. A majority of studies indicate that lignins do not exhibit a general cytotoxicity, but open questions regarding the possibility for lignin-based carrier systems to pass regulatory hurdles remain. It would also be necessary to understand the fate of lignins in front of the human metabolic system. It has been suggested that lignins, used in isolated form to be essentially an excipient, could be treated as fibres from a regulatory point of view, but given the proven activity of lignin in the form of, *e.g*., anti-inflammatory agent, renders this approach challenging. Lignin fractionation seems to be a promising approach to arrive at lignins that might facilitate the regulatory aspects while maintaining the lignin benefits, but yet capsule and particle formation from lignin fractions have been investigated only scarcely [289], disclosing open questions that would need to be answered in order to make progress and move to the next plateau.

Additional challenges connected to the use of lignin in nanoscaled preparations lies in potentially adverse, toxic effects that originate from the nanoscale itself. While eventually non-toxic as bulk material, once concentrated in the form of a nanoparticle of microcapsule, local toxicities can occur due to the unnaturally high concentration of reactive phenolic groups.

In terms of using lignin as the main active, beside challenges similar to those just discussed, more work in terms of structure-activity relationships is needed that might require an innovative *in-silico* description of lignins.

With respect to research targeting the use of lignans and the exploitation of their manifold activities, structures can be described more easily, and studies can relate certain lignans, hence certain structural motifs to observed pharmacological effects. Some lignans are studied for the activity and effects in clinical trials. Yet the problem persists that lignans, as well as lignins, have always more than one activity, so that a recurring and persisting challenge exists in determining the individual importance of the various effects.

CONSENT FOR PUBLICATION

Not applicable.

CONFLICT OF INTEREST

The author declares no conflict of interest, financial or otherwise.

ACKNOWLEDGEMENT

Declared none.

REFERENCES

[1] Lewis, N.G.; Davin, L.B.; Sarkanen, S. Lignin and Lignan Biosynthesis *Distinctions and Reconciliations. ACS Symposium Series, vol. 697***1998**, , 1-27. [http://dx.doi.org/10.1021/bk-1998-0697.ch001]

[2] Aresta, M.; Dibenedetto, A.; Dumeignil, F. Biorefineries, An Introduction. **2015**, [http://dx.doi.org/10.1515/9783110331585]

[3] Glasser, W.G.; Sarkanen, S. Lignin: Properties and Materials. **1989**, [http://dx.doi.org/10.1021/bk-1989-0397]

[4] Lewis, N.G.; Yamamoto, E. Lignin: occurrence, biogenesis and biodegradation. *Annu. Rev. Plant Physiol. Plant Mol. Biol.*, **1990**, *41*(1), 455-496. [http://dx.doi.org/10.1146/annurev.pp.41.060190.002323] [PMID: 11543592]

[5] Sarkanen, K.V.; Ludwig, C.H. Lignins: occurrence, formation, structure and reactions. **1971**,

[6] Adler, E. Lignin chemistry?past, present and future. *Wood Sci. Technol.*, **1977**, *11*(3), 169-218. [http://dx.doi.org/10.1007/BF00365615]

[7] Brunow, G.; Lundquist, K. Functional Groups and Bonding Patterns in Lignin (Including the Lignin-Carbohydrate Complexes). *Lignin and Lignans: Advances in Chemistry.*, **2010**, , 267-299. [http://dx.doi.org/10.1201/EBK1574444865-c7]

[8] Pesquet, E.; Zhang, B.; Gorzsás, A.; Puhakainen, T.; Serk, H.; Escamez, S.; Barbier, O.; Gerber, L.; Courtois-Moreau, C.; Alatalo, E.; Paulin, L.; Kangasjärvi, J.; Sundberg, B.; Goffner, D.; Tuominen, H. Non-cell-autonomous postmortem lignification of tracheary elements in Zinnia elegans. *Plant Cell*, **2013**, *25*(4), 1314-1328. [http://dx.doi.org/10.1105/tpc.113.110593] [PMID: 23572543]

[9] Decou, R.; Serk, H.; Ménard, D.; Pesquet, E. Analysis of Lignin Composition and Distribution Using Fluorescence Laser Confocal Microspectroscopy. **2017**.
[http://dx.doi.org/10.1007/978-1-4939-6722-3_17]

[10] Vanholme, R.; Demedts, B.; Morreel, K.; Ralph, J.; Boerjan, W. Lignin biosynthesis and structure. *Plant Physiol.,* **2010**, *153*(3), 895-905.
[http://dx.doi.org/10.1104/pp.110.155119] [PMID: 20472751]

[11] Boerjan, W.; Ralph, J.; Baucher, M. Lignin Biosynthesis. *Annu. Rev. Plant Biol.,* **2003**, *54*(1), 519-546.
[http://dx.doi.org/10.1146/annurev.arplant.54.031902.134938] [PMID: 14503002]

[12] Donaldson, L.A. Lignification and lignin topochemistry — an ultrastructural view. *Phytochemistry,* **2001**, *57*(6), 859-873.
[http://dx.doi.org/10.1016/S0031-9422(01)00049-8] [PMID: 11423137]

[13] Whetten, R.; Sederoff, R. Lignin Biosynthesis. *Plant Cell,* **1995**, *7*(7), 1001-1013.
[http://dx.doi.org/10.2307/3870053] [PMID: 12242395]

[14] Achnine, L.; Blancaflor, E.B.; Rasmussen, S.; Dixon, R.A. Colocalization of L-phenylalanine ammonia-lyase and cinnamate 4-hydroxylase for metabolic channeling in phenylpropanoid biosynthesis. *Plant Cell,* **2004**, *16*(11), 3098-3109.
[http://dx.doi.org/10.1105/tpc.104.024406] [PMID: 15472080]

[15] Li, L.; Popko, J.L.; Umezawa, T.; Chiang, V.L. 5-hydroxyconiferyl aldehyde modulates enzymatic methylation for syringyl monolignol formation, a new view of monolignol biosynthesis in angiosperms. *J. Biol. Chem.,* **2000**, *275*(9), 6537-6545.
[http://dx.doi.org/10.1074/jbc.275.9.6537] [PMID: 10692459]

[16] Burlat, V.; Kwon, M.; Davin, L.B.; Lewis, N.G. Dirigent proteins and dirigent sites in lignifying tissues. *Phytochemistry,* **2001**, *57*(6), 883-897.
[http://dx.doi.org/10.1016/S0031-9422(01)00117-0] [PMID: 11423139]

[17] Hatfield, R.; Vermerris, W. Lignin formation in plants. The dilemma of linkage specificity. *Plant Physiol.,* **2001**, *126*(4), 1351-1357.
[http://dx.doi.org/10.1104/pp.126.4.1351] [PMID: 11500535]

[18] Ralph, J.; Peng, J.; Lu, F.; Hatfield, R.D.; Helm, R.F. Are lignins optically active? *J. Agric. Food Chem.,* **1999**, *47*(8), 2991-2996.
[http://dx.doi.org/10.1021/jf9901136] [PMID: 10552598]

[19] Davin, L.B.; Lewis, N.G. Lignin primary structures and dirigent sites. *Curr. Opin. Biotechnol.,* **2005**, *16*(4), 407-415.
[http://dx.doi.org/10.1016/j.copbio.2005.06.011] [PMID: 16023847]

[20] Gang, D.R.; Costa, M.A.; Fujita, M.; Dinkova-Kostova, A.T.; Wang, H.B.; Burlat, V.; Martin, W.; Sarkanen, S.; Davin, L.B.; Lewis, N.G. Regiochemical control of monolignol radical coupling: A new paradigm for lignin and lignan biosynthesis. *Chem. Biol.,* **1999**, *6*(3), 143-151.
[http://dx.doi.org/10.1016/S1074-5521(99)89006-1] [PMID: 10074466]

[21] Humphreys, J.M.; Chapple, C. Rewriting the lignin roadmap. *Curr. Opin. Plant Biol.,* **2002**, *5*(3), 224-229.
[http://dx.doi.org/10.1016/S1369-5266(02)00257-1] [PMID: 11960740]

[22] Ralph, J.; Lundquist, K.; Brunow, G.; Lu, F.; Kim, H.; Schatz, P.F.; Marita, J.M.; Hatfield, R.D.; Ralph, S.A.; Christensen, J.H.; Boerjan, W. Lignins: Natural polymers from oxidative coupling of 4-hydroxyphenyl- propanoids. *Phytochem. Rev.,* **2004**, *3*(1-2), 29-60.
[http://dx.doi.org/10.1023/B:PHYT.0000047809.65444.a4]

[23] Karhunen, P.; Rummakko, P.; Sipilä, J.; Brunow, G.; Kilpeläinen, I. Dibenzodioxocins; a novel type of linkage in softwood lignins. *Tetrahedron Lett.,* **1995**, *36*(1), 169-170.
[http://dx.doi.org/10.1016/0040-4039(94)02203-N]

[24] Hatfield, R.; Fukushima, R.S. Can Lignin Be Accurately Measured? *Crop Sci.*, **2005**, *45*(3), 832-839. [http://dx.doi.org/10.2135/cropsci2004.0238]

[25] Lupoi, J.S.; Singh, S.; Parthasarathi, R.; Simmons, B.A.; Henry, R.J. Recent innovations in analytical methods for the qualitative and quantitative assessment of lignin. *Renew. Sustain. Energy Rev.*, **2015**, *49*, 871-906. [http://dx.doi.org/10.1016/j.rser.2015.04.091]

[26] Vaz, S., Jr Analytical techniques for the chemical analysis of plant biomass and biomass products. *Anal. Methods,* **2014**, *6*(20), 8094-8105. [http://dx.doi.org/10.1039/C4AY00388H]

[27] Heitner, C.; Dimmel, D.; Schmidt, J. Lignin and Lignans: Advances in Chemistry. **2010**,

[28] Lange, H.; Schiffels, P.; Sette, M.; Sevastyanova, O.; Crestini, C. Fractional Precipitation of Wheat Straw Organosolv Lignin: Macroscopic Properties and Structural Insights. *ACS Sustain. Chem.& Eng.*, **2016**, *4*(10), 5136-5151. [http://dx.doi.org/10.1021/acssuschemeng.6b01475]

[29] Crestini, C.; Lange, H.; Sette, M.; Argyropoulos, D.S. On the structure of softwood kraft lignin. *Green Chem.*, **2017**, *19*(17), 4104-4121. [http://dx.doi.org/10.1039/C7GC01812F]

[30] Björkman, A. Studies on Finely Divided Wood. Part 1. Extraction of ligin with neutral solvents. *Sven. Papperstidn.*, **1956**, *59*, 477-485.

[31] Guerra, A.; Filpponen, I.; Lucia, L.A.; Argyropoulos, D.S. Comparative evaluation of three lignin isolation protocols for various wood species. *J. Agric. Food Chem.*, **2006**, *54*(26), 9696-9705. [http://dx.doi.org/10.1021/jf062433c] [PMID: 17177489]

[32] McDonough, T.J. The Chemistry of Organosolv Delignification. *Tappi J.*, **1993**, *76*, 186-193.

[33] Pye, E.K.; Lora, J.H. The Alcell Process. A Proven Alternative to Kraft Pulping. *Tappi J.*, **1991**, *74*, 113-118.

[34] Chakar, F.S.; Ragauskas, A.J. Review of current and future softwood kraft lignin process chemistry. *Ind. Crops Prod.*, **2004**, *20*(2), 131-141. [http://dx.doi.org/10.1016/j.indcrop.2004.04.016]

[35] Gierer, J. Chemical aspects of kraft pulping. *Wood Sci. Technol.*, **1980**, *14*(4), 241-266. [http://dx.doi.org/10.1007/BF00383453]

[36] Tomani, P. The LignoBoost Process. *Cellul. Chem. Technol.*, **2010**, *44*, 53-58.

[37] Howard, G.C. Utilization of Sulfite,Liquor. *Ind. Eng. Chem.*, **1934**, *26*(6), 614-617. [http://dx.doi.org/10.1021/ie50294a007]

[38] van Parijs, F.R.D.; Morreel, K.; Ralph, J.; Boerjan, W.; Merks, R.M.H. Modeling lignin polymerization. I. Simulation model of dehydrogenation polymers. *Plant Physiol.*, **2010**, *153*(3), 1332-1344. [http://dx.doi.org/10.1104/pp.110.154468] [PMID: 20472753]

[39] Tuomela, M.; Hatakka, A.; Raiskila, S.; Vikman, M.; Itävaara, M. Biodegradation of radiolabelled synthetic lignin (14 C-DHP) and mechanical pulp in a compost environment. *Appl. Microbiol. Biotechnol.*, **2001**, *55*(4), 492-499. [http://dx.doi.org/10.1007/s002530000513] [PMID: 11398933]

[40] Hatcher, P.G.; Minard, R.D. Comparison of dehydrogenase polymer (DHP) lignin with native lignin from gymnosperm wood by thermochemolysis using tetramethylammonium hydroxide (TMAH). *Org. Geochem.*, **1996**, *24*(6-7), 593-600. [http://dx.doi.org/10.1016/0146-6380(96)00051-4]

[41] Lockhart, J. Altering Lignin Composition to Improve Biofuel Production. *Plant Cell,* **2015**, *27*(8),

2082-2082.
[http://dx.doi.org/10.1105/tpc.15.00668] [PMID: 26265760]

[42] Eudes, A.; Liang, Y.; Mitra, P.; Loqué, D. Lignin bioengineering. *Curr. Opin. Biotechnol.*, **2014**, *26*, 189-198.
[http://dx.doi.org/10.1016/j.copbio.2014.01.002] [PMID: 24607805]

[43] Poovaiah, C.R.; Nageswara-Rao, M.; Soneji, J.R.; Baxter, H.L.; Stewart, C.N., Jr Altered lignin biosynthesis using biotechnology to improve lignocellulosic biofuel feedstocks. *Plant Biotechnol. J.*, **2014**, *12*(9), 1163-1173.
[http://dx.doi.org/10.1111/pbi.12225] [PMID: 25051990]

[44] Verma, S.R.; Dwivedi, U.N. Lignin genetic engineering for improvement of wood quality: Applications in paper and textile industries, fodder and bioenergy production. *S. Afr. J. Bot.*, **2014**, *91*, 107-125.
[http://dx.doi.org/10.1016/j.sajb.2014.01.002]

[45] Baucher, M.; Halpin, C.; Petit-Conil, M.; Boerjan, W. Lignin: genetic engineering and impact on pulping. *Crit. Rev. Biochem. Mol. Biol.*, **2003**, *38*(4), 305-350.
[http://dx.doi.org/10.1080/10409230391036757] [PMID: 14551235]

[46] Baucher, M.; Monties, B.; Montagu, M.V.; Boerjan, W. Biosynthesis and Genetic Engineering of Lignin. *Crit. Rev. Plant Sci.*, **1998**, *17*(2), 125-197.
[http://dx.doi.org/10.1080/07352689891304203]

[47] Boudet, A.; Grima-Pettenati, J. Lignin genetic engineering. *Mol. Breed.*, **1996**, *2*(1), 25-39.
[http://dx.doi.org/10.1007/BF00171349]

[48] Gray, J.; Caparrós-Ruiz, D.; Grotewold, E. Grass phenylpropanoids: Regulate before using! *Plant Sci.*, **2012**, *184*, 112-120.
[http://dx.doi.org/10.1016/j.plantsci.2011.12.008] [PMID: 22284715]

[49] Lundquist, K.; Kirk, T.K. Fractionation-Purification of an Industrial Kraft Lignin. *Tappi J.*, **1980**, *63*, 1.

[50] Schuerch, C. The Solvent Properties of Liquids and Their Relation to the Solubility, Swelling, Isolation and Fractionation of Lignin. *J. Am. Chem. Soc.*, **1952**, *74*(20), 5061-5067.
[http://dx.doi.org/10.1021/ja01140a020]

[51] Mousavioun, P.; Doherty, W.O.S. Chemical and thermal properties of fractionated bagasse soda lignin. *Ind. Crops Prod.*, **2010**, *31*(1), 52-58.
[http://dx.doi.org/10.1016/j.indcrop.2009.09.001]

[52] Cui, C.; Sun, R.; Argyropoulos, D.S. Fractional Precipitation of Softwood Kraft Lignin: Isolation of Narrow Fractions Common to a Variety of Lignins. *ACS Sustain. Chem.& Eng.*, **2014**, *2*(4), 959-968.
[http://dx.doi.org/10.1021/sc400545d]

[53] Thring, R.W.; Vanderlaan, M.N.; Griffin, S.L. Fractionation Of Alcell® Lignin By Sequential Solvent Extraction. *J. Wood Chem. Technol.*, **1996**, *16*(2), 139-154.
[http://dx.doi.org/10.1080/02773819608545815]

[54] Teng, N.Y.; Dallmeyer, I.; Kadla, J.F. Effect of Softwood Kraft Lignin Fractionation on the Dispersion of Multiwalled Carbon Nanotubes. *Ind. Eng. Chem. Res.*, **2013**, *52*(19), 6311-6317.
[http://dx.doi.org/10.1021/ie303261z]

[55] Gosselink, R.J.A.; van Dam, J.E.G.; de Jong, E.; Scott, E.L.; Sanders, J.P.M.; Li, J.; Gellerstedt, G. Fractionation, analysis, and PCA modeling of properties of four technical lignins for prediction of their application potential in binders. *Holzforschung,* **2010**, *64*(2), 193-200.
[http://dx.doi.org/10.1515/hf.2010.023]

[56] Zikeli, F.; Ters, T.; Fackler, K.; Srebotnik, E.; Li, J. Successive and quantitative fractionation and extensive structural characterization of lignin from wheat straw. *Ind. Crops Prod.*, **2014**, *61*, 249-257.
[http://dx.doi.org/10.1016/j.indcrop.2014.07.013]

[57] Duval, A.; Vilaplana, F.; Crestini, C.; Lawoko, M. Solvent screening for the fractionation of industrial kraft lignin. *Holzforschung,* **2016**, *70*(1), 11-20. [http://dx.doi.org/10.1515/hf-2014-0346]

[58] Griffini, G.; Passoni, V.; Suriano, R.; Levi, M.; Turri, S. Polyurethane Coatings Based on Chemically Unmodified Fractionated Lignin. *ACS Sustain. Chem.& Eng.,* **2015**, *3*(6), 1145-1154. [http://dx.doi.org/10.1021/acssuschemeng.5b00073]

[59] Passoni, V.; Scarica, C.; Levi, M.; Turri, S.; Griffini, G. Fractionation of Industrial Softwood Kraft Lignin: Solvent Selection as a Tool for Tailored Material Properties. *ACS Sustain. Chem.& Eng.,* **2016**, *4*(4), 2232-2242. [http://dx.doi.org/10.1021/acssuschemeng.5b01722]

[60] Majdar, R.E.; Crestini, C.; Lange, H. Lignin Fractionation in Segmented Continuous Flow. *ChemSusChem,* **2020**, *13*(17), 4735-4742. [http://dx.doi.org/10.1002/cssc.202001138] [PMID: 32715624]

[61] Gosselink, RJA; Van, DP; Van, E **2015**.

[62] Toledano, A.; García, A.; Mondragon, I.; Labidi, J. Lignin separation and fractionation by ultrafiltration. *Separ. Purif. Tech.,* **2010**, *71*(1), 38-43. [http://dx.doi.org/10.1016/j.seppur.2009.10.024]

[63] Sevastyanova, O.; Helander, M.; Chowdhury, S.; Lange, H.; Wedin, H.; Zhang, L.; Ek, M.; Kadla, J.F.; Crestini, C.; Lindström, M.E. Tailoring the molecular and thermo-mechanical properties of kraft lignin by ultrafiltration. *J. Appl. Polym. Sci.,* **2014**, *131*(18), n/a. [http://dx.doi.org/10.1002/app.40799]

[64] Duval, A.; Molina-Boisseau, S.; Chirat, C. Fractionation of lignosulfonates: comparison of ultrafiltration and ethanol solubility to obtain a set of fractions with distinct properties. *Holzforschung,* **2015**, *69*(2), 127-134. [http://dx.doi.org/10.1515/hf-2014-0082]

[65] Sadeghifar, H.; Ragauskas, A. Perspective on Technical Lignin Fractionation. *ACS Sustain. Chem.& Eng.,* **2020**, *8*(22), 8086-8101. [http://dx.doi.org/10.1021/acssuschemeng.0c01348]

[66] Gigli, M.; Crestini, C. Lignin fractionation: Opportunities and Challenges. *Green Chem.,* **2020**, *22*, 4722-4746. [http://dx.doi.org/10.1039/D0GC01606C]

[67] Teponno, R.B.; Kusari, S.; Spiteller, M. Recent advances in research on lignans and neolignans. *Nat. Prod. Rep.,* **2016**, *33*(9), 1044-1092. [http://dx.doi.org/10.1039/C6NP00021E] [PMID: 27157413]

[68] Umezawa, T. Diversity in lignan biosynthesis. *Phytochem. Rev.,* **2003**, *2*(3), 371-390. [http://dx.doi.org/10.1023/B:PHYT.0000045487.02836.32]

[69] Fuss, E. Lignans in plant cell and organ cultures: An overview. *Phytochem. Rev.,* **2003**, *2*(3), 307-320. [http://dx.doi.org/10.1023/B:PHYT.0000045500.56476.f5]

[70] Sakakibara, N.; Suzuki, S.; Umezawa, T.; Shimada, M. Biosynthesis of yatein in Anthriscus sylvestrisA part of this work was performed as a part of the R & D Project of Industrial Science and Technology Frontier Program supported by NEDO (New Energy and Industrial Technology Development Organization). *Org. Biomol. Chem.,* **2003**, *1*(14), 2474-2485. [http://dx.doi.org/10.1039/b304411d] [PMID: 12956064]

[71] Seidel, V.; Windhövel, J.; Eaton, G.; Alfermann, W.A.; Arroo, R.R.; Medarde, M.; Petersen, M.; Woolley, J.G. Biosynthesis of podophyllotoxin in Linum album cell cultures. *Planta,* **2002**, *215*(6), 1031-1039. [http://dx.doi.org/10.1007/s00425-002-0834-1] [PMID: 12355164]

[72] van Uden, W.; Pras, N.; Homan, B.; Malingré, T.M. Improvement of the production of 5-methoxypodophyllotoxin using a new selected root culture of Linum flavum L. *Plant Cell Tissue Organ Cult.*, **1991**, *27*(2), 115-121.
[http://dx.doi.org/10.1007/BF00041279]

[73] Broomhead, A.J.; Dewick, P.M. Biotransformation of *Podophyllum* lignans in cell suspension cultures of *Forsythia intermedia. Phytochemistry,* **1991**, *30*(5), 1511-1517.
[http://dx.doi.org/10.1016/0031-9422(91)84199-3]

[74] Rahman, M.M.A.; Dewick, P.M.; Jackson, D.E.; Lucas, J.A. Biosynthesis of lignans in Forsythia intermedia. *Phytochemistry,* **1990**, *29*(6), 1841-1846.
[http://dx.doi.org/10.1016/0031-9422(90)85025-B]

[75] Davin, L.B.; Wang, H.B.; Crowell, A.L.; Bedgar, D.L.; Martin, D.M.; Sarkanen, S.; Lewis, N.G. Stereoselective bimolecular phenoxy radical coupling by an auxiliary (dirigent) protein without an active center. *Science,* **1997**, *275*(5298), 362-367.
[http://dx.doi.org/10.1126/science.275.5298.362] [PMID: 8994027]

[76] Davin, L.B.; Lewis, N.G. An historical perspective on lignan biosynthesis: Monolignol, allylphenol and hydroxycinnamic acid coupling and downstream metabolism. *Phytochem. Rev.,* **2003**, *2*(3), 257-288.
[http://dx.doi.org/10.1023/B:PHYT.0000046175.83729.b5]

[77] Moinuddin, S.G.A.; Youn, B.; Bedgar, D.L.; Costa, M.A.; Helms, G.L.; Kang, C.; Davin, L.B.; Lewis, N.G. Secoisolariciresinol dehydrogenase: mode of catalysis and stereospecificity of hydride transfer in Podophyllum peltatum. *Org. Biomol. Chem.,* **2006**, *4*(5), 808-816.
[http://dx.doi.org/10.1039/b516563f] [PMID: 16493463]

[78] von Heimendahl, C.B.I.; Schäfer, K.M.; Eklund, P.; Sjöholm, R.; Schmidt, T.J.; Fuss, E. Pinoresinol–lariciresinol reductases with different stereospecificity from Linum album and Linum usitatissimum. *Phytochemistry,* **2005**, *66*(11), 1254-1263.
[http://dx.doi.org/10.1016/j.phytochem.2005.04.026] [PMID: 15949826]

[79] Okunishi, T.; Sakakibara, N.; Suzuki, S.; Umezawa, T.; Shimada, M. Stereochemistry of matairesinol formation by Daphne secoisolariciresinol dehydrogenase. *J. Wood Sci.,* **2004**, *50*(1), 77-81.
[http://dx.doi.org/10.1007/s10086-003-0516-z]

[80] Xia, Z.Q.; Costa, M.A.; Pélissier, H.C.; Davin, L.B.; Lewis, N.G. Secoisolariciresinol dehydrogenase purification, cloning, and functional expression. Implications for human health protection. *J. Biol. Chem.,* **2001**, *276*(16), 12614-12623.
[http://dx.doi.org/10.1074/jbc.M008622200] [PMID: 11278426]

[81] Dinkova-Kostova, A.T.; Gang, D.R.; Davin, L.B.; Bedgar, D.L.; Chu, A.; Lewis, N.G. (+)-Pinoresinol/(+)-lariciresinol reductase from Forsythia intermedia. Protein purification, cDNA cloning, heterologous expression and comparison to isoflavone reductase. *J. Biol. Chem.,* **1996**, *271*(46), 29473-29482.
[http://dx.doi.org/10.1074/jbc.271.46.29473] [PMID: 8910615]

[82] Lange, H.; Giannì, P.; Crestini, C. Lignin Analytics. *Energy Environ. Ser., Cambridge.,* **2018**, , 413-476.

[83] Lapierre, C. Determining Lignin Structure by Chemical Degradations. *Lignin and Lignans: Advances in Chemistry.,* **2010**, , 11-48.
[http://dx.doi.org/10.1201/EBK1574444865-c2]

[84] Schmidt, J. Electronic Spectroscopy of Lignins. *Lignin and Lignans: Advances in Chemsitry.,* **2010**, , 49-102.
[http://dx.doi.org/10.1201/EBK1574444865-c3]

[85] Argyropoulos, D. Heteronuclear NMR Spectroscopy of Lignins. *Lignin and Lignans: Advances in Chemsitry.,* **2010**, , 245-265.

[http://dx.doi.org/10.1201/EBK1574444865-c6]

[86] Hatakeyama, H.; Hatakeyama, T. Thermal Properties of Isolated and *in situ* Lignin. *Lignin and Lignans: Adcances in Chemistry.*, **2010**, , 301-319. [http://dx.doi.org/10.1201/EBK1574444865-c8]

[87] Zhang, J.; Chen, J.; Liang, Z.; Zhao, C. New lignans and their biological activities. *Chem. Biodivers.*, **2014**, *11*(1), 1-54. [http://dx.doi.org/10.1002/cbdv.201100433] [PMID: 24443425]

[88] Yang, W.J.; Griffiths, P.R.; Byler, D.M.; Susi, H. Protein Conformation by Infrared Spectroscopy: Resolution Enhancement by Fourier Self-Deconvolution. *Appl. Spectrosc.*, **1985**, *39*(2), 282-287. [http://dx.doi.org/10.1366/0003702854248917]

[89] Kauppinen, J.K.; Moffatt, D.J.; Mantsch, H.H.; Cameron, D.G. Fourier Self-Deconvolution: A Method for Resolving Intrinsically Overlapped Bands. *Appl. Spectrosc.*, **1981**, *35*(3), 271-276. [http://dx.doi.org/10.1366/0003702814732634]

[90] Maddams, W.F. The Scope and Limitations of Curve Fitting. *Appl. Spectrosc.*, **1980**, *34*(3), 245-267. [http://dx.doi.org/10.1366/0003702804730312]

[91] Pierce, J.A.; Jackson, R.S.; Van Every, K.W.; Griffiths, P.R.; Gao, H. Combined deconvolution and curve fitting for quantitative analysis of unresolved spectral bands. *Anal. Chem.*, **1990**, *62*(5), 477-484. [http://dx.doi.org/10.1021/ac00204a011]

[92] Hergert, H.L. *An Investigation of the Vibrational Spectra of Lignin Model Compounds.*, **1984**,

[93] Agarwal, U.; Atalla, R. Vibrational Spectroscopy. *Lignin and Lignans: Advances in Chemistry.*, **2010**, , 103-136. [http://dx.doi.org/10.1201/EBK1574444865-c4]

[94] Larsen, K.L.; Barsberg, S. Theoretical and Raman spectroscopic studies of phenolic lignin model monomers. *J. Phys. Chem. B,* **2010**, *114*(23), 8009-8021. [http://dx.doi.org/10.1021/jp1028239] [PMID: 20499919]

[95] Meyer, M.W.; Lupoi, J.S.; Smith, E.A. 1064nm dispersive multichannel Raman spectroscopy for the analysis of plant lignin. *Anal. Chim. Acta,* **2011**, *706*(1), 164-170. [http://dx.doi.org/10.1016/j.aca.2011.08.031] [PMID: 21995924]

[96] Meng, X.; Crestini, C.; Ben, H.; Hao, N.; Pu, Y.; Ragauskas, A.J.; Argyropoulos, D.S. Determination of hydroxyl groups in biorefinery resources *via* quantitative ^{31}P NMR spectroscopy. *Nat. Protoc.*, **2019**, *14*(9), 2627-2647. [http://dx.doi.org/10.1038/s41596-019-0191-1] [PMID: 31391578]

[97] Ralph, J.; Landucci, L. NMR of Lignins. *Lignin and Lignans: Advances in Chemistry.*, **2010**, , 137-243. [http://dx.doi.org/10.1201/EBK1574444865-c5]

[98] Lundquist, K. Proton (1H) NMR Spectroscopy. *Methods in Lignin Chemistry.*, **1992**, , 242-249. [http://dx.doi.org/10.1007/978-3-642-74065-7_17]

[99] Robert, D. Carbon-13 Nuclear Magnetic Resonance Spectrometry. *Methods in Lignin Chemistry.*, **1992**, , 250-273. [http://dx.doi.org/10.1007/978-3-642-74065-7_18]

[100] Leary, G.J.; Newman, R.H. Cross Polarization/Magic Angle Spinning Nuclear Magnetic Resonance (CP/MAS NMR) Spectroscopy. *Methods in Lignin Chemistry.*, **1992**, , 146-161. [http://dx.doi.org/10.1007/978-3-642-74065-7_11]

[101] Peterson, D.J.; Loening, N.M. QQ-HSQC: a quick, quantitative heteronuclear correlation experiment for NMR spectroscopy. *Magn. Reson. Chem.*, **2007**, *45*(11), 937-941. [http://dx.doi.org/10.1002/mrc.2073] [PMID: 17924357]

[102] Hu, K.; Westler, W.M.; Markley, J.L. Simultaneous quantification and identification of individual

chemicals in metabolite mixtures by two-dimensional extrapolated time-zero (1)H-(13)C HSQC (HSQC(0)). *J. Am. Chem. Soc.*, **2011**, *133*(6), 1662-1665. [http://dx.doi.org/10.1021/ja1095304] [PMID: 21247157]

[103] Sette, M.; Wechselberger, R.; Crestini, C. Elucidation of lignin structure by quantitative 2D NMR. *Chemistry,* **2011**, *17*(34), 9529-9535. [http://dx.doi.org/10.1002/chem.201003045] [PMID: 21721058]

[104] Sette, M.; Lange, H.; Crestini, C. Quantitative HSQC Analyses of Lignin: A Practical Comparison. *Comput. Struct. Biotechnol. J.,* **2013**, *6*(7), e201303016. [http://dx.doi.org/10.5936/csbj.201303016] [PMID: 24688724]

[105] Crestini, C.; Melone, F.; Sette, M.; Saladino, R. Milled wood lignin: a linear oligomer. *Biomacromolecules,* **2011**, *12*(11), 3928-3935. [http://dx.doi.org/10.1021/bm200948r] [PMID: 21928799]

[106] Zhang, L.; Gellerstedt, G. Quantitative 2D HSQC NMR determination of polymer structures by selecting suitable internal standard references. *Magn. Reson. Chem.,* **2007**, *45*(1), 37-45. [http://dx.doi.org/10.1002/mrc.1914] [PMID: 17080511]

[107] Saake, B.; Argyropoulos, D.S.; Beinhoff, O.; Faix, O. A comparison of lignin polymer models (DHPs) and lignins by 31P NMR spectroscopy. *Phytochemistry,* **1996**, *43*(2), 499-507. [http://dx.doi.org/10.1016/0031-9422(96)00283-X]

[108] Wroblewski, A.E.; Lensink, C.; Markuszewski, R.; Verkade, J.G. Phosphorus-31 NMR spectroscopic analysis of coal pyrolysis condensates and extracts for heteroatom functionalities possessing labile hydrogen. *Energy Fuels,* **1988**, *2*(6), 765-774. [http://dx.doi.org/10.1021/ef00012a008]

[109] Granata, A.; Argyropoulos, D.S. 2-Chloro-4,4,5,5-tetramethyl-1,3,2-dioxaphospholane, a Reagent for the Accurate Determination of the Uncondensed and Condensed Phenolic Moieties in Lignins. *J. Agric. Food Chem.,* **1995**, *43*(6), 1538-1544. [http://dx.doi.org/10.1021/jf00054a023]

[110] Zhen, L.; Lange, H.; Crestini, C. An Analytical Toolbox for Fast and Straightforward Structural Characterisation of Commercially Available Tannins. *Molecules,* **2021**, *26*(9), 2532. [http://dx.doi.org/10.3390/molecules26092532] [PMID: 33926135]

[111] Crestini, C.; Lange, H.; Bianchetti, G. Detailed Chemical Composition of Condensed Tannins *via* Quantitative ^{31}P NMR and HSQC Analyses: *Acacia catechu*, *Schinopsis balansae*, and *Acacia mearnsii*. *J. Nat. Prod.,* **2016**, *79*(9), 2287-2295. [http://dx.doi.org/10.1021/acs.jnatprod.6b00380] [PMID: 27551744]

[112] Obiaga, T.I.; Wayman, M. Improved calibration procedure for gel permeation chromatography of lignins. *J. Appl. Polym. Sci.,* **1974**, *18*(7), 1943-1952. [http://dx.doi.org/10.1002/app.1974.070180704]

[113] Chen, F.; Li, J. Aqueous Gel Permeation Chromatographic Methods for Technical Lignins. *J. Wood Chem. Technol.,* **2000**, *20*(3), 265-276. [http://dx.doi.org/10.1080/02773810009349636]

[114] Salanti, A.; Zoia, L.; Tolppa, E.L.; Orlandi, M. Chromatographic detection of lignin-carbohydrate complexes in annual plants by derivatization in ionic liquid. *Biomacromolecules,* **2012**, *13*(2), 445-454. [http://dx.doi.org/10.1021/bm2014763] [PMID: 22220942]

[115] Wong, K.K.Y.; de Jong, E. Size-exclusion chromatography of lignin- and carbohydrate-containing samples using alkaline eluents. *J. Chromatogr. A,* **1996**, *737*(2), 193-203. [http://dx.doi.org/10.1016/0021-9673(95)01382-2]

[116] Pellinen, J.; Salkinoja-Salonen, M. Aqueous size exclusion chomatography of industrial lignins. *J. Chromatogr. A,* **1985**, *322*, 129-138.

[http://dx.doi.org/10.1016/S0021-9673(01)97665-4]

[117] Chum, H.L.; Johnson, D.K.; Tucker, M.P.; Himmel, M.E. Some Aspects of Lignin Characterization by High Performance Size Exclusion Chromatography Using Styrene Divinylbenzene Copolymer Gels. *Holzforschung,* **1987**, *41*(2), 97-108. [http://dx.doi.org/10.1515/hfsg.1987.41.2.97]

[118] Bikova, T.; Treimanis, A.; Rossinska, G.; Telysheva, G. On-line study of lignin behaviour in dilute alkaline solution by the SEC-UV method. *Holzforschung,* **2004**, *58*(5), 489-494. [http://dx.doi.org/10.1515/HF.2004.074]

[119] Ringena, O.; Lebioda, S.; Lehnen, R.; Saake, B. Size-exclusion chromatography of technical lignins in dimethyl sulfoxide/water and dimethylacetamide. *J. Chromatogr. A,* **2006**, *1102*(1-2), 154-163. [http://dx.doi.org/10.1016/j.chroma.2005.10.037] [PMID: 16288767]

[120] Gidh, A.V.; Decker, S.R.; Vinzant, T.B.; Himmel, M.E.; Williford, C. Determination of lignin by size exclusion chromatography using multi angle laser light scattering. *J. Chromatogr. A,* **2006**, *1114*(1), 102-110. [http://dx.doi.org/10.1016/j.chroma.2006.02.044] [PMID: 16566937]

[121] Gidh, A.V.; Decker, S.R.; See, C.H.; Himmel, M.E.; Williford, C.W. Characterization of lignin using multi-angle laser light scattering and atomic force microscopy. *Anal. Chim. Acta,* **2006**, *555*(2), 250-258. [http://dx.doi.org/10.1016/j.aca.2005.09.023]

[122] Braaten, S.M.; Christensen, B.E.; Fredheim, G.E. Comparison of Molecular Weight and Molecular Weight Distributions of Softwood and Hardwood Lignosulfonates. *J. Wood Chem. Technol.,* **2003**, *23*(2), 197-215. [http://dx.doi.org/10.1081/WCT-120021925]

[123] Cathala, B.; Saake, B.; Faix, O.; Monties, B. Association behaviour of lignins and lignin model compounds studied by multidetector size-exclusion chromatography. *J. Chromatogr. A,* **2003**, *1020*(2), 229-239. [http://dx.doi.org/10.1016/j.chroma.2003.08.046] [PMID: 14661746]

[124] Fredheim, G.E.; Braaten, S.M.; Christensen, B.E. Molecular weight determination of lignosulfonates by size-exclusion chromatography and multi-angle laser light scattering. *J. Chromatogr. A,* **2002**, *942*(1-2), 191-199. [http://dx.doi.org/10.1016/S0021-9673(01)01377-2] [PMID: 11822385]

[125] Morreel, K.; Dima, O.; Kim, H.; Lu, F.; Niculaes, C.; Vanholme, R.; Dauwe, R.; Goeminne, G.; Inzé, D.; Messens, E.; Ralph, J., Boerjan, W. Mass spectrometry-based sequencing of lignin oligomers. *Plant Physiol.,* **2010**, *153*(4), 1464-1478. [http://dx.doi.org/10.1104/pp.110.156489] [PMID: 20554692]

[126] Richel, A.; Vanderghem, C.; Simon, M.; Wathelet, B.; Paquot, M. Evaluation of matrix-assisted laser desorption/ionization mass spectrometry for second-generation lignin analysis. *Anal. Chem. Insights,* **2012**, *7*, ACI.S10799. [http://dx.doi.org/10.4137/ACI.S10799] [PMID: 23300342]

[127] Araújo, P.; Ferreira, M.S.; de Oliveira, D.N.; Pereira, L.; Sawaya, A.C.H.F.; Catharino, R.R.; Mazzafera, P. Mass spectrometry imaging: an expeditious and powerful technique for fast *in situ* lignin assessment in Eucalyptus. *Anal. Chem.,* **2014**, *86*(7), 3415-3419. [http://dx.doi.org/10.1021/ac500220r] [PMID: 24451041]

[128] Bayerbach, R.; Nguyen, V.D.; Schurr, U.; Meier, D. Characterization of the water-insoluble fraction from fast pyrolysis liquids (pyrolytic lignin). *J. Anal. Appl. Pyrolysis,* **2006**, *77*(2), 95-101. [http://dx.doi.org/10.1016/j.jaap.2006.02.002]

[129] Banoub, J.; Delmas, G.H., Jr; Joly, N.; Mackenzie, G.; Cachet, N.; Benjelloun-Mlayah, B.; Delmas, M. A critique on the structural analysis of lignins and application of novel tandem mass spectrometric strategies to determine lignin sequencing. *J. Mass Spectrom.,* **2015**, *50*(1), 5-48.

[http://dx.doi.org/10.1002/jms.3541] [PMID: 25601673]

[130] Banoub, J.H.; Delmas, M. Structural elucidation of the wheat straw lignin polymer by atmospheric pressure chemical ionization tandem mass spectrometry and matrix-assisted laser desorption/ionization time-of-flight mass spectrometry. *J. Mass Spectrom.*, **2003**, *38*(8), 900-903. [http://dx.doi.org/10.1002/jms.503] [PMID: 12938111]

[131] Gaya, P.; Arqués, J.L.; Medina, M.; Álvarez, I.; Landete, J.M. A New HPLC-PAD/HPLC-ESI-MS Method for the Analysis of Phytoestrogens Produced by Bacterial Metabolism. *Food Anal. Methods*, **2016**, *9*(2), 537-547. [http://dx.doi.org/10.1007/s12161-015-0226-3]

[132] Wang, C.Y.; Lam, S.H.; Tseng, L.H.; Lee, S.S. Rapid screening of lignans from *Phyllanthus myrtifolius* and stilbenoids from *Syagrus romanzoffiana* by HPLC-SPE-NMR. *Phytochem. Anal.*, **2011**, *22*(4), 352-360. [http://dx.doi.org/10.1002/pca.1286] [PMID: 21337650]

[133] Schmidt, T.J.; Hemmati, S.; Fuss, E.; Alfermann, A.W. A combined HPLC-UV and HPLC-MS method for the identification of lignans and its application to the lignans ofLinum usitatissimum L. andL. bienne Mill. *Phytochem. Anal.*, **2006**, *17*(5), 299-311. [http://dx.doi.org/10.1002/pca.918] [PMID: 17019931]

[134] Liu, S.; Chen, K.; Schliemann, W.; Strack, D. Isolation and identification of arctiin and arctigenin in leaves of burdock (Arctium lappa L.) by polyamide column chromatography in combination with HPLC-ESI[sol]MS. *Phytochem. Anal.*, **2005**, *16*(2), 86-89. [http://dx.doi.org/10.1002/pca.816] [PMID: 15881114]

[135] Sicilia, T.; Niemeyer, H.B.; Honig, D.M.; Metzler, M. Identification and stereochemical characterization of lignans in flaxseed and pumpkin seeds. *J. Agric. Food Chem.*, **2003**, *51*(5), 1181-1188. [http://dx.doi.org/10.1021/jf0207979] [PMID: 12590454]

[136] Meagher, L.P.; Beecher, G.R.; Flanagan, V.P.; Li, B.W. Isolation and characterization of the lignans, isolariciresinol and pinoresinol, in flaxseed meal. *J. Agric. Food Chem.*, **1999**, *47*(8), 3173-3180. [http://dx.doi.org/10.1021/jf981359y] [PMID: 10552626]

[137] Pellegrini, N.; Serafini, M.; Colombi, B.; Del Rio, D.; Salvatore, S.; Bianchi, M.; Brighenti, F. Total antioxidant capacity of plant foods, beverages and oils consumed in Italy assessed by three different *in vitro* assays. *J. Nutr.*, **2003**, *133*(9), 2812-2819. [http://dx.doi.org/10.1093/jn/133.9.2812] [PMID: 12949370]

[138] Ou, B.; Huang, D.; Hampsch-Woodill, M.; Flanagan, J.A.; Deemer, E.K. Analysis of antioxidant activities of common vegetables employing oxygen radical absorbance capacity (ORAC) and ferric reducing antioxidant power (FRAP) assays: a comparative study. *J. Agric. Food Chem.*, **2002**, *50*(11), 3122-3128. [http://dx.doi.org/10.1021/jf0116606] [PMID: 12009973]

[139] Da Silva, J.M.R.; Darmon, N.; Fernandez, Y.; Mitjavila, S. Oxygen free radical scavenger capacity in aqueous models of different procyanidins from grape seeds. *J. Agric. Food Chem.*, **1991**, *39*(9), 1549-1552. [http://dx.doi.org/10.1021/jf00009a002]

[140] Rigo, A.; vianello, F.; Clementi, G.; Rossetto, M.; Scarpa, M.; Vrhovšek, U.; Mattivi, F. Contribution of proanthocyanidins to the peroxy radical scavenging capacity of some Italian red wines. *J. Agric. Food Chem.*, **2000**, *48*(6), 1996-2002. [http://dx.doi.org/10.1021/jf991203d] [PMID: 10888488]

[141] Szabo, M.; Idiţoiu, C.; Chambre, D.; Lupea, A. Improved DPPH determination for antioxidant activity spectrophotometric assay. *Chem. Pap.*, **2007**, *61*(3), 214-216. [http://dx.doi.org/10.2478/s11696-007-0022-7]

[142] Serpen, A.; Capuano, E.; Fogliano, V.; Gökmen, V. A new procedure to measure the antioxidant

activity of insoluble food components. *J. Agric. Food Chem.*, **2007**, *55*(19), 7676-7681. [http://dx.doi.org/10.1021/jf071291z] [PMID: 17708649]

[143] Re, R.; Pellegrini, N.; Proteggente, A.; Pannala, A.; Yang, M.; Rice-Evans, C. Antioxidant activity applying an improved ABTS radical cation decolorization assay. *Free Radic. Biol. Med.*, **1999**, *26*(9-10), 1231-1237. [http://dx.doi.org/10.1016/S0891-5849(98)00315-3] [PMID: 10381194]

[144] Lora, J.H.; Glasser, W.G. Recent Industrial Applications of Lignin: A Sustainable Alternative to Nonrenewable Materials. *J. Polym. Environ.*, **2002**, *10*(1/2), 39-48. [http://dx.doi.org/10.1023/A:1021070006895]

[145] Glasser, W.G.; Northey, R.A.; Schultz, T.P., Eds. *Lignin: Historical, Biological, and Materials Perspectives.*, **1999**, *Vol. 742* [http://dx.doi.org/10.1021/bk-2000-0742]

[146] Gil-Chávez, J.; Gurikov, P.; Hu, X.; Meyer, R.; Reynolds, W.; Smirnova, I. Application of novel and technical lignins in food and pharmaceutical industries: structure-function relationship and current challenges. *Biomass Convers. Biorefin.*, **2021**, *11*(6), 2387-2403. [http://dx.doi.org/10.1007/s13399-019-00458-6]

[147] Domínguez-Robles, J.; Cárcamo-Martínez, Á.; Stewart, S.A.; Donnelly, R.F.; Larrañeta, E.; Borrega, M. Lignin for pharmaceutical and biomedical applications – Could this become a reality? *Sustain. Chem. Pharm.*, **2020**, *18*, 100320. [http://dx.doi.org/10.1016/j.scp.2020.100320]

[148] Andrijevic, Lj.; Radotic, K.; Bogdanovic, J.; Mutavdzic, D.; Bogdanovic, G. Antiproliferative effect of synthetic lignin against human breast cancer and normal fetal lung cell lines. Potency of low molecular weight fractions. *J. BUON*, **2008**, *13*(2), 241-244. [PMID: 18555472]

[149] Ugartondo, V.; Mitjans, M.; Vinardell, M.P. Applicability of lignins from different sources as antioxidants based on the protective effects on lipid peroxidation induced by oxygen radicals. *Ind. Crops Prod.*, **2009**, *30*(2), 184-187. [http://dx.doi.org/10.1016/j.indcrop.2009.03.001]

[150] Liu, X.; Wang, J.; Li, S.; Zhuang, X.; Xu, Y.; Wang, C.; Chu, F. Preparation and properties of UV-absorbent lignin graft copolymer films from lignocellulosic butanol residue. *Ind. Crops Prod.*, **2014**, *52*, 633-641. [http://dx.doi.org/10.1016/j.indcrop.2013.11.036]

[151] Ugartondo, V.; Mitjans, M.; Vinardell, M. Comparative antioxidant and cytotoxic effects of lignins from different sources. *Bioresour. Technol.*, **2008**, *99*(14), 6683-6687. [http://dx.doi.org/10.1016/j.biortech.2007.11.038] [PMID: 18187323]

[152] Mikulášová, M.; Košíková, B. Modulation of mutagenicity of various mutagens by lignin derivatives. *Mutat. Res. Genet. Toxicol. Environ. Mutagen.*, **2003**, *535*(2), 171-180. [http://dx.doi.org/10.1016/S1383-5718(02)00319-4] [PMID: 12581535]

[153] Petersen, M.; Alfermann, A.W. The production of cytotoxic lignans by plant cell cultures. *Appl. Microbiol. Biotechnol.*, **2001**, *55*(2), 135-142. [http://dx.doi.org/10.1007/s002530000510] [PMID: 11330705]

[154] Sakagami, H.; Satoh, K.; Aiuchi, T.; Nakaya, K.; Takeda, M. Stimulation of ascorbate-induced hypoxia by lignin. *Anticancer Res.*, **1997**, *17*(2A), 1213-1216. [PMID: 9137474]

[155] Domínguez-Robles, J.; Stewart, S.A.; Rendl, A.; González, Z.; Donnelly, R.F.; Larrañeta, E. Lignin and Cellulose Blends as Pharmaceutical Excipient for Tablet Manufacturing *via* Direct Compression. *Biomolecules*, **2019**, *9*(9), 423. [http://dx.doi.org/10.3390/biom9090423] [PMID: 31466387]

[156] Pishnamazi, M.; Hafizi, H.; Shirazian, S.; Culebras, M.; Walker, G.; Collins, M. Design of Controlled Release System for Paracetamol Based on Modified Lignin. *Polymers (Basel),* **2019**, *11*(6), 1059. [http://dx.doi.org/10.3390/polym11061059] [PMID: 31216694]

[157] Pishnamazi, M.; Iqbal, J.; Shirazian, S.; Walker, G.M.; Collins, M.N. Effect of lignin on the release rate of acetylsalicylic acid tablets. *Int. J. Biol. Macromol.,* **2019**, *124*, 354-359. [http://dx.doi.org/10.1016/j.ijbiomac.2018.11.136] [PMID: 30448498]

[158] Ichimura, T.; Otake, T.; Mori, H.; Maruyama, S. HIV-1 protease inhibition and anti-HIV effect of natural and synthetic water-soluble lignin-like substances. *Biosci. Biotechnol. Biochem.,* **1999**, *63*(12), 2202-2204. [http://dx.doi.org/10.1271/bbb.63.2202] [PMID: 10664853]

[159] Raghuraman, A.; Tiwari, V.; Zhao, Q.; Shukla, D.; Debnath, A.K.; Desai, U.R. Viral inhibition studies on sulfated lignin, a chemically modified biopolymer and a potential mimic of heparan sulfate. *Biomacromolecules,* **2007**, *8*(5), 1759-1763. [http://dx.doi.org/10.1021/bm0701651] [PMID: 17439173]

[160] Tarasov, D.; Leitch, M.; Fatehi, P. Lignin–carbohydrate complexes: properties, applications, analyses, and methods of extraction: a review. *Biotechnol. Biofuels,* **2018**, *11*(1), 269. [http://dx.doi.org/10.1186/s13068-018-1262-1] [PMID: 30288174]

[161] Lawoko, M.; Henriksson, G.; Gellerstedt, G. Structural differences between the lignin-carbohydrate complexes present in wood and in chemical pulps. *Biomacromolecules,* **2005**, *6*(6), 3467-3473. [http://dx.doi.org/10.1021/bm058014q] [PMID: 16283780]

[162] Giummarella, N.; Pu, Y.; Ragauskas, A.J.; Lawoko, M. A critical review on the analysis of lignin carbohydrate bonds. *Green Chem.,* **2019**, *21*(7), 1573-1595. [http://dx.doi.org/10.1039/C8GC03606C]

[163] Oinonen, P.; Zhang, L.; Lawoko, M.; Henriksson, G. On the formation of lignin polysaccharide networks in Norway spruce. *Phytochemistry,* **2015**, *111*, 177-184. [http://dx.doi.org/10.1016/j.phytochem.2014.10.027] [PMID: 25549980]

[164] Spiridon, I. Extraction of lignin and therapeutic applications of lignin-derived compounds. A review. *Environ. Chem. Lett.,* **2020**, *18*(3), 771-785. [http://dx.doi.org/10.1007/s10311-020-00981-3]

[165] Dong, H.; Zheng, L.; Yu, P.; Jiang, Q.; Wu, Y.; Huang, C.; Yin, B. Characterization and Application of Lignin–Carbohydrate Complexes from Lignocellulosic Materials as Antioxidants for Scavenging *In Vitro* and *In Vivo* Reactive Oxygen Species. *ACS Sustain. Chem.& Eng.,* **2020**, *8*(1), 256-266. [http://dx.doi.org/10.1021/acssuschemeng.9b05290]

[166] Niu, H.; Song, D.; Mu, H.; Zhang, W.; Sun, F.; Duan, J. Investigation of three lignin complexes with antioxidant and immunological capacities from Inonotus obliquus. *Int. J. Biol. Macromol.,* **2016**, *86*, 587-593. [http://dx.doi.org/10.1016/j.ijbiomac.2016.01.111] [PMID: 26845476]

[167] Sakagami, H.; Kawano, M.; Thet, M.M.; Hashimoto, K.; Satoh, K.; Kanamoto, T.; Terakubo, S.; Nakashima, H.; Haishima, Y.; Maeda, Y.; Sakurai, K. Anti-HIV and immunomodulation activities of cacao mass lignin-carbohydrate complex. *In Vivo,* **2011**, *25*(2), 229-236. [PMID: 21471539]

[168] Kushida, T.; Makino, T.; Tomomura, M.; Tomomura, A.; Sakagami, H. Enhancement of Dectin-2 gene expression by lignin-carbohydrate complex from Lentinus edodes mycelia extract (LEM) in a mouse macrophage-like cell line. *Anticancer Res.,* **2011**, *31*(4), 1241-1248. [PMID: 21508371]

[169] Sakagami, H.; Kushida, T.; Oizumi, T.; Nakashima, H.; Makino, T. Distribution of lignin–carbohydrate complex in plant kingdom and its functionality as alternative medicine. *Pharmacol. Ther.,* **2010**, *128*(1), 91-105.

[http://dx.doi.org/10.1016/j.pharmthera.2010.05.004] [PMID: 20547183]

[170] Zhang, Y.; But, P.P.H.; Ooi, V.E.C.; Xu, H.X.; Delaney, G.D.; Lee, S.H.S.; Lee, S.F. Chemical properties, mode of action, and *in vivo* anti-herpes activities of a lignin–carbohydrate complex from Prunella vulgaris. *Antiviral Res.*, **2007**, *75*(3), 242-249. [http://dx.doi.org/10.1016/j.antiviral.2007.03.010] [PMID: 17475343]

[171] Sakagami, H.; Hashimoto, K.; Suzuki, F.; Ogiwara, T.; Satoh, K.; Ito, H.; Hatano, T.; Takashi, Y.; Fujisawa, S. Molecular requirements of lignin–carbohydrate complexes for expression of unique biological activities. *Phytochemistry,* **2005**, *66*(17), 2108-2120. [http://dx.doi.org/10.1016/j.phytochem.2005.05.013] [PMID: 15978643]

[172] Ebrahimi Majdar, R.; Ghasemian, A.; Resalati, H.; Saraeian, A.; Crestini, C.; Lange, H. Facile Isolation of LCC-Fraction from Organosolv Lignin by Simple Soxhlet Extraction. *Polymers (Basel),* **2019**, *11*(2), 225. [http://dx.doi.org/10.3390/polym11020225] [PMID: 30960209]

[173] Balakshin, M.; Capanema, E.; Berlin, A. Chapter 4 - Isolation and Analysis of Lignin–Carbohydrate Complexes Preparations with Traditional and Advanced Methods: A Review. In: Atta-ur-Rahman, Ed. Studies in Natural Products Chemistry, Amsterdam: Elsevier; **2014**, *42*, 83-115.

[174] Du, X.; Gellerstedt, G.; Li, J. Universal fractionation of lignin-carbohydrate complexes (LCCs) from lignocellulosic biomass: an example using spruce wood. *Plant J.,* **2013**, *74*(2), 328-338. [http://dx.doi.org/10.1111/tpj.12124] [PMID: 23332001]

[175] Sajjadi, M.; Ahmadpoor, F.; Nasrollahzadeh, M.; Ghafuri, H. Lignin-derived (nano)materials for environmental pollution remediation: Current challenges and future perspectives. *Int. J. Biol. Macromol.,* **2021**, *178*, 394-423. [http://dx.doi.org/10.1016/j.ijbiomac.2021.02.165] [PMID: 33636266]

[176] Liu, R.; Dai, L.; Xu, C.; Wang, K.; Zheng, C.; Si, C. Lignin□Based Micro□ and Nanomaterials and their Composites in Biomedical Applications. *ChemSusChem,* **2020**, *13*(17), 4266-4283. [http://dx.doi.org/10.1002/cssc.202000783] [PMID: 32462781]

[177] Sipponen, M.H.; Lange, H.; Crestini, C.; Henn, A.; Österberg, M. Lignin for Nano□ and Microscaled Carrier Systems: Applications, Trends, and Challenges. *ChemSusChem,* **2019**, *12*(10), 2039-2054. [http://dx.doi.org/10.1002/cssc.201900480] [PMID: 30933420]

[178] Beisl, S.; Miltner, A.; Friedl, A.; Beisl, S.; Miltner, A.; Friedl, A. Lignin from Micro- to Nanosize: Production Methods. *Int. J. Mol. Sci.,* **2017**, *18*(6), 1244. [http://dx.doi.org/10.3390/ijms18061244] [PMID: 28604584]

[179] Beisl, S.; Friedl, A.; Miltner, A.; Beisl, S.; Friedl, A.; Miltner, A. Lignin from Micro- to Nanosize: Applications. *Int. J. Mol. Sci.,* **2017**, *18*(11), 2367. [http://dx.doi.org/10.3390/ijms18112367] [PMID: 29117142]

[180] Ago, M.; Tardy, B.L.; Wang, L.; Guo, J.; Khakalo, A.; Rojas, O.J. Supramolecular assemblies of lignin into nano- and microparticles. *MRS Bull.,* **2017**, *42*(5), 371-378. [http://dx.doi.org/10.1557/mrs.2017.88]

[181] Tang, Q.; Qian, Y.; Yang, D.; Qiu, X.; Qin, Y.; Zhou, M. Lignin-Based Nanoparticles: A Review on Their Preparations and Applications. *Polymers (Basel),* **2020**, *12*(11), 2471. [http://dx.doi.org/10.3390/polym12112471] [PMID: 33113775]

[182] Kai, D.; Ren, W.; Tian, L.; Chee, P.L.; Liu, Y.; Ramakrishna, S.; Loh, X.J. Engineering Poly(lactide)–Lignin Nanofibers with Antioxidant Activity for Biomedical Application. *ACS Sustain. Chem.& Eng.,* **2016**, *4*(10), 5268-5276. [http://dx.doi.org/10.1021/acssuschemeng.6b00478]

[183] Massey-Brooker, A; Vaccaro, M; Scialla, S A consumer goods product comprising chitin, lignin and a polymer or co-polymer. CA2960127A1, **2016**.

[184] Lee, E.S.; Kim, Y.O.; Ha, Y.M.; Lim, D.; Hwang, J.Y.; Kim, J.; Park, M.; Cho, J.W.; Jung, Y.C.

Antimicrobial properties of lignin-decorated thin multi-walled carbon nanotubes in poly(vinyl alcohol) nanocomposites. *Eur. Polym. J.*, **2018**, *105*, 79-84. [http://dx.doi.org/10.1016/j.eurpolymj.2018.05.014]

[185] Saudi, A.; Amini, S.; Amirpour, N.; Kazemi, M.; Zargar Kharazi, A.; Salehi, H.; Rafienia, M. Promoting neural cell proliferation and differentiation by incorporating lignin into electrospun poly(vinyl alcohol) and poly(glycerol sebacate) fibers. *Mater. Sci. Eng. C,* **2019**, *104*, 110005. [http://dx.doi.org/10.1016/j.msec.2019.110005] [PMID: 31499996]

[186] Amini, S.; Saudi, A.; Amirpour, N.; Jahromi, M.; Najafabadi, S.S.; Kazemi, M.; Rafienia, M.; Salehi, H. Application of electrospun polycaprolactone fibers embedding lignin nanoparticle for peripheral nerve regeneration: *In vitro* and *in vivo* study. *Int. J. Biol. Macromol.*, **2020**, *159*, 154-173. [http://dx.doi.org/10.1016/j.ijbiomac.2020.05.073] [PMID: 32416294]

[187] Xiong, F.; Han, Y.; Wang, S.; Li, G.; Qin, T.; Chen, Y.; Chu, F. Preparation and formation mechanism of size-controlled lignin nanospheres by self-assembly. *Ind. Crops Prod.*, **2017**, *100*, 146-152. [http://dx.doi.org/10.1016/j.indcrop.2017.02.025]

[188] Lievonen, M.; Valle-Delgado, J.J.; Mattinen, M.L.; Hult, E-L.; Lintinen, K.; Kostiainen, M.A.; Paananen, A.; Szilvay, G.R.; Setälä, H.; Österberg, M. A simple process for lignin nanoparticle preparation. *Green Chem.*, **2016**, *18*(5), 1416-1422. [http://dx.doi.org/10.1039/C5GC01436K]

[189] Sipponen, M.H.; Smyth, M.; Leskinen, T.; Johansson, L.S.; Österberg, M. All-lignin approach to prepare cationic colloidal lignin particles: stabilization of durable Pickering emulsions. *Green Chem.*, **2017**, *19*(24), 5831-5840. [http://dx.doi.org/10.1039/C7GC02900D]

[190] Li, H.; Deng, Y.; Wu, H.; Ren, Y.; Qiu, X.; Zheng, D.; Li, C.L. Self-assembly of kraft lignin into nanospheres in dioxane-water mixtures. *Holzforschung,* **2016**, *70*(8), 725-731. [http://dx.doi.org/10.1515/hf-2015-0238]

[191] Tian, D.; Hu, J.; Chandra, R.P.; Saddler, J.N.; Lu, C. Valorizing Recalcitrant Cellulolytic Enzyme Lignin *via* Lignin Nanoparticles Fabrication in an Integrated Biorefinery. *ACS Sustain. Chem.& Eng.*, **2017**, *5*(3), 2702-2710. [http://dx.doi.org/10.1021/acssuschemeng.6b03043]

[192] Tian, D.; Hu, J.; Bao, J.; Chandra, R.P.; Saddler, J.N.; Lu, C. Lignin valorization: lignin nanoparticles as high-value bio-additive for multifunctional nanocomposites. *Biotechnol. Biofuels,* **2017**, *10*(1), 192. [http://dx.doi.org/10.1186/s13068-017-0876-z] [PMID: 28747994]

[193] Yearla, S.R.; Padmasree, K. Exploitation of subabul stem lignin as a matrix in controlled release agrochemical nanoformulations: a case study with herbicide diuron. *Environ. Sci. Pollut. Res. Int.*, **2016**, *23*(18), 18085-18098. [http://dx.doi.org/10.1007/s11356-016-6983-8] [PMID: 27259957]

[194] Farooq, M.; Zou, T.; Riviere, G.; Sipponen, M.H.; Österberg, M. Strong, ductile and waterproof cellulose nanofibril composite films with colloidal lignin particles. *Biomacromolecules,* **2019**, *20*(2), 693-704. [http://dx.doi.org/10.1021/acs.biomac.8b01364] [PMID: 30358992]

[195] Leskinen, T.; Smyth, M.; Xiao, Y.; Lintinen, K.; Mattinen, M.L.; Kostiainen, M.A.; Oinas, P.; Österberg, M. Scaling Up Production of Colloidal Lignin Particles. *Nord. Pulp Paper Res. J.*, **2017**, *32*(4), 586-596. [http://dx.doi.org/10.3183/npprj-2017-32-04_p586-596_leskinen]

[196] Li, H.; Deng, Y.; Liu, B.; Ren, Y.; Liang, J.; Qian, Y.; Qiu, X.; Li, C.; Zheng, D. Preparation of Nanocapsules *via* the Self-Assembly of Kraft Lignin: A Totally Green Process with Renewable Resources. *ACS Sustain. Chem.& Eng.*, **2016**, *4*(4), 1946-1953. [http://dx.doi.org/10.1021/acssuschemeng.5b01066]

[197] Cailotto, S.; Gigli, M.; Bonini, M.; Rigoni, F.; Crestini, C. Sustainable Strategies in the Synthesis of

Lignin Nanoparticles for the Release of Active Compounds: A Comparison. *ChemSusChem,* **2020**, *13*(17), 4759-4767.
[http://dx.doi.org/10.1002/cssc.202001140] [PMID: 32697394]

[198] Ago, M.; Huan, S.; Borghei, M.; Raula, J.; Kauppinen, E.I.; Rojas, O.J. High-throughput synthesis of lignin particles (~30 nm to ~2 μm) *via* aerosol flow reactor: Size fractionation and utilization in pickering emulsions. *ACS Appl. Mater. Interfaces,* **2016**, *8*(35), 23302-23310.
[http://dx.doi.org/10.1021/acsami.6b07900] [PMID: 27538013]

[199] Gilca, I.A.; Popa, V.I.; Crestini, C. Obtaining lignin nanoparticles by sonication. *Ultrason. Sonochem.,* **2015**, *23*, 369-375.
[http://dx.doi.org/10.1016/j.ultsonch.2014.08.021] [PMID: 25218770]

[200] Yearla, S.R.; Padmasree, K. Preparation and characterisation of lignin nanoparticles: evaluation of their potential as antioxidants and UV protectants. *J. Exp. Nanosci.,* **2016**, *11*(4), 289-302.
[http://dx.doi.org/10.1080/17458080.2015.1055842]

[201] Sipponen, M.H.; Lange, H.; Ago, M.; Crestini, C. Understanding Lignin Aggregation Processes. A Case Study: Budesonide Entrapment and Stimuli Controlled Release from Lignin Nanoparticles. *ACS Sustain. Chem.& Eng.,* **2018**, *6*(7), 9342-9351.
[http://dx.doi.org/10.1021/acssuschemeng.8b01652] [PMID: 30271691]

[202] Tortora, M.; Cavalieri, F.; Mosesso, P.; Ciaffardini, F.; Melone, F.; Crestini, C. Ultrasound driven assembly of lignin into microcapsules for storage and delivery of hydrophobic molecules. *Biomacromolecules,* **2014**, *15*(5), 1634-1643.
[http://dx.doi.org/10.1021/bm500015j] [PMID: 24720505]

[203] Yiamsawas, D.; Beckers, S.J.; Lu, H.; Landfester, K.; Wurm, F.R. Morphology-Controlled Synthesis of Lignin Nanocarriers for Drug Delivery and Carbon Materials. *ACS Biomater. Sci. Eng.,* **2017**, *3*(10), 2375-2383.
[http://dx.doi.org/10.1021/acsbiomaterials.7b00278] [PMID: 33445295]

[204] Chen, N.; Dempere, L.A.; Tong, Z. Synthesis of pH-Responsive Lignin-Based Nanocapsules for Controlled Release of Hydrophobic Molecules. *ACS Sustain. Chem.& Eng.,* **2016**, *4*(10), 5204-5211.
[http://dx.doi.org/10.1021/acssuschemeng.6b01209]

[205] Pan, J.; Yin, Y.; Gan, M.; Meng, M.; Dai, X.; Wu, R.; Shi, W.; Yan, Y. Fabrication and evaluation of molecularly imprinted multi-hollow microspheres adsorbents with tunable inner pore structures derived from templating Pickering double emulsions. *Chem. Eng. J.,* **2015**, *266*, 299-308.
[http://dx.doi.org/10.1016/j.cej.2014.11.126]

[206] Yang, Y.; Wei, Z.; Wang, C.; Tong, Z. Lignin-based Pickering HIPEs for macroporous foams and their enhanced adsorption of copper(ii) ions. *Chem. Commun. (Camb.),* **2013**, *49*(64), 7144-7146.
[http://dx.doi.org/10.1039/c3cc42270d] [PMID: 23831814]

[207] Bartzoka, E.D.; Lange, H.; Thiel, K.; Crestini, C. Coordination Complexes and One-Step Assembly of Lignin for Versatile Nanocapsule Engineering. *ACS Sustain. Chem.& Eng.,* **2016**, *4*(10), 5194-5203.
[http://dx.doi.org/10.1021/acssuschemeng.6b00904]

[208] Pang, Y.; Qin, Z.; Wang, S.; Yi, C.; Zhou, M.; Lou, H.; Qiu, X. Preparation and application performance of lignin-polyurea composite microcapsule with controlled release of avermectin. *Colloid Polym. Sci.,* **2020**, *298*(8), 1001-1012.
[http://dx.doi.org/10.1007/s00396-020-04664-x]

[209] Caicedo, H.M.; Dempere, L.A.; Vermerris, W. Template-mediated synthesis and bio-functionalization of flexible lignin-based nanotubes and nanowires. *Nanotechnology,* **2012**, *23*(10), 105605.
[http://dx.doi.org/10.1088/0957-4484/23/10/105605] [PMID: 22362196]

[210] Jin, W.; Chen, L.; Hu, M.; Sun, D.; Li, A.; Li, Y. Tween-80 is effective for enhancing steam-exploded biomass enzymatic saccharification and ethanol production by specifically lessening cellulase absorption with lignin in common reed. *Appl. Energy,* **2016**, *175*, 82-90.
[http://dx.doi.org/10.1016/j.apenergy.2016.04.104]

[211] Kirk, T.K. Edr. Lignin Biodegradation: Microbiology, Chemistry and Potential Applications. **1980**,

[212] Li, M.; Miao, H.; Li, Y.; Wang, F.; Xu, J. Protein Engineering of an Artificial P450BM3 Peroxygenase System Enables Highly Selective *O*-Demethylation of Lignin Monomers. *Molecules,* **2022**, *27*(10), 3120.
[http://dx.doi.org/10.3390/molecules27103120] [PMID: 35630597]

[213] Zdarta, J.; Klapiszewski, Ł.; Wysokowski, M.; Norman, M.; Kołodziejczak-Radzimska, A.; Moszyński, D.; Ehrlich, H.; Maciejewski, H.; Stelling, A.; Jesionowski, T. Chitin-lignin material as a novel matrix for enzyme immobilization. *Mar. Drugs,* **2015**, *13*(4), 2424-2446.
[http://dx.doi.org/10.3390/md13042424] [PMID: 25903282]

[214] Gong, W.; Ran, Z.; Ye, F.; Zhao, G. Lignin from bamboo shoot shells as an activator and novel immobilizing support for α-amylase. *Food Chem.,* **2017**, *228*, 455-462.
[http://dx.doi.org/10.1016/j.foodchem.2017.02.017] [PMID: 28317749]

[215] Chen, L.; Zhou, X.; Shi, Y.; Gao, B.; Wu, J.; Kirk, T.B.; Xu, J.; Xue, W. Green synthesis of lignin nanoparticle in aqueous hydrotropic solution toward broadening the window for its processing and application. *Chem. Eng. J.,* **2018**, *346*, 217-225.
[http://dx.doi.org/10.1016/j.cej.2018.04.020]

[216] Capecchi, E.; Piccinino, D.; Delfino, I.; Bollella, P.; Antiochia, R.; Saladino, R. Functionalized Tyrosinase-Lignin Nanoparticles as Sustainable Catalysts for the Oxidation of Phenols. *Nanomaterials (Basel),* **2018**, *8*(6), 438.
[http://dx.doi.org/10.3390/nano8060438] [PMID: 29914085]

[217] Figueiredo, P.; Lintinen, K.; Kiriazis, A.; Hynninen, V.; Liu, Z.; Bauleth-Ramos, T.; Rahikkala, A.; Correia, A.; Kohout, T.; Sarmento, B.; Yli-Kauhaluoma, J.; Hirvonen, J.; Ikkala, O.; Kostiainen, M.A.; Santos, H.A. *In vitro* evaluation of biodegradable lignin-based nanoparticles for drug delivery and enhanced antiproliferation effect in cancer cells. *Biomaterials,* **2017**, *121*, 97-108.
[http://dx.doi.org/10.1016/j.biomaterials.2016.12.034] [PMID: 28081462]

[218] Dai, L.; Liu, R.; Hu, L.Q.; Zou, Z.F.; Si, C.L. Lignin nanoparticle as a novel green carrier for the efficient delivery of resveratrol. *ACS Sustain. Chem.& Eng.,* **2017**, *5*(9), 8241-8249.
[http://dx.doi.org/10.1021/acssuschemeng.7b01903]

[219] Figueiredo, P.; Ferro, C.; Kemell, M.; Liu, Z.; Kiriazis, A.; Lintinen, K.; Florindo, H.F.; Yli-Kauhaluoma, J.; Hirvonen, J.; Kostiainen, M.A.; Santos, H.A. Functionalization of carboxylated lignin nanoparticles for targeted and pH-responsive delivery of anticancer drugs. *Nanomedicine (Lond.),* **2017**, *12*(21), 2581-2596.
[http://dx.doi.org/10.2217/nnm-2017-0219] [PMID: 28960138]

[220] Li, Y.; Qiu, X.; Qian, Y.; Xiong, W.; Yang, D. pH-responsive lignin-based complex micelles: Preparation, characterization and application in oral drug delivery. *Chem. Eng. J.,* **2017**, *327*, 1176-1183.
[http://dx.doi.org/10.1016/j.cej.2017.07.022]

[221] Kim, S.; Fernandes, M.M.; Matamá, T.; Loureiro, A.; Gomes, A.C.; Cavaco-Paulo, A. Chitosan–lignosulfonates sono-chemically prepared nanoparticles: Characterisation and potential applications. *Colloids Surf. B Biointerfaces,* **2013**, *103*, 1-8.
[http://dx.doi.org/10.1016/j.colsurfb.2012.10.033] [PMID: 23178385]

[222] Piombino, C.; Lange, H.; Sabuzi, F.; Galloni, P.; Conte, V.; Crestini, C. Lignosulfonate Microcapsules for Delivery and Controlled Release of Thymol and Derivatives. *Molecules,* **2020**, *25*(4), 866.
[http://dx.doi.org/10.3390/molecules25040866] [PMID: 32079068]

[223] Zou, T.; Sipponen, M.H.; Österberg, M. Natural Shape-Retaining Microcapsules With Shells Made of Chitosan-Coated Colloidal Lignin Particles. *Front Chem.,* **2019**, *7*, 370.
[http://dx.doi.org/10.3389/fchem.2019.00370] [PMID: 31192192]

[224] Zhou, Y.; Han, Y.; Li, G.; Chu, F. Effects of Lignin-Based Hollow Nanoparticle Structure on the

Loading and Release Behavior of Doxorubicin. *Materials (Basel),* **2019**, *12*(10), 1694. [http://dx.doi.org/10.3390/ma12101694] [PMID: 31137707]

[225] Qiu, X.; Li, Y.; Qian, Y.; Wang, J.; Zhu, S. Long-Acting and Safe Sunscreens with Ultrahigh Sun Protection Factor *via* Natural Lignin Encapsulation and Synergy. *ACS Appl. Bio Mater.,* **2018**, *1*(5), 1276-1285. [http://dx.doi.org/10.1021/acsabm.8b00138] [PMID: 34996231]

[226] Sipponen, M.H.; Farooq, M.; Koivisto, J.; Pellis, A.; Seitsonen, J.; Österberg, M. Spatially confined lignin nanospheres for biocatalytic ester synthesis in aqueous media. *Nat. Commun.,* **2018**, *9*(1), 2300. [http://dx.doi.org/10.1038/s41467-018-04715-6] [PMID: 29895870]

[227] Zdarta, J.; Klapiszewski, L.; Jedrzak, A.; Nowicki, M.; Moszynski, D.; Jesionowski, T. Lipase B from Candida antarctica Immobilized on a Silica-Lignin Matrix as a Stable and Reusable Biocatalytic System. *Catalysts,* **2017**, *7*, 1-21.

[228] Li, Y.; Zhou, M.; Pang, Y.; Qiu, X. Lignin-Based Microsphere: Preparation and Performance on Encapsulating the Pesticide Avermectin. *ACS Sustain. Chem.& Eng.,* **2017**, *5*(4), 3321-3328. [http://dx.doi.org/10.1021/acssuschemeng.6b03180]

[229] Deng, Y.; Zhao, H.; Qian, Y.; Lü, L.; Wang, B.; Qiu, X. Hollow lignin azo colloids encapsulated avermectin with high anti-photolysis and controlled release performance. *Ind. Crops Prod.,* **2016**, *87*, 191-197. [http://dx.doi.org/10.1016/j.indcrop.2016.03.056]

[230] Yiamsawas, D.; Baier, G.; Thines, E.; Landfester, K.; Wurm, F.R. Biodegradable lignin nanocontainers. *RSC Advances,* **2014**, *4*(23), 11661-11663. [http://dx.doi.org/10.1039/C3RA47971D]

[231] Richter, A.P.; Bharti, B.; Armstrong, H.B.; Brown, J.S.; Plemmons, D.; Paunov, V.N.; Stoyanov, S.D.; Velev, O.D. Synthesis and characterization of biodegradable lignin nanoparticles with tunable surface properties. *Langmuir,* **2016**, *32*(25), 6468-6477. [http://dx.doi.org/10.1021/acs.langmuir.6b01088] [PMID: 27268077]

[232] Leskinen, T.; Witos, J.; Valle-Delgado, J.J.; Lintinen, K.; Kostiainen, M.; Wiedmer, S.K.; Österberg, M.; Mattinen, M.L. Adsorption of proteins on colloidal lignin particles for advanced biomaterials. *Biomacromolecules,* **2017**, *18*(9), 2767-2776. [http://dx.doi.org/10.1021/acs.biomac.7b00676] [PMID: 28724292]

[233] Zhong, J.F.; Xu, L.; Qin, X.L. Efficient antibacterial silver nanoparticles composite using lignin as a template. *J. Compos. Mater.,* **2015**, *49*(19), 2329-2335. [http://dx.doi.org/10.1177/0021998314545192]

[234] Klapiszewski, Ł.; Rzemieniecki, T.; Krawczyk, M.; Malina, D.; Norman, M.; Zdarta, J.; Majchrzak, I.; Dobrowolska, A.; Czaczyk, K.; Jesionowski, T. Kraft lignin/silica–AgNPs as a functional material with antibacterial activity. *Colloids Surf. B Biointerfaces,* **2015**, *134*, 220-228. [http://dx.doi.org/10.1016/j.colsurfb.2015.06.056] [PMID: 26204502]

[235] Richter, A.P.; Brown, J.S.; Bharti, B.; Wang, A.; Gangwal, S.; Houck, K.; Cohen Hubal, E.A.; Paunov, V.N.; Stoyanov, S.D.; Velev, O.D. An environmentally benign antimicrobial nanoparticle based on a silver-infused lignin core. *Nat. Nanotechnol.,* **2015**, *10*(9), 817-823. [http://dx.doi.org/10.1038/nnano.2015.141] [PMID: 26167765]

[236] Zálešák, F.; Bon, D.J.Y.D.; Pospíšil, J. Lignans and Neolignans: Plant secondary metabolites as a reservoir of biologically active substances. *Pharmacol. Res.,* **2019**, *146*, 104284. [http://dx.doi.org/10.1016/j.phrs.2019.104284] [PMID: 31136813]

[237] Kandar, C.C. Secondary Metabolites from Plant Sources. *Bioactive Natural Products for Pharmaceutical Applications.,* **2021**, , 329-377. [http://dx.doi.org/10.1007/978-3-030-54027-2_10]

[238] Daglia, M. Polyphenols as antimicrobial agents. *Curr. Opin. Biotechnol.,* **2012**, *23*(2), 174-181.

[http://dx.doi.org/10.1016/j.copbio.2011.08.007] [PMID: 21925860]

[239] Dar, A.A.; Arumugam, N. Lignans of sesame: Purification methods, biological activities and biosynthesis – A review. *Bioorg. Chem.,* **2013**, *50*, 1-10. [http://dx.doi.org/10.1016/j.bioorg.2013.06.009] [PMID: 23933354]

[240] López-Biedma, A.; Sánchez-Quesada, C.; Delgado-Rodríguez, M.; Gaforio, J.J. The biological activities of natural lignans from olives and virgin olive oils: A review. *J. Funct. Foods,* **2016**, *26*, 36-47. [http://dx.doi.org/10.1016/j.jff.2016.07.005]

[241] Deyama, T.; Nishibe, S. Pharmacological Properties of Lignans. *Lignin and Lignans: Advances in Chemistry.,* **2010**, , 585-629. [http://dx.doi.org/10.1201/EBK1574444865-c17]

[242] Teodor, E.D.; Moroeanu, V.; Radu, G.L. Lignans from Medicinal Plants and their Anticancer Effect. *Mini Rev. Med. Chem.,* **2020**, *20*(12), 1083-1090. [http://dx.doi.org/10.2174/1389557520666200212110513] [PMID: 32048969]

[243] Ionkova, I. Anticancer lignans--from discovery to biotechnology. *Mini Rev. Med. Chem.,* **2011**, *11*(10), 843-856. [http://dx.doi.org/10.2174/138955711796575425] [PMID: 21762103]

[244] Senizza, A.; Rocchetti, G.; Mosele, J.I.; Patrone, V.; Callegari, M.L.; Morelli, L.; Lucini, L. Lignans and Gut Microbiota: An Interplay Revealing Potential Health Implications. *Molecules,* **2020**, *25*(23), 5709. [http://dx.doi.org/10.3390/molecules25235709] [PMID: 33287261]

[245] Cui, Q.; Du, R.; Liu, M.; Rong, L. Lignans and Their Derivatives from Plants as Antivirals. *Molecules,* **2020**, *25*(1), 183. [http://dx.doi.org/10.3390/molecules25010183] [PMID: 31906391]

[246] Rasouli, H.; Farzaei, M.H.; Khodarahmi, R. Polyphenols and their benefits: A review. *Int. J. Food Prop.,* **2017**, *20*, 1700-1741.

[247] De Silva, S.F.; Alcorn, J. Flaxseed Lignans as Important Dietary Polyphenols for Cancer Prevention and Treatment: Chemistry, Pharmacokinetics, and Molecular Targets. *Pharmaceuticals (Basel),* **2019**, *12*(2), 68. [http://dx.doi.org/10.3390/ph12020068] [PMID: 31060335]

[248] Blitz, C.L.; Murphy, S.P.; Au, D.L.M. Adding lignan values to a food composition database. *J. Food Compos. Anal.,* **2007**, *20*(2), 99-105. [http://dx.doi.org/10.1016/j.jfca.2006.05.006]

[249] Durazzo, A.; Lucarini, M.; Camilli, E.; Marconi, S.; Gabrielli, P.; Lisciani, S.; Gambelli, L.; Aguzzi, A.; Novellino, E.; Santini, A.; Turrini, A.; Marletta, L. Dietary Lignans: Definition, Description and Research Trends in Databases Development. *Molecules,* **2018**, *23*(12), 3251. [http://dx.doi.org/10.3390/molecules23123251] [PMID: 30544820]

[250] Ávila-Gálvez, M.Á.; Giménez-Bastida, J.A.; Espín, J.C.; González-Sarrías, A. Dietary Phenolics against Breast Cancer. A Critical Evidence-Based Review and Future Perspectives. *Int. J. Mol. Sci.,* **2020**, *21*(16), 5718. [http://dx.doi.org/10.3390/ijms21165718] [PMID: 32784973]

[251] Touré, A.; Xueming, X. Flaxseed Lignans: Source, Biosynthesis, Metabolism, Antioxidant Activity, Bio-Active Components, and Health Benefits. *Compr. Rev. Food Sci. Food Saf.,* **2010**, *9*(3), 261-269. [http://dx.doi.org/10.1111/j.1541-4337.2009.00105.x] [PMID: 33467817]

[252] Pan, X.; Ma, X.; Jiang, Y.; Wen, J.; Yang, L.; Chen, D.; Cao, X.; Peng, C. A Comprehensive Review of Natural Products against Liver Fibrosis: Flavonoids, Quinones, Lignans, Phenols, and Acids. *Evid. Based Complement. Alternat. Med.,* **2020**, *2020*, 1-19. [http://dx.doi.org/10.1155/2020/7171498] [PMID: 33082829]

[253] Marcotullio, M.; Pelosi, A.; Curini, M. Hinokinin, an emerging bioactive lignan. *Molecules,* **2014**, *19*(9), 14862-14878.
[http://dx.doi.org/10.3390/molecules190914862] [PMID: 25232707]

[254] Chang, V.C.; Cotterchio, M.; Boucher, B.A.; Jenkins, D.J.A.; Mirea, L.; McCann, S.E.; Thompson, L.U. Effect of dietary flaxseed intake on circulating sex hormone levels among postmenopausal women: A randomized controlled intervention trial. *Nutr. Cancer,* **2019**, *71*(3), 385-398.
[http://dx.doi.org/10.1080/01635581.2018.1516789] [PMID: 30375890]

[255] Barre, D.E.; Mizier-Barre, K.A. Lignans' Potential in Pre and Post-onset Type 2 Diabetes Management. *Curr. Diabetes Rev.,* **2019**, *16*(1), 2-11.
[http://dx.doi.org/10.2174/1573399814666180914094520] [PMID: 30215336]

[256] Buja, A.; Pierbon, M.; Lago, L.; Grotto, G.; Baldo, V. Breast Cancer Primary Prevention and Diet: An Umbrella Review. *Int. J. Environ. Res. Public Health,* **2020**, *17*(13), 4731.
[http://dx.doi.org/10.3390/ijerph17134731] [PMID: 32630215]

[257] Šamec, D.; Karalija, E.; Šola, I.; Vujčić Bok, V.; Salopek-Sondi, B. The Role of Polyphenols in Abiotic Stress Response: The Influence of Molecular Structure. *Plants,* **2021**, *10*(1), 118.
[http://dx.doi.org/10.3390/plants10010118] [PMID: 33430128]

[258] Spano, M.; Di Matteo, G.; Ingallina, C.; Ambroselli, D.; Carradori, S.; Gallorini, M.; Giusti, A.M.; Salvo, A.; Grosso, M.; Mannina, L. Modulatory Properties of Food and Nutraceutical Components Targeting NLRP3 Inflammasome Activation. *Nutrients,* **2022**, *14*(3), 490.
[http://dx.doi.org/10.3390/nu14030490] [PMID: 35276849]

[259] Sharma, A.; Kaur, M.; Katnoria, J.K.; Nagpal, A.K. Polyphenols in Food: Cancer Prevention and Apoptosis Induction. *Curr. Med. Chem.,* **2018**, *25*(36), 4740-4757.
[http://dx.doi.org/10.2174/0929867324666171006144208] [PMID: 28990504]

[260] Su, S.; Wink, M. Natural lignans from Arctium lappa as antiaging agents in Caenorhabditis elegans. *Phytochemistry,* **2015**, *117*, 340-350.
[http://dx.doi.org/10.1016/j.phytochem.2015.06.021] [PMID: 26141518]

[261] Szopa, A.; Dziurka, M.; Warzecha, A.; Kubica, P.; Klimek-Szczykutowicz, M.; Ekiert, H. Targeted Lignan Profiling and Anti-Inflammatory Properties of Schisandra rubriflora and Schisandra chinensis Extracts. *Molecules,* **2018**, *23*(12), 3103.
[http://dx.doi.org/10.3390/molecules23123103] [PMID: 30486445]

[262] Shi, Y.; Wang, J.; Yan, H. Therapeutic potential of naturally occurring lignans as anticancer agents. *Curr. Top. Med. Chem.,* **2022**, *22*(17), 1393-1405.
[http://dx.doi.org/10.2174/1568026622666220511155442] [PMID: 35546769]

[263] Churiyah, ; Pongtuluran, O.B.; Rofaani, E.; Tarwadi, Antiviral and Immunostimulant Activities of Andrographis paniculata. *Hayati J. Biosci.,* **2015**, *22*(2), 67-72.
[http://dx.doi.org/10.4308/hjb.22.2.67]

[264] Mir, M.A.; Hamdani, S.S.; Sheikh, B.A.; Mehraj, U. Recent Advances in Metabolites from Medicinal Plants in Cancer Prevention and Treatment. *Curr. Immunol. Rev.,* **2019**, *15*(2), 185-201.
[http://dx.doi.org/10.2174/1573395515666191102094330]

[265] Paul, S.; Hwang, J.K.; Kim, H.Y.; Jeon, W.K.; Chung, C.; Han, J.S. Multiple biological properties of macelignan and its pharmacological implications. *Arch. Pharm. Res.,* **2013**, *36*(3), 264-272.
[http://dx.doi.org/10.1007/s12272-013-0048-z] [PMID: 23435944]

[266] Pilkington, L. Lignans: A Chemometric Analysis. *Molecules,* **2018**, *23*(7), 1666.
[http://dx.doi.org/10.3390/molecules23071666] [PMID: 29987225]

[267] Larrosa, M.; Luceri, C.; Vivoli, E.; Pagliuca, C.; Lodovici, M.; Moneti, G.; Dolara, P. Polyphenol metabolites from colonic microbiota exert anti-inflammatory activity on different inflammation models. *Mol. Nutr. Food Res.,* **2009**, *53*(8), 1044-1054.
[http://dx.doi.org/10.1002/mnfr.200800446] [PMID: 19557820]

[268] Rodríguez-García, C.; Sánchez-Quesada, C.; Toledo, E.; Delgado-Rodríguez, M.; Gaforio, J. Naturally Lignan-Rich Foods: A Dietary Tool for Health Promotion? *Molecules,* **2019**, *24*(5), 917. [http://dx.doi.org/10.3390/molecules24050917] [PMID: 30845651]

[269] Huang, Y.; Liu, C.; Liu, S.; Liu, Z.; Li, S.; Wang, Y. *In vitro* metabolism of magnolol and honokiol in rat liver microsomes and their interactions with seven cytochrome P substrates. *Rapid Commun. Mass Spectrom.,* **2019**, *33*(2), 229-238. [http://dx.doi.org/10.1002/rcm.8314] [PMID: 30343517]

[270] Patsenker, E.; Chicca, A.; Petrucci, V.; Moghadamrad, S.; de Gottardi, A.; Hampe, J.; Gertsch, J.; Semmo, N.; Stickel, F. 4-O′-methylhonokiol protects from alcohol/carbon tetrachloride-induced liver injury in mice. *J. Mol. Med. (Berl.),* **2017**, *95*(10), 1077-1089. [http://dx.doi.org/10.1007/s00109-017-1556-y] [PMID: 28689299]

[271] Moraes, D.F.C.; de Mesquita, L.S.S.; do Amaral, F.M.M.; de Sousa Ribeiro, M.N.; Malik, S. Anticancer Drugs from Plants. *Biotechnology and Production of Anti-Cancer Compounds.,* **2017**, , 121-142. [http://dx.doi.org/10.1007/978-3-319-53880-8_5]

[272] Hazra, S; Chattopadhyay, S An overview of lignans with special reference to podophyllotoxin, a cytotoxic lignan **2016**, 3-9.

[273] Niedzwiecki, A.; Roomi, M.; Kalinovsky, T.; Rath, M. Anticancer Efficacy of Polyphenols and Their Combinations. *Nutrients,* **2016**, *8*(9), 552. [http://dx.doi.org/10.3390/nu8090552] [PMID: 27618095]

[274] Yeung, A.W.K.; Tzvetkov, N.T.; Balacheva, A.A.; Georgieva, M.G.; Gan, R.Y.; Jozwik, A.; Pyzel, B.; Horbańczuk, J.O.; Novellino, E.; Durazzo, A.; Lucarini, M.; Camilli, E.; Souto, E.B.; Atanasov, A.G.; Santini, A. Lignans: Quantitative Analysis of the Research Literature. *Front. Pharmacol.,* **2020**, *11*, 37. [http://dx.doi.org/10.3389/fphar.2020.00037] [PMID: 32116713]

[275] Zinov'eva, V.N.; Spasov, A.A. Mechanisms of the anticancer effects of plant polyphenols. I. Blockade of initiation of carcinogenesis. *Biochem. Suppl. Ser. B: Biomed. Chem.,* **2011**, *5*(2), 113-123. [http://dx.doi.org/10.1134/S1990750811020181]

[276] Marcotullio, M.; Curini, M.; Becerra, J. An Ethnopharmacological, Phytochemical and Pharmacological Review on Lignans from Mexican *Bursera* spp. *Molecules,* **2018**, *23*(8), 1976. [http://dx.doi.org/10.3390/molecules23081976] [PMID: 30096772]

[277] Lim, S.Y.M.; Chieng, J.Y.; Pan, Y. Recent insights on anti-dengue virus (DENV) medicinal plants: review on *in vitro, in vivo* and in silico discoveries. *Life,* **2021**, *14*, 1-33.

[278] Loaiza-Cano, V.; Monsalve-Escudero, L.M.; Filho, C.S.M.B.; Martinez-Gutierrez, M.; Sousa, D.P. Antiviral Role of Phenolic Compounds against Dengue Virus: A Review. *Biomolecules,* **2020**, *11*(1), 11. [http://dx.doi.org/10.3390/biom11010011] [PMID: 33374457]

[279] Uttekar, M.M.; Das, T.; Pawar, R.S.; Bhandari, B.; Menon, V.; Nutan, ; Gupta, S.K.; Bhat, S.V. Anti-HIV activity of semisynthetic derivatives of andrographolide and computational study of HIV-1 gp120 protein binding. *Eur. J. Med. Chem.,* **2012**, *56*, 368-374. [http://dx.doi.org/10.1016/j.ejmech.2012.07.030] [PMID: 22858223]

[280] Chen, Q.; Zhang, H.; Cao, Y.; Li, Y.; Sun, S.; Zhang, J.; Zhang, G. Schisandrin B attenuates CCl_4-induced liver fibrosis in rats by regulation of Nrf2-ARE and TGF-β/Smad signaling pathways. *Drug Des. Devel. Ther.,* **2017**, *11*, 2179-2191. [http://dx.doi.org/10.2147/DDDT.S137507] [PMID: 28794616]

[281] Yao, Z.; Han, J.; Lou, S.; Jiang, L.; Xu, J.; Zhou, Y.; Fang, W.; Li, X.; Zhou, L.; Qian, Y.; Lou, D. Schisandrin B attenuates lipopolysaccharide-induced activation of hepatic stellate cells through Nrf--activating anti-oxidative activity. *Int. J. Clin. Exp. Pathol.,* **2018**, *11*(10), 4917-4925.

[PMID: 31949567]

[282] Zhang, H.; Chen, Q.; Dahan, A.; Xue, J.; Wei, L.; Tan, W.; Zhang, G. Transcriptomic analyses reveal the molecular mechanisms of schisandrin B alle*via*tes CCl_4-induced liver fibrosis in rats by RNA-sequencing. *Chem. Biol. Interact.,* **2019**, *309*, 108675.
[http://dx.doi.org/10.1016/j.cbi.2019.05.041] [PMID: 31150632]

[283] Elfeky, M.G.; Mantawy, E.M.; Gad, A.M.; Fawzy, H.M.; El-Demerdash, E. Mechanistic aspects of antifibrotic effects of honokiol in Con A-induced liver fibrosis in rats: Emphasis on TGF-β/SMAD/MAPK signaling pathways. *Life Sci.,* **2020**, *240*, 117096.
[http://dx.doi.org/10.1016/j.lfs.2019.117096] [PMID: 31760097]

[284] Zhang, H.; Ju, B.; Zhang, X.; Zhu, Y.; Nie, Y.; Xu, Y.; Lei, Q. Magnolol Attenuates Concanavalin A-induced Hepatic Fibrosis, Inhibits CD4 $^+$ T Helper 17 (Th17) Cell Differentiation and Suppresses Hepatic Stellate Cell Activation: Blockade of Smad3/Smad4 Signalling. *Basic Clin. Pharmacol. Toxicol.,* **2017**, *120*(6), 560-570.
[http://dx.doi.org/10.1111/bcpt.12749] [PMID: 28032440]

[285] Sung, S.H.; Kim, Y.C. Hepatoprotective diastereomeric lignans from Saururus chinensis herbs. *J. Nat. Prod.,* **2000**, *63*(7), 1019-1021.
[http://dx.doi.org/10.1021/np990499e] [PMID: 10924192]

[286] Lee, J.H.; Jang, E.J.; Seo, H.L. Sauchinone attenuates liver fibrosis and hepatic stellate cell activation through TGF-β/Smad signaling pathway. *Chem. Biol. Interact.,* **2014**, *224*, 58-67.
[http://dx.doi.org/10.1016/j.cbi.2014.10.005] [PMID: 25451574]

[287] Kim, Y.W.; Lee, S.M.; Shin, S.M.; Hwang, S.J.; Brooks, J.S.; Kang, H.E.; Lee, M.G.; Kim, S.C.; Kim, S.G. Efficacy of sauchinone as a novel AMPK-activating lignan for preventing iron-induced oxidative stress and liver injury. *Free Radic. Biol. Med.,* **2009**, *47*(7), 1082-1092.
[http://dx.doi.org/10.1016/j.freeradbiomed.2009.07.018] [PMID: 19616619]

[288] Reddy, V.P.; Aryal, P.; Robinson, S.; Rafiu, R.; Obrenovich, M.; Perry, G. Polyphenols in Alzheimer's Disease and in the Gut–Brain Axis. *Microorganisms,* **2020**, *8*(2), 199.
[http://dx.doi.org/10.3390/microorganisms8020199] [PMID: 32023969]

[289] Lee, J.H.; Park, S.Y.; Choi, I.G.; Choi, J.W. Investigation of Molecular Size Effect on the Formation of Lignin Nanoparticles by Nanoprecipitation. *Appl. Sci. (Basel),* **2020**, *10*(14), 4910.
[http://dx.doi.org/10.3390/app10144910]

CHAPTER 8

Semisynthetic Resveratrol-derived Systems: A Synergism between Nature and Organic Synthesis

Antonella Capperucci[1] and **Damiano Tanini**[1,*]

[1] *Department of Chemistry Ugo Schiff, University of Florence, Via della Lastruccia 13, I-50019 Sesto Fiorentino, Italy*

Abstract: Structural modifications of the resveratrol scaffold are valuable tools in order to develop new derivatives with potential biomedical and pharmacological applications. The investigation of the biological properties of resveratrol-derived semisynthetic systems and the study of their structure-activity relationships are attracting growing interest from medicinal chemists and biologists. In this context, the synthesis of novel resveratrol-derived systems characterisaed by elevated molecular complexity is highly sought after. Over the past years, a wide variety of resveratrol derivatives have been prepared and studied for their biological properties. Therefore, a number of stilbenoid-related potential anticancer, antioxidant, antiviral, analgesic, and anti-neurodegenerative systems have been investigated. This chapter focuses on recent studies related to the preparation and the study of semisynthetic resveratrol-derived systems.

Keywords: Antioxidants, Anticancer Agents, Functionalization, Organic Synthesis, Prodrugs, Resveratrol, Stilbenoids, Structural Modifications.

INTRODUCTION

Resveratrol is a polyphenol-based natural product which can be isolated from a broad range of plants, where it has been demonstrated to act as phytoalexin [1]. Resveratrol is widely known because of its occurrence in red wine and its implication in the “French paradox” [2]. Owing to its antioxidant activity, resveratrol prevents the oxidation of LDL *in vitro* and reduces the markers of oxidative stress *in vivoi* [3]. A number of activities, including antioxidant, anti-inflammatory, anticancer, estrogenic, neuroprotective, anti-atherosclerosis, cardioprotective, anti-diabetic, anti-osteoporosis, anti-obesity, and anti-aging properties, have been described for resveratrol. The abundance and the diversity of resveratrol molecular targets reasonably account for the multiplicity of phar-

* **Corresponding author Damiano Tanini:** Department of Chemistry Ugo Schiff, University of Florence, *Via* della Lastruccia 13, I-50019 Sesto Fiorentino, Italy; E-mail: damiano.tanini@unifi.it

macological effects of this stilbenoid. For these reasons, resveratrol and related stilbenoids have been widely studied over the past years. However, the clinical benefits of resveratrol are hampered by unfavourable pharmacokinetic and pharmacodynamics, including poor bioavailability, low aqueous solubility, and chemical instability. In this context, considerable efforts have been devoted to evaluate whether suitable structural modifications could improve or modulate the biological properties of the parent stilbenoid [4, 5]. On the other hand, structural modifications of resveratrol can also be performed in order to improve its metabolic stability and to access new hybrids through the conjugation of two biologically active molecules. Indeed, a number of differently functionalised resveratrol derivatives and resveratrol-based hybrids have been proposed as potential pharmacological tools, exhibiting anticancer [6], antiviral [7], antibacterial [8], analgesic [9] and antioxidant properties [10]. Additionally, resveratrol derivatives have also been studied for their potential role in preventing or treating cardiovascular [11], Alzheimer's, and Parkinson's diseases [12].

This chapter focuses on recent studies on the preparation and the biological properties of semisynthetic resveratrol-derived systems. Only synthetic procedures employing resveratrol as the starting material will be discussed herein. However, several approaches for the preparation of resveratrol-based hybrids rely on the construction of the functionalised resveratrol skeleton through the coupling of suitably decorated and substituted building blocks.

RESVERATROL ETHERS AND RELATED DERIVATIVES

The anticancer activity of a series of resveratrol derivatives, prepared through functionalization of the stilbene double bond and/or protection of phenolic moieties, was reported by Orsini *et al.* [13]. Phenolic groups of resveratrol **1** could be protected as methyl ethers or benzyl ethers to afford compounds **2** and **3** in good yields. Tri-pivaloyl ester and tri-acetyl esters of resveratrol **4** and **5** were, respectively, obtained upon the reaction of resveratrol with pivaloyl chloride or acetyl chloride. Epoxides **6** and **7** were efficiently prepared through the epoxidation of the stilbene double bond of **4** and **5** with *m*-chloroperbenzoic acid (*m*CPBA). Epoxides **6** and **7** could be employed as precursors for a variety of resveratrol derivatives. Ring-opening reaction of **6** with morpholine enabled the formation of regioisomeric amino alcohols **8**,**9** and **10**,**11**. Oxidation of these regioisomeric alcohols under Jones conditions was exploited for the synthesis of functionalised ketones **12**,**13** and **14**,**15** Scheme **(1).**

Resveratrol tri-*O*-methyl ether **2** and tri-*O*-benzyl ether **3** were also employed as substrates for the synthesis of enantio-enriched diols (1*S*,2*S*)-**16** and (1*S*,2*S*)-**17** through asymmetric Sharpless dihydroxylation using AD-mix-α. Similarly, resveratrol-derived enantio-enriched diol (1*R*,2*R*)-**16** was efficiently prepared from **2** by using AD-mix-β. The enantiomeric purity of both enantiomers of **16** was determined by the application of the Mosher method Scheme **(2).** Therefore, ^{1}H and ^{19}F NMR spectra of esters **18** and **19**, were prepared upon the reaction of the aforementioned enantio-enriched diols with (*R*)-α-methoxy, α-trifluoromethyl phenylacetyl chloride, were studied and the optical purity was assessed to be greater than 99%.

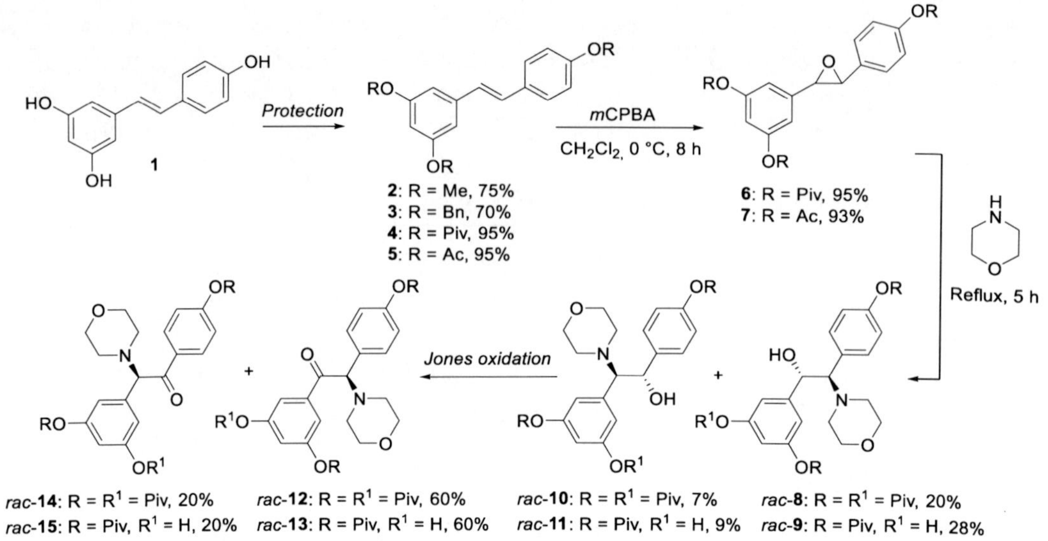

Scheme (1). Synthesis of resveratrol derivatives through the reactivity of resveratrol epoxides.

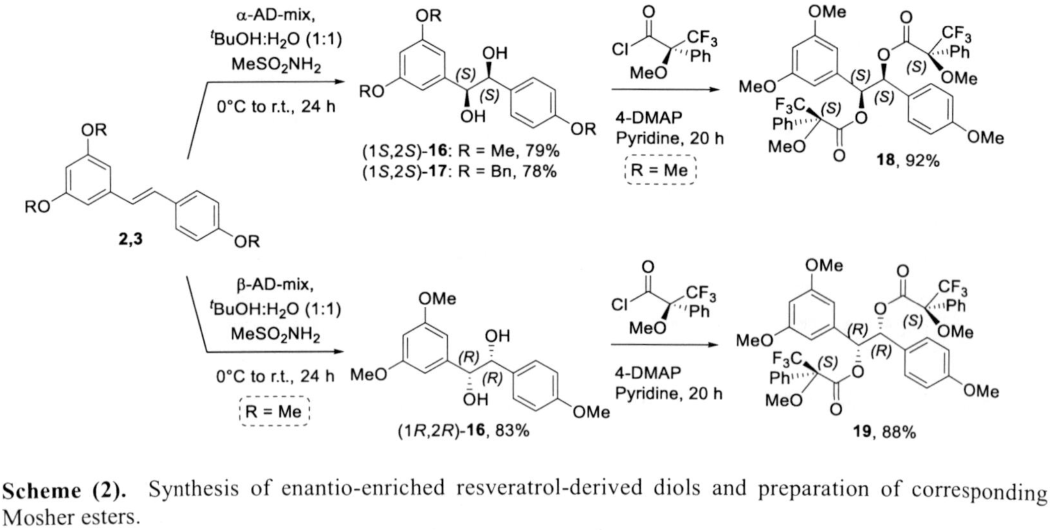

Scheme (2). Synthesis of enantio-enriched resveratrol-derived diols and preparation of corresponding Mosher esters.

A series of nitrogen-containing resveratrol derivatives were also synthesised. The carbonate **20**, easily obtained from the diol (1*S*,2*S*)-**16** and triphosgene, was converted into a regioisomeric mixture of azido alcohols **21** and **22** upon treatment with NaN_3 Scheme **(3).**

Azido alcohols **21** and **22** were efficiently used as precursors of the series of *N*-containing resveratrol derivatives reported in Fig. (**1**) Amino alcohols **23**, **24**, as well as ketoamines **25**, **26** could also be employed for the synthesis of resveratrol-derived nitrogen-containing heterocycles, such as **27** and **28**.

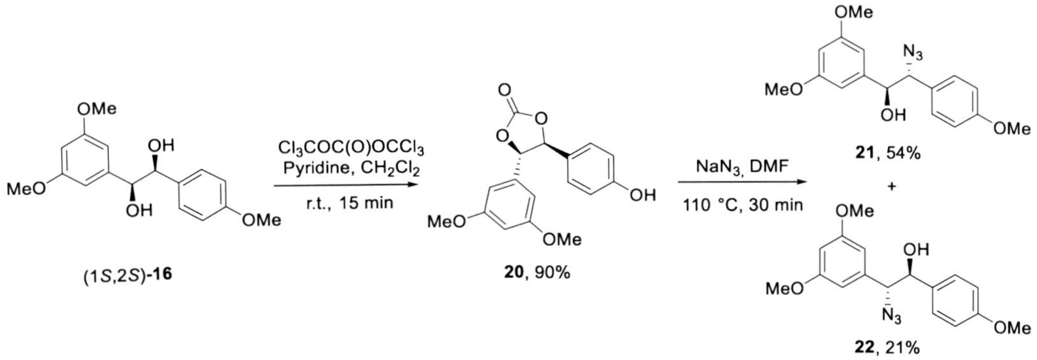

Scheme (3). Synthesis of azido alcohols **21** and **22**.

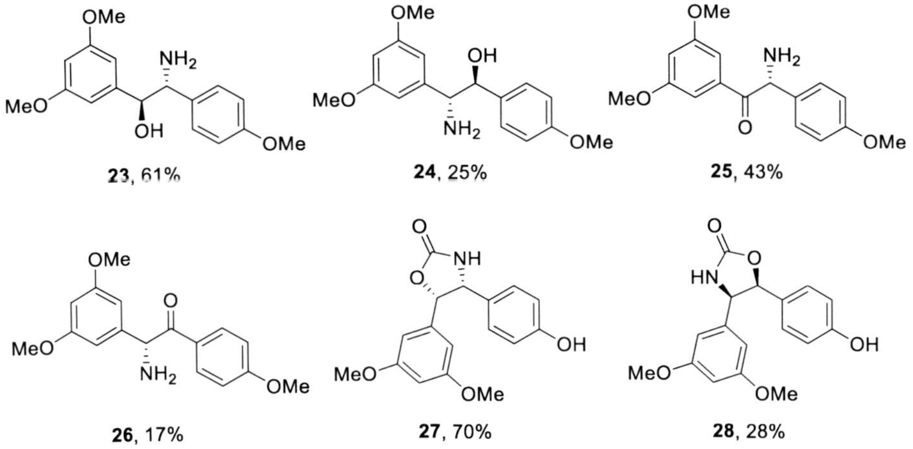

Fig. (1). Nitrogen-containing resveratrol derivatives.

The effect of such resveratrol-derived molecules on carcinogen metabolizing enzymes was studied in order to evaluate their potential chemopreventive activities. The antioxidant and anti-inflammatory activities of such compounds were also investigated according to different assays. Notably, 3,4',5-tri-*O*-methyl resveratrol **2** was about seven-fold more active than resveratrol in inhibiting Cyp1A (cytochrome P450 1A) activity, it was a potent inducer of QR (quinone reductase) activity, and – contrarily to what was observed for resveratrol – exhibited pure anti-estrogenic activity in the human Ishikawa endometrial adenocarcinoma cells. Similarly, aminoalcohols **23** and **24** showed pure anti-estrogenic activity. Interestingly, the epoxide **6** behaved as a potent inducer of phase 2 enzymes concomitant with the inhibition of LPS-mediated iNOS induction. Data related to the effect of selected resveratrol derivatives on carcinogen metabolizing enzymes are reported in Table 1. [13].

The effects on biological activities of above-discussed structural modifications of resveratrol are summarised in Fig. (**2**) [13].

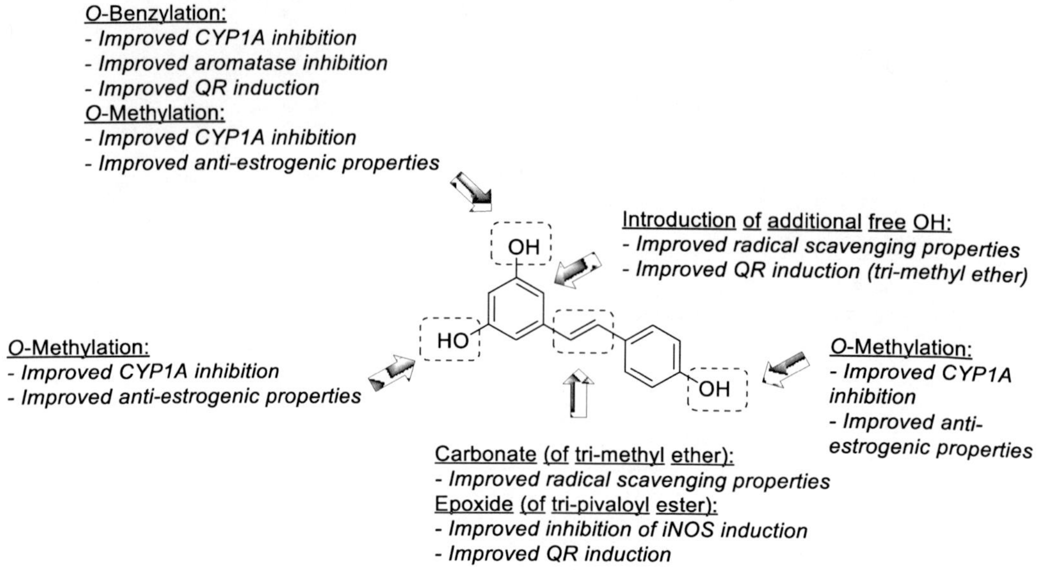

Fig. (2). Structural modification of resveratrol and related effects on biological properties.

Table 1. Inhibitory concentrations of some resveratrol derivatives on carcinogen metabolizing enzymes.

Product	CYP1A	NAD(P)H/QR	
	IC_{50} (μM)[a]	**CD (μM)[b]**	**IC_{50} (μM)[a]**
Resveratrol	0.23	12.4	29.8
2	0.03	>2.6	2.6
3	4.3	>50 (1.4)[c]	>50
6	>5 (49)[d]	0.83	4.2
(1*S*,2*S*)-**16**	>0.5 (15)[d]	>50 (1.5)[c]	>50

(Table 1) cont.....

Product	CYP1A	NAD(P)H/QR	
	IC_{50} (μM)[a]	CD (μM)[b]	IC_{50} (μM)[a]
20	>5 (37)[d]	>50 (1.1)[c]	>50
23 + 24	>5 (40)[d]	>19.2	19.2

[a]IC_{50}: half-maximal inhibitory concentration; [b]CD: concentration required to double the specific activity of QR; [c]values in parentheses indicate the maximum fold induction at the indicated concentration; [d]values in parentheses indicate the percentage of inhibition at the indicated concentration.

Pastorková *et al.* [14] also found that 3,4',5-tri-*O*-methyl resveratrol **2** behaves as a strong activator of human AhR and inducer of CYP1A1 in human hepatoma HepG2. Conversely, resveratrol is a partial agonist of AhR.

Other studies highlighted the interesting anticancer properties of different etherified resveratrol derivatives. Benzyl ethers were demonstrated to possess potential anticancer activity [13, 15]. Hong *et al.* [15] reported that compounds **29** and **30** (Fig. **3**), prepared upon the reaction of resveratrol with benzyl chloride, behaved as strong anticancer agents against different tumor cell lines (A549, LAC, and HeLa). Notably **29** showed an IC_{50} value of 1.41 μM (1.41 ± 3.21 μM) against HeLa cells and was demonstrated to be 90-fold more active than resveratrol (IC_{50} = 98.17 ± 0.54 μM) and almost potent as the reference compound, Adriamycin (IC_{50} = 0.48 ± 0.96 μM).

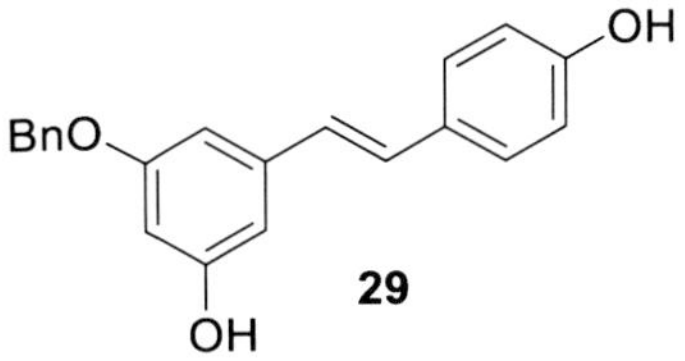

29

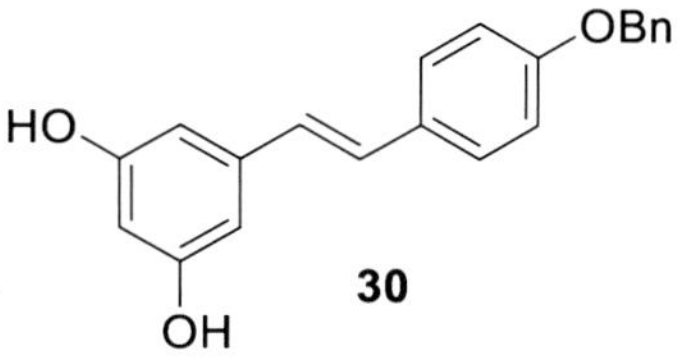

30

Fig. (3). Resveratrol benzyl ether derivatives **29** and **30**.

With the aim of avoiding the low bioavailability and the rapid metabolism of resveratrol, a series of glycosylated prodrugs was also recently developed by Falomir *et al.* [16].

Compounds **31**-**33**, as well as the anti-angiogenic prodrug piceid (Fig. **4**), proved to be cytotoxic against human colon adenocarcinoma HT-29 and breast adenocarcinoma MCF-7 cells. On the other hand, the toxicity of such compounds in non-cancerous HEK-293 cells was lower than that of resveratrol. Additionally, treatment of HT-29 cells with the above-mentioned glucosylated resveratrol derivatives led to a significantly decreased production of vascular endothelial growth factor (VEGF). Such compounds also downregulated the human telomerase reverse transcriptase (*hTERT*) gene by decreasing the transcription of the *c-Myc* gene.

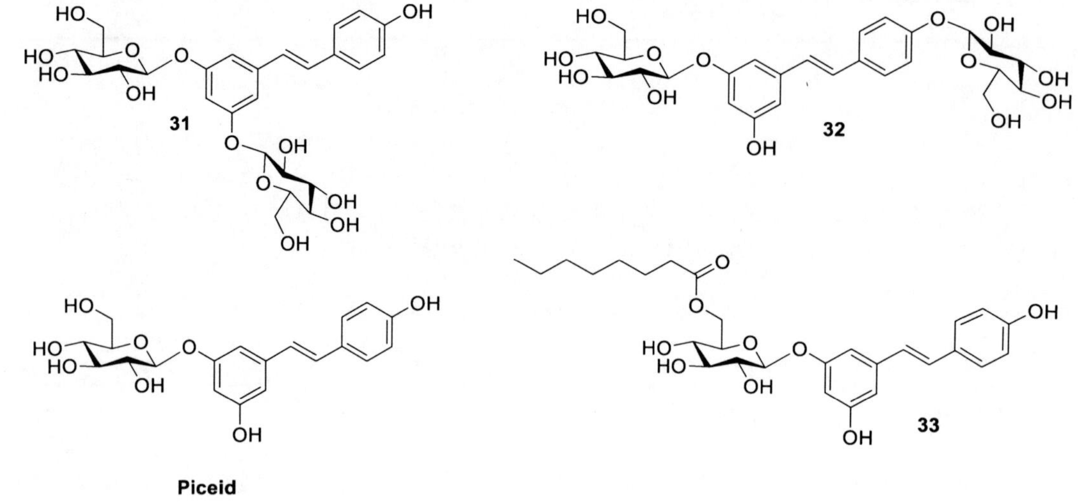

Fig. (4). Structures of resveratrol-derived glucosydes with cytotoxicity against HT-29 and MCF-7 cells.

In this context, it is worth mentioning that stilbenoids, such as piceid, have also been evaluated as antiviral agents exhibiting interesting virus inhibitor properties [7].

Nakao *et al.* [10] reported a study on the modulatory effect on the TRPA1 channel of a series of resveratrol derivatives, easily synthesised as described in Scheme **(4).** in order to develop new analgesic drugs. Notably, some of these simple molecules, such as **2**, have also been demonstrated to possess interesting potential anticancer properties [13].

Owing to their antioxidant properties, a number of resveratrol-derived systems, such as pterostilbene **38** as well as the ether **39** and the sulfur-containing derivative **40** (Fig. **5**), have also been reported as potential agents in the prevention and treatment of cardiovascular disease (CVD) [11, 17, 18].

Importantly, a number of resveratrol ethers and related derivatives, including piceid and pterostilbene, have also been studied as potential drugs against Alzheimer's and Parkinson's diseases [12].

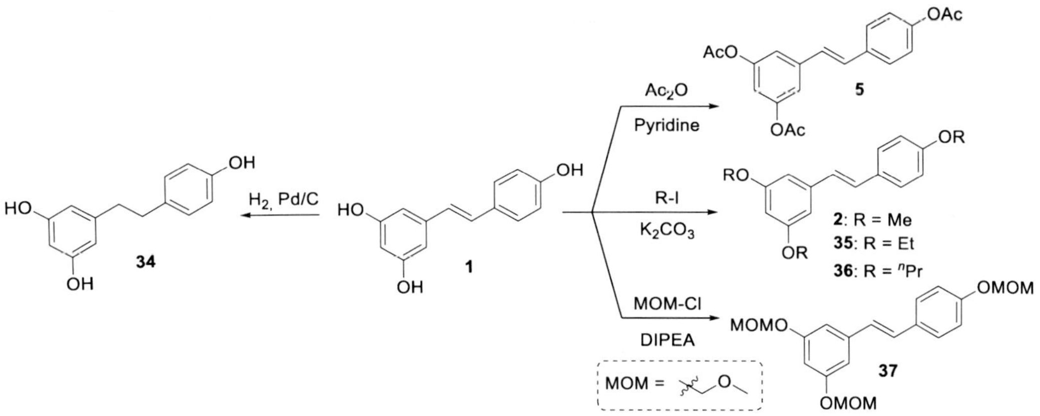

Scheme (4). Synthesis of resveratrol derivatives **2**, **5**, **34-37**.

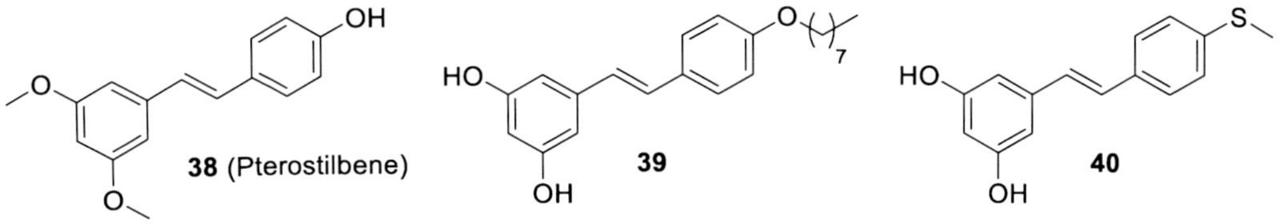

Fig. (5). Structures of resveratrol derivatives **38** (pterostilbene), **39**, and **40**.

Resveratryl Esters and Related Derivatives

As mentioned above, besides the etherification of phenolic moieties of resveratrol, also their esterification represents a rewarding strategy in order to develop new semisynthetic resveratrol derivatives with anticancer properties. Chelsky *et al.* [19] described the *in vitro* antitumor activity of the resveratrol-derived acetate **41** (Fig. **6**) against different human tumor cell lines including human glioma (U251MG), human breast (MDA-MB-231 and MCF-7), and pancreatic (Panc-1). IC_{50} values ranged between 6 and 19 μM. The activity of **41** against human U251MG glioblastoma is related to the dose-dependent suppression of Stat3 tyrosine705 phosphorylation and the induction of Stat3 serine727 phosphorylation.

In this context, 4'-pivaloyl- and 4'-butyroyl-resveratrol derivatives **42** and **43** (Fig. **6**) were demonstrated to reduce the cell *Via*bility of MDA-MB-231 human breast cancer cells through the activation of the pro-apoptotic calcium signalling pathway and the inhibition of plasma membrane Ca^{2+}-ATPase proteins [20].

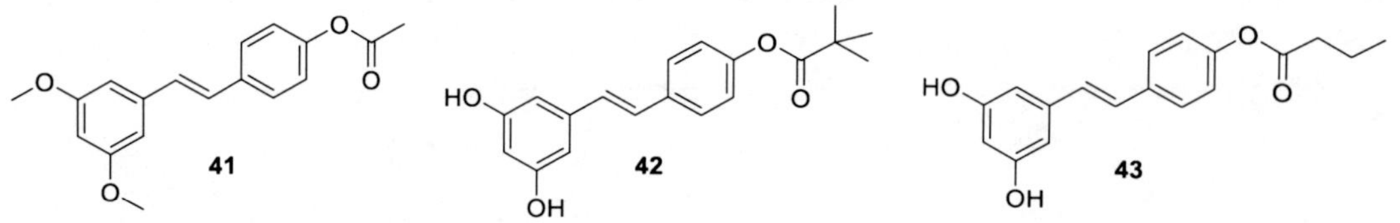

Fig. (6). Structure of resveratrol-derived esters **41-43**.

The antitumor activity against cisplatin-resistant oral squamous cells (CAR) of a series of resveratrol-derived esters was investigated by Hsieh *et al.* [21] Notably, exhibiting higher activity than pterostilbene, resveratrol, and cisplatin against CAR cells, **44** (Fig. 7) behaved as the most effective compound among the studied derivatives, exhibiting IC_{50} values at 48 h and 72 h of 73.25 ± 4.20 μM and 38. 58 ± 2.39 μM, respectively. *In vivoi* studies also highlighted the antitumor activity of compound **44**.

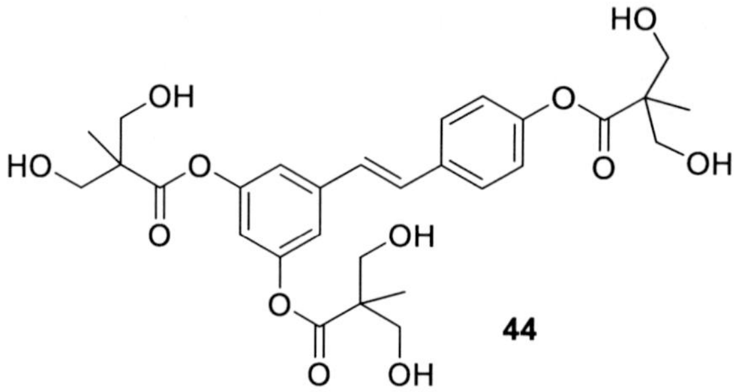

Fig. (7). Structure of resveratrol-derived ester **44**.

A wide variety of resveratrol-derived esters characterised by a high molecular diversity were synthesised by Urbaniak *et al.* [22] through a microwave-assisted direct approach using acyl chlorides. Selected examples of such compounds are reported in Scheme **(5).** The anticancer activity of resveratrol-derived esters against primary acute lymphoblastic leukemia (ALL) cells was evaluated and found to be strongly influenced by the nature of the acyl moiety. Particularly, the shortest carbon chain-substituted derivatives such as those of resveratryl tri-acetate **5** and tri-isobutyrate **45** were demonstrated to be correlated with higher activity and displayed more potency than resveratrol. IC_{50} values of selected compounds from Urbaniak's work are reported in Scheme. **(5)** [23].

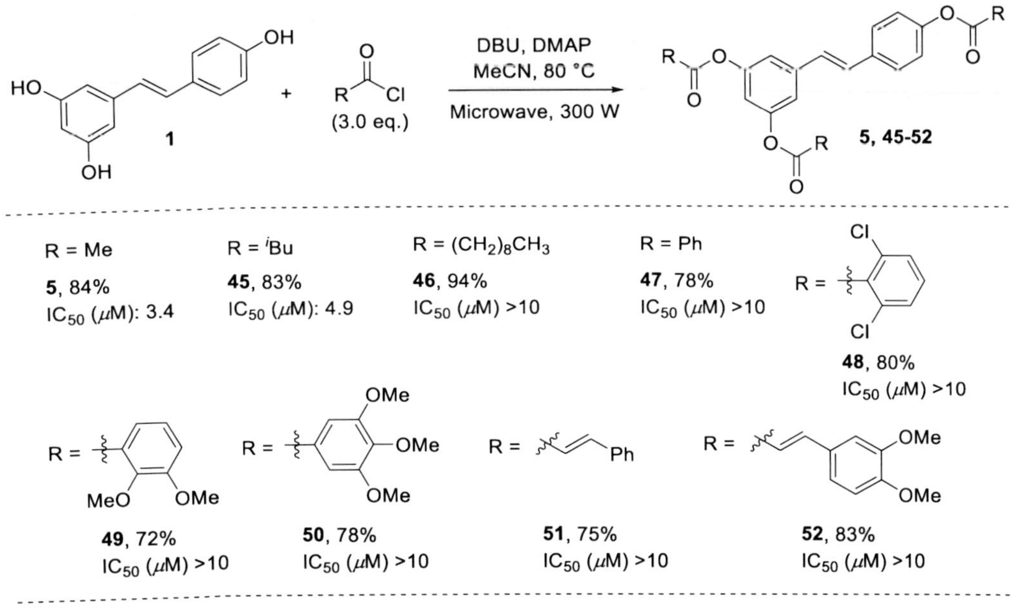

Scheme (5). Microwave-assisted synthesis of resveratrol-derived esters. Selected examples and related IC_{50} values against ALL primary cancer cells [22, 23].

The anticancer properties of resveratryl triacetate **5**, easily obtained upon treatment of resveratrol with acetic anhydride and pyridine, have also been reported by Hong *et al.* [15] Indeed, **5** exhibited remarkable cytotoxicity against A549 (lung adenocarcinoma) and HeLa (cervical cancer) cell lines. Additionally, compound **5** has also been recently studied as a potential therapeutic agent for the treatment of pancreatic cancer. The anticancer activity of **5** seems to be due to the inhibition of the formation of colony and the induction of apoptosis through activation of caspase-3 in human pancreatic cancer AsPC-1 and PANC-1 cells. No effect was observed on human pancreatic normal ductal epithelial cells (HPNE). Furthermore, resveratryl triacetate **5** also exhibited important biological effects, such as the inhibition of the Zeb1 3'UTR-luciferase activity by upregulating miRNA-200, through the suppression of the Sonic Hedgehog (Shh) pathway [24].

Resveratrol-derived esters generally exhibit higher fat solubility and permeability when compared with resveratrol. For these reasons, resveratryl esters can be regarded as interesting prodrugs, undergoing hydrolysis by the activity of esterases in blood, liver, and other tissues. In order to conjugate two potentially active systems, Jin *et al.* [25] studied a series of new derivatives obtained through esterification of resveratrol with 2-furoyl- and 2-thiophenecarbonyl-chlorides. 2-Furoic acid and 2-thiophenecarboxylic acid are respectively an antibiotic and a key precursor of the anticancer raltitrexed. Notably, the 2-thienyl-substituted derivative **53** exhibited an interesting *in vitro* antitumor activity against cervical cancer HeLa cells, proving to be significantly more active than resveratrol (Fig. **8**).

In this context, the synthesis of a larger series of heteroaryl-substituted resveratrol-derived esters was recently reported by the same group in order to develop new anticancer systems with improved chemical and metabolic stability with respect to resveratrol [26]. Mono-, di-, or tri-esters of resveratrol could be achieved upon the reaction of **1** with heteroaromatic carboxylic acids under 1-ethyl-3-(3-dimethylaminopropyl)carbodiimide hydrochloride and 4-dimethylaminopyridine (EDC•HCl/DMAP) conditions. Furthermore, mono-, di-, or tri-sulfonate esters of resveratrol were prepared through the reaction of **1** with sulfonyl chlorides in the presence of triethylamine Scheme **(6).** The study also suggests the role of some structural modifications, such as the introduction of heterocyclic-containing moieties at a selected position, on modulating the cytotoxicity of resveratrol-derived esters and sulfonates against breast cancer cells. In Scheme **(6).** are reported the IC_{50} values of resveratrol-derived esters **54**, **55**, and **56** which, within the studied series, exhibited the highest anti-breast cancer activity [26].

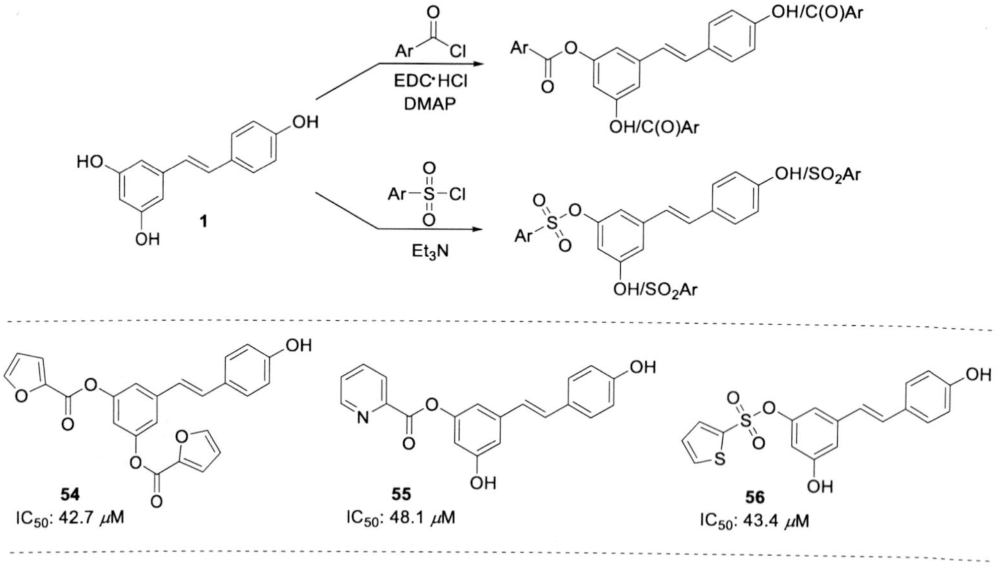

Scheme (6). Synthesis of heterocycle-substituted resveratryl esters and sulfonate esters. The IC_{50} value against MCF-7 cancer cells (breast) of selected examples is reported [26].

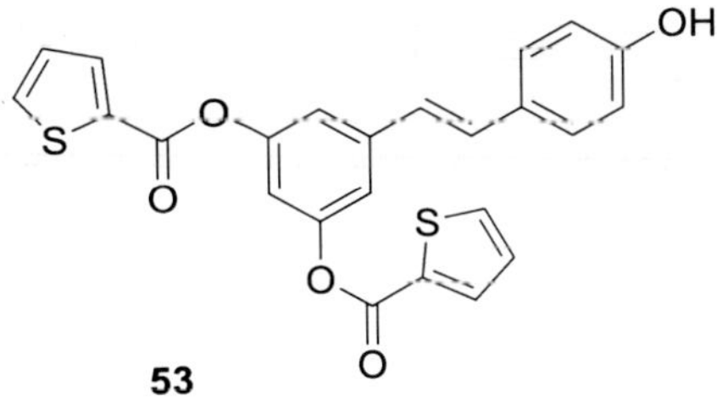

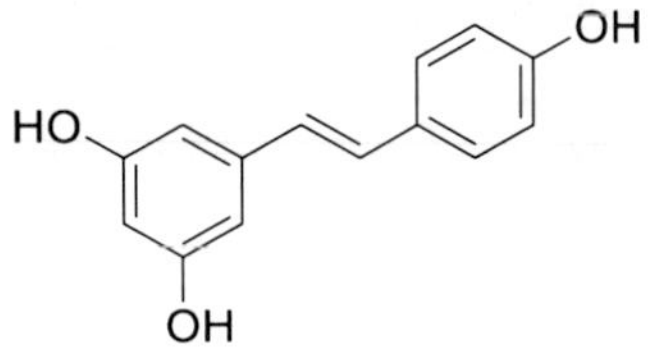

53
IC_{50}: 26.7 μM

1, Resveratrol
IC_{50}: 112 μM

Fig. (8). 2-thiophenecarboxylic acid-derived resveratryl ester **53** and resveratrol **1**. IC_{50} values refer to the cytotoxicity against cervical cancer HeLa cells [25].

The anticancer properties of sulfonate esters were also reported by Hong *et al.* [15]. Compounds **57** and **58**, bearing one and two sulfonate moieties respectively, exhibited remarkable cytotoxicity against three cancer cell lines (A549, LAC, and HeLa). Notably, the anticancer activity of sulfonate **58** proved to be 15-fold higher than that of resveratrol itself (Fig. **9**).

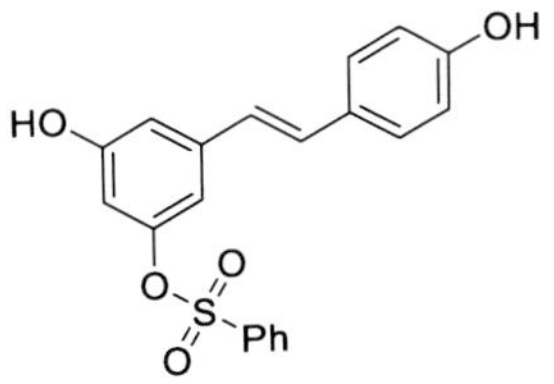

57
IC_{50} (A549): 4.38 ± 0.71 μM
IC_{50} (LAC): 10.19 ± 0.37 μM
IC_{50} (HeLa): 8.16 ± 0.95 μM

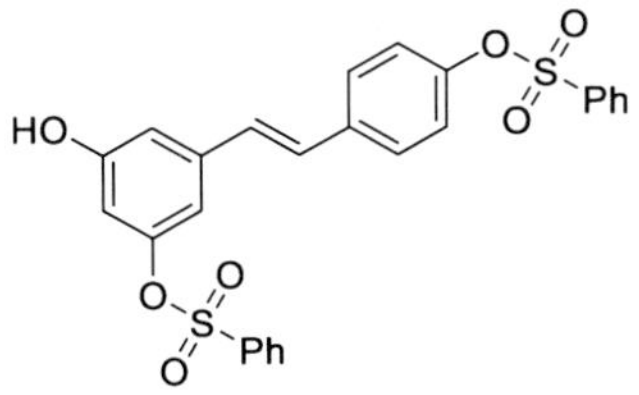

58
IC_{50} (A549): 4.90 ± 1.18 μM
IC_{50} (LAC): 5.55 ± 1.07 μM
IC_{50} (HeLa): 6.48 ± 1.56 μM

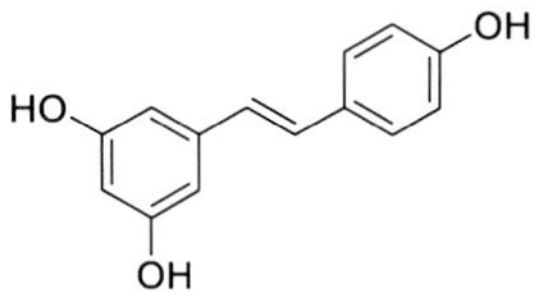

Resveratrol, **1**
IC_{50} (A549): 66.25 ± 2.07 μM
IC_{50} (LAC): 24.89 ± 1.40 μM
IC_{50} (HeLa): 98.17 ± 0.54 μM

Fig. (9). Structure and cytotoxicity of compounds **57** and **58** against three different cancer cell lines.

Similarly, resveratrol-derived sulfates were also studied by Falomir *et al.* [16]. For example, compound **60**, efficiently synthesised from the resveratrol silyl ether **59** upon treatment with SO_3•NMe_3 and final protodesilylation reaction, exhibited significant cytotoxicity against MCF-7 cells while proving to be less toxic than resveratrol in HEK-293 normal cells Scheme **(7).** Notably, **60** is not involved in the downregulation of the c-Myc gene expression and exhibits a reduction in the gene expression of hTERT in HT-29 cells. These results provide evidence that the resveratrol derivative **60** acts through a different mechanism with respect to that of resveratrol and does not behave simply as a resveratrol precursor.

Liu *et al.* [27] reported a study on the eight-arm-polyethylene glycol resveratrol-derived prodrug **61** (Fig. **10**)., easily synthesised through the esterification of the hydroxyl moiety of pterostilbene, a dimethyl-substituted analogue of resveratrol, with the carboxylic group of eight-arm-polyethylene glycol carboxylic acid. The esterification reaction was performed under 1-ethyl -3-(3- dimethylaminopropyl) carbodiimide hydrochloride and 4-dimethylaminopyridine (EDC•HCl/DMAP) conditions. PEG-pterostilbene derivatives proved to possess interesting anticancer properties, which were demonstrated to be higher with respect to those of pterostilbene. Furthermore, such compounds exhibited moderate systemic toxicity.

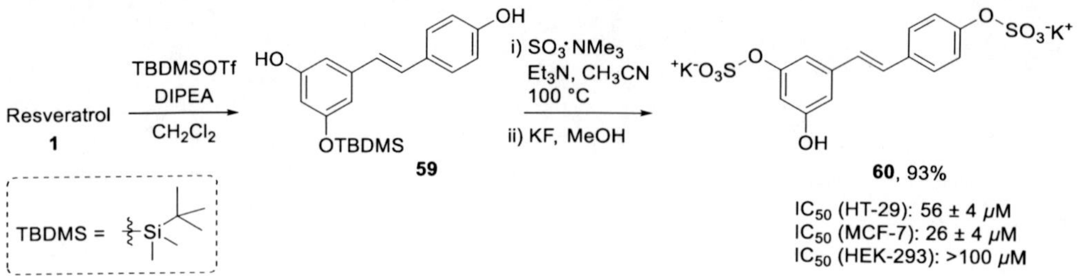

Scheme (7). Synthesis and *in vitro* cytotoxicity of resveratrol sulfate derivative **60**.

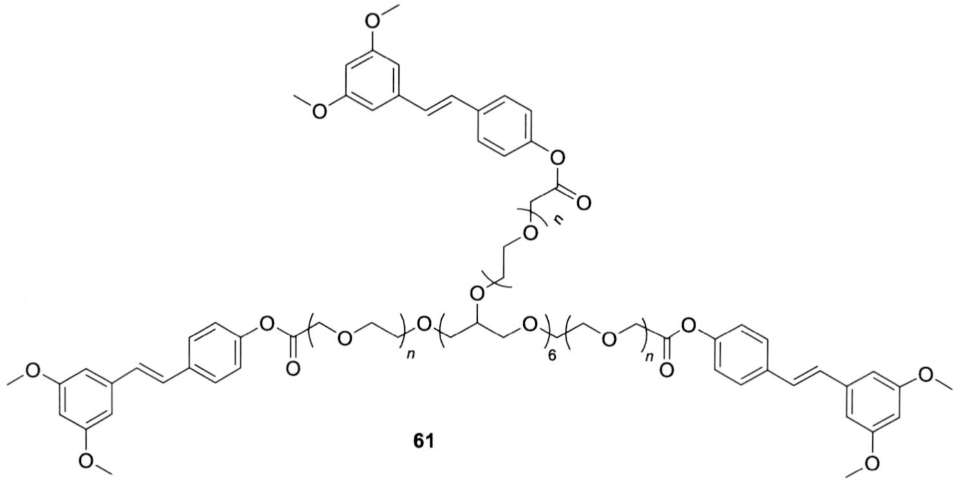

Fig. (10). Eight-arm-polyethylene glycol pterostilbene-derived prodrug **61**.

Selenium-containing Resveratrol Derivatives

The introduction of chalcogen atoms into natural products is emerging as a rewarding strategy in order to conjugate the biological activities of chalcogens with those of the functionalised substrate [28 - 30]. For example, sulfur-, selenium-, and tellurium-containing natural-products-derived systems, including resveratrol [10], eugenol [31, 32], limonene [31, 32], tocopherols [33, 34], and L-ascorbic acid [35, 36] derivatives, exhibited interesting antioxidant properties. In this context, the synthesis of a novel class of resveratrol derivatives featuring a 2-

phenylbenzoselenophene skeleton was reported. Benzoselenophene **64** as well as its monochloro- and dichloro-substituted derivatives **65** and **66** were achieved upon the reaction of resveratrol with elemental selenium and sulfuryl chloride [10]. The reaction involves the electrophilic aromatic substitution of the resorcin moiety of resveratrol with *in situ* generated $SeCl_2$ to yield **62**, which undergoes intramolecular addition to the double bond to give **63** and further HCl elimination to provide **64** Scheme **(8).** Monochloro- and dichloro-substituted benzoselenophenes **65** and **66** are reasonably formed through chlorination reactions with Cl_2, generated by dismutation of SO_2Cl_2. Remarkably, a judicious tuning of the reaction stoichiometry enabled a selective entry to compounds **64-66**. All the novel resveratrol-derived benzoselenophenes proved to behave as effective antioxidants, being more efficient than resveratrol and exhibiting both GPx-like properties and chain-breaking antioxidant activity [10].

Notably, the antioxidant activity of benzoselenofenes **64-66** in intestinal myofibroblast and osteocyte cell lines in which the oxidative stress was induced by GSH depletion or starvation was demonstrated to be higher than that of resveratrol itself. Owing to their structural features, resveratrol-derived benzoselenophenes exhibited different antioxidant capacity in myofibroblasts and in osteocytes. Such a different activity might also be due to the diverse degree of oxidative stress [37]. Furthermore, resveratrol-derived benzoselenophenes **64-66** were also demonstrated to possess interesting carbonic anhydrase inhibitor activities [38].

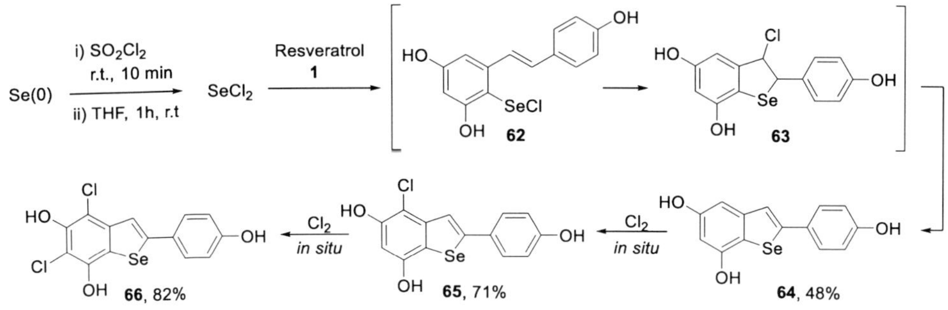

Scheme (8). Synthesis of resveratrol-derived benzoselenophenes.

In order to evaluate the possibility to conjugate the biological and pharmacological activities of resveratrol (*i.e.,* inhibition of cancer cells cycle progression) with those of ebselen-like systems (*i.e.,* inhibition of thioredoxin reductase, GPx-like properties), Yan *et al.* [39] reported the synthesis and the study of a series of benzoselenazole-stilbene hybrids (Fig. **11**). Such conjugate systems exhibited remarkable antiproliferative activity against non-small-cell lung cancer (A549), liver carcinoma (Bel-7402), epithelial cervical cancer (HeLa), and breast cancer (MCF-7) [39].

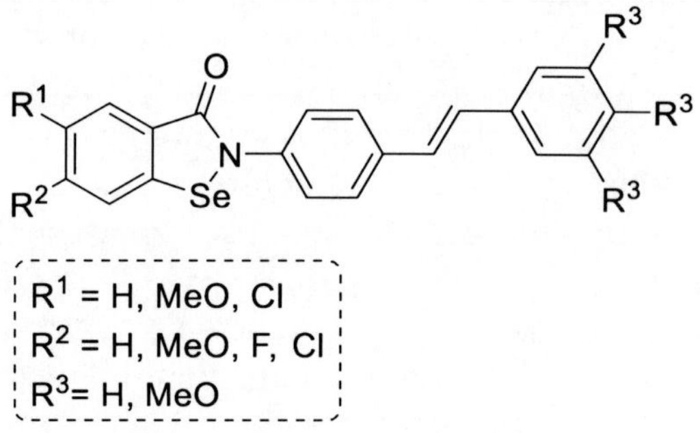

Fig. (11). General structure of benzoselenazole-stilbene ebselen-like hybrids.

Resveratrol-Derived Hybrids and Other Conjugates

Conjugation of resveratrol with peptides has also been exploited in order to develop novel potential anticancer compounds with improved solubility and bioavailability. Mrkus *et al.* [40] reported a study on functionalised peptidyl derivatives where a portion of the peptide is linked to a natural antioxidant polyphenol, such as quercetin and resveratrol. The mixed anhydride method with isobutylchloroformate in DMF with NMM and DMAP was employed for the synthesis of different functionalised and protected peptidyl derivatives through a simple condensation reaction, followed by a deprotection step. Notably, all quercetin- or resveratrol-derived esters of Leu/Met-enkephalin and tetrapeptide Leu-Ser-Lys-Leu (LSKL) exhibited remarkable antioxidant properties. Significant anticancer activity was obtained for LSKL-based derivatives. Particularly, the LSKL-resveratrol conjugate **67** (Fig. **12**) was found to possess growth inhibitory activity against HCT116 (colon), MCF-7 (breast), and H460 (lung) carcinoma cells. The mean values of the corresponding IC_{50} ranged from 41 and 78 mM [40].

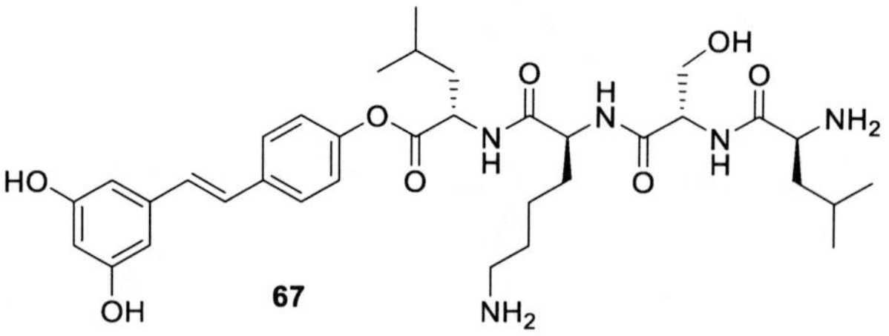

67

Fig. (12). Resveratrol-functionalised tetrapeptide Leu-Ser-Lys-Leu (LSKL) **67**.

A series of novel amphiphilic resveratrol derivatives were synthesised and studied by Chillemi *et al.* [41]. Phosphoramidites **68-71** (Fig. **13**) prepared from resveratrol through multi-steps procedures, often involving enzymatic reactions, were used as precursors of derivatives **72-76**.

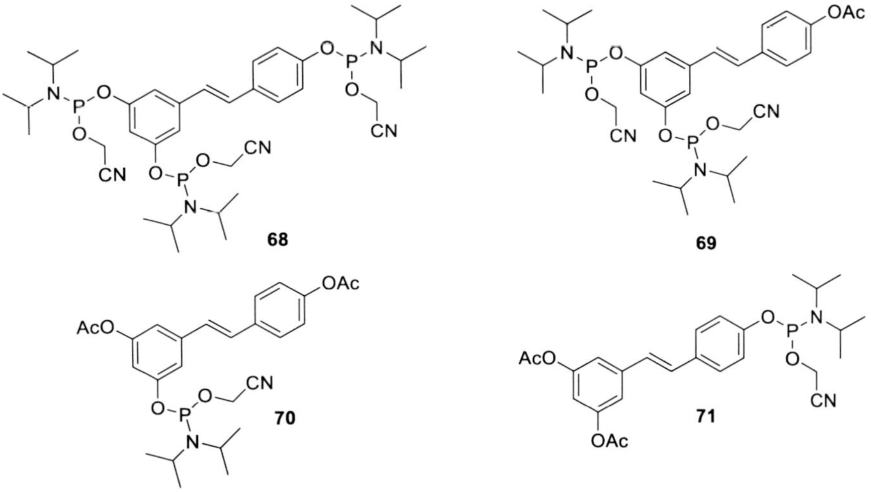

Fig. (13). Structures of resveratrol phosphoramidites **68-71** employed as precursors for the synthesis of amphiphilic resveratrol derivatives.

Indeed, conjugation of **68-71** with cholesterol or with the appropriate 1,2-di-*O*-acylglycerol could be easily achieved by employing the phosphoramidite chemistry. Selected examples of amphiphilic lipoconjugates of resveratrol, bearing the lipophilic moiety anchored through a phosphate bridge, are reported in the Scheme **(9).** The newly synthesised compounds exhibited remarkable anticancer activity against neuroblastoma SH-SY5Y cell line. Particularly, di-palmitoyl derivative **74** (IC_{50} – 8.4 μM) proved to be the most active compound within the studied series. Notably, the activity of unconjugated resveratrol against SH-SY5Y cells was considerably lower (IC_{50} > 50 μM) [41].

The synthesis of resveratrol-Aspirin regioisomeric hybrids **78** and **79** has been reported by Zhu *et al.* through the esterification of resveratrol with the Aspirin-derived chloride **77** under Et_3N conditions Scheme **(10)** [42]. Such hybrids behave as prodrugs capable of releasing the anti-inflammatory drug and the resveratrol molecule. Notably, while the anticancer activity of Aspirin is retained, the side effect of gastrointestinal ulceration is reduced. The anticancer activity of **78** and **79** against human colon cancer cells HT-29 and HCT-116 was evaluated, demonstrating that the acylation of Aspirin with resveratrol results in improved anticancer activity with respect to the use of physical mixtures of the two bioactive molecules. Compound **78** proved to be more active than the regioisomer

79. Additionally, methylation reactions performed on **78** demonstrated that the hydroxyl moieties play a key role in determining the activity of the hybrid [42].

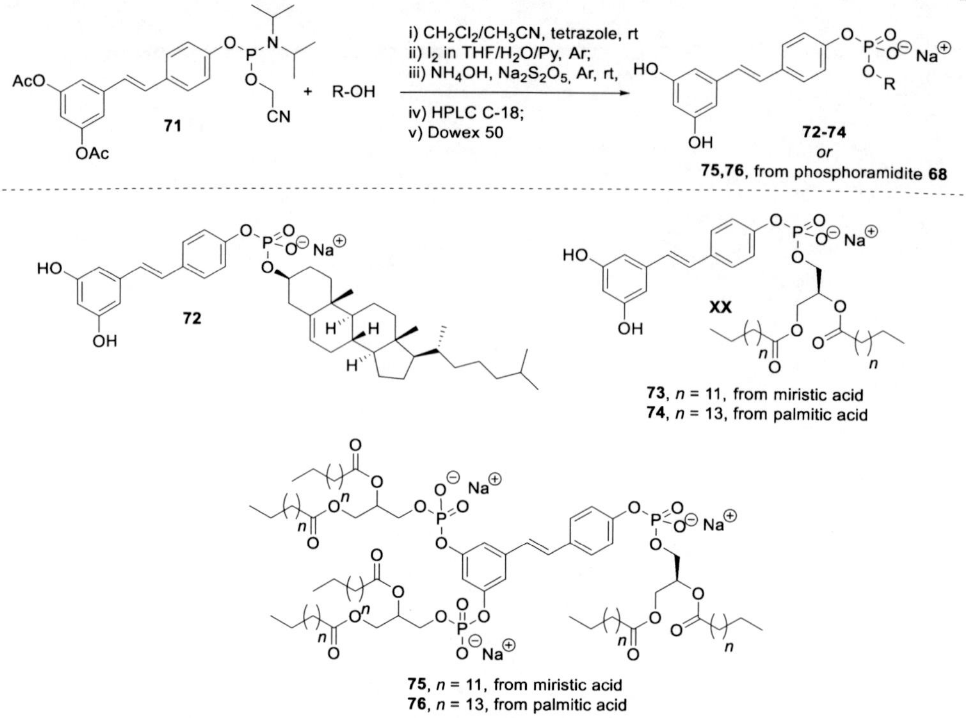

Scheme (9). Synthesis of resveratrol amphiphilic derivatives from phosphoramidites (selected examples).

Zhang *et al.* [43] exploited the molecular hybridization strategy to conjugate podophyllotoxin **80** with pterostilbene **38** and to develop the resveratrol-related potential multifunctional antineoplastic agent **82**. Reaction of pterostilbene **38** with the chloroacetate **81** in the presence of K_2CO_3 and KI afforded compound **82**. Chloride **81** was prepared upon reaction of podophyllotoxin with chloroacetyl chloride in the presence of Et_3N Scheme **(11)**.

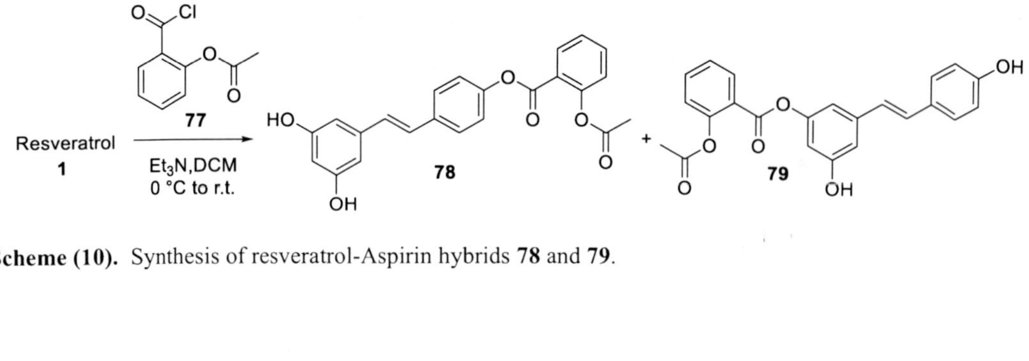

Scheme (10). Synthesis of resveratrol-Aspirin hybrids **78** and **79**.

Studies performed using human uveal melanoma cells (MUM-2B) demonstrate that **82** possesses antimigratory activity and is involved in the induction of cell cycle arrest at the S phase and in the apoptosis. Additionally, **82** was found to inhibit the expression of DNA topoisomerase IIα and IIβ through the simultaneous suppression of ERK1/2 and AKT pathways [43].

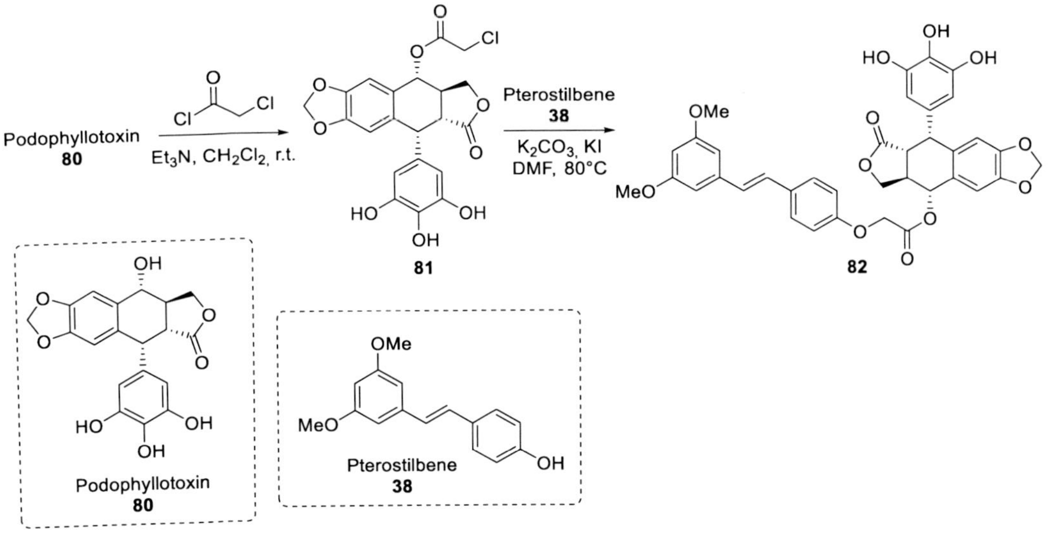

Scheme (11). Synthesis of resveratrol-related Podophyllotoxin-pterostilbene conjugate **82**.

An interesting semi-synthetic resveratrol derivative (structure **84**) with remarkable activity against human colorectal cancer HCT116 cells was recently reported by Okamoto *et al.* [44]. Compound **84** (named UHA6052), easily synthesised from caffeic acid **83** and resveratrol **1** in the presence of phosphoric acid Scheme **(12).**, exhibited almost the same inhibitory efficacy of 5-fluorouracil, a conventional anticancer drug. Notably, the IC_{50} value of **84** in inhibiting the proliferation of HCT116 cell spheroids in three-dimensional cultures (3DC) was determined to be 9.52 μM. The anti-colorectal cancer activity of **84**, about four-times higher than resveratrol, is related with the inhibition of an oncogenic KRAS-mediated signalling pathway.

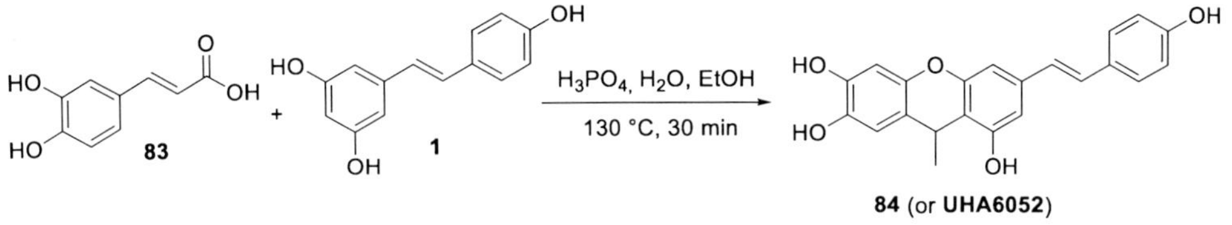

Scheme (12). Synthesis of resveratrol-caffeic acid conjugate **84**.

CONCLUSION

Stilbenoid-derived molecules and, more specifically, resveratrol-based compounds, represent an attractive and versatile tool in order to develop new potentially useful therapeutic agents.

Unfavourable pharmacokinetic and pharmacodynamic properties – including poor bioavailability, low aqueous solubility, and chemical instability – represent a significant hurdle for the clinical application of resveratrol. A broad range of structural modifications of resveratrol have been accomplished in order to modulate or enhance its properties and activities. The effect of several functionalisations, including the protection of phenolic groups (*i.e.*, etherification, esterification, glycosylation), the elaboration of the stilbene double bond (*i.e.*, epoxidation, epoxidation-ring-opening-based sequences, selenylation), and the introduction of additional substituents (*i.e.*, hydroxylation) onto the resorcin moiety of resveratrol has been investigated over the past decade. The conjugation of resveratrol with bio-active molecules enables to obtain new hybrids (*i.e.*, ebselen-like-resveratrol hybrids, aspirin-resveratrol hybrids) incorporating additional pharmacophores. A number of functionalised resveratrol-based compounds and resveratrol-derived hybrids have been developed as potential drug candidates with anticancer, antiviral, antibacterial, analgesic and antioxidant properties. The potential role of certain resveratrol derivatives in preventing or treating cardiovascular, Alzheimer's, and Parkinson's diseases has also been investigated.

In this *scenario*, several challenges, including the synthesis and the study of more complex polyfunctionalised structures, as well as the investigation of new hybrids of resveratrol with biologically active molecules and pharmacophores, remain ahead.

CONFLICT OF INTEREST

None Declared.

ACKNOWLEDGEMENT

None Declared.

CONSENT OF PUBLICATION

None

REFERENCES

[1] Kennedy, D.O. Polyphenols and the human brain: plant "secondary metabolite" ecologic roles and endogenous signaling functions drive benefits. *Adv. Nutr.*, **2014**, *5*(5), 515-533. [http://dx.doi.org/10.3945/an.114.006320] [PMID: 25469384]

[2] Renaud, S.; de Lorgeril, M. Wine, alcohol, platelets, and the French paradox for coronary heart disease. *Lancet,* **1992**, *339*(8808), 1523-1526. [http://dx.doi.org/10.1016/0140-6736(92)91277-F] [PMID: 1351198]

[3] Baur, J.A.; Sinclair, D.A. Therapeutic potential of resveratrol: the in vivo evidence. *Nat. Rev. Drug Discov.,* **2006**, *5*(6), 493-506. [http://dx.doi.org/10.1038/nrd2060] [PMID: 16732220]

[4] Biasutto, L.; Mattarei, A.; Azzolini, M.; La Spina, M.; Sassi, N.; Romio, M.; Paradisi, C.; Zoratti, M. Resveratrol derivatives as a pharmacological tool. *Ann. N. Y. Acad. Sci.,* **2017**, *1403*(1), 27-37. [http://dx.doi.org/10.1111/nyas.13401] [PMID: 28675763]

[5] Keylor, M.H.; Matsuura, B.S.; Stephenson, C.R.J. Chemistry and Biology of Resveratrol-Derived Natural Products. *Chem. Rev.,* **2015**, *115*(17), 8976-9027. [http://dx.doi.org/10.1021/cr500689b] [PMID: 25835567]

[6] Ahmadi, R.; Ebrahimzadeh, M.A. Resveratrol – A comprehensive review of recent advances in anticancer drug design and development. *Eur. J. Med. Chem.,* **2020**, *200*112356 [http://dx.doi.org/10.1016/j.ejmech.2020.112356] [PMID: 32485531]

[7] Mattio, L.M.; Catinella, G.; Pinto, A.; Dallavalle, S. Natural and nature-inspired stilbenoids as antiviral agents. *Eur. J. Med. Chem.,* **2020**, *202*112541 [http://dx.doi.org/10.1016/j.ejmech.2020.112541] [PMID: 32652408]

[8] Mattio, L.M.; Dallavalle, S.; Musso, L.; Filardi, R.; Franzetti, L.; Pellegrino, L.; D'Incecco, P.; Mora, D.; Pinto, A.; Arioli, S. Antimicrobial activity of resveratrol-derived monomers and dimers against foodborne pathogens. *Sci. Rep.,* **2019**, *9*(1), 19525. [http://dx.doi.org/10.1038/s41598-019-55975-1] [PMID: 31862939]

[9] Nakao, S.; Mabuchi, M.; Wang, S.; Kogure, Y.; Shimizu, T.; Noguchi, K.; Tanaka, A.; Dai, Y. Synthesis of resveratrol derivatives as new analgesic drugs through desensitization of the TRPA1 receptor. *Bioorg. Med. Chem. Lett.,* **2017**, *27*(14), 3167-3172. [http://dx.doi.org/10.1016/j.bmcl.2017.05.025] [PMID: 28576617]

[10] Tanini, D.; Panzella, L.; Amorati, R.; Capperucci, A.; Pizzo, E.; Napolitano, A.; Menichetti, S.; d'Ischia, M. Resveratrol-based benzoselenophenes with an enhanced antioxidant and chain breaking capacity. *Org. Biomol. Chem.,* **2015**, *13*(20), 5757-5764. [http://dx.doi.org/10.1039/C5OB00193E] [PMID: 25902184]

[11] Ruan, B.F.; Lu, X.Q.; Song, J.; Zhu, H.L. Derivatives of resveratrol: potential agents in prevention and treatment of cardiovascular disease. *Curr. Med. Chem.,* **2012**, *19*(24), 4175-4183. [http://dx.doi.org/10.2174/092986712802430054] [PMID: 22830334]

[12] Arbo, B.D.; André-Miral, C.; Nasre-Nasser, R.G.; Schimith, L.E.; Santos, M.G.; Costa-Silva, D.; Muccillo-Baisch, A.L.; Hort, M.A. Resveratrol derivatives as potential treatments for Alzheimer's and Parkinson's disease. *Front. Aging Neurosci.,* **2020**, *12*, 103. [http://dx.doi.org/10.3389/fnagi.2020.00103] [PMID: 32362821]

[13] Orsini, F.; Verotta, L.; Klimo, K.; Gerhäuser, C. Synthesis of resveratrol erivatives and *in vitro* screening for potential cancer chemopreventive activities. *Arch. Pharm. (Weinheim),* **2016**, *349*(6), 414-427. [http://dx.doi.org/10.1002/ardp.201600022] [PMID: 27159630]

[14] Pastorková, B.; Vrzalová, A.; Bachleda, P.; Dvořák, Z. Hydroxystilbenes and methoxystilbenes activate human aryl hydrocarbon receptor and induce CYP1A genes in human hepatoma cells and human hepatocytes. *Food Chem. Toxicol.,* **2017**, *103*, 122-132.

[http://dx.doi.org/10.1016/j.fct.2017.03.008] [PMID: 28279696]

[15] Hong, T.; Jiang, W.; Dong, H.M.; Qiu, S.X.; Lu, Y. Synthesis and cytotoxic activities of *E*-resveratrol derivatives. *Chin. J. Nat. Med.*, **2015**, *13*(5), 375-382.
[http://dx.doi.org/10.1016/S1875-5364(15)30029-7] [PMID: 25986287]

[16] Falomir, E.; Lucas, R.; Peñalver, P.; Martí-Centelles, R.; Dupont, A.; Zafra-Gómez, A.; Carda, M.; Morales, J.C. Cytotoxic, antiangiogenic and antitelomerase activity of glucosyl- and acyl- resveratrol prodrugs and resveratrol sulfate metabolites. *ChemBioChem*, **2016**, *17*(14), 1343-1348.
[http://dx.doi.org/10.1002/cbic.201600084] [PMID: 27147200]

[17] Das, J.; Pany, S.; Majhi, A. Chemical modifications of resveratrol for improved protein kinase C alpha activity. *Bioorg. Med. Chem.*, **2011**, *19*(18), 5321-5333.
[http://dx.doi.org/10.1016/j.bmc.2011.08.008] [PMID: 21880495]

[18] Yang, H.; Baur, J.A.; Chen, A.; Miller, C.; Sinclair, D.A.; Kisielewski, A.; Howitz, K.T.; Zipkin, R.E.; Sinclair, D.A. Design and synthesis of compounds that extend yeast replicative lifespan. *Aging Cell*, **2007**, *6*(1), 35-43.
[http://dx.doi.org/10.1111/j.1474-9726.2006.00259.x] [PMID: 17156081]

[19] Chelsky, Z.L.; Yue, P.; Kondratyuk, T.P.; Paladino, D.; Pezzuto, J.M.; Cushman, M.; Turkson, J. A Resveratrol analogue promotes ERKMAPK–dependent Stat3 serine and tyrosine phosphorylation alterations and antitumor effects *in vitro* against human tumor cells. *Mol. Pharmacol.*, **2015**, *88*(3), 524-533.
[http://dx.doi.org/10.1124/mol.115.099093] [PMID: 26138072]

[20] Peterson, J.; Doughty, H.; Eells, A.; Johnson, T.; Hastings, J.; Crowther, C.; Andrus, M.; Kenealey, J. The effects of 4′-esterified resveratrol derivatives on calcium dynamics in breast cancer cells. *Molecules*, **2017**, *22*(11), 1968.
[http://dx.doi.org/10.3390/molecules22111968] [PMID: 29135943]

[21] Hsieh, M.T.; Huang, L.J.; Wu, T.S.; Lin, H.Y.; Morris-Natschke, S.L.; Lee, K.H.; Kuo, S.C. Synthesis and antitumor activity of bis(hydroxymethyl)propionate analogs of pterostilbene in cisplatin-resistant human oral cancer cells. *Bioorg. Med. Chem.*, **2018**, *26*(14), 3909-3916.
[http://dx.doi.org/10.1016/j.bmc.2018.06.011] [PMID: 29908756]

[22] Kacprzak, K.; Urbaniak, A.; Warżajtis, B.; Rychlewska, U. Microwave-assisted synthesis of aromatic and aliphatic triesters of resveratrol. *Synthesis*, **2016**, *48*(7), 1002-1010.
[http://dx.doi.org/10.1055/s-0035-1561325]

[23] Urbaniak, A.; Delgado, M.; Kacprzak, K.; Chambers, T.C. Activity of resveratrol triesters against primary acute lymphoblastic leukemia cells. *Bioorg. Med. Chem. Lett.*, **2017**, *27*(12), 2766-2770.
[http://dx.doi.org/10.1016/j.bmcl.2017.04.066] [PMID: 28499732]

[24] Fu, J.; Shrivastava, A.; Shrivastava, S.; Srivastava, R.; Shankar, S. Triacetyl resveratrol upregulates miRNA□200 and suppresses the Shh pathway in pancreatic cancer: A potential therapeutic agent. *Int. J. Oncol.*, **2019**, *54*(4), 1306-1316.
[http://dx.doi.org/10.3892/ijo.2019.4700] [PMID: 30720134]

[25] Jin, L.; Ren, Y.J.; Du, C. Synthesis and antitumor activities of resveratrol derivatives on cervical cancer Hela cells. *Chem. Nat. Compd.*, **2015**, *51*(4), 652-655.
[http://dx.doi.org/10.1007/s10600-015-1377-6]

[26] Du, C.; Dong, M.H.; Ren, Y.J.; Jin, L.; Xu, C. Design, synthesis and antibreast cancer MCF-7 cells biological evaluation of heterocyclic analogs of resveratrol. *J. Asian Nat. Prod. Res.*, **2017**, *19*(9), 890-902.
[http://dx.doi.org/10.1080/10286020.2016.1250747] [PMID: 27809606]

[27] Liu, K.; Li, C.; Dai, L.; Liu, J.; Wang, L.; Lei, J.; Guo, L. Design, synthesis and in vivo antitumor efficacy of novel eight-arm-polyethylene glycol–pterostilbene prodrugs. *RSC Advances*, **2015**, *5*(64), 51592-51599.
[http://dx.doi.org/10.1039/C5RA06253E]

[28] Singh, V.P.; Poon, J.; Engman, L. Catalytic antioxidants: regenerable tellurium analogues of vitamin E. *Org. Lett.*, **2013**, *15*(24), 6274-6277.
[http://dx.doi.org/10.1021/ol403131t] [PMID: 24279415]

[29] Vraka, P.S.; Drouza, C.; Rikkou, M.P.; Odysseos, A.D.; Keramidas, A.D. Synthesis and study of the cancer cell growth inhibitory properties of α-, γ-tocopheryl and γ-tocotrienyl 2-phenylselenyl succinates. *Bioorg. Med. Chem.*, **2006**, *14*(8), 2684-2696.
[http://dx.doi.org/10.1016/j.bmc.2005.11.045] [PMID: 16378730]

[30] Fonseca, S.F.; Lima, D.B.; Alves, D.; Jacob, R.G.; Perin, G.; Lenardão, E.J.; Savegnago, L. Synthesis, characterization and antioxidant activity of organoselenium and organotellurium compound derivatives of chrysin. *New J. Chem.*, **2015**, *39*(4), 3043-3050.
[http://dx.doi.org/10.1039/C4NJ02329C]

[31] Tanini, D.; Degl'Innocenti, A.; Capperucci, A. Degl'Innocenti, A. Bis-(trimethylsilyl)selenide in the selective synthesis of β-hydroxy, β-mercapto, and β-amino diorganyl diselenides and selenides through ring opening of strained heterocycles. *Eur. J. Org. Chem.*, **2015**, *2015*(2), 357-369.
[http://dx.doi.org/10.1002/ejoc.201403015]

[32] Tanini, D.; Ricci, L.; Capperucci, A. Rongalite□promoted *on water* synthesis of functionalised tellurides and ditellurides. *Adv. Synth. Catal.*, **2020**, *362*(6), 1323-1332.
[http://dx.doi.org/10.1002/adsc.201901536]

[33] Viglianisi, C.; Vasa, K.; Tanini, D.; Capperucci, A.; Amorati, R.; Valgimigli, L.; Baschieri, A.; Menichetti, S. Ditocopheryl sulfides and disulfides: synthesis and antioxidant profile. *Chemistry,* **2019**, *25*(38), 9108-9116.
[http://dx.doi.org/10.1002/chem.201901537] [PMID: 31017702]

[34] Viglianisi, C.; Bonardi, C.; Ermini, E.; Capperucci, A.; Menichetti, S.; Tanini, D. Selenosilane-promoted selective mild transformation of *N*-thiophthalimides into symmetric disulfides. *Synthesis,* **2019**, *51*(8), 1819-1824.
[http://dx.doi.org/10.1055/s-0037-1610354]

[35] Tanini, D.; Lupori, B.; Malevolti, G.; Ambrosi, M.; Nostro, P.L.; Capperucci, A. Direct biocatalysed synthesis of first sulfur-, selenium- and tellurium- containing L -ascorbyl hybrid derivatives with radical trapping and GPx-like properties. *Chem. Commun. (Camb.),* **2019**, *55*(40), 5705-5708.
[http://dx.doi.org/10.1039/C9CC02427A] [PMID: 31033970]

[36] Tanini, D.; Scarpelli, S.; Ermini, E.; Capperucci, A. Seleno-Michael reaction of stable functionalised alkyl selenols: A versatile tool for the synthesis of acyclic and cyclic unsymmetrical alkyl and vinyl selenides. *Adv. Synth. Catal.*, **2019**, *361*(10), 2337-2346.
[http://dx.doi.org/10.1002/adsc.201900168]

[37] Domazetovic, V.; Fontani, F.; Tanini, D.; D'Esopo, V.; Viglianisi, C.; Marcucci, G.; Panzella, L.; Napolitano, A.; Brandi, M.L.; Capperucci, A.; Menichetti, S.; Vincenzini, M.T.; Iantomasi, T. Protective role of benzoselenophene derivatives of resveratrol on the induced oxidative stress in intestinal myofibroblasts and osteocytes. *Chem. Biol. Interact.*, **2017**, *275*, 13-21.
[http://dx.doi.org/10.1016/j.cbi.2017.07.015] [PMID: 28735861]

[38] Angeli, A.; Tanini, D.; Viglianisi, C.; Panzella, L.; Capperucci, A.; Menichetti, S.; Supuran, C.T. Evaluation of selenide, diselenide and selenoheterocycle derivatives as carbonic anhydrase I, II, IV, VII and IX inhibitors. *Bioorg. Med. Chem.*, **2017**, *25*(8), 2518-2523.
[http://dx.doi.org/10.1016/j.bmc.2017.03.013] [PMID: 28302505]

[39] Yan, J.; Guo, Y.; Wang, Y.; Mao, F.; Huang, L.; Li, X. Design, synthesis, and biological evaluation of benzoselenazole-stilbene hybrids as multi-target-directed anti-cancer agents. *Eur. J. Med. Chem.*, **2015**, *95*, 220-229.
[http://dx.doi.org/10.1016/j.ejmech.2015.03.030] [PMID: 25817772]

[40] Mrkus, L.; Batinić, J.; Bjeliš, N.; Jakas, A. Synthesis and biological evaluation of quercetin and resveratrol peptidyl derivatives as potential anticancer and antioxidant agents. *Amino Acids,* **2019**,

51(2), 319-329.
[http://dx.doi.org/10.1007/s00726-018-2668-6] [PMID: 30392096]

[41] Chillemi, R.; Cardullo, N.; Greco, V.; Malfa, G.; Tomasello, B.; Sciuto, S. Synthesis of amphiphilic resveratrol lipoconjugates and evaluation of their anticancer activity towards neuroblastoma SH-SY5Y cell line. *Eur. J. Med. Chem.*, **2015**, *96*, 467-481.
[http://dx.doi.org/10.1016/j.ejmech.2015.04.038] [PMID: 25932501]

[42] Zhu, Y.; Fu, J.; Shurlknight, K.L.; Soroka, D.N.; Hu, Y.; Chen, X.; Sang, S. Novel resveratrolbased aspirin prodrugs: synthesis, metabolism, and anticancer activity. *J. Med. Chem.*, **2015**, *58*(16), 6494-6506.
[http://dx.doi.org/10.1021/acs.jmedchem.5b00536] [PMID: 26204233]

[43] Zhang, L.; Wang, J.; Liu, L.; Zheng, C.; Wang, Y.; Chen, Y.; Wei, G. Podophyllotoxin–pterostilbene fused conjugates as potential multifunctional antineoplastic agents against human uveal melanoma cells. *RSC Advances*, **2017**, *7*(17), 10601-10608.
[http://dx.doi.org/10.1039/C6RA28832D]

[44] Okamoto, H.; Matsukawa, T.; Doi, S.; Tsunoda, T.; Sawata, Y.; Naemura, M.; Ohnuki, K.; Shirasawa, S.; Kotake, Y. A novel resveratrol derivative selectively inhibits the proliferation of colorectal cancer cells with KRAS mutation. *Mol. Cell. Biochem.*, **2018**, *442*(1-2), 39-45.
[http://dx.doi.org/10.1007/s11010-017-3191-x] [PMID: 28936721]

CHAPTER 9

Aurone Scaffold and Structural Analogues for the Development of Monoamine Oxidase (MAO) Inhibitors

Paolo Guglielmi[1], Virginia Pontecorvi[1,*] and Atilla Akdemir[2]

[1] *Department of Drug Chemistry and Technologies, Sapienza University of Rome, P.le A. Moro 5, 00185Rome, Italy*

[2] *Computer-aided Drug Discovery Laboratory, Department of Pharmacology, Bezmialem Vakif University, Fatih, Istanbul 34093, Turkey*

Abstract: Continuous efforts in the development of monoamine oxidase inhibitors prompted the search for effective strategies for the design of novel drugs candidate. Thankfully, nature often provides scaffolds useful for the promotion of novel exploitable chemical entities. In this regard, aurones (a class of uncommon flavonoids) and their structural related analogues may play an important role in the development of monoamine oxidase inhibitors. The target prediction of the simplest aurone (2-benzylidenebenzofuran-3(2*H*)-one) clearly suggests that this compound probably affects MAO (monoamine oxidase) enzymes, which is in accordance with the recently reported literature. The current chapter reports the recent discoveries involving aurones and their structurally related analogues as MAO inhibitors, describing detailed structure-activity relationships (SARs) for each subgroup of compounds.

Keywords: Aurones, Homoisoflavonoids, Indanones, MAO inhibitors, Monoamine oxidase, Neurodegenerative diseases, Tetralones.

INTRODUCTION

Human monoamine oxidases (hMAOs) are flavoenzymes that catalyze the oxidative deamination of dietary amines, monoamine neurotransmitters and hormones [1, 2]. The common substrates for MAO include important monoamine neurotransmitters such as dopamine, noradrenaline, adrenaline and serotonin [3]; this leads MAOs to play an important role in behavioral, cognitive, and endocrine regulation [4]. The specificity of MAO for its substrate depends on the concentration, affinity, and turnover rate of the substrate as well as the conc-

* **Corresponding author Paolo Guglielmi Ph.D:** Department of Drug Chemistry and Technologies, Sapienza University of Rome, P.le A. Moro 5, 00185 Rome, Italy; E-mail: paolo.guglielmi@uniroma1.it

Simone Carradori (Ed.)

entration of the enzyme [5]. Two human isoforms have been proposed and discovered, i.e., hMAO-A and hMAO-B. They are characterized by structural homology, active site differences and catalytic efficiency, tissue localization, substrate and inhibitor selectivity [6]. The two isoforms are quite similar, sharing ~70% overall sequence identity [7].

These enzymes are bound to the mitochondrial intermembrane *via* their transmembrane (TM) domains and their catalytic domain is located in the cytosol (Fig. **1**). They have subunit molecular weights of 59,700 (hMAO-A) and 58,000 (hMAO-B), consisting of 527 and 520 amino acids, respectively [3]. The (dimeric) holoenzyme has a covalently bound flavin adenine dinucleotide (FAD) cofactor for each subunit, which interacts with Cys406 of hMAO-A or Cys397 of hMAO-B, and an 'aromatic cage' which is the site where the amine group of the substrate binds and undergoes oxidation [3, 4, 7].

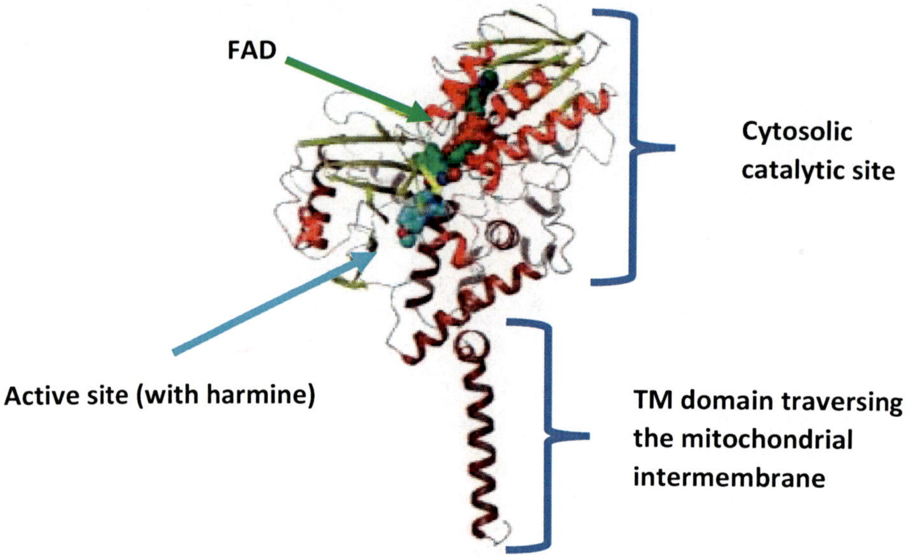

Fig. (1). The overall 3D structure of human MAO-A in complex with FAD (green CPK) and harmine (turquoise CPK). The cytosolic catalytic domain and the transmembrane (TM) domain that traverses the mitochondrial intermembrane are indicated.

The covalent binding of FAD seems to act as a structural core for the active conformation instead of being required for catalytic activity [5]. Both the isoforms share a substrate binding cavity of ~400 Å^3. hMAO-B is also endowed with a hydrophobic cavity of 290 Å^3, the "entrance cavity", which works as a "gate" for the "closed" or "open" conformations [7]. It has been discovered that aromatic and aliphatic residues seem to contribute to substrate selectivity of hMAO-A and hMAO-B [5].

The substrate binding site is located adjacent to the FAD binding site and consists of the conserved residues Tyr69, Tyr197, Phe208, Phe352, Tyr407, Trp441 and Tyr444 (Fig. **2**). Also conserved in both isozymes are Phe112, Trp128, Leu176 and Phe177, however, these residues have a significantly different conformation in hMAO-A and hMAO-B (Fig. **2**). The amino acids Ala111, Phe173, Ile180, Asn181 and Ile335 in hMAO-A are not conserved and their hMAO-B counterparts are Pro102, Leu164, Leu171, Cys172 and Tyr326. This changes the shape and binding characteristics of the substrate binding sites.

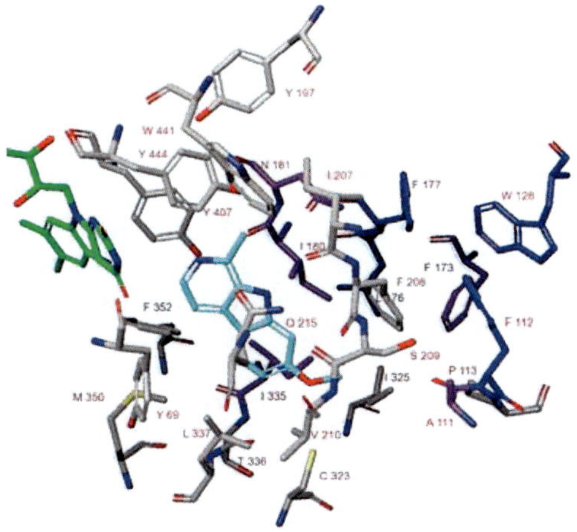

Fig. (2). The active site of hMAO-A in complex with harmine (pdb: 2z5y). The conserved amino acids are indicated in light grey. The amino acids that are different in hMAO-B are indicated in purple (A111, F173, I180, N181 and I335). The amino acids that are conserved but have different conformations are indicated in dark blue (F112, W128, L176 and F177). FAD is indicated in green and only partly shown for clarity reasons. The ligand harmine is indicated in turquoise.

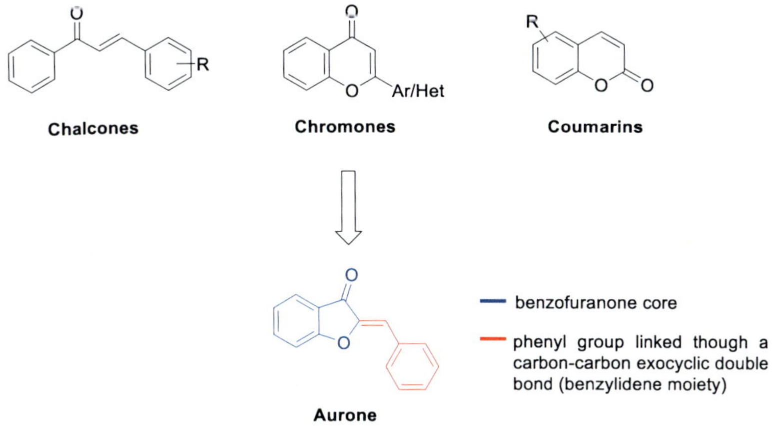

Fig. (3). Structure of chalcones, chromones and coumarins. Structural correlation between flavonoids and aurones.

The products derived from hMAO enzymatic activity are aldehydes and ammonium ion [8]; the flavin, which undergoes a two-electron reduction with substrate oxidation, is re-oxidized by molecular oxygen to generate hydrogen peroxide as a by-product. For each equivalent of substrate oxidized by MAO, one equivalent of hydrogen peroxide is produced [4]. The abnormal expression or increased activity of hMAOs leads to the excessive production of H_2O_2 that can expose cells to oxidative damage [8]. In fact, it has been proposed that hydrogen peroxide generated by MAO in the brain may react with ferrous ion (Fe^{2+}) in the Fenton reaction leading to hydroxyl radical, which reacts with biomolecules causing its damage [4]. For this reason, MAO-mediated oxidative stress has been associated with different neurodegenerative pathologies as well as cardiomyopathies [8]. The presence of MAO in most tissues appears to reflect a functional need: MAO-A is the dominant isoform in the gastrointestinal tract, placenta and heart, while MAO-B predominates in platelets and glial cells in the brain [4, 5]. The distribution of MAO-A and -B in the brain is related to their difference in substrate specificities [4]: while MAO-A is predominantly found in catecholaminergic neurons, MAO-B is the most abundant form in serotonergic and histaminergic neurons and is mostly expressed in the *substantia nigra* and periventricular region of the hypothalamus [5, 9]. The two MAO enzymes share similar affinity for dopamine, noradrenaline, adrenaline, and tyramine. MAO-A preferential substrates are serotonin, noradrenaline, and adrenaline; clorgyline is a selective MAO-A inhibitor. Instead, MAO-B prefers PEA (β-phenylethylamine) and benzylamine as a substrate and is inactivated by deprenyl, as a selective inhibitor [3, 8, 9]. Recent studies revealed that the inhibitors of MAO-A and -B should contain one or more hydrophobic rings, preferably aromatic or heteroaromatic nuclei, hydrogen bond acceptors and hydrogen bond donors [10]. The inhibition of hMAO, especially of hMAO-B, has been demonstrated to confer neuroprotection through anti-apoptotic mechanisms, reduction of reactive oxygen species production and stabilization of the mitochondrial membrane [9]. This suggests how MAO inhibitors may have a role as protective and therapeutic agents. Many scaffolds, synthetic or naturally occurring, have been proposed as effective inhibitors of these enzymes [10 - 14]. Among the preferred ones, almost three come from natural compounds: chalcones, coumarins and 4*H*-chromen-4-one (chromones) which are the central nucleus of flavonoids and isoflavonoids [15, 16] (Fig. **3**). These scaffolds have inspired the production of effective hMAOs inhibitors; furthermore, when properly decorated, also multitarget directed ligands (MTDLs) useful for neurodegenerative disorders such as Alzheimer's or Parkinson's diseases (AD and PD, respectively), have been developed based on these structural motifs [17 - 26]. In the last years, another uncommon flavonoid is fascinating as a valid structure to develop effective hMAO inhibitors: aurone (Fig. **3**).

AURONES AND THEIR STRUCTURAL-RELATED COMPOUNDS

Aurones are structural isomers of the well-known flavones, comprising a benzofuran-3(*2H*)-one (benzofuranone) core and a phenyl group linked through a carbon-carbon exocyclic double bond (benzylidene moiety). Such compounds, along with chalcones, dihydrochalcones, flavanones and dihydroflavonols possess a limited abundance in nature: in fact they are considered as minor flavonoids [27]. Although aurones have been mainly found in eudicots, specifically *Anacardiaceae*, *Asteraceae*, *Gesneriaceae*, *Fabaceae*, *Oxalidaceae*, *Plumbaginaceae*, *Rubiaceae*, *Rhamnaceae*, *Rosaceae*, *Cactaceae*, *Moraceae* or *Plantaginaceae* families, some of them were also isolated from advanced monocots, such as *Cyperaceae*. By performing the target prediction, using the freely-available web-tool SwissTargetPrediction for the simplest aurone (2-benzylidenebenzofuran-3(*2H*)-one), it turns out that MAOs are the enzymes with a putative probability of been affected by this compound (Fig. **4**) [28].

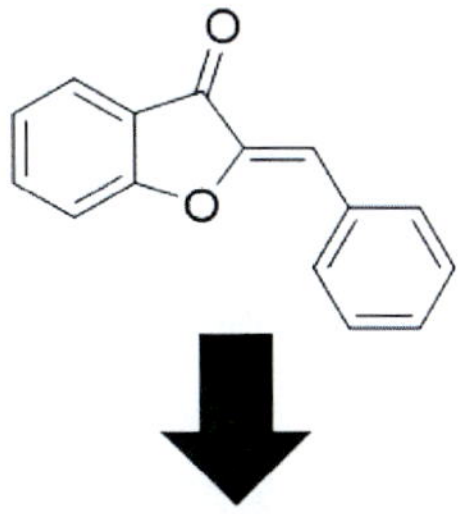

Target	Common name	Uniprot ID	ChEMBL ID	Target Class	Probability*	Known actives (3D/2D)
Monoamine oxidase B	MAOB	P27338	CHEMBL2039	Oxidoreductase		272 / 90
Monoamine oxidase A	MAOA	P21397	CHEMBL1951	Oxidoreductase		129 / 28
Leukocyte elastase	ELANE	P08246	CHEMBL248	Protease		107 / 10
Vascular endothelial growth factor receptor 2	KDR	P35968	CHEMBL279	Kinase		85 / 2
Stem cell growth factor receptor	KIT	P10721	CHEMBL1936	Kinase		5 / 1
Glycogen synthase kinase-3 beta	GSK3B	P49841	CHEMBL262	Kinase		52 / 3
Serine/threonine-protein kinase Aurora-C	AURKC	Q9UQB9	CHEMBL3935	Kinase		0 / 1

Fig. (4). Prediction of putative targets of the simplest aurone obtained with the web-tool SwissTargetPrediction platform [28].

For this reason, an increasing number of works are focusing on this scaffold for the development of effective MAO inhibitors or MTDL analogues. Taking advantage by pharmaceutical chemistry approaches such as isosteric replacement as well as ring expansion, a series of analogues related to the aurone scaffold have been developed (Fig. **5**). This chapter reports the works published in the last five years describing the employment of the aurones and their structurally related analogues, indanones, tetralones and 3-benzylidenechroman-4-ones (homoisoflavonoids), as monoamine oxidase inhibitors. Chalcones should be considered as the opened analogues of aurones, as well; however, they have been extensively reviewed recently and will not deepened furtherly [7].

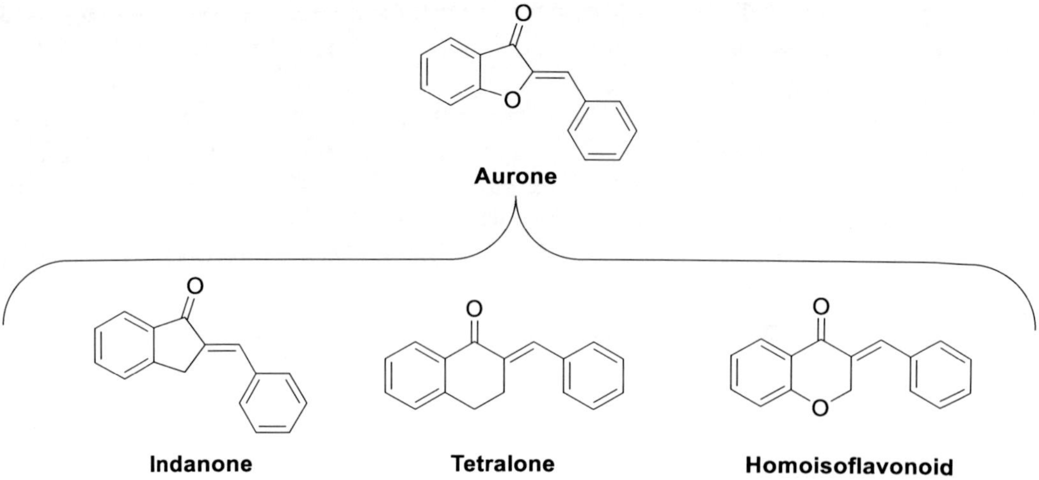

Fig. (5). Aurone and its structural related scaffolds.

Aurones

Aurones can be considered as the closed analogues coming from cyclization of 2-hydroxychalcones, whose ability to inhibit MAO enzymes has been widely reported (Fig. **6**) [7, 29]. On the basis of this concept, Morales-Camilo and colleagues developed a library of aurones starting from the corresponding "opened" analogues, i.e. chalcones, and evaluated them against rat monoamine oxidases A and B (rMAO-A and rMAO-B) (Fig. **6**), **II**) [30]. This was the first work reporting the employment of the aurone scaffold for the inhibition of MAOs even if the inhibition data were not remarkable. Eight aurones endowed with different substituents were screened against rMAO isoforms at 10 μM concentration, at first, exhibiting preference for the B isoform. However, only four compounds with appreciable inhibition rate were further investigated for IC_{50} evaluation (Fig. **6**), **II**), exhibiting micromolar inhibition of rMAO-B ($11.6 < IC_{50}$ (μM) < 26.3). The effects of substituents on the benzylidene moiety phenyl ring did not exhibit a clear correlation or trend. However, crowded phenyl ring containing two or more substituents was well tolerated by the scaffold. The presence of substituents, as well as their position on the benzofuran-3(2*H*)-one core, plays an important role influencing activity and selectivity of the aurones. In this regard, methoxy group placed on the benzofuran-3(2*H*)-one core was better tolerated in position 5 instead of 4 (Fig. **6**), **II**).

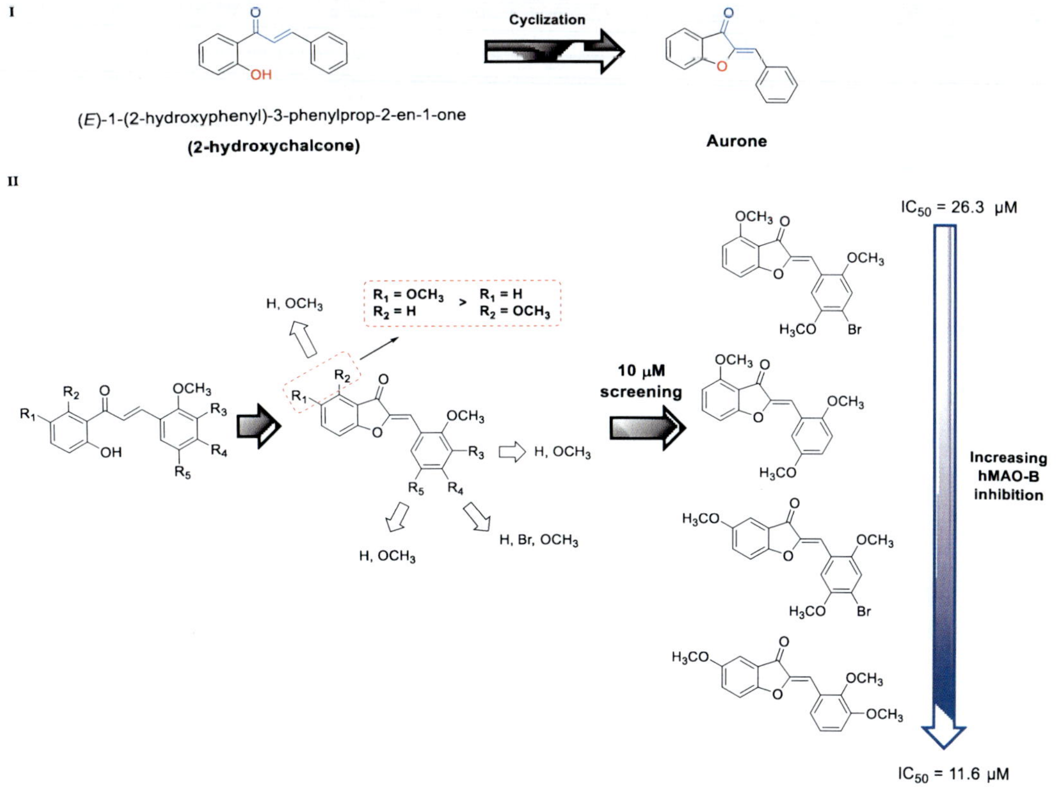

Fig. (6). I) Structural correlation between 2-hydoxychalcone and aurone scaffold. **II)** SAR of the first MAO inhibitors based on aurone motif.

The introduction of a 6-OH group on the benzofuran-3(2*H*)-one core seems to positively affect the activity and selectivity against MAO-A. As a matter of fact, the natural derived compounds hispidol and sulfuretin, endowed with this molecular attribute, exhibited selectivity against this isoform Table **1**. A similar behaviour was also shown by aurones developed by Li and colleagues (see below) [31, 32].

Hispidol and sulfuretin were extracted from *Glycine max* Merrill and *Toxicodendron vernicifluum*, respectively, and purified for evaluation against hMAOs. Both the analogues inhibited preferentially the A isoform and possessed hydroxy-substituted benzylidene phenyl ring. Interestingly, the addition of a second OH group on this moiety (sulfuretin) led to the drop of the inhibitory activity against both the isoforms, although with a minor extent for hMAO-A, thus increasing the selectivity against this isoform. Hispidol exhibited a reversible inhibition (with 80% of the activity recovered after dialysis) and a competitive mechanism of action against both the hMAOs.

Table 1. Structure and inhibitory activity of hispidol and sulfuretin. Selectivity Index (SI) is defined as the IC_{50} ratio between hMAO-B/hMAO-A.

Name	Structure	IC_{50} (μM)		SI
		hMAO-A	hMAO-B	
Hispidol	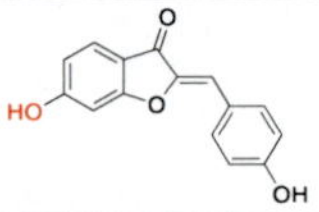	0.26	2.45	9.4
Sulfuretin	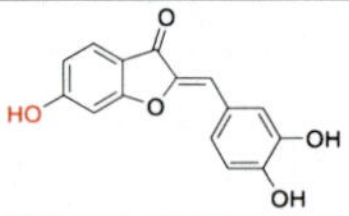	4.16	> 80	> 19.2

With the aim of developing multifunctional agents for AD, Li and co-workers investigated a small library of 4-hydroxyl aurones gifted with different substituents to assure anti A*β*-aggregation, hMAO inhibition, antioxidant and biometal chelating properties [32]. In addition to the hydroxyl group kept constant at position 4 of all the compounds, the position 6 of benzofuranone core was decorated with three different substituents: hydroxy, methoxy and dimethylamino group (Fig. 7). Moreover, a series of aliphatic and cycloaliphatic amines were evaluated as substituents of the phenyl ring. The initial screening performed against the two hMAO isoforms evidenced a different selectivity depending on the substituent placed at position 6 of the benzofuranone ring. The presence of 6-OH, in addition to the one placed at position 4, favoured the selectivity against hMAO-A (as previously observed for hispidol and sulfuretin). The presence of 6-OCH_3, instead, moved the selectivity towards hMAO-B. This behaviour is addressable, mainly, to the effect of OH/OCH_3 substitutions on hMAO-A inhibition. In general, the hydroxy group sited at position 6 clearly improved inhibitory activity against both the isoforms, particularly promoting the hMAO-A inhibition. On the contrary, 6-OCH_3 slightly increased the affinity against hMAO-B while leading to a clear decrease in the inhibitory activity against the A isoform. The evaluation of the dimethylamino group as a substituent at position 6 of the benzofuranone ring, did not show noteworthy results, being the only analogue endowed with this attribute inactive against both the isoforms (IC_{50} > 10 μM). Similarly, the derivatives obtained through the benzylidene double bond reduction were ineffective, not reaching the 50% inhibition limit of the initial screening performed at the concentration of 10 μM (Fig. 7). The addition of substituents on the benzylidene phenyl ring led to outcomes that did not display a general inhibitory activity trend. The hMAO-B inhibition was impaired by introducing dimethylamino group, regardless of the substitution of the benzofuranone core. In the presence of the 6-OH-benzofuran-3(2*H*)-one ring, the cyclic aliphatic amines favoured hMAO-B selectivity, while the non-cyclic amines moved the preference against the A isoform, with the dimethylethylamino group promoting the best hMAO-A inhibition (IC_{50} hMAO-A = 0.0279 μM, SI > 0.035).

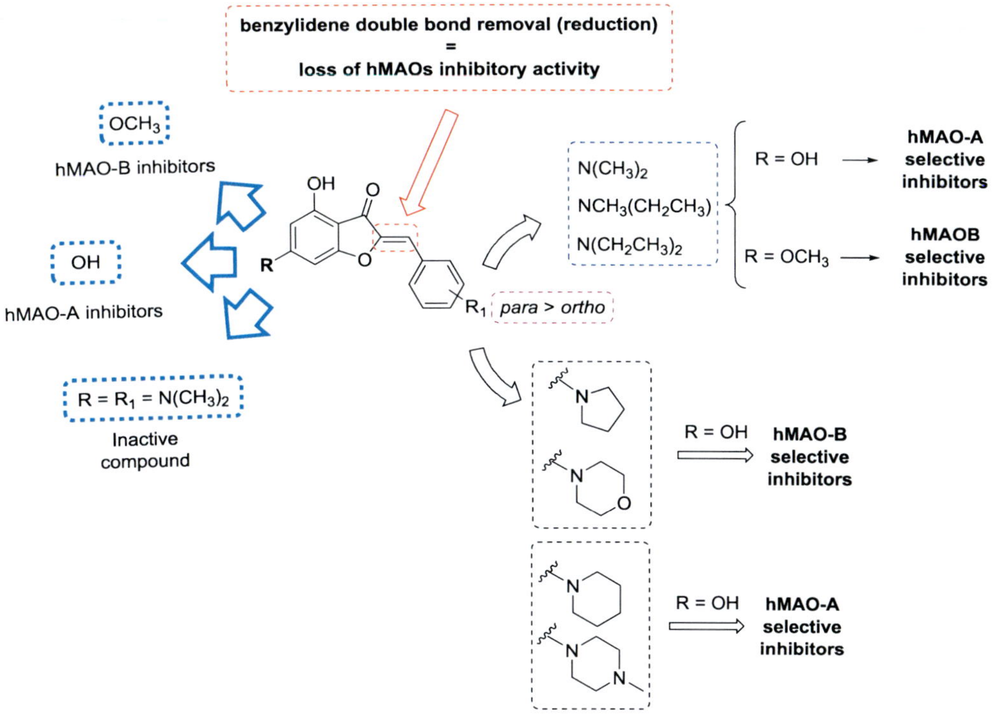

Fig. (7). Structure and SAR of the multitarget aurones developed by Li and co-workers [32].

The best hMAO-B inhibitor of this library was obtained through the substitution of the 6th position of the benzofuran-3(2*H*)-one moiety with methoxy group along the benzylidene endowed with 4-piperidine moiety (IC_{50} hMAO-B = 0.226 μM, SI > 44.248). This compound was also investigated by parallel artificial membrane permeability assay (PAMPA-BBB) to evaluate its ability to cross the blood brain barrier (BBB), showing that it should be able to reach CNS (central nervous system). Docking studies performed for the two hMAO isoforms with non-selective and hMAO-B selective inhibitors, respectively, demonstrated that the distribution inside the active sites was similar, with the benzofuranone ring accommodated next to the FAD cofactor, establishing parallel π-π interactions with Tyr326. On the contrary, the benzylidene moiety was distributed in the entrance cavity proving π-π interactions with Phe208. The reasons of the different selectivity between the two compounds have to be searched in the different hydrogen bond network that takes place inside the two hMAO isoforms, depending on the inhibitor's substituents.

A similar approach was employed by Liew and colleagues that developed six small libraries of compounds differing for the substituents placed on the benzofuran-3(2*H*)-one ring as well as the benzylidene/arylidene one (Fig. **8**) [33]. After screening at the concentration of 50 μM, only the analogues exhibiting more than 75% inhibition were evaluated in further deepening. All the compounds were devoid of noteworthy affinity against hMAO-A (% hMAO-A inhibition $< 75\%$ at 50 μM), while some analogues inhibited hMAO-B in the micromolar range ($0.895 < IC_{50}$ (μM) < 13.3).

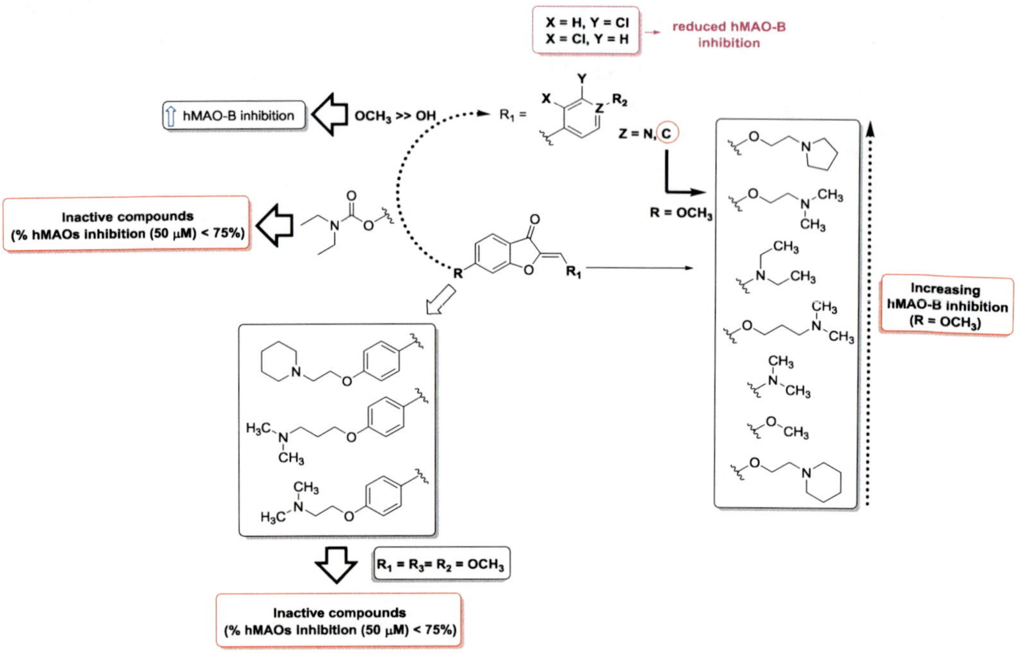

Fig. (8). Structure and SAR of the multitarget aurones developed by Liew and colleagues [33].

As already observed for Li's compounds, the substitution of the benzofuranone core at the position 6 with the methoxy group elicited, compared to the hydroxyl one, the improvement of the hMAO-B inhibition. The best inhibitor of the series belonged to the analogues endowed with this molecular attribute along with 2-(pyrrolidin-1-yl)ethanol moiety bound at the *para* position of the benzylidene phenyl ring (IC_{50} hMAO-B = 0.895 μM) (Fig. **8**). The introduction of chlorine atom at the positions 2 or 3 of the same ring was not tolerated leading to the loss of affinity against hMAO-B. The replacement of the 6-methoxy group with the bulkier carbamoyl one led to weak inhibitors, not achieving the 75% inhibition limit. It has been also assessed the challenge to "reverse" the substitution pattern by distributing the methoxy group on benzylidene phenyl ring, thus displacing the amine substituents on the benzofuranone. However, this attempt was ineffective leading to few compounds with acceptable hMAO-B inhibitory activity.

Takao and co-workers developed a series of aurone derivatives containing (un)substituted indole ring as the arylidene part and bound to (un)substituted benzofuran-3(*2H*)-one core (Fig. **8**) [34]. Apart from the derivative substituted at the position 5 of benzofuranone ring with OCH_3, exhibiting micromolar inhibition against hMAO-A (K_i = 14 μM), all the derivatives were ineffective against this isoform (K_i > 100 μM), regardless the substituents. On the contrary, these compounds were effective sub-micromolar inhibitors of hMAO-B (0.12 ≤K_i (μM) ≤ 0.0026), except for the analogue unsubstituted at the benzofuran core and binding 3-methyl indole, resulting inactive against both the isoforms (K_i hMAO-A/B > 100 μM) (Fig. **8**). For the other compounds with unsubstituted benzofuranone ring, the insertion of methyl group at the position 5 of the indanone moiety led to a slight increase of the activity (K_i hMAO-B = 0.032 μM); the same group placed at the position 6 was also tolerated, maintaining the inhibitory activity similar to the unsubstituted one (K_i hMAO-B = 0.039 μM).

The addition of methoxy group at position 6 of the benzofuranone core, positively affected the hMAO-B inhibitory activity leading to 15-fold reduction of the K_i (K_i hMAO-B = 0.0026 μM) if compared to the compound bearing unsubstituted indole (K_i hMAO-B = 0.039 μM) and to 2-fold reduction if compared to the K_i of the ones bearing 5-CH_3 and 4-OCH_3 (Fig. **9**).

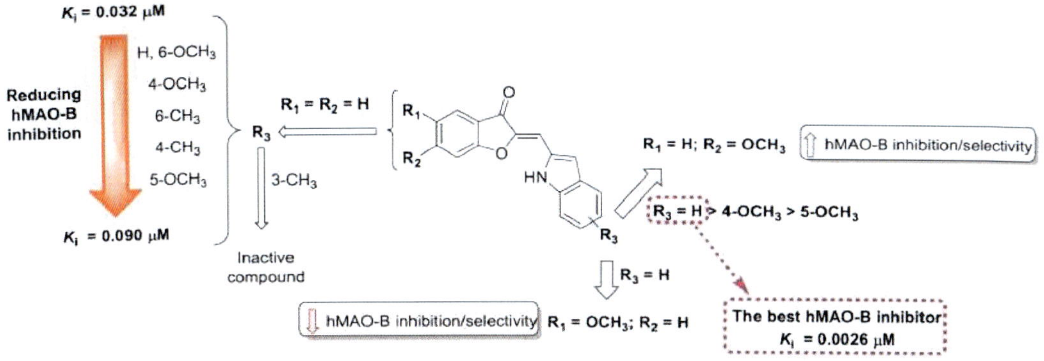

Fig. (9). Structure and SAR of the indole-aurones.

The same effect was not obtained by placing the methoxy group at the position 5 of the benzofuranone ring, leading to a very weak inhibition of hMAO-A and reducing the affinity against hMAO-B (K_i hMAO-A = 14 μM; K_i hMAO-B = 0.15 μM).

Indanone and Tetralone Derivatives

Indanone scaffolds come from the isosteric replacement of the oxygen atom of the aurone core with the methylene group (Fig. **5**). In two different works Petzer and co-workers evaluated the ability of compounds based on this scaffold to inhibit both the hMAO isoforms [35, 36]. One of the two works focused on 2-benzylidene-1-indanones, bearing substituents on the 2,3-dihydro-1*H*-inden-1-one system (also reported in this text as indanone core) as well as benzylidene phenyl ring [35] Fig. (**10,I**). These compounds inhibited preferentially hMAO-B, although most of them exhibited micromolar/sub-micromolar inhibitory activity against the A isoform. In general, the substitution of the indanone core with hydroxy or methoxy group at different positions, elicited effects on both inhibitory activity and selectivity. The hydroxyl group placed at position 6 promoted the hMAO-A selectivity, while the same group moved at position 5, shifted the selectivity to the B isoform, also improving the inhibitory activity with respect to the unsubstituted one (Fig. **10**, **I**, R = H). Regarding hMAO-B inhibition, the methoxy substitution of the indanone ring at position 5 promoted the best effects, effectively increasing inhibitory activity and selectivity (IC_{50} hMAO-B = 0.0092 μM, SI > 10.870). All these SAR results have been obtained for compounds lacking substituents on the benzylidene phenyl ring Fig. (**10, II**). Even though 5-OCH_3 substitution gave the best hMAO-B inhibition results, most of the derivatives of this series were gifted with 5-OH on the 2,3-dihydro-1*H*-inden-1-one. These compounds were provided of substituents placed at different positions of the benzylidene phenyl ring, thus allowing SAR expansion. In general, the introduction of substituents on the phenyl ring positively affected the affinity against hMAO-B, if compared to the unsubstituted compound. Lipophilic groups placed at the *para* position elicited nanomolar inhibitory activity against hMAO-B, as observed for 4-CH_3 (IC_{50} hMAO-B = 0.0052 μM, SI = 619) as well as 4-Br (IC_{50} hMAO-B = 0.0053 μM, SI = 198) substituted compounds, these last ones being the best hMAO-B inhibitors of the library (Fig. **10**, **I**). These substitutions also influenced the hMAO-A inhibitory activity, impaired in a major extent by the 4-CH_3 group, thus justifying the higher selectivity index against hMAO-B. The same groups placed at different positions of the phenyl ring, still increased the hMAO-B inhibitory activity albeit in a lesser degree.

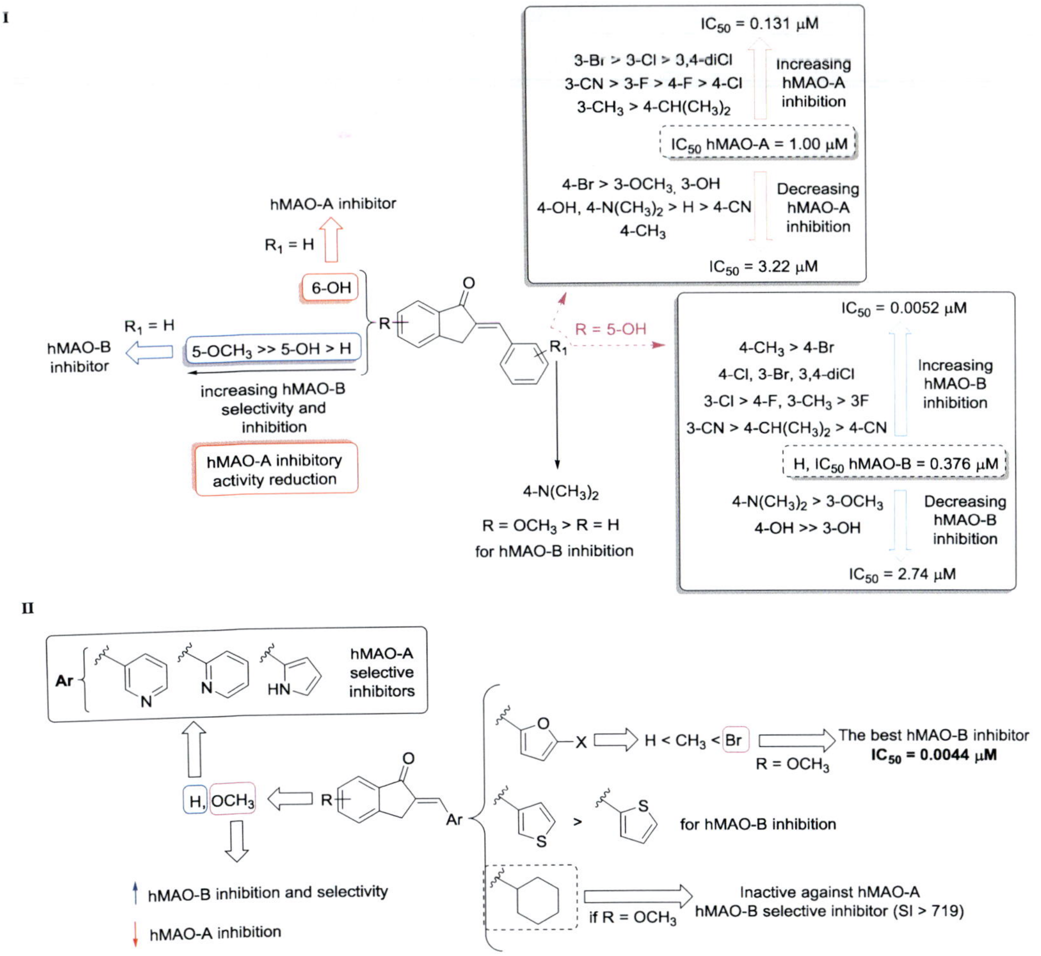

Fig. (10). Structure and SAR of (I) 2-benzylidene-indanones and (II) 2-heteroarylidene-indanones.

The insertion of substituents like CN or the bulkier $CH(CH_3)_2$ at the *para* position led to weakly improvement of the inhibitory activity against both isoforms, while the 4-F substitution slightly increased the hMAO-B affinity, reducing the hMAO-A one. The hydrophilic electron donating group OH was not tolerated by this scaffold, leading to the loss of activity against the hMAO-A and B isoforms, regardless the bound position.

The second set of compounds developed by the same research group was based on analogues that undergone the replacement of the phenyl ring with heterocycles or cycloalkanes [36]. Most of these derivatives still maintained a preference for hMAO-B albeit some of them were selective sub-micromolar inhibitors of hMAO-A. In this regard, the best results were obtained with 2-pyridyl (IC_{50} hMAO-A = 0.853 μM, SI = 0.56) and 3-pyridyl ring (IC_{50} hMAO-A = 0.061 μM, SI = 0.05) bound to unsubstituted indanone core; indeed, the presence of the methoxy group at position 5 of indanone improved the activity and selectivity against hMAO-B also impairing the affinity towards hMAO-A (Fig. **10**, **II**). Among the evaluated heterocycles, the best results were obtained with the furan one, especially if substituted with lipophilic groups. As a matter of fact, the best hMAO-B inhibitor of this library was provided of this characteristic, containing the 5-bromofuran as arylidene part (IC_{50} hMAO-B = 0.0044 μM, SI = 42); similarly, the presence of a methyl group in the same position of the furan ring was beneficial for hMAO-B inhibition (even if in a minor extent) and led to a 4-fold increase of selectivity (IC_{50} hMAO-B = 0.026 μM, SI = 182). In this regard, the most selective derivative was obtained through the insertion of the cyclohexyl moiety bound to 5-OCH_3 substituted 2,3-dihydro-1*H*-inden-1-one ring, albeit showing moderate inhibitory activity (IC_{50} hMAO-B = 0.139 μM, SI > 719)

Fig. (**10**, **II**). The compounds belonging to both the libraries were investigated through docking analysis to understand the binding mode inside the hMAO active site. These studies demonstrated that these derivatives distributed preferentially the indanone core close to the FAD cofactor, establishing interaction with Tyr398 and Tyr435 by means of π- π inter actions. In contrast, the benzylidene / heteroarylidene ring is in the entrance cavity, a hydrophobic space that should justify the reason why the addition of lipophilic groups on phenyl/heteroaryl ring usually led to the increase of the inhibitory activity.

Affini and colleagues designed a series of multi-targeting directed ligands (MTDLs) based on indanone motif, able to affect hMAO-B as well as H_3 receptors (H_3R) for PD treatment Fig. (**11**, **I**) [37]. The authors explored three different strategies based on the introduction of H_3R structural elements on the indanone scaffold selected to assure hMAO-B inhibition. In the first strategy the attachment of the H_3R motif (piperidine- or pyrrolidine(alkyloxy)) at positions 5 or 6 of the indanone core was evaluated (not shown). The other two sets of compounds were obtained by linking the H_3R pharmacophore, the piperidine-alkyloxy moiety, on the 2-benzylidene-1-indanone scaffold either on the indanone core or on the benzylidene phenyl ring. All the obtained analogues were screened at a fixed concentration (10 μM) against the hMAO isoforms, evidencing hMAO-B selectivity (Fig. **11**, **I**). Most of them did not reach the threshold value of 75% inhibition except the three of them endowed with this potency and further explored for IC_{50} evaluation. However, some information can be obtained from the screening performed at 10 μM, too. For the compounds bearing the H_3R motif bound on the indanone core emerged as the length of the chain influenced the affinity against hMAO-B. The increase of the alkyl chain length from ethylene to propylene one, led to hMAO-B inhibition impairment, while the change of the H_3R moiety position (5 and 6 on the indanone core) maintaining the same chain dimension (n = 3), was tolerated giving similar results Fig. (**11, I**).

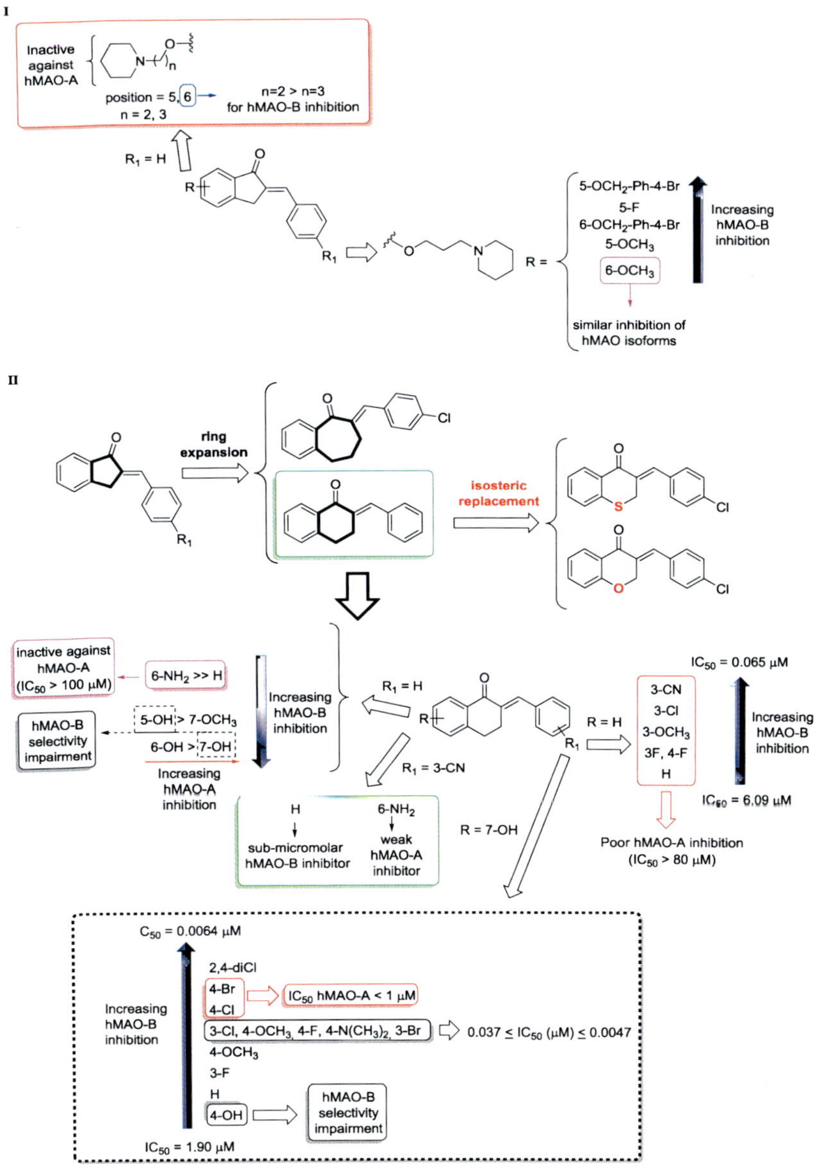

Fig. (11). Structure and SAR of **(I)** multi-targeting directed indanones, **(II)** tetralone-based hMAO-B inhibitors.

Concerning the compounds binding the H_3R moiety on the benzylidene phenyl ring, the piperidine-propyloxy as H_3R pharmacophore was selected, introducing substituents at different positions (5 or 6) of the indanone core. The same substituents gave better results when placed at position 5 than 6, particularly with methoxy and 4-bromobenzyloxy groups. The best hMAO-B inhibitors of this library were endowed with 5-F (IC_{50} = 1.93 μM; after 30' preincubation, IC_{50} = 0.54 μM) and 5-(4-bromobenzyloxy) (IC_{50} = 0.276 μM; after 30' preincubation, IC_{50} = 0.262 μM) substituted indanone (Fig. **11**, **I**), the former also showing 3.5-fold shift of IC_{50} value towards nanomolar concentration after incubation, thus accounting for a slow reversible or tight binding inhibition mode in the conditions used for the tests.

The tetralone scaffold came from the ring expansion of the indanone one Fig. (**3**). This structure was explored for its ability to inhibit hMAO enzymes by Petzer and collaborators that examined a series of changes based on ring expansion and isosteric replacement performed on the 2-benzylidene-1-indanone motif Fig. (**11**, **II**) [38]. Among the modifications attempted, only the one affording the 4-chromanone scaffold led to the improvement of hMAO-B inhibitory activity (all the compounds were selective hMAO-B inhibitors), being all the others weaker inhibitors than the indanone one.

However, to expand the knowledge and perform SAR studies, a series of derivatives based on the tetralone scaffold was developed and evaluated for their inhibitory activity against hMAO enzymes Fig. (**11**, **II**). All the tetralone analogues were selective hMAO-B inhibitors, regardless of the bound substituents. The tetralone moiety was unchanged (R = H, Fig. **11**, **II**) or substituted with NH_2, OH or OCH_3 at positions 5, 6 and 7. In the presence of unsubstituted benzylidene moiety, the affinity against hMAO-B was increased mainly by the hydroxyl group, particularly when placed at position 6. The amino group bound at position 6 of the tetralone ring linked to unsubstituted benzylidene moiety, led to a completely inactive molecule against hMAO-A (IC_{50} hMAO-A > 100 μM); however, the 3-CN substitution of the benzylidene phenyl ring completely reversed the activity, producing weak but selective hMAO-A inhibitor (IC_{50} hMAO-B > 100 μM). A small library of analogues bearing 7-OH substituted tetralone core was synthesised with the aim to evaluate the effects of different substituents on the benzylidene phenyl ring Fig. (**11**, **II**). The best hMAO-B inhibitory activity results were exhibited by halogens, particularly if placed at the *para* position, promoting sub-micromolar inhibition of the hMAO-A, too. Consequently, the best hMAO-B inhibitor of the library was the one gifted with 3,4-dichloro phenyl ring (IC_{50} = 0.0064 μM). In general, lipophilic substituents positively affected the affinity against hMAO-B, while hydrophilic groups as the hydroxy one bound at the *para* position were not tolerated.

Similar to indanones, the tetralone analogues were investigated through docking studies to understand the distribution inside the active site of the hMAO-B, revealing a similarity between the two models. Indeed, both the scaffolds located the bicyclic system (indanone or tetralone) close to the FAD by interacting with the Tyr398 and Tyr435 through stacking π-π interactions. Furthermore, the benzylidene phenyl moiety is positioned in the entrance cavity where it can establish van der Waals interactions, explaining the improving effects elicited by lipophilic substituents placed on the benzylidene phenyl ring.

The tetralone scaffold was also investigated for the development of multifunctional compounds for the treatment of AD [39]. A library of 33 derivatives were synthesised and evaluated against rMAO enzymes, over than cholinesterase ones, exhibiting moderate inhibition of both rMAO isoforms with a slight preference for the B one Fig. (**12**).

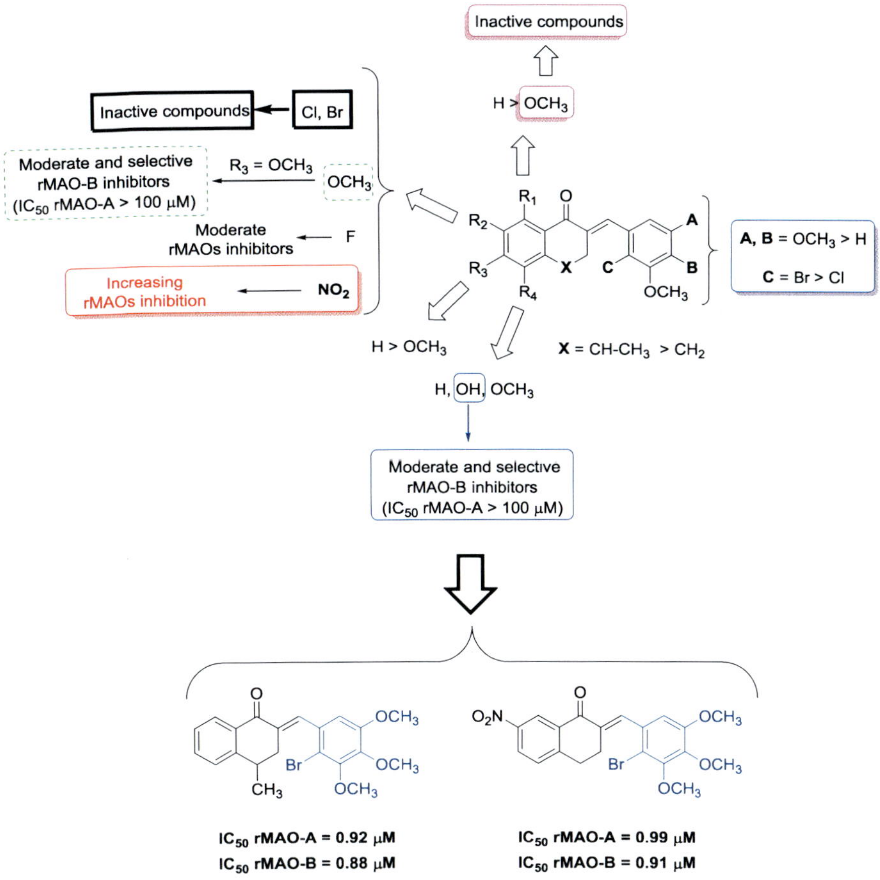

Fig. (12). Structure and SAR of multifunctional tetralones.

Most of the compounds exhibited rMAO-B inhibitory activity in the micromolar range and only few analogues shown $IC_{50} < 1$ μM, however lacking selectivity. The tetralone core was gifted at different positions with substituents like OCH_3, Cl, Br, F, NO_2, while the benzylidene phenyl ring was gifted with OCH_3, Cl and Br. The proposed molecular arrangements, however, were not beneficial: most of the proposed compounds were poor inhibitors of rMAOs. For example, all the derivatives bearing OCH_3 bound at the position 8 of the tetralone ring, were ineffective towards both the isoforms, regardless of the substituents placed on the benzylidene phenyl ring (Fig. **12**). Similarly, the presence of 7-Cl substituted tetralone led to inactive compounds with $IC_{50} > 100$ μM. The substitution of positions 5 or 6 of the tetralone core was better tolerated, producing a series of molecules (bearing different substitution patterns of the benzylidene phenyl ring) devoid of activity against rMAO-A ($IC_{50} > 100$ μM) and provided of weak inhibitory activity toward rMAO-B ($2.9 < IC_{50}$ (μM) < 78.9). A similar behaviour was observed also for analogues endowed with 7-Br or 5-OH substituted tetralone, exhibiting no affinity for rMAO-A and poor inhibitory activity against rMAO-B. Only two compounds displayed sub-micromolar affinity towards both the rMAO-isoforms, underlying the effectiveness of the methyl substitution in cyclohexanone ring of tetralone moiety as well as the nitro substitution on phenyl moiety of the tetralone ring system Fig. (**12**). Furthermore, the two compounds also shared the same crowded substitution pattern of the benzylidene phenyl ring, thus enforcing the importance of these substituents.

Homoisoflavonoids Derivatives (3-Benzylidenechroman-4-ones)

Homoisoflavonoids are natural compounds, subclass of the flavonoid group, produced by a limited number of plant families (Hyacinthaceae, Liliaceae, Asparagaceae, Fabaceae, Agavaceae, and Polygonaceae). They have been investigated for their wide functions, spanning from antidiabetic to antibacterial activity. Among others, also hMAOs inhibition has been described and various strategies have been developed to create synthetic homoisoflavonoids endowed with increased inhibitory activity and selectivity against one of the two hMAO isoforms. Wang and colleagues developed a series of dual functional cholinesterase and hMAO inhibitors useful for the treatment of Alzheimer's disease [40] (Fig. **11, I**). The approach used to develop these compounds focused on the insertion of structural elements that allow the binding with the target enzymes. The main 3-benzylidenechroman-4-one core, able to establish interactions with hMAO enzymes and the peripheral anionic site (PAS) of the acetylcholinesterase (AChE), was added to a series of alkyloxy chains of different dimensions bearing (cyclo)aliphatic amines in order to gain the interaction with the AChE catalytic active site (CAS). Focusing our attention on the hMAOs inhibitory activity, these compounds exhibited marked selectivity against hMAO-

B, although inhibited this isoform weakly. Indeed, only one compound of the library, endowed with pentyloxypiperidine moiety bound at position 6 of the 3,4-dihydronaphthalen-1(2*H*)-one ring Fig. (**13**, **I**), exhibited sub-micromolar inhibition of the hMAO-B (IC_{50} = 0.65 μM), the others possessing IC_{50} values spanning from 1.06 μM to 24.75 μM.

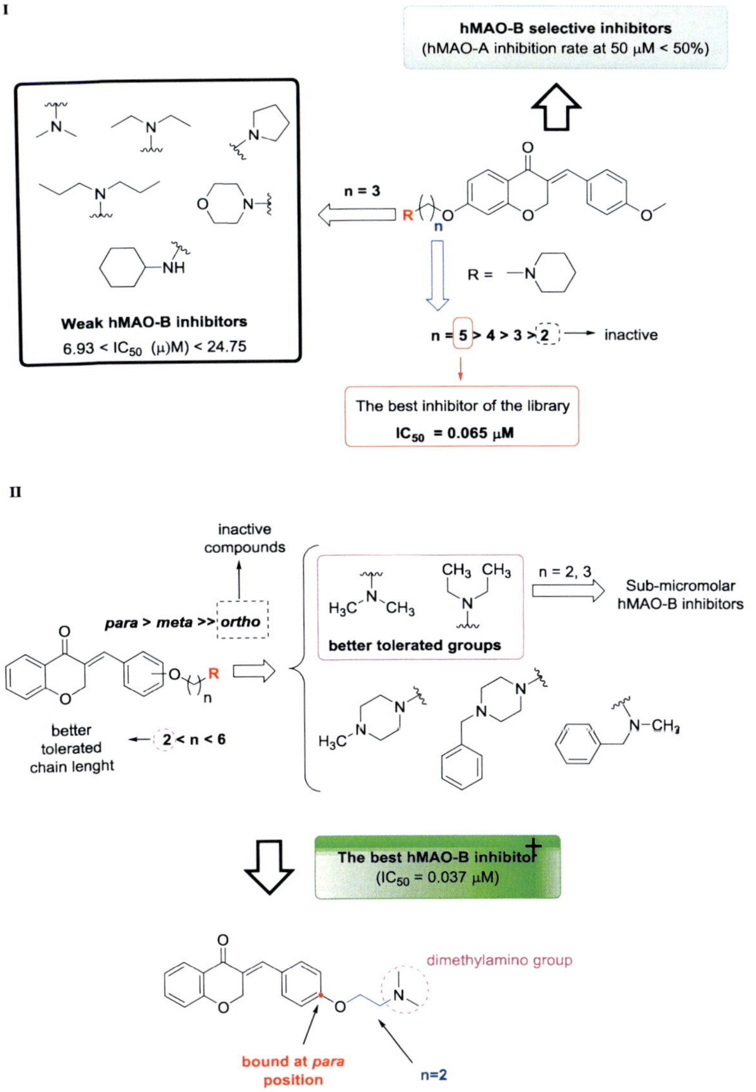

Fig. (13). Structure and SAR of multifunctional homoisoflavonoids bearing alkyloxy chain-amine moiety on the **(I)** 3,4-dihydronaphthalen-1(2*H*)-one core or on the **(II)** benzylidene phenyl ring.

With a similar purpose, a series of derivatives were developed by maintaining the homoisoflavonoid core for the binding with PAS of the AChE enzyme and hMAO-B, while displacing the alkyloxy chain bearing the amine moiety for the interaction with the CAS of AChE on the benzylidene phenyl ring [41] Fig. (**13, II**). A library of 45 derivatives were produced changing the dimensions of the alkyl chain (from 2 to 6 carbon atom chain), the binding position on the phenyl ring (*ortho*, *meta* and *para*) as well as the nature of the nitrogen containing moiety. All the compounds were selective inhibitors of hMAO-B, almost all being devoid of activity against hMAO-A or exhibiting a very poor affinity (IC_{50} > 37.8 μM). The replacement of the dimethyl/diethylamino fraction with other nitrogen-containing moieties negatively affected the activity; in a similar manner, the excessive increase of alkyl chain dimensions was detrimental for the inhibitory activity of hMAO-B. The most active compound of the library Fig. (**13, II**), was further investigated showing its interaction with the hMAO-B in a reversible manner through a non-competitive mechanism, nd also displaying the ability to cross the BBB.

In order to develop a series of MTDLs useful for AD treatment, Li and colleagues proposed a multitarget drug design strategy taking advantage of the molecular attributes of Donepezil, a well-known cholinesterases inhibitor, and phenolic Mannich bases, possessing different biological activities (antioxidant, anti-inflammatory and AChE inhibitory activity) Fig. (**14, I**) [42]. These compounds were selective hMAO-B inhibitors, not reaching 50% inhibition rate of hMAO-A at 20 μM. The nature and position of the nitrogen-containing moiety bound on the benzylidene phenyl ring influenced the inhibitory activity of these compounds Fig. (**14, I**). This scaffold afforded effective micromolar/sub-micromolar hMAO-B inhibitors when the amine group was placed at the *para* position of the benzylidene phenyl ring. The displacement of this moiety at the *ortho* position, maintaining the hydroxyl group at the *meta* one, led to the complete loss of the inhibitory activity. Among the amines evaluated, the better tolerated groups were the dimethylamino, pyrrolidine and *N*-methylpiperazino ones leading to sub-micromolar hMAO-B inhibitors. All the other evaluated nitrogen-containing moieties (such as morpholino, cyclohexylamino, ecc.) led to less effective inhibitors. The derivative exhibiting the better MTDL profile ((*E*)-3-(3-hydr-xy-4-(piperidin-1-ylmethyl)benzylidene)-6,7-dimethoxychroman-4-one, IC_{50} = 1.74 μM) was also investigated to determine its cytotoxicity on PC-12 cells at three concentration levels (1, 10 and 100 μM) demonstrating a decrease in cell *via*bility only at the higher concentration, revealing its wide therapeutic safety.

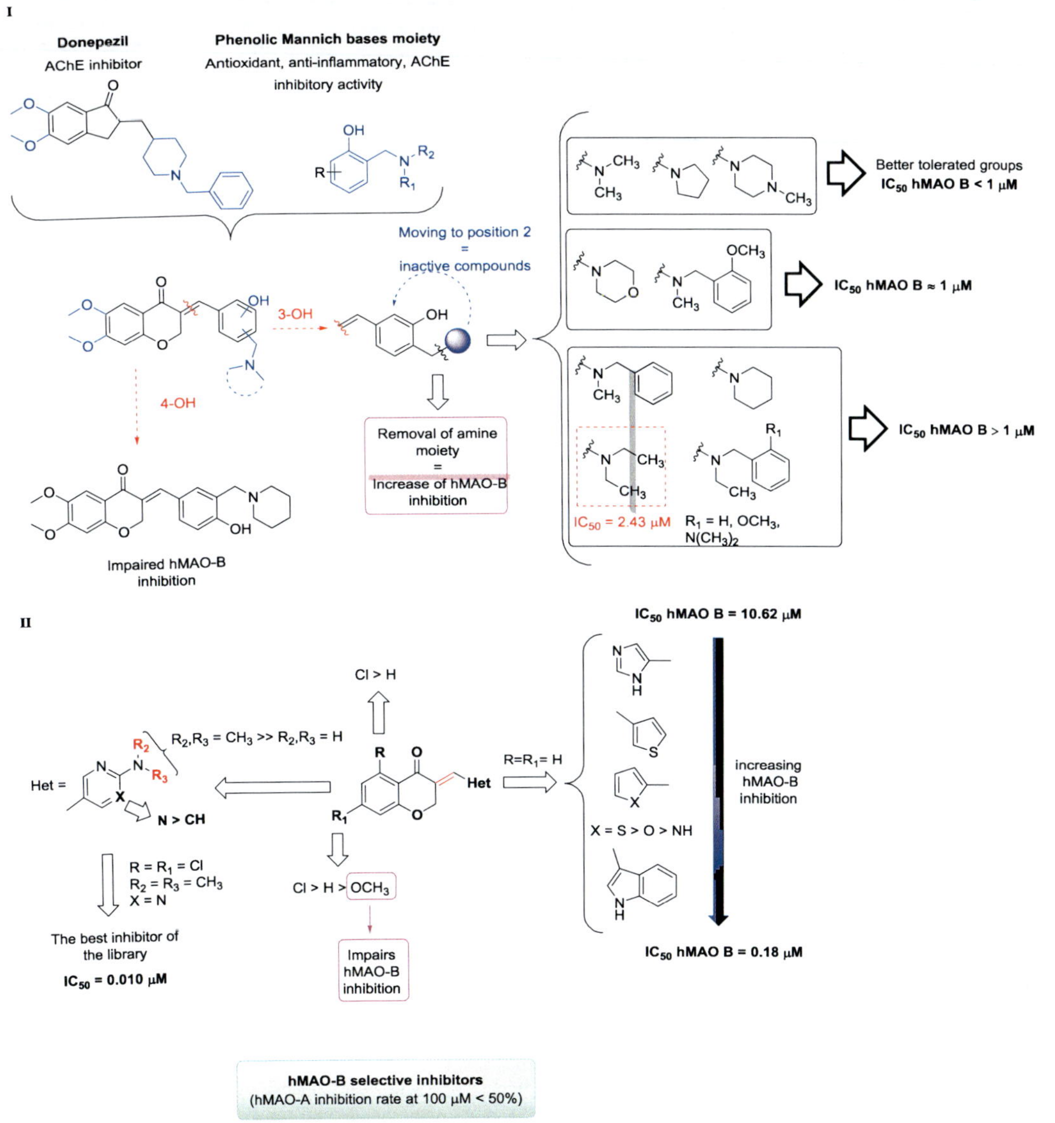

Fig. (14). Structure and SAR of (I) multifunctional homoisoflavonoids containing Donepezil and phenolic Mannich bases motifs; (II) heteroarylidene-homoisoflavonoids developed by Desideri and colleagues [43].

Better results were obtained by Desideri and colleagues who, through the introduction of heterocycles, developed a library of heteroarylidenechroman--one derivatives [43]. All the compounds were selective inhibitors of hMAO-B, being devoid of appreciable affinity for hMAO-A (IC_{50} > 100 μM). The analogues bearing 6-member nitrogen containing heterocycles in the arylidene part, were the best inhibitors of the series showing hMAO-B inhibitory activity in the nanomolar range Fig. (**14**, **I** and **II**). The presence of pyrimidin-5-yl ring was effective particularly if substituted at position 2 with dimethylamino group and if combined with unsubstituted 3,4-dihydronaphthalen-1(2*H*)-one core (R = R_1 = H, IC_{50} hMAO-B = 0.241 μM), or better, with 6,8-dichloro substituted one, leading to the best inhibitor of the library (R = R_1 = Cl, IC_{50} hMAO-B = 0.010 μM). This compound was a partially reversible inhibitor of hMAO-B. On the contrary, *N,N*-dimethylpyrimidin-2-amino ring was poor tolerated if the 3,4-dihydronaphthale--1(2*H*)-one core was substituted at position 6 with OCH_3 group, leading to micromolar inhibitor of hMAO-B.

The removal of one of the two nitrogen atoms of the pyrimidine ring to obtain the pyridine core was tolerated for the unsubstituted dihydronaphthalen-1(2*H*)-one core, while led to an impressive loss of inhibitory activity in the presence of 6,8-dichloro substitution (Fig. **14**, **I** and **II**).

Noteworthy results were also obtained by increasing the dimensions of the aryl moiety, as observed for the derivative bearing the indole core that exhibited sub-micromolar hMAO-B inhibition. The reduction of the ring dimensions instead, seemed to be detrimental for inhibitory activity, mainly for the nitrogen containing heterocycles. Replacing the nitrogen atom with the oxygen or sulfur one to obtain furan and thiophene, respectively, favored an improvement of inhibitory activity in the low micromolar range ($1.13 < IC_{50}$ (μM) < 3.77).

CONCLUSION

Aurones (2-benzylidenebenzofuran-3(2*H*)-ones), a class of uncommon flavonoids, have been described and reported to be endowed with broad spectrum of biological activities, including hMAOs inhibition. Taking advantage of the precise selection of the substituents placed on the aurone ring, is possible to obtain potent and selective inhibitors of one of the two hMAO isoforms. Usually, hydroxyl group placed at the position 6 of the benzofuranone ring promotes hMAO-A selectivity, while its replacement with the methoxy group moves the selectivity against the B isoform. However, a general trend and behaviour are hard to be defined due to the influence exerted by the substituents placed on the benzylidene phenyl ring. The presence of lipophilic substituents on this part seems to promote the interaction with the hMAOs active site, especially for hMAO-B. Docking studies suggest that the reason of this beneficial effect is related to the hydrophobic nature of the entrance cavity of hMAO-B, where the benzylidene phenyl ring would be displaced. The modification of the aurone scaffold can lead to a series of analogues coming from isosteric replacement (indanones) as well as ring expansion (homoisoflavonoids) or both (tetralones). These compounds often exhibited ameliorated activity and selectivity than the parent drugs, albeit also in this case, the substituents strongly influenced the inhibitory profile.

In conclusion, all the outcomes described in this chapter emphasised the different ability of the aurones and their analogues, to inhibit hMAO enzymes. The SAR analysis demonstrated that did not exist a "magic" substituent for the bicyclic (benzofuranone, indanone, chromanone) as well as the benzylidene/arylidene part able to increase MAO inhibition. On the contrary, is the fine regulation of the physical-chemical properties through the proper choice of the substituent groups, that led to effective inhibitors.

CONSENT FOR PUBLICATION

Not applicable.

CONFLICT OF INTEREST

The author declares no conflict of interest, financial or otherwise.

ACKNOWLEDGEMENT

Declared none.

REFERENCES

[1] Bortolato, M.; Chen, K.; Shih, J.C. Monoamine oxidase inactivation: From pathophysiology to therapeutics. *Adv. Drug Deliv. Rev.,* **2008**, *60*(13-14), 1527-1533. [http://dx.doi.org/10.1016/j.addr.2008.06.002] [PMID: 18652859]

[2] De Monte, C.; D'Ascenzio, M.; Guglielmi, P.; Mancini, V.; Carradori, S. Opening new scenarios for human MAO inhibitors. *Cent. Nerv. Syst. Agents Med. Chem.,* **2016**, *16*(2), 98-104. [http://dx.doi.org/10.2174/1871524915666150831141705] [PMID: 26320583]

[3] Nagatsu, T. Progress in monoamine oxidase (MAO) research in relation to genetic engineering. *Neurotoxicology,* **2004**, *25*(1-2), 11-20. [http://dx.doi.org/10.1016/S0161-813X(03)00085-8] [PMID: 14697876]

[4] Carradori, S.; Secci, D.; Petzer, J.P. MAO inhibitors and their wider applications: a patent review. *Expert Opin. Ther. Pat.,* **2018**, *28*(3), 211-226. [http://dx.doi.org/10.1080/13543776.2018.1427735] [PMID: 29324067]

[5] Shih, J.C.; Chen, K.; Ridd, M.J. Monoamine oxidase: from genes to behavior. *Annu. Rev. Neurosci.,* **1999**, *22*(1), 197-217. [http://dx.doi.org/10.1146/annurev.neuro.22.1.197] [PMID: 10202537]

[6] Guglielmi, P.; Carradori, S.; Poli, G. Design, synthesis, docking studies and monoamine oxidase inhibition of a small library of 1-acetyl- and 1-thiocarbamoyl-3,5-diphenyl-4,5-dihydro-(1*H*)-pyrazoles. *Molecules,* **2019**, *24*(3), 484. [http://dx.doi.org/10.3390/molecules24030484] [PMID: 30700029]

[7] Guglielmi, P.; Mathew, B.; Secci, D.; Carradori, S. Chalcones: unearthing their therapeutic possibility as monoamine oxidase b inhibitors. Eur. J. Med. Chem. **2020**, , 112650.

[8] Guglielmi, P.; Secci, D.; Petzer, A. Benzo[*b*]tiophen-3-ol derivatives as effective inhibitors of human

monoamine oxidase: design, synthesis, and biological activity. *J. Enzyme Inhib. Med. Chem.*, **2019**, *34*(1), 1511-1525.
[http://dx.doi.org/10.1080/14756366.2019.1653864] [PMID: 31422706]

[9] Carradori, S.; D'Ascenzio, M.; Chimenti, P.; Secci, D.; Bolasco, A. Selective MAO-B inhibitors: a lesson from natural products. *Mol. Divers.*, **2014**, *18*(1), 219-243.
[http://dx.doi.org/10.1007/s11030-013-9490-6] [PMID: 24218136]

[10] Mathew, B.; Carradori, S.; Guglielmi, P.; Uddin, M.S.; Kim, H. New aspects of monoamine oxidase b inhibitors: the key role of halogens to open the golden door. *Curr. Med. Chem.*, **2020**, *28*(2), 266-283.
[http://dx.doi.org/10.2174/0929867327666200121165931] [PMID: 31965939]

[11] Guglielmi, P.; Carradori, S.; Ammazzalorso, A.; Secci, D. Novel approaches to the discovery of selective human monoamine oxidase-B inhibitors: is there room for improvement? *Expert Opin. Drug Discov.*, **2019**, *14*(10), 995-1035.
[http://dx.doi.org/10.1080/17460441.2019.1637415] [PMID: 31268358]

[12] Chimenti, F.; Secci, D.; Bolasco, A. Synthesis, molecular modeling studies, and selective inhibitory activity against monoamine oxidase of N,N′-bis[2-oxo-2H-benzopyran]-3-carboxamides. *Bioorg. Med. Chem. Lett.*, **2006**, *16*(15), 4135-4140.
[http://dx.doi.org/10.1016/j.bmcl.2006.04.026] [PMID: 16759860]

[13] Secci, D.; Carradori, S.; Petzer, A. 4-(3-Nitrophenyl)thiazol-2-ylhydrazone derivatives as antioxidants and selective hMAO-B inhibitors: synthesis, biological activity and computational analysis. *J. Enzyme Inhib. Med. Chem.*, **2019**, *34*(1), 597-612.
[http://dx.doi.org/10.1080/14756366.2019.1571272] [PMID: 30727777]

[14] Carradori, S.; Gidaro, M.C.; Petzer, A.; Costa, G.; Guglielmi, P.; Chimenti, P.; Alcaro, S.; Petzer, J.P. Inhibition of human monoamine oxidase: biological and molecular modeling studies on selected natural flavonoids. *J. Agric. Food Chem.*, **2016**, *64*(47), 9004-9011.
[http://dx.doi.org/10.1021/acs.jafc.6b03529] [PMID: 27933876]

[15] Huang, J.; Chen, X.; Chang, Z.; Xiao, C.; Najafi, M. Boosting anti-tumour immunity using adjuvant apigenin. *Anticancer. Agents Med. Chem.*, **2022**, *22*
[http://dx.doi.org/10.2174/1871520622666220523151409] [PMID: 35616683]

[16] Turkmenoglu, F.; Baysal, İ.; Ciftci-Yabanoglu, S. Flavonoids from sideritis species: human monoamine oxidase (hMAO) inhibitory activities, molecular docking studies and crystal structure of xanthomicrol. *Molecules,* **2015**, *20*(5), 7454-7473.
[http://dx.doi.org/10.3390/molecules20057454] [PMID: 25915461]

[17] Farina, R.; Pisani, L.; Catto, M. Structure-based design and optimization of multitarget-directed 2*H*-chromen-2-one derivatives as potent inhibitors of monoamine oxidase b and cholinesterases. *J. Med. Chem.*, **2015**, *58*(14), 5561-5578.
[http://dx.doi.org/10.1021/acs.jmedchem.5b00599] [PMID: 26107513]

[18] He, Q.; Liu, J.; Lan, J.S. Coumarin-dithiocarbamate hybrids as novel multitarget AChE and MAO-B inhibitors against Alzheimer's disease: Design, synthesis and biological evaluation. *Bioorg. Chem.*, **2018**, *81*, 512-528.
[http://dx.doi.org/10.1016/j.bioorg.2018.09.010] [PMID: 30245233]

[19] Pisani, L.; Farina, R.; Catto, Exploring basic tail modifications of coumarin-based dual acetylcholinesterase-monoamine oxidase b inhibitors: identification of water-soluble, brain-permeant neuroprotective multitarget agents. *J. Med. Chem.*, **2016**, *59*(14), 6791-6806.
[http://dx.doi.org/10.1021/acs.jmedchem.6b00562] [PMID: 27347731]

[20] De Sanctis, J.B.; Charris, J.; Blanco, Z.; Ramírez, H.; Martínez, G.P.; Mijares, M.R. Molecular Mechanisms of Chloroquine and Hydroxychloroquine use in Cancer Therapy. *Anticancer. Agents Med. Chem.*, **2022**, *22*
[http://dx.doi.org/10.2174/1871520622666220519102948] [PMID: 35598250]

[21] Pisani, L.; Iacobazzi, R.M.; Catto, M. Investigating alkyl nitrates as nitric oxide releasing precursors of

multitarget acetylcholinesterase-monoamine oxidase B inhibitors. *Eur. J. Med. Chem.*, **2019**, *161*, 292-309.
[http://dx.doi.org/10.1016/j.ejmech.2018.10.016] [PMID: 30366255]

[22] Pisani, L.; Farina, R.; Soto-Otero, R. Searching for multi-targeting neurotherapeutics against alzheimer's: discovery of potent AChE-MAO B inhibitors through the decoration of the 2h-chrome--2-one structural motif. *Molecules,* **2016**, *21*(3), 362.
[http://dx.doi.org/10.3390/molecules21030362] [PMID: 26999091]

[23] Xiao, G.; Li, Y.; Qiang, X. Design, synthesis and biological evaluation of 4′-aminochalcon--rivastigmine hybrids as multifunctional agents for the treatment of Alzheimer's disease. *Bioorg. Med. Chem.*, **2017**, *25*(3), 1030-1041.
[http://dx.doi.org/10.1016/j.bmc.2016.12.013] [PMID: 28011206]

[24] Wang, M.; Qin, H.L.; Leng, J. Synthesis and biological evaluation of new tetramethylpyrazine-based chalcone derivatives as potential anti-Alzheimer agents. *Chem. Biol. Drug Des.*, **2018**, *92*(5), 1859-1866.
[http://dx.doi.org/10.1111/cbdd.13355] [PMID: 29923315]

[25] Oh, J.M.; Rangarajan, T.M.; Chaudhary, R.; Singh, R.P.; Singh, M.; Singh, R.P.; Tondo, A.R.; Gambacorta, N.; Nicolotti, O.; Mathew, B.; Kim, H. Novel class of chalcone oxime ethers as potent monoamine oxidase-b and acetylcholinesterase inhibitors. *Molecules,* **2020**, *25*(10), 2356.
[http://dx.doi.org/10.3390/molecules25102356] [PMID: 32443652]

[26] Tian, C.; Qiang, X.; Song, Q. Flurbiprofen-chalcone hybrid Mannich base derivatives as balanced multifunctional agents against Alzheimer's disease: Design, synthesis and biological evaluation. *Bioorg. Chem.*, **2020**, *94*103477
[http://dx.doi.org/10.1016/j.bioorg.2019.103477] [PMID: 31818478]

[27] Bohm, B.A. The minor flavonoids. *The Flavonoids: Advances in Research since 1980.*, **1988**, 329-388.
[http://dx.doi.org/10.1007/978-1-4899-2913-6_9]

[28] Daina, A.; Michielin, O.; Zoete, V. SwissTargetPrediction: updated data and new features for efficient prediction of protein targets of small molecules. *Nucleic Acids Res.*, **2019**, *47*(W1), W357-W364.
[http://dx.doi.org/10.1093/nar/gkz382] [PMID: 31106366]

[29] Chimenti, F.; Fioravanti, R.; Bolasco, A.; Chimenti, P.; Secci, D.; Rossi, F.; Yáñez, M.; Orallo, F.; Ortuso, F.; Alcaro, S. Chalcones: a valid scaffold for monoamine oxidases inhibitors. *J. Med. Chem.*, **2009**, *52*(9), 2818-2824.
[http://dx.doi.org/10.1021/jm801590u] [PMID: 19378991]

[30] Morales-Camilo, N.; Salas, C.O.; Sanhueza, C.; Espinosa-Bustos, C.; Sepúlveda-Boza, S.; Reyes-Parada, M.; Gonzalez-Nilo, F.; Caroli-Rezende, M.; Fierro, A. Synthesis, Biological evaluation, and molecular simulation of chalcones and aurones as selective MAO-B Inhibitors. *Chem. Biol. Drug Des.*, **2015**, *85*(6), 685-695.
[http://dx.doi.org/10.1111/cbdd.12458] [PMID: 25346162]

[31] Baek, S.C.; Lee, H.W.; Ryu, H.W. Selective inhibition of monoamine oxidase A by hispidol. *Bioorg. Med. Chem. Lett.*, **2018**, *28*(4), 584-588.
[http://dx.doi.org/10.1016/j.bmcl.2018.01.049] [PMID: 29395970]

[32] Li, Y.; Qiang, X.; Luo, L.; Li, Y.; Xiao, G.; Tan, Z.; Deng, Y. Synthesis and evaluation of 4-hydroxyl aurone derivatives as multifunctional agents for the treatment of Alzheimer's disease. *Bioorg. Med. Chem.*, **2016**, *24*(10), 2342-2351.
[http://dx.doi.org/10.1016/j.bmc.2016.04.012] [PMID: 27079124]

[33] Liew, K.F.; Lee, E.H.C.; Chan, K.L.; Lee, C.Y. Multi-targeting aurones with monoamine oxidase and amyloid-beta inhibitory activities: Structure-activity relationship and translating multi-potency to neuroprotection. *Biomed. Pharmacother.*, **2019**, *110*(110), 118-128.
[http://dx.doi.org/10.1016/j.biopha.2018.11.054] [PMID: 30466001]

[34] Takao, K.; U, S.; Kamauchi, H.; Sugita, Y. Design, synthesis and evaluation of 2-(indolylmethylidene)-2,3-dihydro-1-benzofuran-3-one and 2-(indolyl)-4*H*-chromen-4-one derivatives as novel monoamine oxidases inhibitors. *Bioorg. Chem.,* **2019**, *87*(January), 594-600. [http://dx.doi.org/10.1016/j.bioorg.2019.03.042] [PMID: 30933784]

[35] Nel, M.S.; Petzer, A.; Petzer, J.P.; Legoabe, L.J. 2-Benzylidene-1-indanone derivatives as inhibitors of monoamine oxidase. *Bioorg. Med. Chem. Lett.,* **2016**, *26*(19), 4599-4605. [http://dx.doi.org/10.1016/j.bmcl.2016.08.067] [PMID: 27578245]

[36] Nel, M.S.; Petzer, A.; Petzer, J.P.; Legoabe, L.J. 2-Heteroarylidene-1-indanone derivatives as inhibitors of monoamine oxidase. *Bioorg. Chem.,* **2016**, *69*, 20-28. [http://dx.doi.org/10.1016/j.bioorg.2016.09.004] [PMID: 27662218]

[37] Affini, A.; Hagenow, S.; Zivkovic, A.; Marco-Contelles, J.; Stark, H. Novel indanone derivatives as MAO B/H_3R dual-targeting ligands for treatment of Parkinson's disease. *Eur. J. Med. Chem.,* **2018**, *148*, 487-497. [http://dx.doi.org/10.1016/j.ejmech.2018.02.015] [PMID: 29477889]

[38] Amakali, K.T.; Legoabe, L.J.; Petzer, A.; Petzer, J.P. Synthesis and evaluation of 2-benzylidene-1-tetralone derivatives for monoamine oxidase inhibitory activity. *Cent. Nerv. Syst. Agents Med. Chem.,* **2018**, *18*(2), 136-149. [http://dx.doi.org/10.2174/1871524918666180501121638] [PMID: 29714148]

[39] Leng, J.; Qin, H.L.; Zhu, K.; Jantan, I.; Hussain, M.A.; Sher, M.; Amjad, M.W.; Naeem-ul-Hassan, M.; Ahmad, W.; Bukhari, S.N.A. Evaluation of multifunctional synthetic tetralone derivatives for treatment of Alzheimer's disease. *Chem. Biol. Drug Des.,* **2016**, *88*(6), 889-898. [http://dx.doi.org/10.1111/cbdd.12822] [PMID: 27434226]

[40] Wang, Y.; Sun, Y.; Guo, Y.; Wang, Z.; Huang, L.; Li, X. Dual functional cholinesterase and MAO inhibitors for the treatment of Alzheimer's disease: synthesis, pharmacological analysis and molecular modeling of homoisoflavonoid derivatives. *J. Enzyme Inhib. Med. Chem.,* **2016**, *31*(3), 389-397. [PMID: 25798687]

[41] Liu, Q.H.; Wu, J.J.; Li, F. Synthesis and pharmacological evaluation of multi-functional homoisoflavonoid derivatives as potent inhibitors of monoamine oxidase B and cholinesterase for the treatment of Alzheimer's disease. *MedChemComm,* **2017**, *8*(7), 1459-1467. [http://dx.doi.org/10.1039/C7MD00199A] [PMID: 30108857]

[42] Li, Y.; Qiang, X.; Luo, L.; Yang, X. Multitarget drug design strategy against Alzheimer's disease: Homoisoflavonoid Mannich base derivatives serve as acetylcholinesterase and monoamine oxidase B dual inhibitors with multifunctional properties. *Bioorg. Med. Chem.,* **2017**, *25*(2), 714-726. [http://dx.doi.org/10.1016/j.bmc.2016.11.048] [PMID: 27923535]

[43] Desideri, N.; Proietti Monaco, L.; Fioravanti, R.; Biava, M.; Yáñez, M.; Alcaro, S.; Ortuso, F. (*E*)---Heteroarylidenechroman-4-ones as potent and selective monoamine oxidase-B inhibitors. *Eur. J. Med. Chem.,* **2016**, *117*, 292-300. [http://dx.doi.org/10.1016/j.ejmech.2016.03.081] [PMID: 27135371]

Medicinal Chemistry Lessons From Nature, 2022, *Vol. 1*, 298-329

CHAPTER 10

Coumarins as Carbonic Anhydrase Inhibitors

Claudiu T. Supuran[1,*]

[1] *Department of NEUROFARBA, Section of Pharmaceutical and Nutraceutical Sciences, Pharmaceutical and Nutraceutical Section, University of Florence, via U. Schiff 6, 50019 Sesto Fiorentino, Firenze, Italy*

Abstract: Carbonic anhydrases (CAs, EC 4.2.1.1) are metalloenzymes and relevant drug targets with many medicinal chemistry applications. Their classes of inhibitors are in clinical use as diuretics, or drugs for the management of glaucoma, epilepsy, obesity, tumors and infectious diseases. Among the inhibitors discovered so far, coumarins constitute an interesting class. They undergo CA-catalyzed hydrolysis and act as "prodrug inhibitors", forming 2-hydroxy-cinnamic acids, which bind at the entrance of the enzyme active site, which has a relevant variability of amino acid residues among the different CA isoforms present in mammals, humans included. Coumarins act as isoform-selective CA inhibitors against pharmacologically relevant enzymes, such as the tumor-associated CA IX and XII. Coumarins present as metabolites in many species of bacteria, fungi, plants and ascidians showed relevant CA inhibitory properties and were used as leads for obtaining synthetic derivatives with enhanced enzyme inhibitory action belonging to a variety of classes, such as polysubstituted coumarins on both rings, thiocoumarins, thioxocoumarins, sulfocoumarins, *etc.*

Keywords: Carbonic Anhydrase, Coumarin, Prodrug Inhibitor, Sulfocoumarins, Thioxocoumarins, Tumors.

CARBONIC ANHYDRASE INHIBITORS AND ACTIVATORS

Carbonic anhydrases (CAs, EC 4.2.1.1) are metalloenzymes present in organisms throughout the life kingdoms (Prokaryotes and Eukaryotes), being encoded by eight genetically diverse families [1 - 10]. They catalyze the carbon dioxide hydration to bicarbonate and H^+ ions. This is a simple reaction but crucial for a variety of processes, both physiologic and pathologic, due to the fact that CO_2 and water, two neutral molecules, generate a weak base, bicarbonate, and a strong acid, and as a consequence, this enzyme plays a key role in acid-base equilibria, pH regulation and metabolism [1, 11 - 15].

* **Corresponding author Claudiu T. Supuran:** Department of NEUROFARBA, Section of Pharmaceutical and Nutraceutical Sciences, Pharmaceutical and Nutraceutical Section, University of Florence, *via* U. Schiff 6, 50019 Sesto Fiorentino, Firenze, Italy; Tel: +39-055-4573729; Fax: +39-055-4573385; E-mail: claudiu.supuran@unifi.it

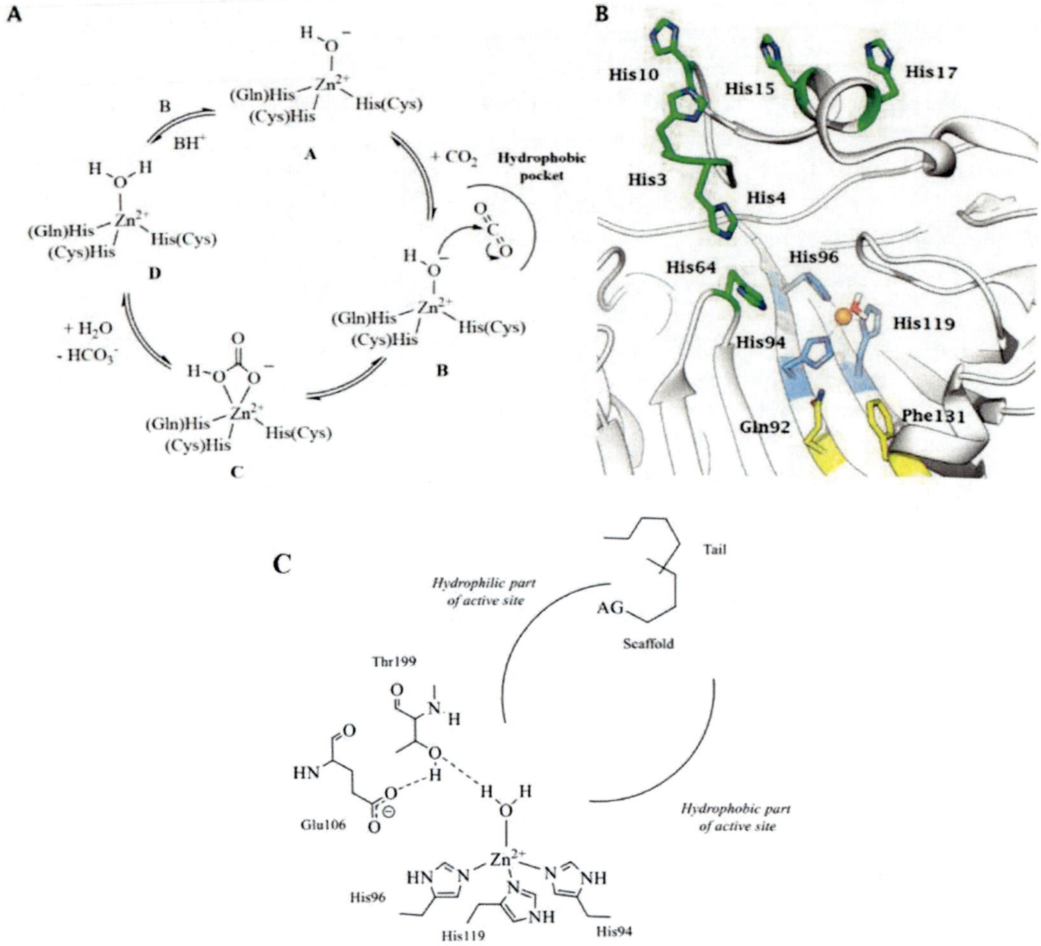

Fig. (1). A. CA catalytic cycle for the CO_2 hydration/bicarbonate dehydration reaction. **B**. α-CA (hCA II) active site, with the zinc ion and its ligands (His94, 96, and 119) as well as His residues involved in proton shuttling. **C**. α-CA inhibition mechanism by occlusion of the active site entrance [16].

The metal ion is usually zinc(II) coordinated by three amino acid residues and a water molecule/hydroxide ion, acting s a nucleophile in the catalytic cycle – (Fig. **1A**) [1 - 9, 16]. The species with zinc hydroxide within the active site is the nucleophilic, catalytically active one, which converts CO_2 bound within the enzyme active site cleft to bicarbonate, originally coordinated to the metal and then released in solution, with the formation of the acidic species, with water coordinated to the zinc. Fig. (**1A**). This form must lose a proton, a process which is achieved by the so-called proton shuttling residues, usually, His residues, shown in Fig. (**1B**) [1 - 9, 16]. This is also the rate-limiting step of the catalytic cycle, but CAs are among the fastest and most effective enzymes known to date [16].

This reaction is crucial for a host of physiologic functions connected to pH regulation processes in all types of organisms and cells [17 - 21]. For this reason, modulating CA activity by using inhibitors and activators, leads to pharmacological applications for the treatment of multiple human diseases. The CA inhibitors (CAIs) are used as diuretics since the '50s [22 - 24], as anti-glaucoma agents [25, 26], antiepileptic drugs [27, 28], antiobesity agents [29, 30], and for the management of metastatic, hypoxic tumors [31 - 36]. The CA activators (CAAs) [37 - 39] started to be used for pharmacological applications more recently, initially for memory therapy [40], or for the modulation of emotional memory, but they may show other applications in areas such as generalised anxiety, post-traumatic stress, phobias, as well as obsessive-compulsive disorders [41, 42].

Among the four CA inhibition mechanisms reported to date for α-CAs [16, 43 - 45], the compounds which occlude the entrance to the active site Fig. (**1C**). will be discussed. These CAIs bind far away from the catalytic metal ion (> 10 Å away from it), in a region that is rather variable among the many mammalian isoforms, which also favoured the discovery of isoform-selective CAIs [16, 43 - 45]. Coumarins were the first compounds for which this inhibition mechanism has been disclosed by Quinn's group [46], both from the inhibition mechanism and drug design viewpoints. In fact, the discovery of coumarins as CAIs and their particular inhibition mechanism [46, 47] allowed for a rational drug design campaign of a large number of isoform-selective inhibitor classes for many catalytically active human (h) CA isoforms (of the 15 hCA isoforms present in humans, 12 possess catalytic activity, with isoforms VIII, X and XI being devoid of it [1]).

COUMARINS WITH CA INHIBITORY ACTION

Natural Product Coumarins

Among the many natural products that are widespread in organisms all over the phylogenetic tree [48], coumarins play a relevant role in medicinal chemistry due to their multiple pharmacologic applications [49 - 55]. They show a variety of biological activities, such as the anticoagulant effects [55], inhibitors of monoamine oxidase (MAO) [52, 53], antibacterial, antifungal and antiviral actions [51, 54], antioxidant activity [50, 54], antitumor effects [51, 54], as well as anti-inflammatory action [50, 51, 54]. The precise mechanisms of action of coumarins against so many different targets are poorly understood, except for the MAO inhibition and anticoagulant activities [53 - 55]. Coumarins incorporate two annulated 6-ring aromatic cycles, possessing one endocyclic and one exocyclic oxygen atom, which form a cyclic lactone, as shown in Fig. (**2**) for the simplest derivative, coumarin **1**. Being lactones, most coumarins may be hydrolysed with the formation of the 2-hydroxy-cinnamic acid **2** (in the case of the simplest derivative **1** mentioned above). Such compounds are *set al* as sodium salts (normally as the *trans* isomer), but in an acidic medium, they are easily recycled , with the re-formation of the original coumarin, losing a water molecule and reforming the aromatic highly *et al* conjugated ring system [49 - 54]. The chemistry of this class of organic compounds was thoroughly reviewed and will not be discussed in detail here [49, 50].

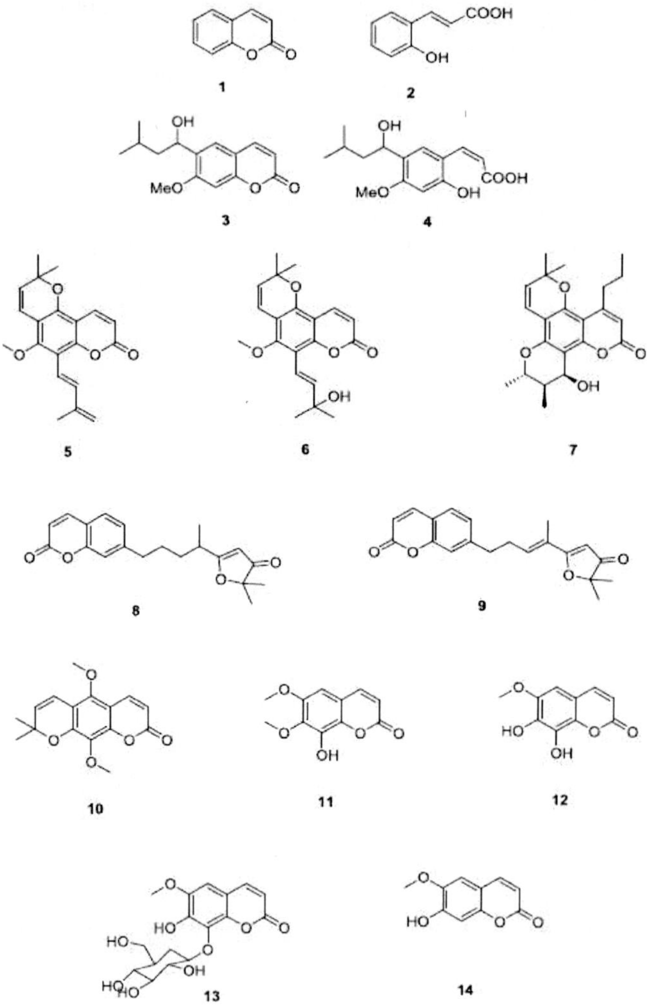

Fig. (2). Simple coumarins, such as derivative **1** and its hydrolysis product **2**, and natural product coumarins **3-14** for which the CA inhibitory activities were reported [47, 57, 58].

Quinn's group first reported in a library of Australian natural products coumarin **3** to act as a CA inhibitor [46]. Shortly thereafter, we demonstrated that the CA inhibition mechanism is rather complex [47]. Indeed, when coumarin **3** (present in the Australian plant *Leionema ellipticum*) is incubated for 15-30 min with the enzyme (when measuring the inhibitory activity), rather weak, micromolar activities were measured, which is also similar to other derivatives, *e.g.*, **1** [47]. However, after incubation periods of 6 h, quite diverse (i.e., much higher) inhibitory activity was measured, with a differentiated structure-activity relationship (SAR) for various derivatives, for example the natural products shown in Fig. (**2**) [47, 57, 58]. Indeed, by means of X-ray crystallography and mass spectrometry, it was possible to evidence that the real inhibitor is the *cis*--hydroxy-cinnamic acid **4** Fig. (**2**). which binds to the enzyme as shown in Fig. (**3**). Furthermore, the hydrolysed coumarin binding site is in fact identical to the CA activator binding site explored earlier [37 - 39].

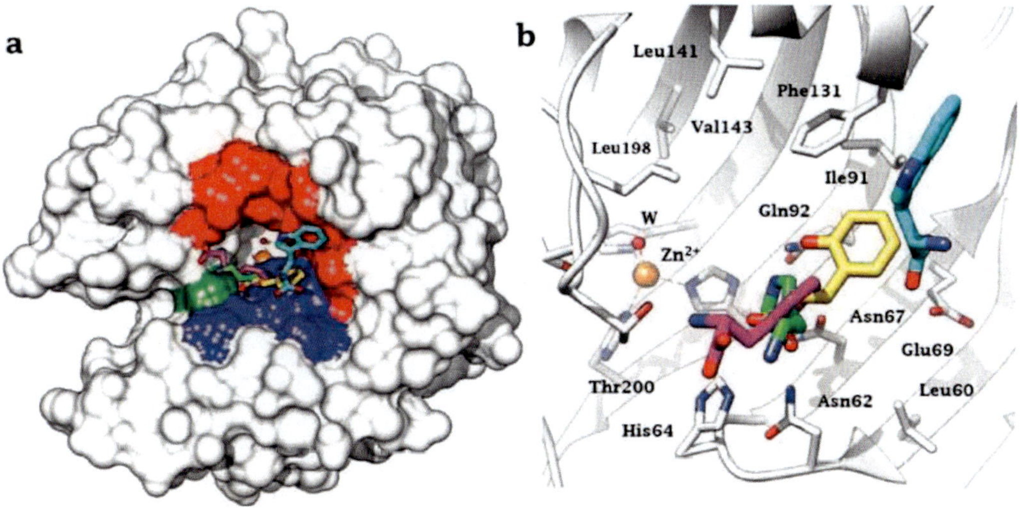

Fig. (3). hCA II complexed with **2** (hydrolysis product of coumarin **1**) and CAAs. The Zn(II) ion is shown as a golden sphere with its three His residues His94, 96 and 119. Red spheres represent water molecules involved in the binding of the inhibitor/activators. Compound **2** is shown in yellow (PDB 5BNL [57]), histamine (CAA) in green (PDB 1AVN [38]), D-Phe in magenta (PDB 2EZ7 [59]), D-Trp in cyan (PDB 3EFI [60]). **a.** Overall view of the superimposition of the ligand-enzyme complexes, with the hydrophobic half of the hCA II active site shown in red, and the hydrophilic one in blue. His64, the proton shuttling residue is shown in green; **b.** Enlarged view of the active site with the superimposition of the four ligands shown in **a.**

In this way, the hydrolyzed coumarin blocks the entrance of the active site cavity, the adduct being stabilized by the formation of many favorable polar and hydrophobic interactions with water molecules and the amino acid residues shown in Fig. (**3b**). As mentioned above, due to the fact that this region is rather variable among the mammalian CA isoforms, the hydrolyzed coumarin is able to interact differently with the diverse isoforms, which are inhibited in some cases in a selective manner [47, 57, 58]. It should be also noted that although the unsubstituted 2-hydroxy-cinnamic acid **2** binds to the enzyme in its *trans* geometry, the bulkier derivative **4**, which is the hydrolysis product of the natural product coumarin **3** was observed, again by X-ray crystallography, bound in the same active site region as derivative **2**, but in its less *set al cis* geometry [47]. Coumarins are thus acting as suicide inhibitors, undergoing hydrolysis due to the esterase CA activity, and generating the 2-hydroxy-cinnamic acids which bind at the entrance of the enzyme active site, a region where only activators have been observed earlier, as mentioned above [37, 38, 47, 57 - 60].

Other natural product coumarins (NPCs) acting as CAIs were thereafter reported by Davis *et al.* [58] (Fig. **2**, compounds **5-14** and Fig. **4**, compounds **15-35**). These coumarins were isolated from plants or ascidians and were investigated as inhibitors of six hCAs *et al.* **1**, i.e., hCA I, II, VII, IX, XII and XIII [58]. The scaffolds of these compounds are variable, ranging from simple coumarins with compact substituents (**11**, **12**, **14**, **17**, **33**) to bulky and complex substituents in diverse positions of the two rings, as well as annulation with other ring systems (**5-7**, **19**, **20**, **24**, **25**, **26**, **34**, **35**) [58].

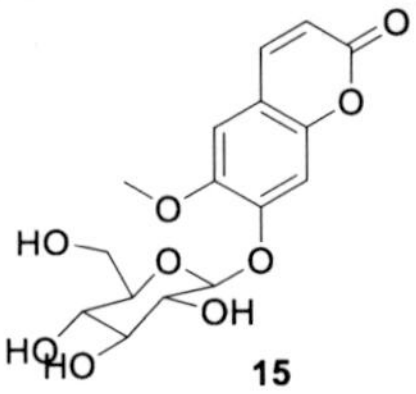

15

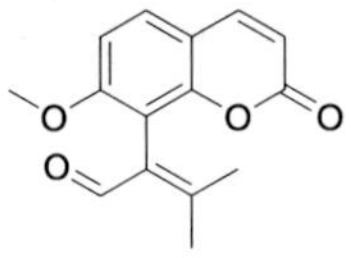

16

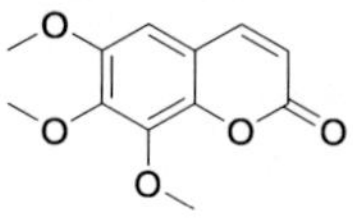

17

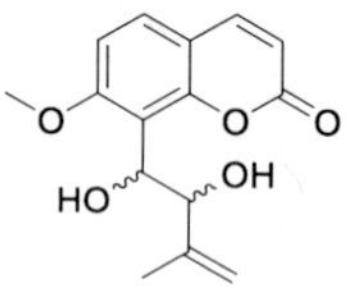

18

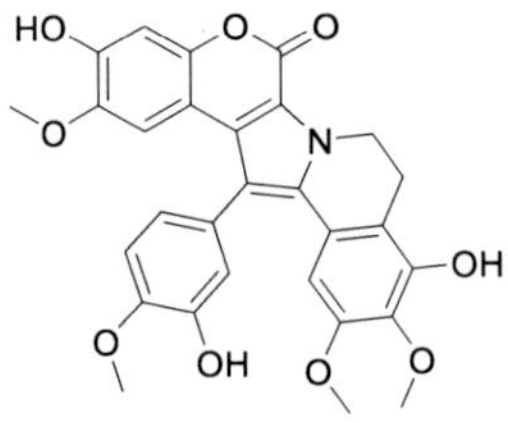

19

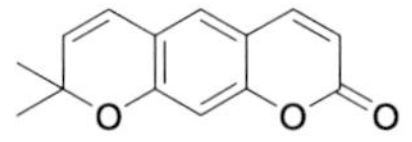

20

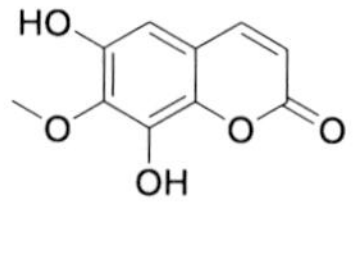

21

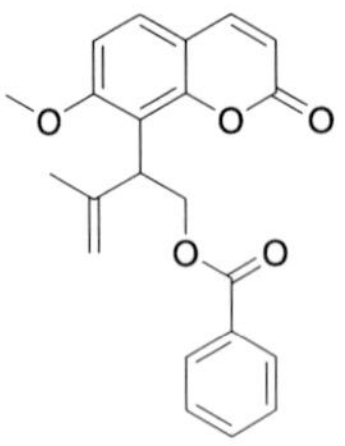

22

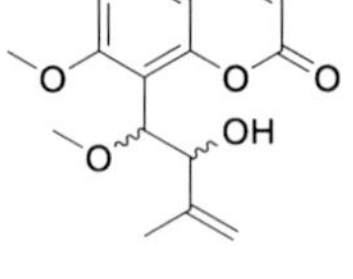

23

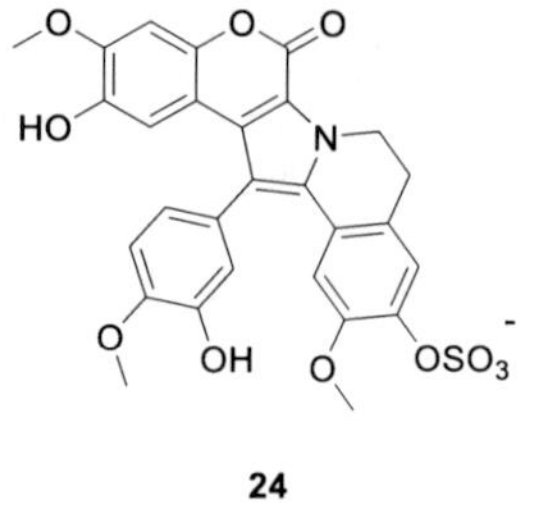

24

(Fig. 4) contd.....

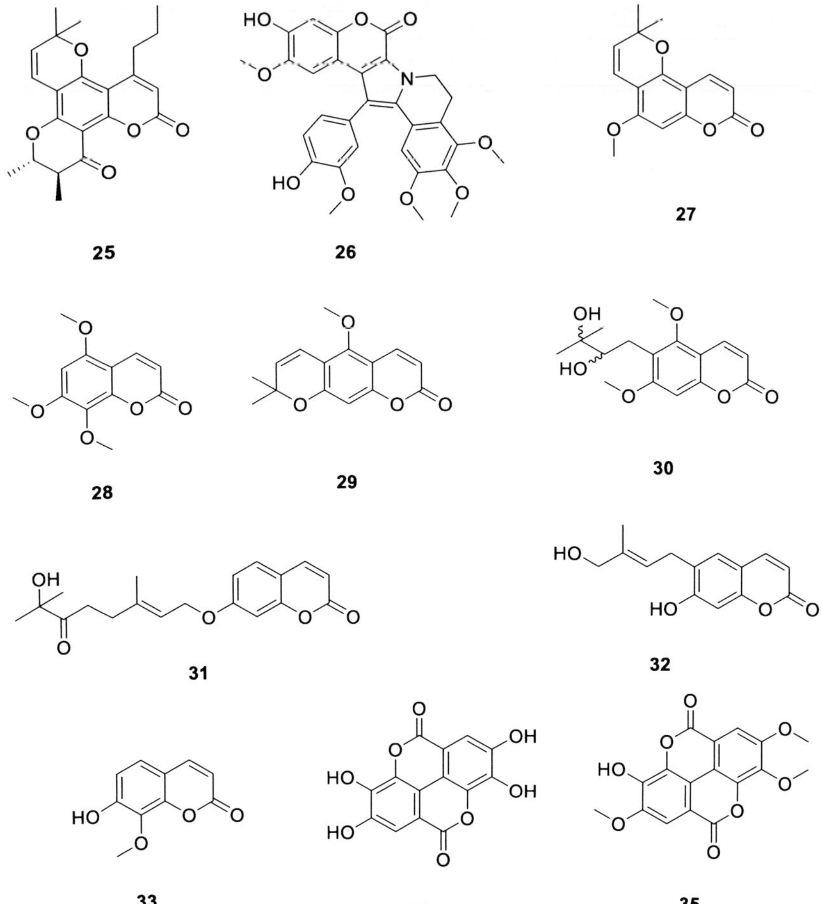

Fig. (4). Natural product coumarins **15-35** investigated as CAIs against six CA isoforms [58].

Table 1. Inhibition data against six CA isoforms (hCA I, II, VII, IX, XII and XIII) with coumarins 5-35.

Compound	K_I (µM)*					
	hCA I	hCA II	hCA VII	hCA IX	hCA XII	hCA XIII
5	7.66	>100	0.65	0.62	0.79	45.0
6	8.46	>100	8.98	0.78	0.77	29.3
7	9.31	50.7	8.87	0.83	0.81	21.0
8	59.2	63.4	9.03	0.89	0.60	27.4
9	9.75	>100	7.82	0.60	0.83	9.62
10	9.21	49.3	9.31	0.86	8.35	>100
11	9.89	>100	5.56	0.85	7.84	95.7

(Table 1) cont.....

Compound	K_I (μM)*					
	hCA I	hCA II	hCA VII	hCA IX	hCA XII	hCA XIII
12	4.86	94.3	4.32	0.61	7.70	9.73
13	5.04	>100	3.87	0.37	7.45	9.80
14	10.56	>100	8.71	0.96	4.05	17.8
15	5.93	>100	9.11	8.72	0.78	8.43
16	9.11	>100	8.85	8.12	7.44	8.89
17	**9.7 nM**	>100	9.28	6.58	18.2	4.24
18	8.43	>100	29.7	3.35	8.91	4.75
19	6.45	>100	14.5	3.22	9.07	4.63
20	21.5	>100	9.18	7.51	25.7	8.36
21	14.0	>100	23.8	7.37	4.14	5.27
22	5.84	>100	>100	0.67	7.39	4.06
23	7.41	>100	>100	0.68	0.76	3.28
24	6.55	>100	78.4	3.27	1.79	4.24
25	8.32	>100	4.15	8.38	0.87	6.26
26	40.1	>100	58.3	6.33	8.51	3.70
27	5.60	>100	8.11	3.50	9.10	5.91
28	4.31	9.65	7.01	0.76	0.83	3.32
29	7.71	>100	6.27	0.74	0.96	3.15
30	2.07	>100	3.34	7.85	0.84	3.48
31	7.81	>100	3.69	4.03	0.70	6.10
32	7.52	78.9	6.92	9.75	0.77	6.35
33	36.4	>100	4.53	0.85	9.12	7.26
34	68.2	>100	8.79	79.8	8.15	4.24
35	44.1	>100	8.58	17.4	7.42	5.97

Coumarins **5-35** show different types of inhibitory activities: most derivatives were ineffective or poorly effective as hCA II inhibitors, whereas they showed more efficient (sometimes micro- or even sub-micromolar inhibition) against isoforms hCA I, VII, IX, XII and XIII. Derivative **17** was a low nanomolar hCA I inhibitor, being the most interesting case studied in this work [58] *et al.* **1**. hCA IX and XII were better inhibited by **5-35** compared to other CA isoforms [58]. The SAR was rather obvious: the position and nature of substituents on both aromatic rings were the most relevant factors influencing CA inhibitory efficacy [58].

In the study by Fois *et al.* [61] coumarins isolated from the Sardinian plant *Magydaris pastinacea* Fig. (**5**) were observed to efficiently inhibit isoforms hCA IX and XII, which are tumor-associated enzymes, whereas the cytosolic isoforms hCA I and II were not inhibited or were weakly inhibited by these compounds *et al* **2**.

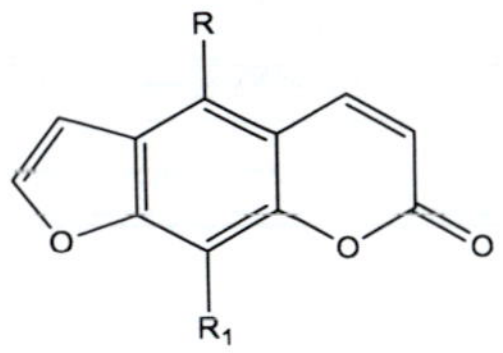

36 R= OCH_3 R_1= H
37 R= H R_1= OCH_3
38 R = OCH_3 R_1 = OCH_3

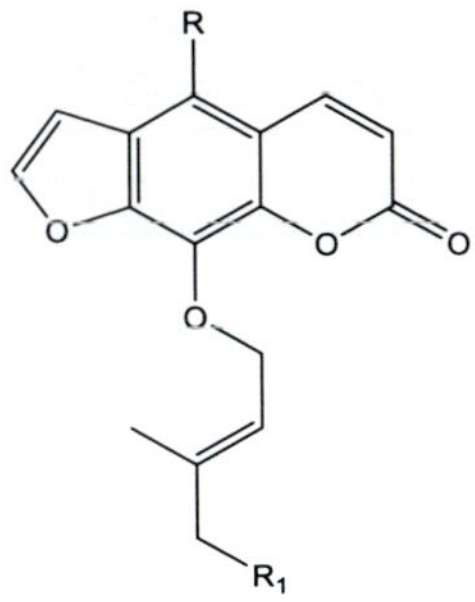

39 R = H R_1 = OH
40 R = OCH_3 R_1 = OH
41 R = H R_1 = H
42 R = OCH_3 R_1 = H

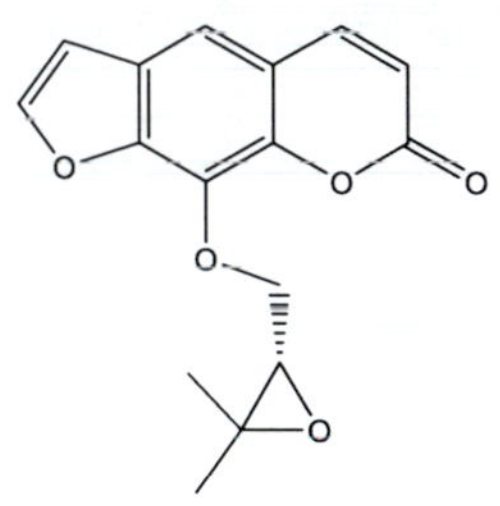

43

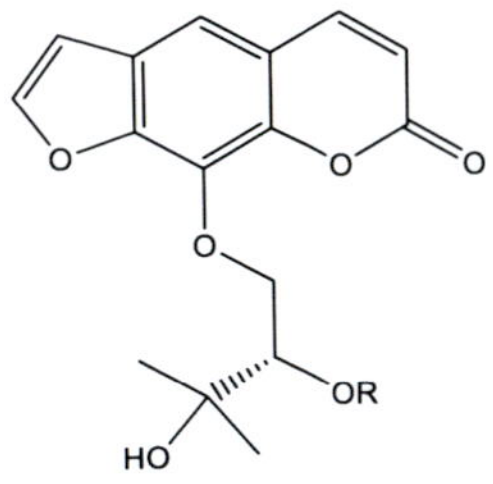

44 R = H
45 R = $COCH_3$

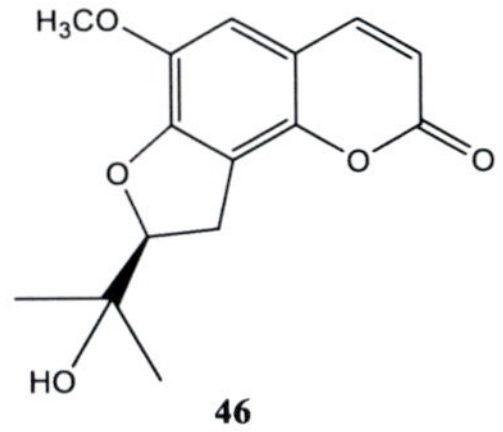

46

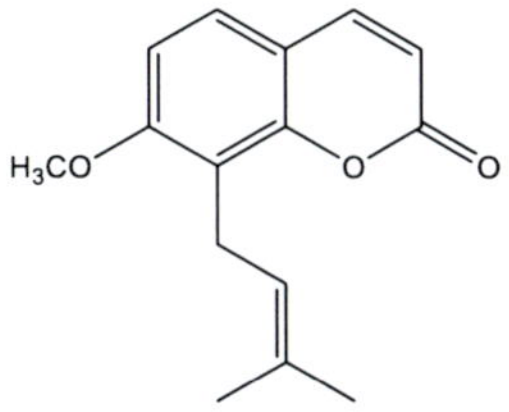

47

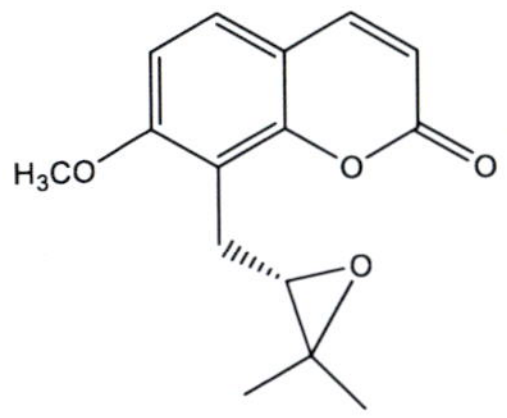

48

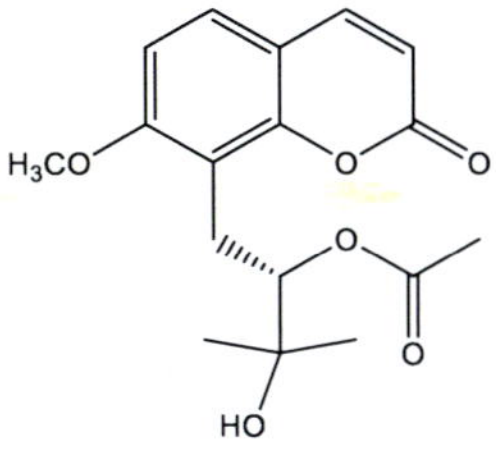

49

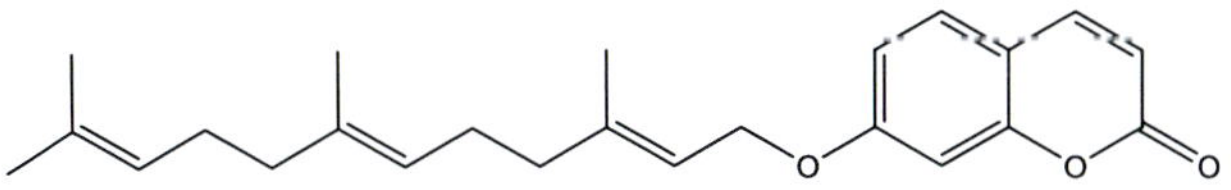

50

Fig. (5). NPCs **36–50** isolated from the *Magydaris pastinacea* and investigated as CAIs.

Table 2. Inhibition data with coumarins 36-50 against isoforms hCA I, II, IX, and XII [61].

NPC	K_I (nM)			
	hCA I	hCA II	hCA IX	hCA XII
36	>10000	>10000	1953	855.1
37	>10000	>10000	194.8	876.3
38	>10000	>10000	159.8	590.1
39	>10000	>10000	2339	550.0

(Table 2) cont.....

NPC	K_I (nM)			
	hCA I	hCA II	hCA IX	hCA XII
40	>10000	>10000	1501	63.5
41	>10000	>10000	221.4	832.9
42	>10000	>10000	201.9	786.9
43	>10000	>10000	162.5	835.6
44	>10000	>10000	27.5	813.8
45	>10000	>10000	192.5	>10000
46	>10000	>10000	150.9	623.0
47	>10000	>10000	2471	74.5
48	>10000	>10000	1888	>10000
49	>10000	>10000	>10000	290.9
50	>10000	>10000	266.4	5.8

Compounds **36-45** are psoralens (furocoumarins), incorporating a tricyclic ring system in which the furan heterocycle is also present. Psoralens are in fact present in many plants [62]. Many of these derivatives also incorporate isoprenyl-, hydrated isoprenyl- or polyprenylated moieties, found in many NPs [61]. Compounds **36-45** were again ineffective as hCA I/II inhibitors, as many coumarins investigated earlier [47, 57, 58], but they effectively inhibited (however, in the high nanomolar range) the tumor-associated hCA IX and XII enzymes *et al* **2** [61].

Melis *et al.* [62] investigated other NCPs and psoralens of types **51-58**. Such compounds also had carboxylic ester/acid moieties in their molecules, and their inhibition was measured against four isoforms, hCA I, II, IX and XII *et al* **3**. Psoralens may show photo-activatable antitumor properties, due to the presence of the furocoumarin ring system in their molecules [62].

Table 3. NPCs/psoralens 51-58 investigated as hCA I, II, IX and XII inhibitors [62].

NPC	R	K_I (nM)			
		hCA I	hCA II	hCA IX	hCA XII
51	Cl	>10000	>10000	23.6	446.6
52	Me	>10000	>10000	122.8	56.6
53	H	>10000	>10000	89.7	72.5
54	F	>10000	>10000	84.7	250.0
55	Cl	>10000	>10000	94.7	9.3
56	Me	>10000	>10000	23.0	9.1
57	H	>10000	>10000	17.5	9.4
58	F	>10000	>10000	17.7	7.4

Table 4. NPCs/psoralens 59-66 investigated as hCA I, II, IX and XII inhibitors [63].

NPC	R	K_i (nM)*			
		hCA I	hCA II	hCA IX	hCA XII
59	4-CH_3	>10000	>10000	247.7	350.3
60	4-OCH_3	>10000	>10000	352.7	324.2
61	4-F	>10000	>10000	239.5	257.1
62	4-C_6H_5	>10000	>10000	135.2	283.1
63	4-CH_3	>10000	>10000	467.3	758.1
64	4-OCH_3	>10000	>10000	489.3	859.4
65	4-F	>10000	>10000	379.7	460.0
66	4-C_6H_5	>10000	>10000	397.7	550.0

More recently, the same group reported hCA I, II, IX and XII inhibition data with other NPCs and psoralens, of type **59-66** [63]. Also, these derivatives incorporating ester or carboxylic acid moieties, were not inhibitory against the cytosolic isoforms hCA I and II, and showed a moderate, submicromolar inhibitory action against the tumor-associated enzymes hCA IX and XII *et al***4** [63].

Synthetic Coumarins

A large number of simple, variously substituted coumarins were investigated as CAIs [64, 65]. Among them, compounds **66-72**, which incorporate hydroxyl, chlorine and/or chloromethyl moieties, were ineffective hCA II inhibitors, and showed a rather high micromolar hCA I inhibitory activity, but were effective, in the low micromolar or submicromolar range against hCA IX and XII, the tumor-associated enzymes, proving that these scaffolds (especially the umbelliferone one, **69**) are quite promising for obtaining CAIs with effective inhibitory power [64, 65] *et al.*

Table 5. Inhibition data of coumarins 66-72 against cytosolic and membrane-associated CA isoforms hCA I, II, IX and XII [64].

Compound	K_I (μM)			
	hCA I	hCA II	hCA IX	hCA XII
66	79.4	> 100	0.51	9.60
67	95.0	> 100	0.42	6.30
68	> 100	> 100	0.20	0.68
69	58.4	> 100	0.48	0.75
70	> 100	> 100	0.48	8.02
71	72.8	> 100	0.36	0.73
72	86.9	> 100	4.92	7.03

In another study, Maresca *et al.* [66] showed that the substitution pattern of the isomeric 6,7- and 7,8-

disubstituted coumarins obtained starting from umbelliferone **69**, of types **77-95**, greatly influences the CA inhibitory properties. The compounds were obtained by using the Fries rearrangement of acylated umbelliferones **75** and **76** in the presence of $AlCl_3$, which afforded the isomeric phenolic ketone pairs **77**, **79** and **78**, **80**, respectively, which in turn were transformed to phenolic ethers by reaction with alcohols Scheme (**1**). The CA inhibitory activity of these compounds against the four mentioned isoforms is shown in *et al***6**.

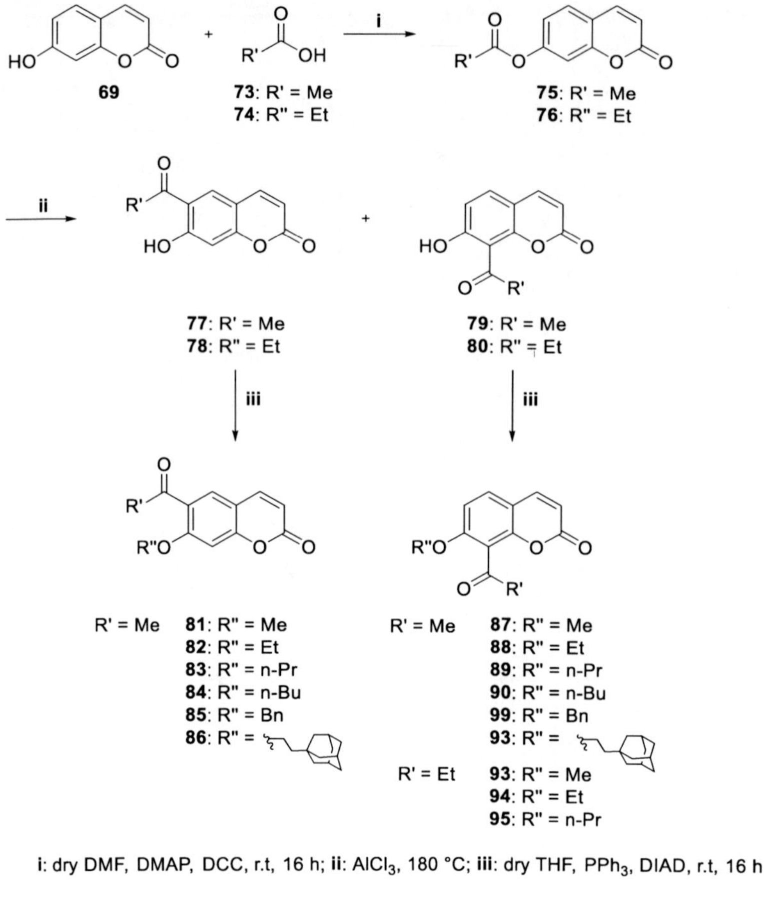

Scheme (1). Preparation of 6,7- and 7,8-disubstituted coumarins by using the Fries rearrangement reaction [66].

Table 6. hCA I, II, IX and XII inhibition data with coumarins 77-95, by a stopped-flow, CO_2 hydration assay method (6 h incubation time between enzyme and coumarin).

Compound	K_I			
	hCA I (µM)	hCA II (µM)	hCA IX (nM)	hCA XII (nM)
77	> 100	> 100	8030	>100000
78	> 100	> 100	8015	>100000
79	> 100	> 100	73.0	61.9
80	> 100	> 100	58.2	61.7

(Table 6) cont.....

Compound	K_I			
	hCA I (μM)	hCA II (μM)	hCA IX (nM)	hCA XII (nM)
81	> 100	> 100	7800	6540
82	> 100	> 100	7400	>100000
83	> 100	> 100	7580	>100000
84	> 100	> 100	>100000	>100000
85	> 100	> 100	>100000	>100000
86	> 100	> 100	>100000	77700
87	> 100	> 100	78.3	60.9
88	> 100	> 100	70.8	1.0
89	> 100	> 100	56.7	0.98
90	> 100	> 100	61.2	8.8
91	> 100	> 100	72.3	22.4
92	> 100	> 100	63.9	31.5
93	> 100	> 100	37.8	26.3
94	> 100	> 100	46.7	33.2
95	> 100	> 100	50.2	38.4

It was quite interesting to note that all these new coumarins were ineffective as inhibitors of the cytosolic isoforms hCA I and II (with inhibition constants > 100 μM). The compounds with the 6,7-substitution pattern were generally also ineffective or poorly effective hCA IX and XII inhibitors (except **79** and **80** which showed K_Is in the range of 58.2–73.0 nM). However, the 7,8-disubstituted derivatives **87-95** showed a much more effective inhibitory activity against the tumor-associated isoforms compared to their corresponding 6,7-regioisomers, possessing K_Is in the range of 0.98–78.3 nM, and being also isoform-selective for the transmembrane *versus* the cytosolic CA isoforms [66]. This is one of the first drug design studies of coumarins acting as highly effective and also isoform-selective CAIs, using as lead umbelliferone **69**, a natural product coumarin with the modest CA inhibitory action [64].

Carta *et al.* [67] reported and investigated CAIs coumarins and 2-thioxo-coumarins of type **96-117** *et al.* which incorporate *tert*-butyl-dimethyl-silyl, propenyl, hydroxymethyl as well as other such simple moieties in 4, 6 and or 7 positions of the coumarin ring.

Table 7. hCA I, II, IX and XII inhibition data against with (thio)coumarins 96-117 by a stopped-flow CO_2 hydrase assay (incubation time of enzyme with inhibitor for 6 h).

96-113 114-117						
Compound	**X**	**R**	**K_I (μM)**			
			hCA I	**hCA II**	**hCA IX**	**hCA XII**
96	O	H (6)	>100	>100	0.19	0.68
97	O	H (7)	58.4	>100	0.48	0.75

(Table 7) cont.....

96-113 114-117						
Compound	**X**	**R**	**K_I (μM)**			
			hCA I	**hCA II**	**hCA IX**	**hCA XII**
98	O	H (4)	95.0	>100	0.41	6.30
99	O	6-*t*-Bu(Me_2)Si	8.78	>200	0.80	0.28
100	S	6-*t*-Bu(Me_2)Si	7.57	>200	0.86	0.31
101	S	H (6)	7.17	>200	0.80	0.34
102	O	6-*t*-Bu(Me_2)Si	8.32	>200	0.85	0.83
103	S	6-*t*-Bu(Me_2)Si	8.18	>200	0.96	0.35
104	S	H (7)	8.02	>200	0.78	0.32
105	O	6-CH_2=CH-CH_2	30.3	>200	0.93	0.80
106	O	7-CH_2=CH-CH_2	72.9	>200	0.73	0.64
107	O	4-CH_2=CH-CH_2	43.2	>200	0.21	0.88
108	S	6-CH_2=CH-CH_2	8.51	>200	3.26	1.25
109	S	7-CH_2=CH-CH_2	7.60	>200	3.23	2.83
110	S	4-CH_2=CH-CH_2	9.24	>200	3.04	1.27
111	O	6-$HOCH_2CH_2$	24.4	>200	0.92	0.63
112	O	6-Ts-OCH_2CH_2	66.3	>200	0.53	0.90
113	O	6-FCH_2CH_2	42.9	>200	0.68	0.59
114	O	H	5.56	>200	7.64	9.13
115	O	Ac	47.7	>200	0.39	0.91
116	O	3,5-$Me_2C_6H_3$NHCO	38.8	>200	0.61	0.64
117	O	*t*-Bu-OCO	91.7	>200	0.97	0.58
1		-	3.1	9.2	>200	>200

For the relatively non-bulky substituents present in these derivatives, again there was no significant inhibition of the cytosolic isoforms, and effective submicromolar inhibition against the tumor-associated ones, but with quite small variations in potency for the various derivatives. This is probably explainable by the relatively small volume of the substituents present in the various positions of the coumarin ring in these derivatives [67].

Bonneau *et al.* [68] used a similar strategy to obtain metronidazole conjugates of 5- and 6-hydroxy-4-methyl-coumarin, as shown in Scheme (**2**). These two compounds (**121** and **123**) as well as 3-cyano-7-hydroxy-coumarin (**123**), reported to act as monocarboxylate transporter (MCT) inhibitors [68], were investigated for the inhibition of 11 human isoforms shown in *et al***8**.

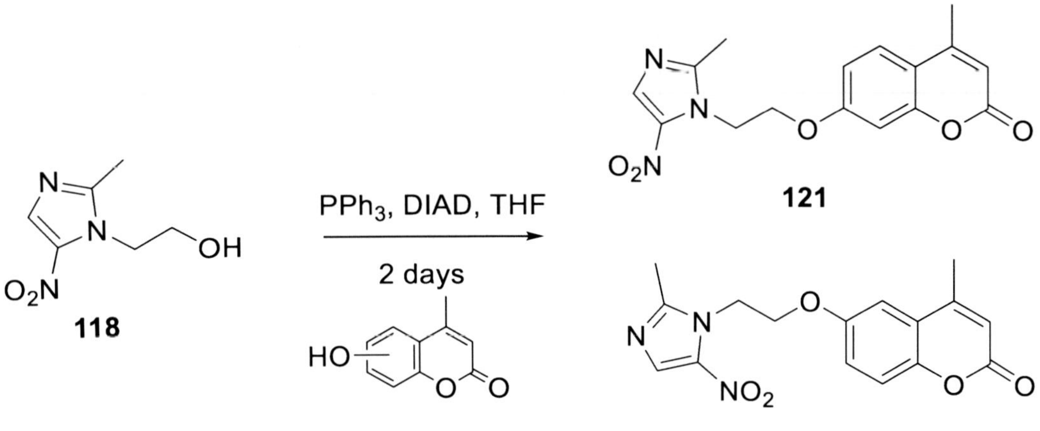

Scheme (2). Preparation of metronidazole-coumarin conjugates **121** and **122** [68].

Table 8. Inhibition of human (h) CA isoforms hCA I-hCA XIV with compounds 121, 122, 123 and the sulfonamide inhibitor acetazolamide 124 (AAZ).

CA Isoform	121	122	123	124
	K_I (μM)			
hCA I	>200	>200	104	0.25
hCA II	>200	>200	>200	0.012
hCA IV	>200	>200	>200	0.074
hCA VA	0.84	2.63	2.27	0.063
hCA VB	0.38	0.43	1.87	0.054
hCA VI	0.46	0.47	0.37	0.011
hCA VII	0.42	0.80	2.98	0.0025
hCA IX	0.37	0.40	0.24	0.025
hCA XII	0.39	53	7.11	0.0057
hCA XIII	>200	>200	5.34	0.017
hCA XIV	0.93	0.82	6.25	0.041

It may be observed that isoforms hCA I, II, IV and XIII are poorly inhibited by these compounds (except **124** against hCA XIII, which acts as a micromolar inhibitor), whereas the remaining isoforms are much better inhibited by all these derivatives, in the micro- or submicromolar range of inhibition constants [68].

Table 9. Inhibition of all human catalytically active isoforms with compounds 125 and 126.

125 126		
CA isoform	125	126
	K_I (nM)	

(Table 9) cont.....

125 126		
CA isoform	**125**	**126**
	K_I (nM)	
hCA I	6120	5560
hCA II	> 10000	> 10000
hCA III	3950	8440
hCA IV	9495	> 10000
hCA VA	904	7810
hCA VI	3900	5695
hCA VII	480	185
hCA IX	124	7640
hCA XII	16.1	9130
hCA XIII	3810	7830
hCA XIV	510	188

7-Amino-3,4-dihydro-1*H*-quinolin-2-one **125**, which has a binuclear ring system similar to one of the coumarins and incorporates a lactam instead of the lactone ring, was investigated together with the structurally related 4-methyl-7-amino coumarins as an inhibitor of all catalytically active hCA isoforms *et al* [69]. The best inhibition was observed for isoforms hCA IX and XII with the lactam **125** and for the brain-associated cytosolic isoform hCA VII with the aminocoumarin **126**, in the nanomolar range. The other isoforms were either not inhibited (hCA II and hCA IV with **126**) or were inhibited in the micromolar range [69].

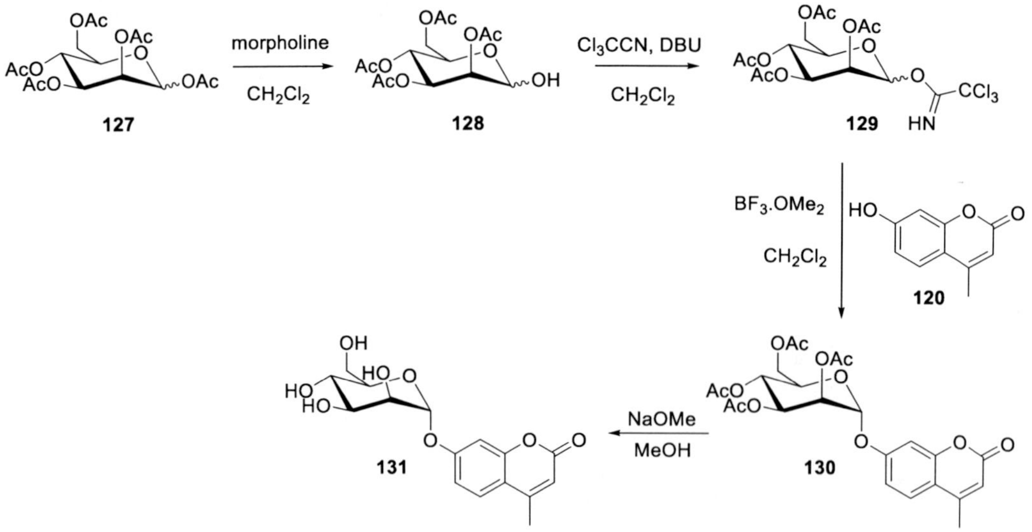

Scheme (3). Synthesis of glycosylated coumarins [70].

Touisini *et al.* [70] reported a series of 7-glycosylated coumarins of type **131** incorporating various mono- and disaccharides the glycosyl derivative synthesis is shown in Scheme (**3**).

Table 10. hCA I, II, IX and XII inhibition data with glycosylcoumarins 131-137.

Compound (sugar)	K_I (μM)			
	hCA I	hCA II	hCA IX	hCA XII
131 (glucose)	1.0	> 100	0.37	54 nM
132 (xylose)	3.4	> 100	0.35	105 nM
133 (galactose)	0.59	77	93 nM	8.5 nM
134 (mannose)	> 100	> 100	9.2 nM	43 nM
135 (rhamnose)	> 100	> 100	201 nM	184 nM
136 (melibiopyranose)	0.88	0.59	0.82	101 nM
137 (ribose)	> 100	> 100	3.2	53 nM

Depending on the nature of the sugar, some of these compounds were low nanomolar CA IX/XII inhibitors and also showed significant anti-tumor effects in a murine model of breast cancer. Their inhibitory effects against hCA I and II were modest or absent, as seen in *et al***10**.

5- and/or 6-membered (thio)lactones were shown to possess similar activities as the coumarins, through a simplification of the pharmacophore, which is in these cases monocyclic, but the activity was reduced compared to the bicyclic corresponding derivatives [71]. However, an interesting X-ray crystal structure of 6-hydroxy-2-thioxocoumarin (compound **101**) bound to hCA II afforded an explanation for the inhibition mechanism with these derivatives. As shown in Fig. (**6**), the exocyclic sulfur atom is anchored to the zinc-coordinated water molecule; this inhibition mechanism is thus diverse of those of the coumarins, which bind towards a more external part of the active site, as discussed above [72].

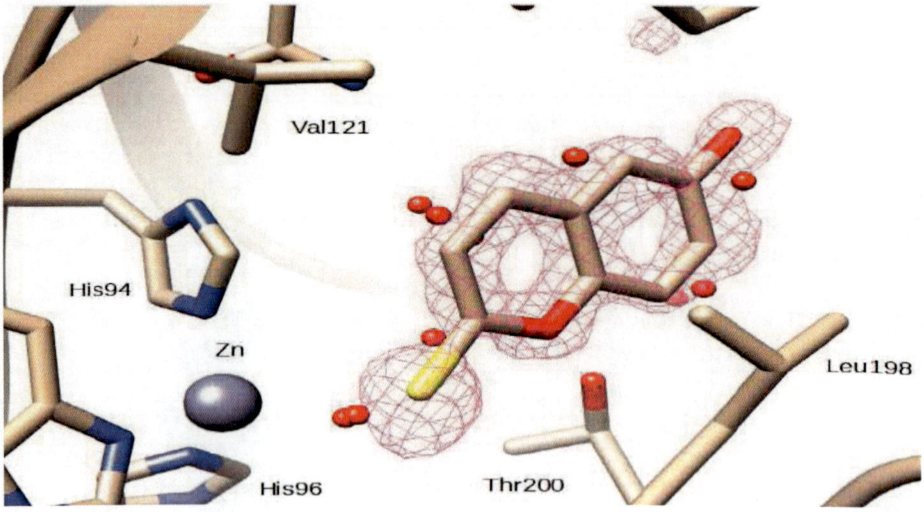

Fig. (6). Binding of 6-hydroxy-2-thioxo-coumarin **101** to hCA II as determined by X-ray crystallography. The zinc ion, its His ligands and the inhibitor (electronic density) are shown in detail. The water molecules are represented as red spheres [72].

One of the most interesting developments in the field was probably the report of coumarin derivatives conjugated with carboxylic acids of the non-steroidal anti-inflammatory drug (NSAID) type – Scheme **4**, compounds **141** and **142** [73].

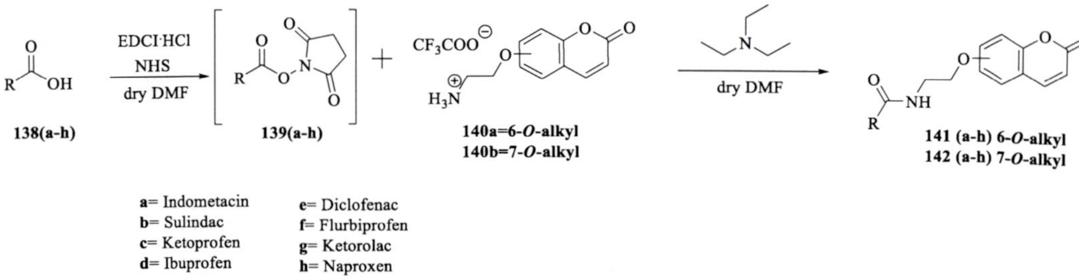

Scheme (4). Synthesis of coumarin–NSAID conjugates **141** and **142**.

Carboxylic moieties of NSAIDs such as indomethacin, sulindac, ketoprofen, ibuprofen, diclofenac, flurbiprofen, ketorolac and naproxen were activated with *N*-hydroxy-succinimide and coupled with the aminoethyloxy-coumarins **140a,b** leading to the desired conjugates **141** and **142** [73]. The obtained compounds are shown in Fig. **(7)**.

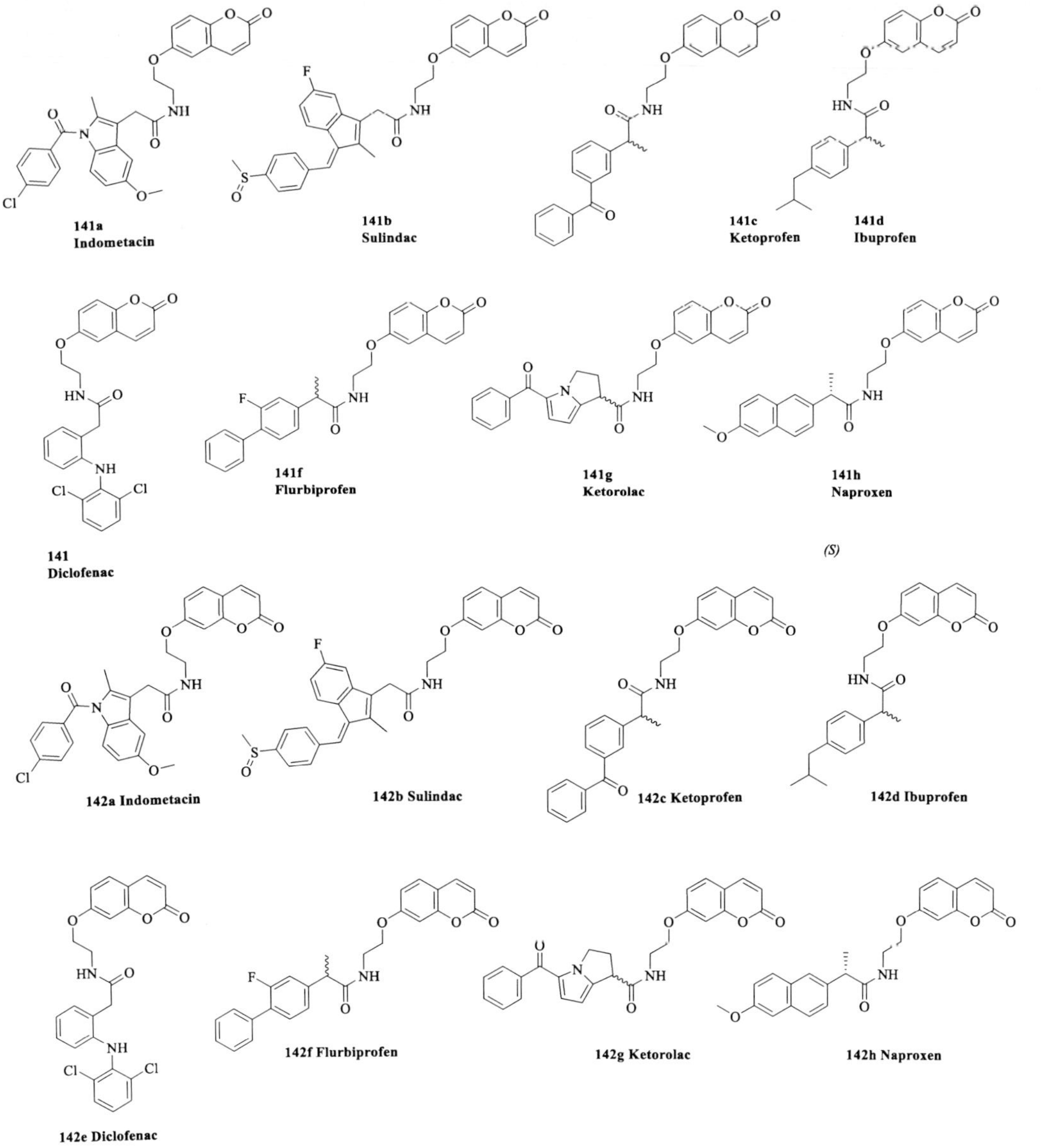

Fig. (7). Coumarin–NSAIDs conjugates **141** and **142**.

Table 11. hCA I, II, IV, VII, IX, and XII inhibition data with compounds 141(a-h) and 142(a-h).

Compound	K_I (nM)					
	hCA I	hCA II	hCA IV	hCA VII	hCA IX	hCA XII
141a	>100	>100	2.6	>100	31.3	59.1

(Table 11) cont.....

Compound	K_I (nM)					
	hCA I	hCA II	hCA IV	hCA VII	hCA IX	hCA XII
141b	>100	>100	7.5	>100	30.8	81.7
141c	>100	>100	4.4	>100	54.7	>100
141d	>100	>100	0.44	>100	>100	>100
141e	>100	>100	5.6	>100	28.9	92.6
141f	>100	>100	0.81	>100	23.5	5.9
141g	>100	>100	0.79	>100	31.8	>100
141h	>100	>100	0.73	>100	>100	>100
142a	>100	>100	8.3	>100	20.1	6.5
142b	>100	>100	9.0	>100	27.9	7.7
142c	>100	85.4	9.5	>100	>100	57.8
142d	>100	>100	9.1	>100	>100	39.0
142e	>100	>100	9.1	>100	89.7	80.8
142f	>100	>100	8.8	>100	>100	>100
142g	>100	>100	9.4	>100	>100	>100
142h	>100	>100	9.8	>100	>100	80.7

These conjugates were not inhibitory against the cytosolic isoforms hCA I, II and VII; but showed a rather effective inhibition against the membrane-bound (CA IV) or transmembrane isoforms (hCA IX and XII), which are involved among others in tumorigenesis and rheumatoid arthritis [73]. Indeed, some of the best among these derivatives, which had nanomolar affinity against these isoforms, were also shown to possess significant anti-inflammatory action (much better than the original NSAID from which they were derived) in an animal model of rheumatoid arthritis [73]. A multitude of other drug design studies of coumarin derivatives of this and other types were reported in the last period, which are not discussed in detail here due to limited space [74 - 78].

Other Drug Design Studies using Coumarins as Lead Molecules

Fig. (**8**) shows some of the new chemotypes that have been investigated as CAIs using coumarins as lead molecules [16], many of which have been discussed in the preceding paragraphs.

However, one of the most interesting chemotypes is constituted by the so-called sulfocoumarins, which are in fact 1,2-benzoxathiine 2,2-dioxides, which were reported by Zalubovskis' group [79]. They were designed by a bioisosteric replacement of the carbonyl moiety from coumarins by a SO_2 functionality. A large variety of such compounds were reported to date [80 - 88], as well as their inhibition mechanism [79].

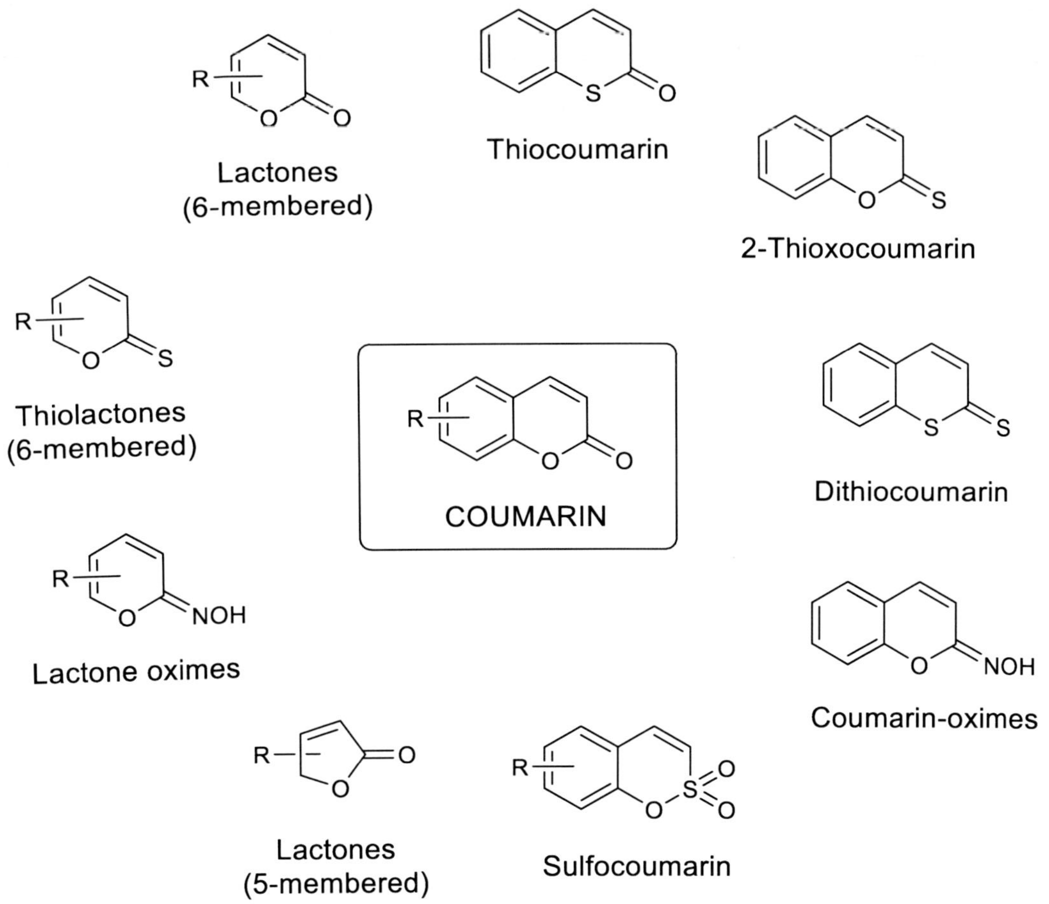

Fig. (8). The main new chemotypes discovered to act as CAIs, using the coumarin scaffold as a lead.

Indeed, by means of X-ray crystallography, it has been observed that the 6-bromo-sulfocoumarin **143** is hydrolysed by the sulfatase CA activity with the formation of presumably the *cis*-sulfonic acid **144**, which is further isomerized to the more s*et al trans*-isomer **145**, observed to be bound within the CA active site cavity, anchored to the zinc coordinated water molecule [79]. In Fig. (**9**), a superimposition with the X-ray structure of the hydrolyzed coumarin **1** (compound **2**) is also shown, in order to note that the hydrolyzed coumarin and the hydrolyzed sulfocoumarin bind in a different mode to the enzyme: the first is observed towards the external art of the active site, occluding its entrance, whereas the second one is bound more internally, by anchoring to the zinc-coordinated water, as thioxocoumarin **101** shown in Fig. (**6**).

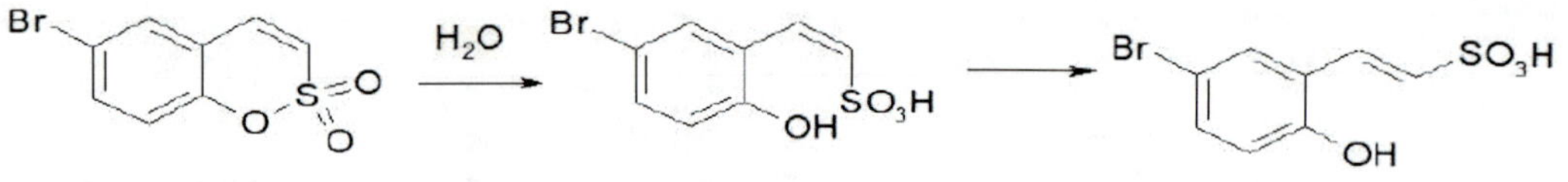

143 **144** **145**

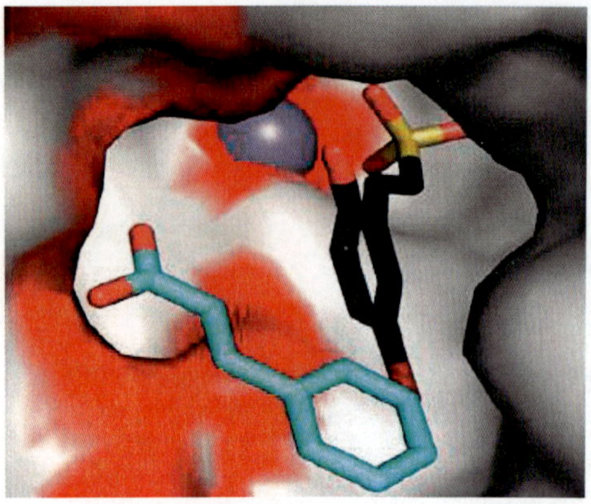

Fig. (9). Overlay of the hydrolyzed sulfocoumarin **145** (black) bound to hCA II and the coumarin **1** (blue sky) hydrolyzed to the *trans*-hydroxycinnamic acid **2**, bound within the enzyme active site, as revealed by X-ray crystallography [57, 79]. The metal ion is shown as the gray sphere with the hydrophobic residues shown in red, and the hydrophilic one in gray.

Some sulfocoumarins reported in this paper [79] have been tested against various CA isoforms and the results are shown in *et al.* The simple derivatives of types **143**, **146–152**, which incorporate either one or two substituents in position(s) 6-, 5,6- and or 6,8- were generally ineffective or poorly effective as inhibitors of the cytosolic isoforms hCA I and II (similar to the coumarins, as discussed in detail above), but they showed low micromolar or submicromolar inhibition against the cancer-associated isoforms hCA IX/XII. The amine **151** was converted to the corresponding azide and used in "click" chemistry for obtaining compounds of types **153-162**, by reactions with various alkynes. These derivatives with a bulkier substitution pattern in position 6, due to the presence of the substituted triazole moieties, showed much more effective inhibitory power against all investigated CA isoforms: they were low micromolar inhibitors of hCA I and II, and nanomolar (in some cases low nanomolar) hCA IX and XII inhibitors. Consequently, a huge number of such derivatives incorporating either substituted triazole, tetrazole, carboxamide, *etc.* moieties in positions 6 or 7 of the sulfocoumarin ring were subsequently prepared and tested for CA inhibitory action, showing rather similar effects to the compounds discussed here [80 - 83].

Table 12. Inhibition of human (h) isozymes hCA I, II, IX, XII and a CA II/IX active site mimic with sulfocoumarins 143, 146-152, by a stopped-flow, CO_2 hydration assay method [79].

143, 146-152 153-162					
Compound	**R**	**K_I (μM)**			
		hCA I	**hCA II**	**hCA IX**	**hCA XII**
143	6-Br	>100	>100	6.83	4.51
146	6-OH	91	>100	0.300	0.234
147	6-$MeSO_3$	99	>100	0.324	0.254
148	6-BnO	93	>100	0.275	0.219
149	5,6-Benzo	>100	>100	0.375	0.717
150	6-O_2N	92	>100	3.77	3.16
151	6-H_2N	6.78	8.89	0.046	0.023
152	6,8-Cl_2	>100	>100	3.26	2.93
153	Ph	6.86	7.76	0.029	0.032
154	COOMe	8.05	6.33	0.95	0.012
155	COOEt	8.88	9.21	0.086	0.013
156	Me_3Si	6.00	7.20	0.060	0.009
157	$HOCH_2$	7.20	9.29	0.058	0.016
158	Et_2NCH_2	8.11	9.37	0.025	0.007
159	4-F_3CO-C_6H_4	8.43	9.64	0.074	0.014
160	4-MeO-C_6H_4	8.93	9.35	0.018	0.039
161	3-F_3C-C_6H_4	6.71	7.72	0.048	0.013
162	3-MeO-C_6H_4	7.47	8.61	0.049	0.021

The derivatives incorporating a 7-membered first ring (3*H*-1,2-benzoxathiepine 2,2-dioxides), also called homosulfocoumarins, were also reported and showed excellent CA IX/XII inhibition, similar to the corresponding sulfocoumarins [84 - 86]. Some of the sulfocoumarins reported ultimately also showed thioredoxin reductase inhibitory action in addition to their CA inhibitory power [87, 88], making them of great interest in conditions in which both enzymes are hyper-expressed (*e.g.*, some types of tumors) [87, 88].

Heterocoumarins, incorporating other chalcogens, such as Se and Te were also recently reported to act as CAIs [89], whereas the coumarin-binding site was observed by means of X-ray crystallography to accommodate the antiepileptic drug lacosamide, structurally very diverse of the coumarins, which showed moderate CA inhibitory properties [90].

CONCLUSIONS

Coumarins and their derivatives are highly abundant natural products [48] and show a variety of biological activities, which explain their multiple pharmacologic applications [91 - 93]. The discovery of their CA inhibitory activity in 2008-2009 constituted the beginning of a new scientific prolific field, which was possible due to the comprehensive explanation of their enzymatic inhibition mechanism, which is quite different from all other CA inhibitory phenomena known earlier. Indeed, as shown in detail here, the coumarins and some of their derivative possess a very particular interaction with these enzymes, as they bind to the active site cleft and first undergo a hydrolytic process that generates rather bulky 2-hydroxy-cinnamic acids which are unable to bind in the neighbourhood of the catalytic metal ion, deep within the active site. Thus, they move and bind steadfastly at the entrance of the cavity, where only CA activators were observed earlier. In this way, they occlude the entrance to the active site cavity and block the catalytic process. Many new chemotypes possessing such properties or similar inhibition mechanisms have been developed in the last decade starting from these discoveries, and nowadays a huge number of such compounds belonging to more than 10 different classes have been evaluated in detail, as outlined here. Thus, the monocyclic 5- and 6-ring lactones and thiolactones, thio- and 2-thioxo-coumarins, quinoline-2-ones, sulfocoumarins, homosulfocoumarins, and hetero-(seleno/telluro) coumarins were investigated so far. Thus, the type of prodrug CAI inspired also research in the field of anti-infectives [91], but mainly anti-tumor [92, 93] and anti-inflammatory derivatives [73] based on such CAIs. Only the human α-class CAs were investigated for the moment for their interaction with coumarins and their derivatives, but these enzymes are also present in pathogenic bacteria, protozoans, fungi, and worms [94 - 101], and investigation of coumarin inhibitors for the potential inhibition of such enzymes may lead to relevant developments in the fight against infections produced by pathogens.

CONSENT FOR PUBLICATION

Not applicable.

CONFLICT OF INTEREST

The author declares no conflict of interest, financial or otherwise.

ACKNOWLEDGEMENT

Declared none.

REFERENCES

[1] Supuran, C.T. Carbonic anhydrases: novel therapeutic applications for inhibitors and activators. *Nat. Rev. Drug Discov.*, **2008**, *7*(2), 168-181.
[http://dx.doi.org/10.1038/nrd2467] [PMID: 18167490]

[2] Supuran, C.T. Structure and function of carbonic anhydrases. *Biochem. J.*, **2016**, *473*(14), 2023-2032.
[http://dx.doi.org/10.1042/BCJ20160115] [PMID: 27407171]

[3] Supuran, C.; Capasso, C. An overview of the bacterial carbonic anhydrases. *Metabolites*, **2017**, *7*(4), 56.
[http://dx.doi.org/10.3390/metabo7040056] [PMID: 29137134]

[4] Capasso, C.; Supuran, C.T. An overview of the alpha-, beta- and gamma-carbonic anhydrases from *Bacteria* : can bacterial carbonic anhydrases shed new light on evolution of bacteria? *J. Enzyme Inhib. Med. Chem.*, **2015**, *30*(2), 325-332.
[http://dx.doi.org/10.3109/14756366.2014.910202] [PMID: 24766661]

[5] Del Prete, S.; Nocentini, A.; Supuran, C.T.; Capasso, C. Bacterial ι-carbonic anhydrase: a new active class of carbonic anhydrase identified in the genome of the Gram-negative bacterium *Burkholderia territorii*. *J. Enzyme Inhib. Med. Chem.*, **2020**, *35*(1), 1060-1068.
[http://dx.doi.org/10.1080/14756366.2020.1755852] [PMID: 32314608]

[6] Güzel-Akdemir, Ö.; Carradori, S.; Grande, R.; Demir-Yazıcı, K.; Angeli, A.; Supuran, C.T.; Akdemir, A. Development of Thiazolidinones as Fungal Carbonic Anhydrase Inhibitors. *Int. J. Mol. Sci.*, **2020**, *21*(8), 2960.
[http://dx.doi.org/10.3390/ijms21082960] [PMID: 32331447]

[7] Supuran, C.T.; Capasso, C. Biomedical applications of prokaryotic carbonic anhydrases. *Expert Opin. Ther. Pat.*, **2018**, *28*(10), 745-754.
[http://dx.doi.org/10.1080/13543776.2018.1497161] [PMID: 29973089]

[8] Nocentini, A.; Supuran, C.T. Advances in the structural annotation of human carbonic anhydrases and impact on future drug discovery. *Expert Opin. Drug Discov.*, **2019**, *14*(11), 1175-1197.
[http://dx.doi.org/10.1080/17460441.2019.1651289] [PMID: 31436118]

[9] Del Prete, S.; Vullo, D.; Fisher, G.M.; Andrews, K.T.; Poulsen, S.A.; Capasso, C.; Supuran, C.T. Discovery of a new family of carbonic anhydrases in the malaria pathogen *Plasmodium falciparum*—The η-carbonic anhydrases. *Bioorg. Med. Chem. Lett.*, **2014**, *24*(18), 4389-4396.
[http://dx.doi.org/10.1016/j.bmcl.2014.08.015] [PMID: 25168745]

[10] Alterio, V.; Langella, E.; Viparelli, F.; Vullo, D.; Ascione, G.; Dathan, N.A.; Morel, F.M.M.; Supuran, C.T.; De Simone, G.; Monti, S.M. Structural and inhibition insights into carbonic anhydrase CDCA1 from the marine diatom *Thalassiosira weissflogii*. *Biochimie*, **2012**, *94*(5), 1232-1241.
[http://dx.doi.org/10.1016/j.biochi.2012.02.013] [PMID: 22381359]

[11] Supuran, C.T.; Capasso, C. Antibacterial carbonic anhydrase inhibitors: an update on the recent literature. *Expert Opin. Ther. Pat.*, **2020**, *30*(12), 963-982.
[http://dx.doi.org/10.1080/13543776.2020.1811853] [PMID: 32806966]

[12] Supuran, C.T. Carbonic anhydrase inhibitors and their potential in a range of therapeutic areas. *Expert Opin. Ther. Pat.*, **2018**, *28*(10), 709-712.
[http://dx.doi.org/10.1080/13543776.2018.1523897] [PMID: 30217119]

[13] McDonald, P.C.; Chafe, S.C.; Brown, W.S. Regulation of pH by carbonic anhydrase 9 mediates survival of pancreatic cancer cells with activated KRAS in response to hypoxia. *Gastroenterology*, **2019**, *157*(3), 823-837.
[http://dx.doi.org/10.1053/j.gastro.2019.05.004] [PMID: 31078621]

[14] Berrino, E.; Carradori, S.; Angeli, A. Dual Carbonic Anhydrase IX/XII Inhibitors and Carbon Monoxide Releasing Molecules Modulate LPS-Mediated Inflammation in Mouse Macrophages. *Antioxidants*, **2021**, *10*(1), 56.

[http://dx.doi.org/10.3390/antiox10010056] [PMID: 33466457]

[15] Berrino, E.; Supuran, C.T. Novel approaches for designing drugs that interfere with pH regulation. *Expert Opin. Drug Discov.*, **2019**, *14*(3), 231-248. [http://dx.doi.org/10.1080/17460441.2019.1567488] [PMID: 30681011]

[16] Supuran, C.T. How many carbonic anhydrase inhibition mechanisms exist? *J. Enzyme Inhib. Med. Chem.*, **2016**, *31*(3), 345-360. [http://dx.doi.org/10.3109/14756366.2015.1122001] [PMID: 26619898]

[17] Supuran, C.T. Carbonic anhydrase inhibitors as emerging agents for the treatment and imaging of hypoxic tumors. *Expert Opin. Investig. Drugs,* **2018**, *27*(12), 963-970. [http://dx.doi.org/10.1080/13543784.2018.1548608] [PMID: 30426805]

[18] Neri, D.; Supuran, C.T. Interfering with pH regulation in tumours as a therapeutic strategy. *Nat. Rev. Drug Discov.*, **2011**, *10*(10), 767-777. [http://dx.doi.org/10.1038/nrd3554] [PMID: 21921921]

[19] Supuran, C.; Vullo, D.; Manole, G.; Casini, A.; Scozzafava, A. Designing of novel carbonic anhydrase inhibitors and activators. *Curr. Med. Chem. Cardiovasc. Hematol. Agents,* **2004**, *2*(1), 49-68. [http://dx.doi.org/10.2174/1568016043477305] [PMID: 15328829]

[20] Supuran, C.T. Carbon- *versus* sulphur-based zinc binding groups for carbonic anhydrase inhibitors? *J. Enzyme Inhib. Med. Chem.*, **2018**, *33*(1), 485-495. [http://dx.doi.org/10.1080/14756366.2018.1428572] [PMID: 29390912]

[21] Provensi, G.; Carta, F.; Nocentini, A.; Supuran, C.T.; Casamenti, F.; Passani, M.B.; Fossati, S. A new kid on the block? Carbonic anhydrases as possible new targets in Alzheimer's disease. *Int. J. Mol. Sci.*, **2019**, *20*(19), 4724. [http://dx.doi.org/10.3390/ijms20194724] [PMID: 31554165]

[22] Supuran, C.T. Applications of carbonic anhydrases inhibitors in renal and central nervous system diseases. *Expert Opin. Ther. Pat.*, **2018**, *28*(10), 713-721. [http://dx.doi.org/10.1080/13543776.2018.1519023] [PMID: 30175635]

[23] Supuran, C.T. Drug interaction considerations in the therapeutic use of carbonic anhydrase inhibitors. *Expert Opin. Drug Metab. Toxicol.*, **2016**, *12*(4), 423-431. [http://dx.doi.org/10.1517/17425255.2016.1154534] [PMID: 26878088]

[24] Temperini, C.; Cecchi, A.; Scozzafava, A.; Supuran, C.T. Carbonic anhydrase inhibitors. Sulfonamide diuretics revisited—old leads for new applications? *Org. Biomol. Chem.*, **2008**, *6*(14), 2499-2506. [http://dx.doi.org/10.1039/b800767e] [PMID: 18600270]

[25] Supuran, C.T. The management of glaucoma and macular degeneration. *Expert Opin. Ther. Pat.*, **2019**, *29*(10), 745-747. [http://dx.doi.org/10.1080/13543776.2019.1674285] [PMID: 31566015]

[26] Supuran, C.T.; Altamimi, A.S.A.; Carta, F. Carbonic anhydrase inhibition and the management of glaucoma: a literature and patent review 2013-2019. *Expert Opin. Ther. Pat.*, **2019**, *29*(10), 781-792. [http://dx.doi.org/10.1080/13543776.2019.1679117] [PMID: 31596641]

[27] Di Fiore, A.; De Simone, G.; Alterio, V.; Riccio, V.; Winum, J.Y.; Carta, F.; Supuran, C.T. The anticonvulsant sulfamide JNJ-26990990 and its S,S-dioxide analog strongly inhibit carbonic anhydrases: solution and X-ray crystallographic studies. *Org. Biomol. Chem.*, **2016**, *14*(21), 4853-4858. [http://dx.doi.org/10.1039/C6OB00803H] [PMID: 27151329]

[28] Aggarwal, M.; Kondeti, B.; McKenna, R. Anticonvulsant/antiepileptic carbonic anhydrase inhibitors: a patent review *Expert Opin. Ther. Pat.*, **2013**, *23*(6), 717-724. [http://dx.doi.org/10.1517/13543776.2013.782394] [PMID: 23514045]

[29] Scozzafava, A.; Supuran, C.T.; Carta, F. Antiobesity carbonic anhydrase inhibitors: a literature and patent review *Expert Opin. Ther. Pat.*, **2013**, *23*(6), 725-735.

[http://dx.doi.org/10.1517/13543776.2013.790957] [PMID: 23607332]

[30] Supuran, C.T.; Fiore, A.D.; Simone, G.D. Carbonic anhydrase inhibitors as emerging drugs for the treatment of obesity. *Expert Opin. Emerg. Drugs,* **2008**, *13*(2), 383-392. [http://dx.doi.org/10.1517/14728214.13.2.383] [PMID: 18537527]

[31] Kuchuk, O.; Tuccitto, A.; Citterio, D.; Huber, V.; Camisaschi, C.; Milione, M.; Vergani, B.; Villa, A.; Alison, M.R.; Carradori, S.; Supuran, C.T.; Rivoltini, L.; Castelli, C.; Mazzaferro, V. pH regulators to target the tumor immune microenvironment in human hepatocellular carcinoma. *OncoImmunology,* **2018**, *7*(7)e1445452 [http://dx.doi.org/10.1080/2162402X.2018.1445452] [PMID: 29900055]

[32] Tanini, D.; Carradori, S.; Capperucci, A. Chalcogenides-incorporating carbonic anhydrase inhibitors concomitantly reverted oxaliplatin-induced neuropathy and enhanced antiproliferative action. *Eur. J. Med. Chem.,* **2021**, *225*113793 [http://dx.doi.org/10.1016/j.ejmech.2021.113793] [PMID: 34507012]

[33] Nocentini, A.; Supuran, C.T. Carbonic anhydrase inhibitors as antitumor/antimetastatic agents: a patent review (2008–2018). *Expert Opin. Ther. Pat.,* **2018**, *28*(10), 729-740. [http://dx.doi.org/10.1080/13543776.2018.1508453] [PMID: 30074415]

[34] D'Ambrosio, K.; Carradori, S.; Cesa, S.; Angeli, A.; Monti, S.M.; Supuran, C.T.; De Simone, G. Catechols: a new class of carbonic anhydrase inhibitors. *Chem. Commun. (Camb.),* **2020**, *56*(85), 13033-13036. [http://dx.doi.org/10.1039/D0CC05172A] [PMID: 33000794]

[35] Angeli, A.; Carta, F.; Nocentini, A. Carbonic anhydrase inhibitors targeting metabolism and tumor microenvironment. *Metabolites,* **2020**, *10*(10), 412. [http://dx.doi.org/10.3390/metabo10100412] [PMID: 33066524]

[36] Supuran, C.T. Experimental carbonic anhydrase inhibitors for the treatment of hypoxic tumors. *J. Exp. Pharmacol.,* **2020**, *12*, 603-617. [http://dx.doi.org/10.2147/JEP.S265620] [PMID: 33364855]

[37] Supuran, C.T. Carbonic anhydrase activators. *Future Med. Chem.,* **2018**, *10*(5), 561-573. [http://dx.doi.org/10.4155/fmc-2017-0223] [PMID: 29478330]

[38] Angeli, A.; Berrino, E.; Carradori, S. Amine- and Amino Acid-Based Compounds as Carbonic Anhydrase Activators. *Molecules,* **2021**, *26*(23), 7331. [http://dx.doi.org/10.3390/molecules26237331] [PMID: 34885917]

[39] Temperini, C.; Scozzafava, A.; Vullo, D.; Supuran, C.T. Carbonic anhydrase activators. Activation of isozymes I, II, IV, VA, VII, and XIV with l- and d-histidine and crystallographic analysis of their adducts with isoform II: engineering proton-transfer processes within the active site of an enzyme. *Chemistry,* **2006**, *12*(27), 7057-7066. [http://dx.doi.org/10.1002/chem.200600159] [PMID: 16807956]

[40] Mollica, A.; Macedonio, G.; Stefanucci, A.; Carradori, S.; Akdemir, A.; Angeli, A.; Supuran, C. Five- and Six-Membered Nitrogen-Containing Compounds as Selective Carbonic Anhydrase Activators. *Molecules,* **2017**, *22*(12), 2178. [http://dx.doi.org/10.3390/molecules22122178] [PMID: 29232847]

[41] Blandina, P.; Provensi, G.; Passani, M.B.; Capasso, C.; Supuran, C.T. Carbonic anhydrase modulation of emotional memory. Implications for the treatment of cognitive disorders. *J. Enzyme Inhib. Med. Chem.,* **2020**, *35*(1), 1206-1214. [http://dx.doi.org/10.1080/14756366.2020.1766455] [PMID: 32401069]

[42] Schmidt, S.D.; Costa, A.; Rani, B. The role of carbonic anhydrases in extinction of contextual fear memory. *Proc. Natl. Acad. Sci. USA,* **2020**, *117*(27), 16000-16008. [http://dx.doi.org/10.1073/pnas.1910690117] [PMID: 32571910]

[43] Supuran, C.T. Advances in structure-based drug discovery of carbonic anhydrase inhibitors. *Expert*

Opin. Drug Discov., **2017**, *12*(1), 61-88.
[http://dx.doi.org/10.1080/17460441.2017.1253677] [PMID: 27783541]

[44] De Simone, G.; Alterio, V.; Supuran, C.T. Exploiting the hydrophobic and hydrophilic binding sites for designing carbonic anhydrase inhibitors. *Expert Opin. Drug Discov.,* **2013**, *8*(7), 793-810.
[http://dx.doi.org/10.1517/17460441.2013.795145] [PMID: 23627619]

[45] Supuran, C.T. Exploring the multiple binding modes of inhibitors to carbonic anhydrases for novel drug discovery. *Expert Opin. Drug Discov.,* **2020**, *15*(6), 671-686.
[http://dx.doi.org/10.1080/17460441.2020.1743676] [PMID: 32208982]

[46] Vu, H.; Pham, N.B.; Quinn, R.J. Direct screening of natural product extracts using mass spectrometry. *SLAS Discov.,* **2008**, *13*(4), 265-275.
[http://dx.doi.org/10.1177/1087057108315739] [PMID: 18349420]

[47] Maresca, A.; Temperini, C.; Vu, H. Non-zinc mediated inhibition of carbonic anhydrases: coumarins are a new class of suicide inhibitors. *J. Am. Chem. Soc.,* **2009**, *131*(8), 3057-3062.
[http://dx.doi.org/10.1021/ja809683v] [PMID: 19206230]

[48] Atanasov, A.G.; Zotchev, S.B.; Dirsch, V.M.; Supuran, C.T. Natural products in drug discovery: advances and opportunities. *Nat. Rev. Drug Discov.,* **2021**, *20*(3), 200-216.
[http://dx.doi.org/10.1038/s41573-020-00114-z] [PMID: 33510482]

[49] Sethna, S.M.; Shah, N.M. The chemistry of coumarins. *Chem. Rev.,* **1945**, *36*(1), 1-62.
[http://dx.doi.org/10.1021/cr60113a001]

[50] Riveiro, M.; De Kimpe, N.; Moglioni, A. Coumarins: old compounds with novel promising therapeutic perspectives. *Curr. Med. Chem.,* **2010**, *17*(13), 1325-1338.
[http://dx.doi.org/10.2174/092986710790936284] [PMID: 20166938]

[51] Pereira, T.M.; Franco, D.P.; Vitorio, F.; Kummerle, A.E. Coumarin compounds in medicinal chemistry: Some important examples from the last years. *Curr. Top. Med. Chem.,* **2018**, *18*(2), 124-148.
[http://dx.doi.org/10.2174/1568026618666180329115523] [PMID: 29595110]

[52] Stefanachi, A.; Leonetti, F.; Pisani, L.; Catto, M.; Carotti, A. Coumarin: A natural, privileged and versatile scaffold for bioactive compounds. *Molecules,* **2018**, *23*(2), 250.
[http://dx.doi.org/10.3390/molecules23020250] [PMID: 29382051]

[53] Carradori, S.; Secci, D.; Petzer, J.P. MAO inhibitors and their wider applications: a patent review. *Expert Opin. Ther. Pat.,* **2018**, *28*(3), 211-226.
[http://dx.doi.org/10.1080/13543776.2018.1427735] [PMID: 29324067]

[54] Menezes, J.C.J.M.D.S.; Diederich, M. Translational role of natural coumarins and their derivatives as anticancer agents. *Future Med. Chem.,* **2019**, *11*(9), 1057-1082.
[http://dx.doi.org/10.4155/fmc-2018-0375] [PMID: 31140865]

[55] Lippi, G.; Gosselin, R.; Favaloro, E.J. Current and emerging direct oral anticoagulants: State-of-t-e-art. *Semin. Thromb. Hemost.,* **2019**, *45*(5), 490-501.
[http://dx.doi.org/10.1055/s-0039-1692703] [PMID: 31216588]

[56] Supuran, C.T. Coumarin carbonic anhydrase inhibitors from natural sources. *J. Enzyme Inhib. Med. Chem.,* **2020**, *35*(1), 1462-1470.
[http://dx.doi.org/10.1080/14756366.2020.1788009] [PMID: 32779543]

[57] Maresca, A.; Temperini, C.; Pochet, L.; Masereel, B.; Scozzafava, A.; Supuran, C.T. Deciphering the mechanism of carbonic anhydrase inhibition with coumarins and thiocoumarins. *J. Med. Chem.,* **2010**, *53*(1), 335-344.
[http://dx.doi.org/10.1021/jm901287j] [PMID: 19911821]

[58] Davis, R.A.; Vullo, D.; Maresca, A.; Supuran, C.T.; Poulsen, S.A. Natural product coumarins that inhibit human carbonic anhydrases. *Bioorg. Med. Chem.,* **2013**, *21*(6), 1539-1543.
[http://dx.doi.org/10.1016/j.bmc.2012.07.021] [PMID: 22892213]

[59] Temperini, C.; Scozzafava, A.; Vullo, D.; Supuran, C.T. Carbonic anhydrase activators. Activation of isoforms I, II, IV, VA, VII, and XIV with L- and D-phenylalanine and crystallographic analysis of their adducts with isozyme II: stereospecific recognition within the active site of an enzyme and its consequences for the drug design. *J. Med. Chem.*, **2006**, *49*(10), 3019-3027. [http://dx.doi.org/10.1021/jm0603320] [PMID: 16686544]

[60] Temperini, C.; Innocenti, A.; Scozzafava, A.; Supuran, C.T. Carbonic anhydrase activators: Kinetic and X-ray crystallographic study for the interaction of d- and l-tryptophan with the mammalian isoforms I–XIV. *Bioorg. Med. Chem.*, **2008**, *16*(18), 8373-8378. [http://dx.doi.org/10.1016/j.bmc.2008.08.043] [PMID: 18774300]

[61] Fois, B.; Distinto, S.; Meleddu, R. Coumarins from *Magydaris pastinacea* as inhibitors of the tumour-associated carbonic anhydrases IX and XII: isolation, biological studies and in silico evaluation. *J. Enzyme Inhib. Med. Chem.*, **2020**, *35*(1), 539-548. [http://dx.doi.org/10.1080/14756366.2020.1713114] [PMID: 31948300]

[62] Carradori, S. Selective carbonic anhydrase IX inhibitors based on coumarin scaffold as promising antimetastatic agents: WO2012070024. *Expert Opin. Ther. Pat.*, **2013**, *23*(6), 751-756. [http://dx.doi.org/10.1517/13543776.2013.769523] [PMID: 23387899]

[63] Gidaro, M.C.; Alcaro, S.; Secci, D. Identification of new anti- *Candida* compounds by ligand-based pharmacophore virtual screening. *J. Enzyme Inhib. Med. Chem.*, **2016**, *31*(6), 1703-1706. [http://dx.doi.org/10.3109/14756366.2016.1156103] [PMID: 26985772]

[64] Maresca, A.; Supuran, C.T. Coumarins incorporating hydroxy- and chloro-moieties selectively inhibit the transmembrane, tumor-associated carbonic anhydrase isoforms IX and XII over the cytosolic ones I and II. *Bioorg. Med. Chem. Lett.*, **2010**, *20*(15), 4511-4514. [http://dx.doi.org/10.1016/j.bmcl.2010.06.040] [PMID: 20580555]

[65] Sharma, A.; Tiwari, M.; Supuran, C.T. Novel coumarins and benzocoumarins acting as isoform-selective inhibitors against the tumor-associated carbonic anhydrase IX. *J. Enzyme Inhib. Med. Chem.*, **2014**, *29*(2), 292-296. [http://dx.doi.org/10.3109/14756366.2013.777334] [PMID: 23488741]

[66] Maresca, A.; Scozzafava, A.; Supuran, C.T. 7,8-Disubstituted- but not 6,7-disubstituted coumarins selectively inhibit the transmembrane, tumor-associated carbonic anhydrase isoforms IX and XII over the cytosolic ones I and II in the low nanomolar/subnanomolar range. *Bioorg. Med. Chem. Lett.*, **2010**, *20*(24), 7255-7258. [http://dx.doi.org/10.1016/j.bmcl.2010.10.094] [PMID: 21067924]

[67] Carta, F.; Maresca, A.; Scozzafava, A.; Supuran, C.T. Novel coumarins and 2-thioxo-coumarins as inhibitors of the tumor-associated carbonic anhydrases IX and XII. *Bioorg. Med. Chem.*, **2012**, *20*(7), 2266-2273. [http://dx.doi.org/10.1016/j.bmc.2012.02.014] [PMID: 22377674]

[68] Bonneau, A.; Maresca, A.; Winum, J.Y.; Supuran, C.T. Metronidazole-coumarin conjugates and 3-cyano-7-hydroxy-coumarin act as isoform-selective carbonic anhydrase inhibitors. *J. Enzyme Inhib. Med. Chem.*, **2013**, *28*(2), 397-401. [http://dx.doi.org/10.3109/14756366.2011.650692] [PMID: 22299576]

[69] Vullo, D.; Isik, S.; Bozdag, M.; Carta, F.; Supuran, C.T. 7-Amino-3,4-dihydro-1H-quinolin-2-one, a compound similar to the substituted coumarins, inhibits **α** -carbonic anhydrases without hydrolysis of the lactam ring. *J. Enzyme Inhib. Med. Chem.*, **2015**, *30*(5), 773-777. [http://dx.doi.org/10.3109/14756366.2014.970185] [PMID: 25672528]

[70] Mathew, B.; Carradori, S.; Guglielmi, P.; Uddin, M.S.; Kim, H. New Aspects of Monoamine Oxidase B Inhibitors: The Key Role of Halogens to Open the Golden Door. *Curr. Med. Chem.*, **2020**, *28*(2), 266-283. [http://dx.doi.org/10.2174/0929867327666200121165931] [PMID: 31965939]

[71] Mathew, B.; Parambi, D.G.T.; Mathew, G.E.; Uddin, M.S.; Inasu, S.T.; Kim, H.; Marathakam, A.;

Unnikrishnan, M.K.; Carradori, S. Emerging therapeutic potentials of dual-acting MAO and AChE inhibitors in Alzheimer's and Parkinson's diseases. *Arch. Pharm. (Weinheim),* **2019**, *352*(11)1900177 [http://dx.doi.org/10.1002/ardp.201900177] [PMID: 31478569]

[72] Ferraroni, M.; Carta, F.; Scozzafava, A.; Supuran, C.T. Thioxocoumarins show an alternative carbonic anhydrase inhibition mechanism compared to coumarins. *J. Med. Chem.,* **2016**, *59*(1), 462-473. [http://dx.doi.org/10.1021/acs.jmedchem.5b01720] [PMID: 26688270]

[73] Bua, S.; Di Cesare Mannelli, L.; Vullo, D. Design and synthesis of novel nonsteroidal anti-inflammatory drugs and carbonic anhydrase inhibitors hybrids (NSAIDs-CAIs) for the treatment of rheumatoid arthritis. *J. Med. Chem.,* **2017**, *60*(3), 1159-1170. [http://dx.doi.org/10.1021/acs.jmedchem.6b01607] [PMID: 28075587]

[74] Peperidou, A.; Bua, S.; Bozdag, M.; Hadjipavlou-Litina, D.; Supuran, C. Novel 6- and 7-substituted coumarins with inhibitory action against lipoxygenase and tumor-associated carbonic anhydrase IX. *Molecules,* **2018**, *23*(1), 153. [http://dx.doi.org/10.3390/molecules23010153] [PMID: 29329232]

[75] Buran, K.; Bua, S.; Poli, G.; Önen Bayram, F.E.; Tuccinardi, T.; Supuran, C.T. Novel 8-substituted coumarins that selectively inhibit human carbonic anhydrase IX and XII. *Int. J. Mol. Sci.,* **2019**, *20*(5), 1208. [http://dx.doi.org/10.3390/ijms20051208] [PMID: 30857344]

[76] Kartsev, V.; Geronikaki, A.; Bua, S. Extending the inhibition profiles of coumarin-based compounds against human carbonic anhydrases: Synthesis, biological, and *in silico* evaluation. *Molecules,* **2019**, *24*(19), 3580. [http://dx.doi.org/10.3390/molecules24193580] [PMID: 31590289]

[77] Teodori, E.; Braconi, L.; Bua, S. Dual P-glycoprotein and CA XII inhibitors: A new strategy to reverse the P-gp mediated Multidrug Resistance (MDR) in cancer cells. *Molecules,* **2020**, *25*(7), 1748. [http://dx.doi.org/10.3390/molecules25071748] [PMID: 32290281]

[78] Aspatwar, A.; Berrino, E.; Bua, S. Toxicity evaluation of sulfamides and coumarins that efficiently inhibit human carbonic anhydrases. *J. Enzyme Inhib. Med. Chem.,* **2020**, *35*(1), 1765-1772. [http://dx.doi.org/10.1080/14756366.2020.1822829] [PMID: 32942905]

[79] Tars, K.; Vullo, D.; Kazaks, A.; Leitans, Sulfocoumarins (1,2-benzoxathiine-2,2-dioxides): a class of potent and isoform-selective inhibitors of tumor-associated carbonic anhydrases. *J. Med. Chem.,* **2013**, *56*(1), 293-300. [http://dx.doi.org/10.1021/jm301625s] [PMID: 23241068]

[80] Grandane, A.; Tanc, M.; Zalubovskis, R.; Supuran, C.T. Synthesis of 6-tetrazolyl-substituted sulfocoumarins acting as highly potent and selective inhibitors of the tumor-associated carbonic anhydrase isoforms IX and XII. *Bioorg. Med. Chem.,* **2014**, *22*(5), 1522-1528. [http://dx.doi.org/10.1016/j.bmc.2014.01.043] [PMID: 24513186]

[81] Grandane, A.; Tanc, M.; Zalubovskis, R.; Supuran, C.T. 6-Triazolyl-substituted sulfocoumarins are potent, selective inhibitors of the tumor-associated carbonic anhydrases IX and XII. *Bioorg. Med. Chem. Lett.,* **2014**, *24*(5), 1256-1260. [http://dx.doi.org/10.1016/j.bmcl.2014.01.076] [PMID: 24518190]

[82] Grandane, A.; Tanc, M.; Žalubovskis, R.; Supuran, C.T. Synthesis of 6-aryl-substituted sulfocoumarins and investigation of their carbonic anhydrase inhibitory action. *Bioorg. Med. Chem.,* **2015**, *23*(7), 1430-1436. [http://dx.doi.org/10.1016/j.bmc.2015.02.023] [PMID: 25753329]

[83] Grandane, A.; Tanc, M.; Di Cesare Mannelli, L. 6-Substituted sulfocoumarins are selective carbonic anhdydrase IX and XII inhibitors with significant cytotoxicity against colorectal cancer cells. *J. Med. Chem.,* **2015**, *58*(9), 3975-3983. [http://dx.doi.org/10.1021/acs.jmedchem.5b00523] [PMID: 25875209]

[84] Pustenko, A.; Stepanovs, D.; Žalubovskis, R.; Vullo, D.; Kazaks, A.; Leitans, J.; Tars, K.; Supuran,

C.T. 3 *H* -1,2-benzoxathiepine 2,2-dioxides: a new class of isoform-selective carbonic anhydrase inhibitors. *J. Enzyme Inhib. Med. Chem.*, **2017**, *32*(1), 767-775.
[http://dx.doi.org/10.1080/14756366.2017.1316720] [PMID: 28537099]

[85] Pustenko, A.; Nocentini, A.; Balašova, A.; Alafeefy, A.; Krasavin, M.; Žalubovskis, R.; Supuran, C.T. Aryl derivatives of 3H-1,2-benzoxathiepine 2,2-dioxide as carbonic anhydrase inhibitors. *J. Enzyme Inhib. Med. Chem.*, **2020**, *35*(1), 245-254.
[http://dx.doi.org/10.1080/14756366.2019.1695795] [PMID: 31790605]

[86] Pustenko, A.; Nocentini, A.; Balašova, A.; Krasavin, M.; Žalubovskis, R.; Supuran, C.T. 7-Acylamino-3H-1,2-benzoxathiepine 2,2-dioxides as new isoform-selective carbonic anhydrase IX and XII inhibitors. *J. Enzyme Inhib. Med. Chem.*, **2020**, *35*(1), 650-656.
[http://dx.doi.org/10.1080/14756366.2020.1722658] [PMID: 32079427]

[87] Krasavin, M.; Žalubovskis, R.; Grandāne, A.; Domračeva, I.; Zhmurov, P.; Supuran, C.T. Sulfocoumarins as dual inhibitors of human carbonic anhydrase isoforms IX/XII and of human thioredoxin reductase. *J. Enzyme Inhib. Med. Chem.*, **2020**, *35*(1), 506-510.
[http://dx.doi.org/10.1080/14756366.2020.1712596] [PMID: 31928252]

[88] Krasavin, M.; Sharonova, T.; Sharoyko, V. Combining carbonic anhydrase and thioredoxin reductase inhibitory motifs within a single molecule dramatically increases its cytotoxicity. *J. Enzyme Inhib. Med. Chem.*, **2020**, *35*(1), 665-671.
[http://dx.doi.org/10.1080/14756366.2020.1734800] [PMID: 32131646]

[89] Angeli, A.; Trallori, E.; Carta, F.; Di Cesare Mannelli, L.; Ghelardini, C.; Supuran, C.T. Heterocoumarins are selective carbonic anhydrase IX and XII inhibitors with cytotoxic effects against cancer cells lines. *ACS Med. Chem. Lett.*, **2018**, *9*(9), 947-951.
[http://dx.doi.org/10.1021/acsmedchemlett.8b00362] [PMID: 30258546]

[90] Temperini, C.; Innocenti, A.; Scozzafava, A.; Parkkila, S.; Supuran, C.T. The coumarin-binding site in carbonic anhydrase accommodates structurally diverse inhibitors: the antiepileptic lacosamide as an example and lead molecule for novel classes of carbonic anhydrase inhibitors. *J. Med. Chem.*, **2010**, *53*(2), 850-854.
[http://dx.doi.org/10.1021/jm901524f] [PMID: 20028100]

[91] D'Agostino, I.; Mathew, G.E.; Angelini, P. Biological investigation of *N* -methyl thiosemicarbazones as antimicrobial agents and bacterial carbonic anhydrases inhibitors. *J. Enzyme Inhib. Med. Chem.*, **2022**, *37*(1), 986-993.
[http://dx.doi.org/10.1080/14756366.2022.2055009] [PMID: 35322729]

[92] Grande, R.; Carradori, S.; Puca, V. Selective Inhibition of *Helicobacter pylori* Carbonic Anhydrases by Carvacrol and Thymol Could Impair Biofilm Production and the Release of Outer Membrane Vesicles. *Int. J. Mol. Sci.*, **2021**, *22*(21), 11583.
[http://dx.doi.org/10.3390/ijms222111583] [PMID: 34769015]

[93] Monte, C.; Carradori, S.; Gentili, A.; Mollica, A.; Trisciuoglio, D.; Supuran, C. Dual Cyclooxygenase and Carbonic Anhydrase Inhibition by Nonsteroidal Anti-Inflammatory Drugs for the Treatment of Cancer. *Curr. Med. Chem.*, **2015**, *22*(24), 2812-2818.
[http://dx.doi.org/10.2174/0929867322666150716113501] [PMID: 26180003]

[94] Bonardi, A.; Nocentini, A.; Osman, S.M. Inhibition of α-, β- and γ-carbonic anhydrases from the pathogenic bacterium *Vibrio cholerae* with aromatic sulphonamides and clinically licenced drugs – a joint docking/molecular dynamics study. *J. Enzyme Inhib. Med. Chem.*, **2021**, *36*(1), 469-479.
[http://dx.doi.org/10.1080/14756366.2020.1862102] [PMID: 33472446]

[95] Campestre, C.; De Luca, V.; Carradori, S.; Grande, R.; Carginale, V.; Scaloni, A.; Supuran, C.T.; Capasso, C. Carbonic Anhydrases: New Perspectives on Protein Functional Role and Inhibition in *Helicobacter pylori*. *Front. Microbiol.*, **2021**, *12*629163
[http://dx.doi.org/10.3389/fmicb.2021.629163] [PMID: 33815311]

[96] Modak, J.K.; Tikhomirova, A.; Gorrell, R.J.; Rahman, M.M.; Kotsanas, D.; Korman, T.M.; Garcia-

Bustos, J.; Kwok, T.; Ferrero, R.L.; Supuran, C.T.; Roujeinikova, A. Anti- *Helicobacter pylori* activity of ethoxzolamide. *J. Enzyme Inhib. Med. Chem.,* **2019**, *34*(1), 1660-1667. [http://dx.doi.org/10.1080/14756366.2019.1663416] [PMID: 31530039]

[97] Ronci, M.; Del Prete, S.; Puca, V.; Carradori, S.; Carginale, V.; Muraro, R.; Mincione, G.; Aceto, A.; Sisto, F.; Supuran, C.T.; Grande, R.; Capasso, C. Identification and characterization of the α-CA in the outer membrane vesicles produced by *Helicobacter pylori. J. Enzyme Inhib. Med. Chem.,* **2019**, *34*(1), 189-195. [http://dx.doi.org/10.1080/14756366.2018.1539716] [PMID: 30734607]

[98] Angeli, A.; Pinteala, M.; Maier, S.S.; Del Prete, S.; Capasso, C.; Simionescu, B.C.; Supuran, C.T. Inhibition of α-, β-, γ-, δ-, ζ- and η-class carbonic anhydrases from bacteria, fungi, algae, diatoms and protozoans with famotidine. *J. Enzyme Inhib. Med. Chem.,* **2019**, *34*(1), 644-650. [http://dx.doi.org/10.1080/14756366.2019.1571273] [PMID: 30727781]

[99] Angeli, A.; Pinteala, M.; Maier, S.S.; Simionescu, B.C.; Da'dara, A.A.; Skelly, P.J.; Supuran, C.T. Sulfonamide Inhibition Studies of an α-Carbonic Anhydrase from *Schistosoma mansoni*, a Platyhelminth Parasite Responsible for Schistosomiasis. *Int. J. Mol. Sci.,* **2020**, *21*(5), 1842. [http://dx.doi.org/10.3390/ijms21051842] [PMID: 32155992]

[100] Da'dara, A.A.; Angeli, A.; Ferraroni, M.; Supuran, C.T.; Skelly, P.J. Crystal structure and chemical inhibition of essential schistosome host-interactive virulence factor carbonic anhydrase SmCA. *Commun. Biol.,* **2019**, *2*(1), 333. [http://dx.doi.org/10.1038/s42003-019-0578-0] [PMID: 31508507]

[101] Ferraroni, M.; Angeli, A.; Carradori, S.; Supuran, C.T. Inhibition of *Schistosoma mansoni* carbonic anhydrase by the antiparasitic drug clorsulon: X-ray crystallographic and *in vitro* studies. *Acta Crystallogr. D Struct. Biol.,* **2022**, *78*(3), 321-327. [http://dx.doi.org/10.1107/S2059798322000079] [PMID: 35234146]

Medicinal Chemistry Lessons From Nature, 2022, *Vol. 1*, 330-383

CHAPTER 11

Phenols and Polyphenols as Carbonic Anhydrase Inhibitors

Alessandro Bonardi[1], Claudiu T. Supuran[1] and Alessio Nocentini[1,*]

[1] *Department of NEUROFARBA, Section of Pharmaceutical and Nutraceutical Sciences, Pharmaceutical and Nutraceutical Section, University of Florence, Via U. Schiff 6, 50019 Sesto Fiorentino, Firenze, Italy*

Abstract: Thousands of phenolic derivatives have been identified in the plant kingdom, which exert crucial roles in plant physiology. Many such derivatives were shown to produce pharmacological effects in humans which address their use in medicine as antiaging, anti-inflammatory, antioxidant, antidiabetic, and antiproliferative agents among others. Numerous such pharmacological activities are likely to derive from the inhibition of human carbonic anhydrase (CAs, EC 4.2.1.1) isoforms. Phenols, in fact, are able to anchor to the zinc-bound nucleophile present in the enzyme active site, blocking the catalytic action of CAs in humans and/or encoded in various microorganisms. This chapter discusses natural, semisynthetic and synthetic phenol derivatives that exhibited a CA inhibitory action. The discussion over the CA inhibition profiles is categorized as the inhibition of human CAs and inhibition of CAs from microorganisms. Multiple types of inhibition mechanisms by phenolic derivatives are discussed according to X-ray crystallographic resolutions and *in silico* studies.

Keywords: Antitumor, Antibiotic, Anti-infective, Bacteria, Carbonic anhydrase, Enzymology, Fungi, Inhibitor, *In silico*, Phenol, Polyphenol, Protozoa.

PHENOLS AND POLYPHENOLS

Since ancient times, *Homo sapiens* have been using plants and herbal extracts as natural medicines to treat health issues. In modern medicine, the research for natural derivatives as precursors for the development of drugs has spread considerably [1].

More than five thousand phenol and polyphenol derivatives have been identified in plants. They play key roles as structural polymers (*i.e.* lignin), antioxidants, UV screens (*i.e.* flavonoids), signal compounds (*i.e.* flavonoids and salicylic acid),

* **Corresponding author Alessio Nocentini:** Department of NEUROFARBA, Section of Pharmaceutical and Nutraceutical Sciences, Pharmaceutical and Nutraceutical Section, University of Florence, *via* U. Schiff 6, 50019 Sesto Fiorentino, Firenze, Italy; E-mail: alessio.nocentini@unifi.it

Simone Carradori (Ed.)

attractants to accelerate pollination (*i.e.* flavonoids and carotenoids), and defense response chemicals (*i.e.* tannins and phytoalexins), such as coloring for camouflage and defense against herbivores, as well as antibacterials and antifungals [2 - 4].

Numerous phenol derivatives are actively used nowadays in medicine according to demonstrated anti-aging [5], anti-inflammatory [6], antioxidant [7], anti-diabetic (*i.e.* stilbenoids) [8, 9], and antiproliferative activities (*i.e.* flavonoids, phenolic alcohols, lignans, and secoiroides) [10, 11]. Other polyphenol derivatives, such as resveratrol, have been demonstrated to prevent cardiovascular diseases by improving the function of the endothelial tissue, inhibiting platelet aggregation and reducing blood pressure and flogosis [12 - 17].

Carbonic Anhydrases

The superfamily of metalloenzymes carbonic anhydrases (CAs, EC 4.2.1.1) is widely expressed among all life kingdoms. Eight distinct classes are encoded by eight evolutionarily unrelated gene families: α-, β-, γ-, δ-, ζ-, η-, θ- and ι-CAs [18 - 29]. The CAs chiefly catalyze the reversible hydration of carbon dioxide (CO_2) to bicarbonate (HCO_3^-) and proton (H^+). This reaction is physiologically crucial for all living beings as it is involved in respiration, pH and CO_2 homeostasis, transport of CO_2/HCO_3^- and a multitude of biosynthetic reactions [18 - 21]. Fifteen α-class CA isoforms are encoded in humans and are implicated in numerous physiological processes such as electrolytes secretion, metabolic reactions (*i.e.* gluconeogenesis, lipogenesis, ureagenesis), bone resorption, and calcification [29 - 39]. An anomalous expression and/or activity of specific human CA isoforms was observed in a multitude of human pathological processes. Hence, many such diseases can be pharmacologically treated with CA inhibitors (CAIs) or activators (CAAs) [18].

Also human pathogens, among which bacteria, protozoa, and fungi, encode for α-, β-, γ- and η-CAs. In fact, CAs are crucial for the parasite virulence, growth or acclimatization in the hosts. The inhibition of these CAs produces growth impairment and defects in the pathogen, being a promising strategy for anti-infective intervention [39, 40].

CA Inhibition Mechanism of Phenol Derivatives

The mechanisms through which CAs are inhibited or activated have been studied for decades and are well-understood processes [18, 19, 41]. To date, four inhibition mechanisms have been discovered and characterized:

1. The zinc-binders, which include inorganic anions, sulfonamides and their bioisosteres (sulfamates, sulfamides), dithiocarbamates (and bioisosteres), hydroxamates, carboxylic acids, phosphates, benzoxaboroles, selenols, phosphonamidates [42 - 50].
2. Compounds that anchor to the zinc-bound water molecule/hydroxide ion, such as phenols, polyamines, sulfocoumarins, and thioxocoumarins [51 - 55].
3. Compounds that occlude the entrance of the active site, that are coumarins and their bioisosteres [56 - 58].
4. Compounds binding out of the active site, that is 2-(benzylsulfonyl)-benzoic acid [42, 59].

The CA inhibition mechanism of phenolic derivatives was described for the first time in 1994 by Nair *et al.* [51], which solved the crystal structure of hCA II in adduct with phenol **1** (Fig. **1A-B**). Successively, Lomelino *et al.* reported an analogous binding mode to hCA II for resorcinol **3** (pdb 4E49) and hydroquinone **4** (pdb 4E3H) (Fig. **1C-D**) [60]. The phenol OH group anchors to the zinc-bound water molecule/hydroxide through an H-bond as a donator, while it receives a second H-bond by the NH backbone of Thr199, a conserved amino acid in the active site of all α-CAs. The benzene ring accommodates within the active site forming hydrophobic interactions with Val121, Val143, Leu198, and Trp209 (Fig. **1**). The *m*-OH group of resorcinol **3** formed a water-bridged H-bond with Gln92. In contrast, two coexisting binding orientations were found for hydroxyquinone **4** within hCA II active site which differ from the orientation of the *p*-OH group. In only one of these, the *p*-OH formed an H-bond with Gln92 side chain NH_2.

Lately, in 2020 a new inhibition mechanism was reported crystallographically by D'Ambrosio *et al.* for catechols [61], which are 1,2-dihydroxybenzene derivatives. Multiple crystallization experiments were conducted on hCA II and chlorogenic acid **49** as CAI produced analogues, *i.e.* the shape of the ligand electron density within the active site was not compatible with **49**, but well matched with its hydrolysis product caffeic acid **42** (Fig. **2**). The authors demonstrated that **49** is hydrolyzed to **42** only in the simultaneous presence of hCA II and the crystallization buffer. Thus, under physiological conditions, this molecule does not act as a suicide inhibitor as coumarins or sulfocoumarins did instead. In detail, **42** is anchored to the enzyme by means of the two OH groups of the catechol which are H-bonded to both the zinc-bound nucleophile and to another water molecule characteristic of α-CAs active site, that is named "deep water" (W_d in Fig. (**2**). One of these OH groups is also at H-bond distances from the Thr200 side chain OH and Thr199 amide NH. The organic scaffold of the inhibitor establishes several hydrophobic interactions with residues Val121, Phe131 and Leu198, whereas the carboxylate functionality points towards the protein surface and does not interact with any protein residue.

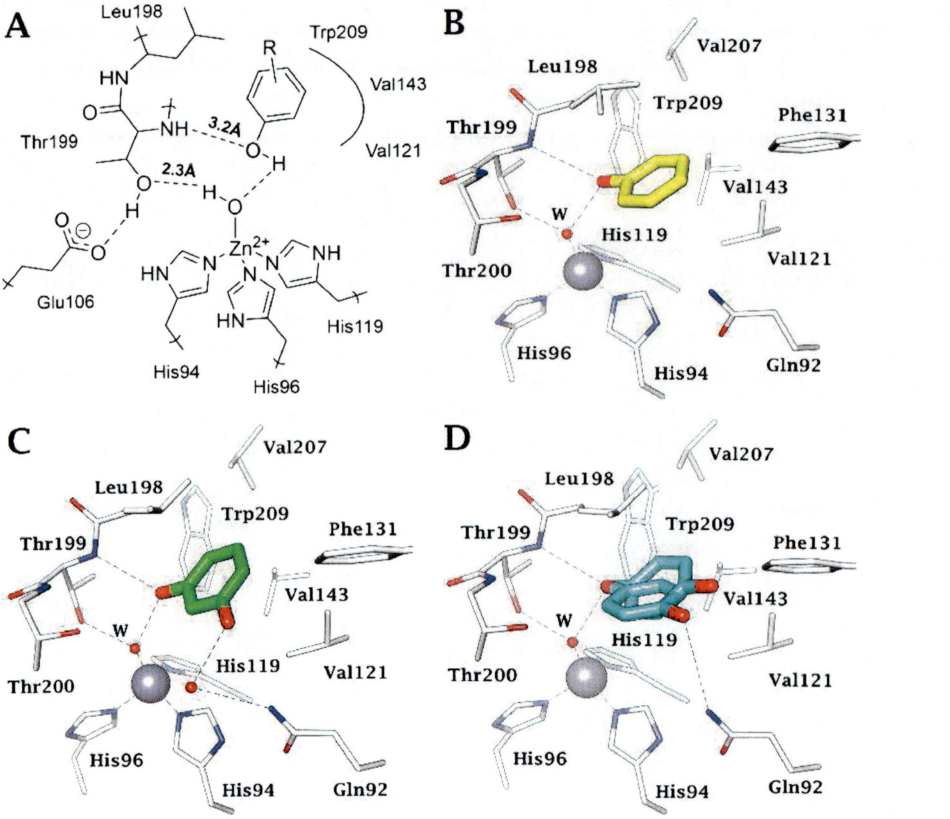

Fig. (1). A) 2D Representation of the binding mode of phenols to hCA II active site. Active site view of hCA II adducts with B) phenol **1**, C) resorcinol **3** (pdb 4E49) and D) hydroxyquinone **4** (pdb 4E3H).

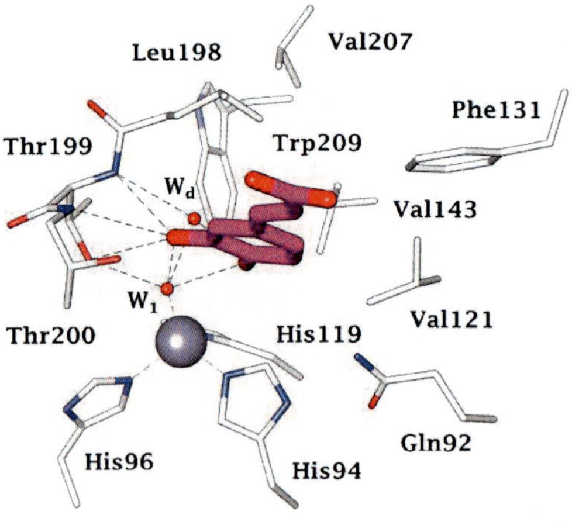

Fig. (2). Active site view of the hCA II/caffeic acid **42** complex (pdb 6YRI) [61].

It should be noted that another catechol was cocrystallized with hCA II, namely L-adrenaline, which has been however described as a CA activator [62]. In fact, L-adrenaline binds in a completely different region of the active site, that is the CA activators binding site, probably due to its positive charge at the experiments pH, whereas **42** is negatively charged.

The succeeding paragraphs report on natural, semisynthetic and synthetic phenol derivatives that possess a CA inhibitory action. The discussion over the CA inhibition profiles is categorized as the inhibition of human CAs (of the α-class, paragraph 1.4) and inhibition of CAs from microorganisms (of the β-, γ, δ-, and η-classes, paragraph 1.5). Additionally, the numerous derivatives were grouped into subsets to ease the discussion over the structure-activity relationship (SAR).

Phenolic Derivatives Inhibit Human CAs

Phenol **1** and many other simply substituted phenol derivatives showed significant efficacy in inhibiting several hCAs - *i.e.* the natural compounds pyrocatechol **2**, resorcinol **3**, hydroquinone **4**, pyrogallol **5**, hydroxyquinol **6**, guaiacol **7**, salicylic acid **8**, *m*-hydroxybenzoic acid **9**, *p*-hydroxybenzoic acid **10**, 3-methylcatechol **11**, 3-methoxycatechol **12**, 4-methylcatechol **13**, protocatechuic acid **14**, 2,4-dihydroxybenzoic acid **15**, 2,5-dihydroxybenzoic acid **16**, 2,6-dihydroxybenzoic acid **17**, 4-methyl guaiacol **18**, vanillin **19**, vanillic acid **20**, 3,5-dihydroxybenzoic acid **21**, gallic acid **22**, syringaldehyde **23**, and syringic acid **24** and carvacrol **25**, and the synthetic derivatives *m*-aminophenol **26**, *p*-aminophenol **27**, the antipyretic drug paracetamol **28**, and *p*-benzonitrile **29**, 2,5-difluorophenol **30**, 3,5-difluorophenol **31**, 2,4,6-trifluorophenol **32**, 3-amino-4-chlorophenol **33** and 4-amino-3-chlorophenol **34** (Fig. **3**)

The inhibition profiles of phenols **1-34** available against more or less extended sets of hCAs were assessed by a stopped-flow CO_2 hydrase assay [63] and are gathered in Table **1.** as K_I values (μM) (or IC_{50} in μg/mL for compound **20**). The clinically used sulfonamide acetazolamide (**AAZ**) is reported as a comparison. Overall, phenols **1-34** inhibited hCAs with K_I values spanning in a wide range (0.09–4003 μM). hCA III only was inhibited more intensively by derivatives **1-34** (K_Is of 0.71–13.0 μM) than by **AAZ** (K_I of 200 μM), with the exception of resorcinol **3** (K_I = 605 μM) and salicylic acid **8** (K_I = 885 μM). Numerous compounds showed a greater CA inhibitory action than the lead phenol **1** against hCA I (K_Is of 0.55–7.5 μM *vs* a K_I of 10.2 μM), II (K_Is of 0.090–4.7 μM *vs* a K_I of 5.5 μM), VA (K_Is of 4.08–65.0 μM *vs* a K_I of 218 μM), VB (K_Is of 4.2–98.4 μM *vs* a K_I of 543 μM), VI (K_Is of 0.52–90.6 μM *vs* a K_I of 208 μM), VII (K_Is of 4.08–644 μM *vs* a K_I of 710 μM), IX (K_Is of 3.73–8.20 μM *vs* a K_I of 8.8 μM), XII (K_Is of 4.09–9.01 μM *vs* a K_I of 9.2 μM), mXIII (K_Is of 7.79–84.2 μM *vs* a K_I

of 697 μM), and XIV (K_Is of 0.65–10.7 μM *vs* a K_I of 11.5 μM). Derivatives **31** and **10** only inhibited hCA III (K_I of 0.71 μM *vs* K_I of 2.7 μM) and hCA IV (K_I of 7.78 μM *vs* K_I of 9.5 μM) more than phenol **1,** respectively.

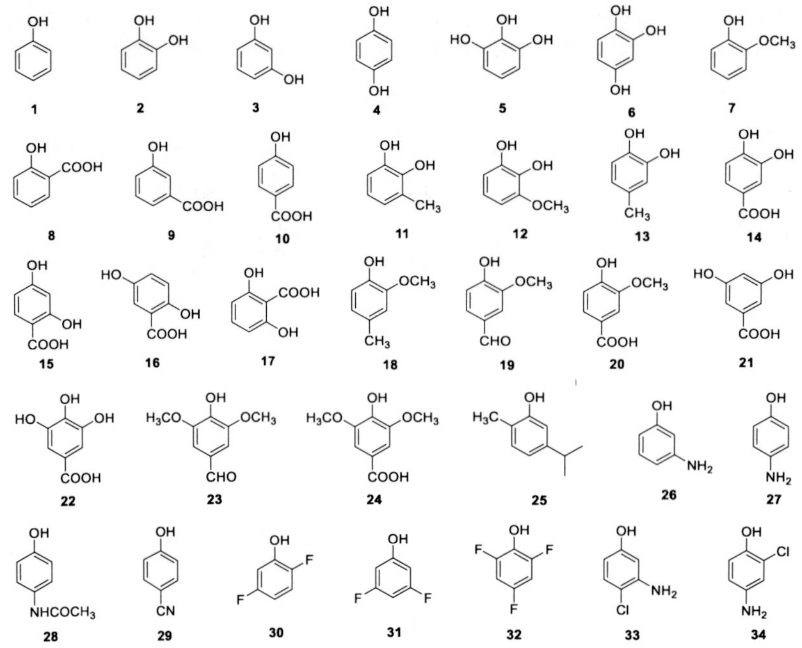

Fig. (3). Chemical structure of phenols **1-34**.

Table 1. Inhibition data of hCAs I-XII and XIV and mCA XIII with phenols 1-34 and the standard sulfonamide inhibitor acetazolamide (AAZ) by a stopped-flow CO_2 hydrase assay [63].

cmpd	K_I^a (μM)												Ref.
	hCA												
	I	II	III	IV	VA	VB	VI	VII	IX	XII	mXIII	XIV	
1	10.2	5.5	2.7	9.5	218	543	208	710	8.8	9.2	697	11.5	[64 - 68]
2	4003	9.91	13.0	10.9	55.1	4.2	606	714	115	8.9	12.2	48.9	[65, 67 - 69]
3	795	7.7	605	570	8.7	7.1	550	644	69.7	7.5	62.6	10.7	[65, 67, 69]
4	10.7	0.09	8.2	10.8	14.1	12.5	521	883	32.5	7.8	74.3	42.0	[65, 69]
5	7.41	0.54	63.7^b	-	-	-	0.52	-	-	-	-	-	[64, 69, 70]
6	>100	>100	-	-	-	-	-	-	-	-	-	-	[71]
7	7.50	5.63	-	-	-	-	-	-	9.98	9.83	-	-	[72]
8	9.9	7.1	885	11.1	678	355	11.9	82.1	78.7	8.8	67	49.8	[65]
9	2.37	0.60	-	-	-	-	3.17	-	4.53	3.53	-	-	[69, 73, 74]

(Table 1) cont.....

cmpd	K_I^a (μM)												Ref.
	hCA												
	I	II	III	IV	VA	VB	VI	VII	IX	XII	mXIII	XIV	
10	9.8	10.6	6.61	7.78	9.2	10.5	11.4	4.08	3.73	6.27	7.79	6.16	[65, 68, 69, 75]
11	5.95	4.69	-	-	-	-	-	-	9.55	7.22	-	-	[72]
12	6.32	2.20	-	-	-	-	-	-	7.83	7.53	-	-	[72]
13	6.16	2.76	-	-	-	-	-	-	8.11	6.58	-	-	[72]
14	1.08	0.47	-	-	-	-	4.72	7.87	4.45	4.09	-	0.69	[69, 73 - 75]
15	5.2	4.9	-	-	-	-	-	72	68	7.5	-	70	[74, 75]
16	4.2	4.1	-	-	-	-	-	68	6.6	7.3	-	67	[75]
17	5.7	5.2	-	-	-	-	-	6.6	5.9	7.2	-	6.5	[76]
18	9.15	7.74	-	-	-	-	-	-	9.89	8.55	-	-	[72]
19	11.37	7.15	-	-	-	-	-	-	9.81	8.39	-	-	[72]
20	0.47[c]	0.42[c]	-	-	-	-	-	-	-	-	-	-	[73]
21	0.55	0.51	-	-	-	-	1.78	7.17	4.41	3.67	-	0.65	[69, 75]
22	3.20	2.25	7.49	9.80	4.08	9.97	6.13	6.07	6.99	7.78	9.86	7.03	[64, 68, 69]
23	10.92	6.68	-	-	-	-	-	-	9.11	7.70	-	-	[71]
24	4.15	3.19	8.58	10.6	6.34	35.4	7.55	7.81	8.20	9.01	11.0	9.14	[64, 68]
25	79.6	84.8	-	-	-	-	-	-	-	-	-	-	[76]
26	4.9	4.7	-	-	-	-	-	-	-	-	-	-	[71]
27	159	752	9.5	743	867	649	23.5	1359	517	479	657	10.1	[65]
28	10.0	6.2	7 1	11.4	802	296	658	9.1	70.7	4.1	30.3	10.6	[65]
29	131	0.10	6.7	634	520	557	13.7	777	56.0	9.2	45	29.1	[65]
30	134	870	10.8	426	12.0	51.2	90.6	554	68.7	598	69.5	34.0	[65]
31	38.8	33.9	0.71	10.7	65.0	98.4	82.6	163	9.4	70.2	84.2	10.6	[65, 77]
32	>100	>100	-	-	-	-	-	-	-	-	-	-	[71]
33	6.3	4.9	-	-	-	-	-	-	-	-	-	-	[71]
34	57.8	57.5	-	-	-	-	-	-	-	-	-	-	[71]
AAZ	0.250	0.012	200	0.074	0.063	0.054	0.011	0.0025	0.025	0.0057	0.017	0.041	[18]

[a]Mean from 3 different assays, by a Stopped-Flow technique (errors were in the range of ± 5-10% of the reported values); [b]CA III from bovine. [c]Data reported as IC_{50} (μg/mL). m = murine; - = not available data.

Another set of phenolic derivatives assayed for CA inhibition is depicted in Fig. **(4)**. It gathers the synthetic compounds 4-(hydroxymethyl)phenol **35** and tyrosol **36**, the olive oil component 2-(4-hydroxyphenyl)acetic acid **37** and its derivative

38, propylparaben **39**, *p*-coumaric acid **40**, *o*-coumaric acid **41**, caffeic acid **42**, ferulic acid **43**, 4-propylguaiacol **44**, the spicy zingerone **45**, the anesthetic eugenol **46** and its isomer isoeugenol **47**, the stilbenoid resveratrol **48**, the natural ester between caffeic and astringent L-quinic acid, chlorogenic acid **49**, curcumin **50**, the spicy capsaicin **51**, dodoneine **52**, extracted from African mistletoe *Agelanthus dodoneifolius*, the central analeptic cardiovascular drug dobutamine **53**, the estrogens α-estradiol **54** and estrone **55**, the plant secondary metabolites endiandrins A **56** and B **57** and (-)-dihydroguaiaretic acid **58**, ellagic acid **59**, xanthones **60** and **61**, and the marine ascidian-derived alkaloids polyandrocarpamines A **62** and B **63**.

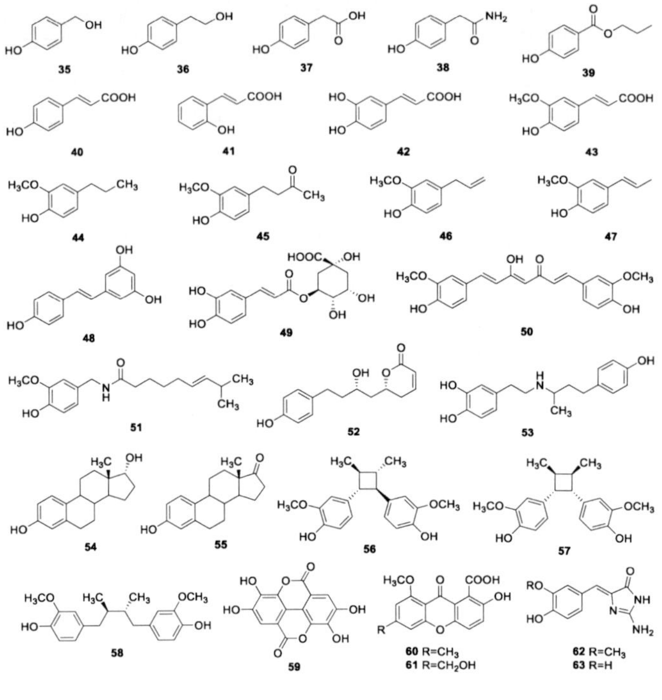

Fig. (4). Chemical structure of phenols **35-63**.

The CA inhibition profiles of this second set of phenols against the fifteen hCA isoforms are reported in Table **2.** in comparison with acetazolamide (**AAZ**) and the simple phenol **1** as references. Overall, the K_I values spanned again in a wide range from 0.069 to more than1000 μM [63]. All compounds exerted a weaker hCA III inhibition (K_Is of 7.40– >1000 μM) with respect to phenol **1**, but were more active than **AAZ** with the exception of derivative **41** (K_I >1000 μM). It should be noted that most compounds within this set showed potent inhibitory activity against the mitochondrial isoforms hCA VA (K_Is of 0.085–10.25 μM) and VB (K_Is of 0.069–12.7 μM). Notably, compounds **36-38**, **56-58**, and **60-63** acted as low nanomolar inhibitors *versus* both hCA VA (K_I = 0.085–0.101 µM) and VB (K_I = 0.069–0.107 µM) and showed selectivity of action against these two CA isoforms over most remaining ones.

Table 2. Inhibition data of hCAs I-XIV with phenols 35-63, standard phenol 1, and the standard sulfonamide inhibitor acetazolamide (AAZ) by a stopped-flow CO_2 hydrase assay [63].

cmpd	K_I[a] (µM)												Ref.
	hCA												
	I	II	III	IV	VA	VB	VI	VII	IX	XII	XIII	XIV	
1	10.2	5.5	2.7	9.5	218	543	208	710	8.8	9.2	697 (m)	11.5	[46 - 68]
35	68.9	95.3	-	-	-	-	-	-	-	-	-	-	[71]
36	430	8.7	-	-	0.101	0.105	-	-	-	-	-	-	[78]
37	309	10.3	-	-	0.099	0.107	-	-	-	-	-	-	[78]
38	309	11.2			0.092	0.081							[78]
39	0.84[b]	0.82[b]	-	-	-	-	-	-	-	-	-	-	[73]
40	1.07	0.98	7.57	9.60	5.96	7.76	6.72	5.23	5.33	8.01	10.1 (m)	6.68	[64, 68, 75]
41	3.1	9.2	>1000	62.3	>1000	5.78	>1000	>1000	>1000	>1000	>1000	>1000	[66, 73, 74]
42	2.38	1.61	10.0	10.1	6.49	9.08	7.33	6.42	7.87	9.06	10.9 (m)	8.71	[69]
43	2.89	2.40	11.1	10.8	7.04	10.5	8.45	7.41	9.87	9.78	12.2 (m)	9.43	[64, 68]
44	10.34	8.51	-	-	-	-	-	-	9.01	9.12	-	-	[72]
45	72.18	74.88	-	-	-	-	-	-	-	-	-	-	[76]
46	8.32	7.27	-	-	-	-	-	-	9.62	8.89	-	-	[72]
47	10.29	6.73	-	-	-	-	-	-	9.32	9.13	-	-	72]
48	2.21	2.77	9.09	4.47	4.75	4.64	8.07	4.35	0.81	0.95	4.09	0.83	[66, 68, 79]
49	0.98[b]	0.88[b]	-	-	-	-	-	-	-	-	-	-	[73]
50	2.41	0.38	11.30	4.97	10.25	9.46	9.94	9.30	4.05	3.48	6.85	11.73	[66, 68, 79]
51	696.1	208.4	-	-	-	-	-	-	-	-	-	-	[80]
52	5.48	>100	10.35	9.61	>100	>100	>100	>100	>100	>100	9.27 (m)	9.34	[81]
53	1.92	0.48	7.40	8.98	0.73	0.89	9.47	4.30	9.82	4.35	9.53	12.02	[66, 68, 79]
54	87.8	40.4	-	>100	-	-	-	-	49.6	-	-	-	[82]
55	>100	50.8	-	>100	-	-	-	-	71.4	-	-	-	[82]
56	368	11.7	-	-	0.091	0.069	-	-	-	-	-	-	[78, 79]

(Table 2) cont.....

cmpd	K_I[a] (μM)												Ref.
	hCA												
	I	II	III	IV	VA	VB	VI	VII	IX	XII	XIII	XIV	
57	354	12.1	-	-	0.098	0.079	-	-	-	-	-	-	[78]
58	307	230	-	-	0.085	0.071	-	-	-	-	-	-	[78]
59	2.32	2.18	10.5	9.08	7.59	12.7	7.06	6.32	9.37	10.1	10.3 (m)	8.91	[68]
60	201	8.4	-	-	0.093	0.103	-	-	-	-	-	-	[78]
61	374	9.2	-	-	0.094	0.102	-	-	-	-	-	-	[78]
62	10.5	9.6	-	-	0.099	0.070	-	-	-	-	-	-	[78]
63	355	13.1	-	-	0.101	0.076	-	-	-	-	-	-	[78]
AAZ	0.250	0.012	200	0.074	0.063	0.054	0.011	0.0025	0.025	0.0057	0.017 (m)	0.041	[18]

[a]Mean from 3 different assays, by a Stopped-Flow technique (errors were in the range of ± 5-10% of the reported values); [b]Data reported as IC_{50} (μg/mL). [c]Inhibition data measured by the 4-nitrophenylacetate esterase assay [83]. m = murine; - = not available data.

(Fig. **5**) . gathers the chemical structures of another subset of CAI phenol derivatives, *i.e.* the endophytic fungal metabolite (-)-xylariamide A **64**, including its synthetic derivatives (+)-xylariamide A **65**, and compounds **66-69**, the bromophenols vidalol B **70** and compound **71** from red algae of the family Rhodomelaceae, the aromatic plants derivatives sal*Via*nolic acid A **72**, sal*Via*nolic acid B **73**, lithospermic acid **74** and rosmarinic acid **75**, and the antifungal drug clioquinol **76**. The structure of polyphenol tannic acid **77**, the decagalloyl glucose, is shown in Fig. (**6**).

The hCA inhibition data of derivatives **64-77** are collected in Table **3**. The K_I values spanned over a wide low nanomolar to high micromolar range (0.004–369 μM). Interestingly, all compounds induced a better inhibition of isoforms hCA IV-XIV (K_Is of 0.004–16.0 μM) with respect to the reference phenol **1**. Additionally, derivatives **72** and **74** (hCA IV K_Is of 0.066 and 0.065 μM, respectively) were better hCA IV inhibitors than **AAZ** (hCA IV K_I = 0.074 μM). Compound **73** inhibited hCA XII (K_I of 0.004 μM) better than **AAZ** (K_I of 0.0057 μM).

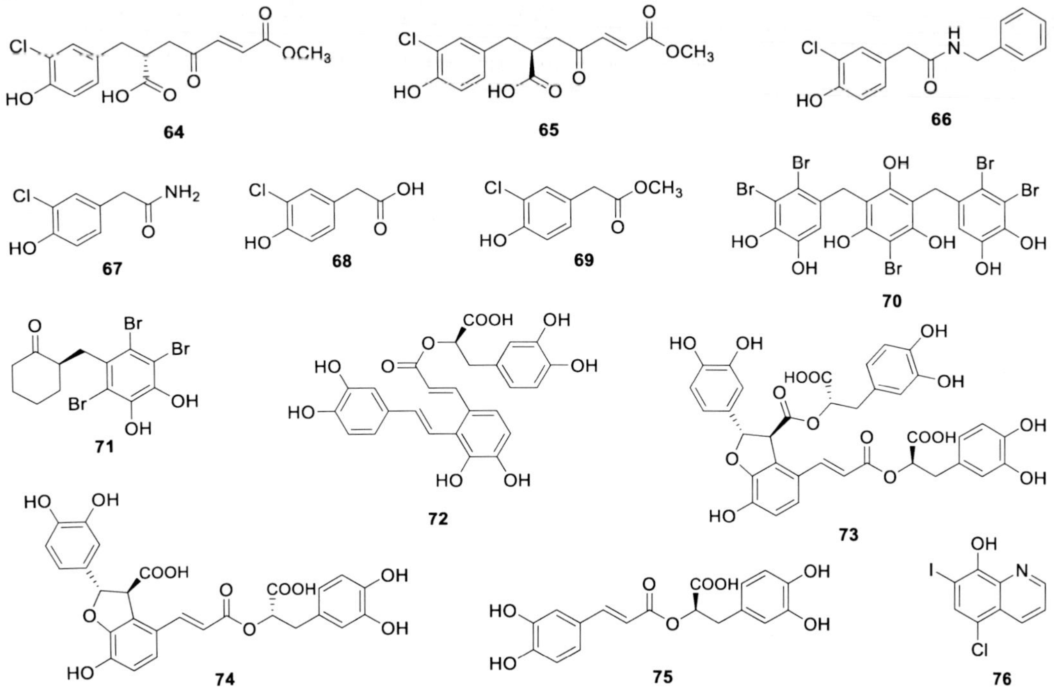

Fig. (5). Chemical structure of phenols **64-76**.

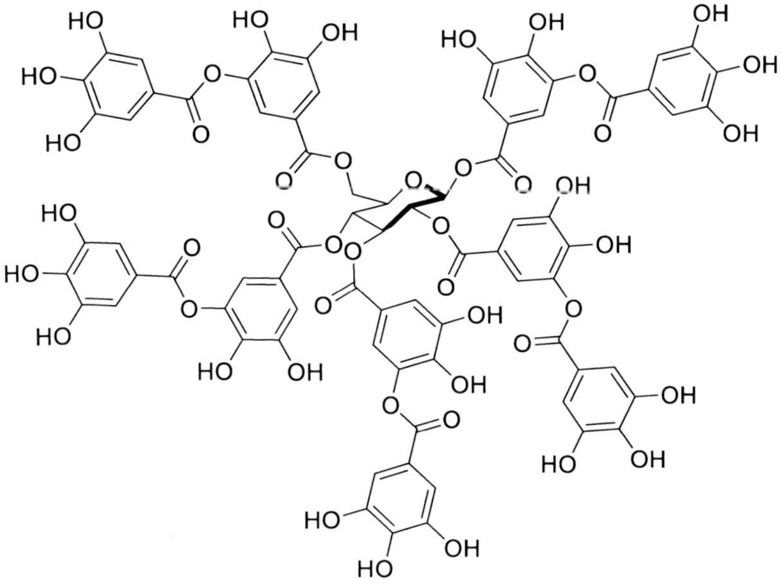

77

Fig. (6). Chemical structure of polyphenol tannic acid **77**.

Table 3. Inhibition data of hCAs I-XIV with phenols 64-77, the reference phenol 1, and the standard sulfonamide inhibitor acetazolamide (AAZ) by a stopped-flow CO_2 hydrase assay [63].

cmpd	K_I^a (μM)												Ref.
	hCA												
	I	II	III	IV	VA	VB	VI	VII	IX	XII	XIII	XIV	
1	10.2	5.5	2.7	9.5	218	543	208	710	8.8	9.2	697 (m)	11.5	[64 - 68]
64	239	8.3	-	-	0.095	0.114	-	-	-	-	-	-	[78]
65	231	8.0	-	-	0.108	0.102	-	-	-	-	-	-	[78]
66	10.5	11.4	-	-	0.096	0.085	-	-	-	-	-	-	[78]
67	237	131	-	-	0.110	0.106	-	-	-	-	-	-	[78]
68	265	8.6	-	-	0.100	0.118	-	-	-	-	-	-	[78]
69	369	10.7	-	-	0.109	0.125	-	-	-	-	-	-	[78]
70	12.2[b]	1.13[b]	-	1.84[b]	-	-	3.41[b]	-	-	-	-	-	[84]
71	1.67[b]	0.56[b]	-	1.08[b]	-	-	0.59[b]	-	-	-	-	-	[85]
72	>10	9.594	-	0.066	-	-	-	0.071	-	0.039	-	-	[86]
73	>10	>10	-	0.101	-	-	-	0.268	-	0.004	-	-	[86]
74	>10	>10	-	0.065	-	-	-	0.035	-	0.453	-	-	[86]
75	86.0[b]	57.0[b]	-	-	-	-	-	-	4.63	4.71	-	-	[87, 88]
76	6.6	6.5	3.3	5.4	8.3	-	5.3	16.0	5.6	8.1	4.9 (m)	5.0	[77]
77	36.2	0.37	-	-	-	-	0.34	-	-	-	-	-	[69]
AAZ	0.250	0.012	200	0.074	0.063	0.054	0.011	0.0025	0.025	0.0057	0.017 (m)	0.041	[18]

[a]Mean from 3 different assays, by a Stopped-Flow technique (errors were in the range of ± 5-10% of the reported values); m = murine; - = not available data. b. Inhibition data measured by the 4-nitrophenylacetate esterase assay [83].

A large number of polyphenols belonging to the class of flavonoids were tested as hCAs inhibitors. Among these are the flavanols catechin **78** and epicatechin **79**, flavones chrysin **80**, apigenin **81**, luteolin **82** and diosmetin **83**, isoflavones biochanin A **84**, daidzein **85** and puerarin **86**, prenyl isoflavones osajin **87** and pomiferin **88**, flavanonols taxifolin **89**, silychristin A **90** and silymarin **91**, flavanones naringenin **92**, the aglicone of naringin **93**, eriodictyol **94**, the aglicone of eriocitrin **95**, hesperitin **96**, the aglicone of hesperidin **97**, anthocyanin callistephin **98**, oenin **99** and malvin **100** (Fig. 7), and flavonols galangin **101**, kaempferol **102**, kaempferol-3-*O*-glucoside **103**, tiliroside **104**, kaempferol-3-*O*-(2",6"-di-*E*-*p*-coumaroyl)-β-glucopyranoside **105**, kaempferol-3-*O*-(3",4--diacetyl-2",6"-di-*E*-*p*-coumaroyl)-β-glucopyranoside **106**, fisetin **107**, quercetin **108**, quercetin-3-*O*-glucoside **109**, quercetin-3-*O*-rhamnoside **110**, rutin **111**, rhamnetin **112**, isorhamnetin **113** and morin **114** (Fig. **8**).

Their CA inhibition data are collected in Table **4**. Again, a range of action spanning from 0.003 to 235.7 μM was detected. Flavonoids **78-114** are generally more active against hCA IV-XIV than the reference phenol **1**. In particular, polyphenols **94**, **106**, and **110** (K_Is of 0.072, 0.062 and0.067 μM) were even more efficient than AAZ as hCA IV inhibitors. Compound **103** inhibited hCA XII more than **AAZ** (K_I of 0.004 μM *vs* 0.0057). Moreover, this fourth set of compounds showed a better inhibition profile against hCA III (K_Is of 0.004–235.7 μM) than **AAZ**. Only polyphenol **81** showed a lower K_I value (2.21 μM) than phenol **1**. It is very relevant that a significant subset of derivatives (*i.e.***82**, **85**, **92**, **94**, **96**, **104**, **106**, **109**, **110**, **113**) showed a K_I value against hCA VII, CNS-related hCA, comparable to that of **AAZ** in a single-digit nanomolar range.

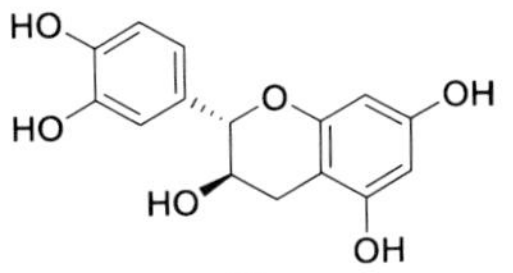

78

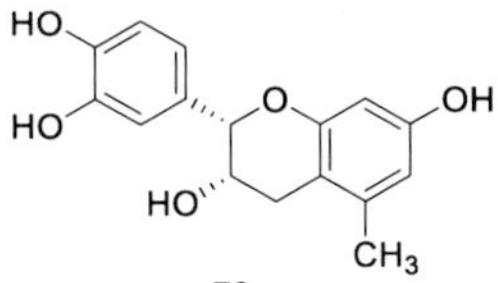

79

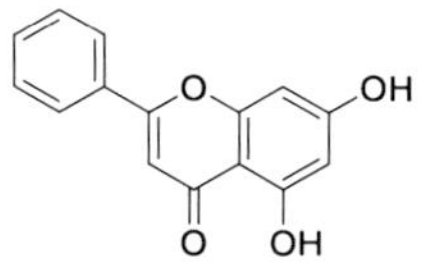

80

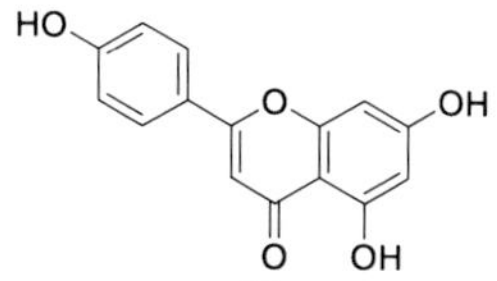

81

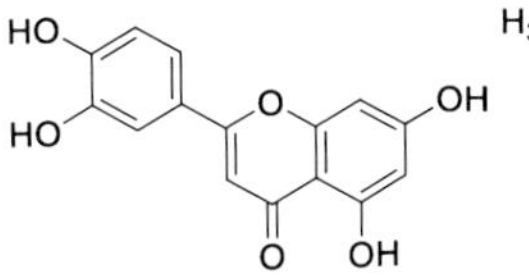

82

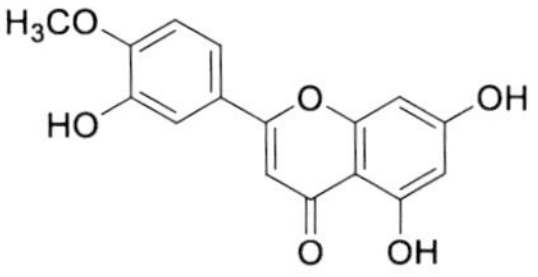

83

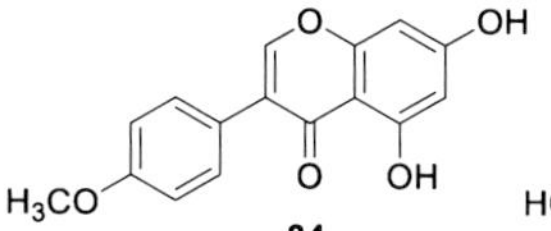

84

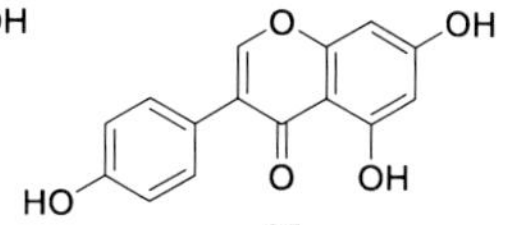

85

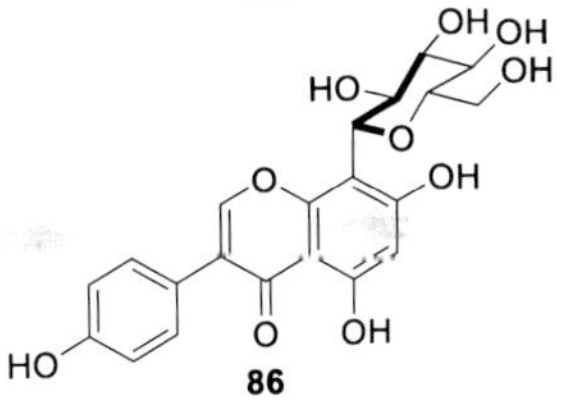

86

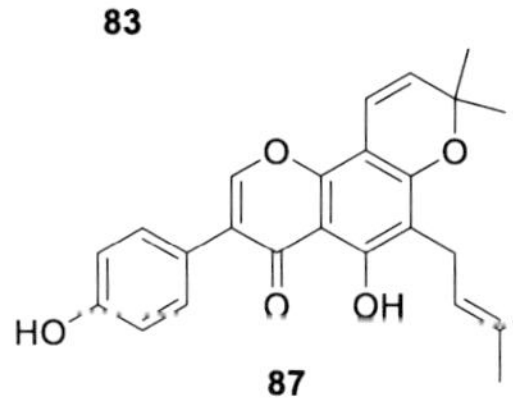

87

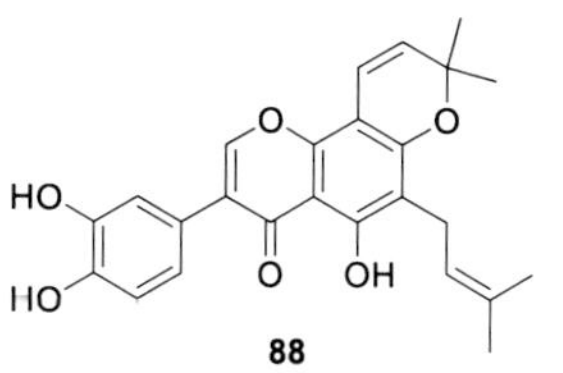

88

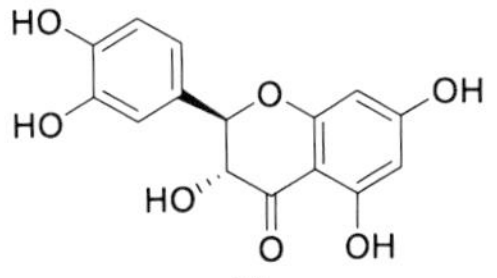

89

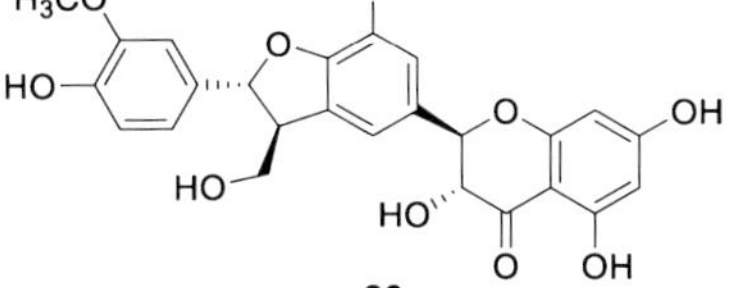

90

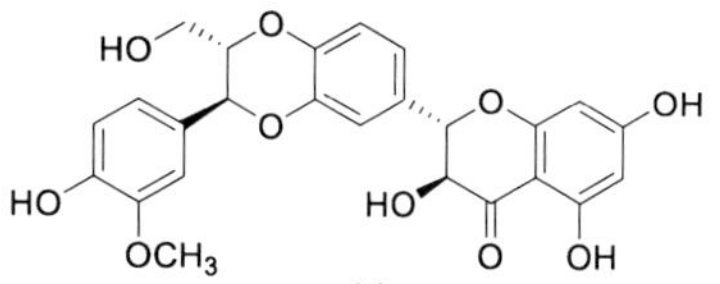

91

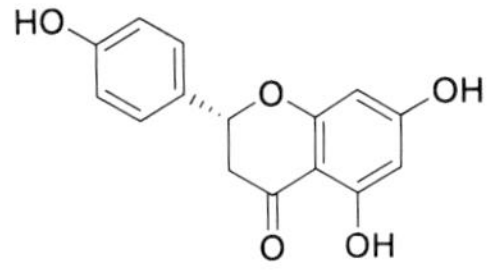

92

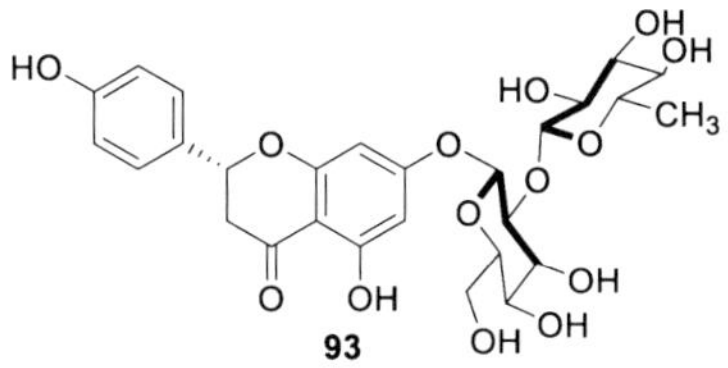

93

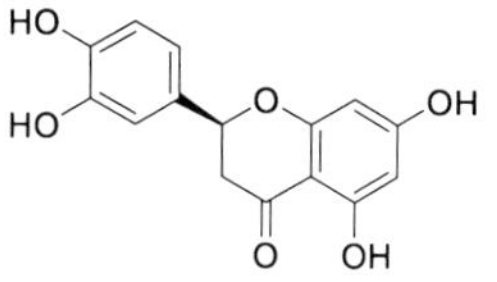

94

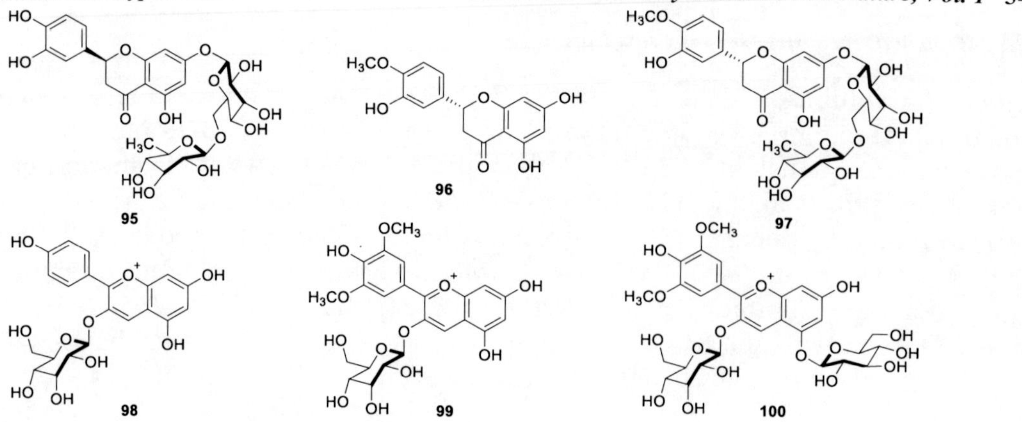

Fig. (7). Chemical structure of polyphenols **78-100**.

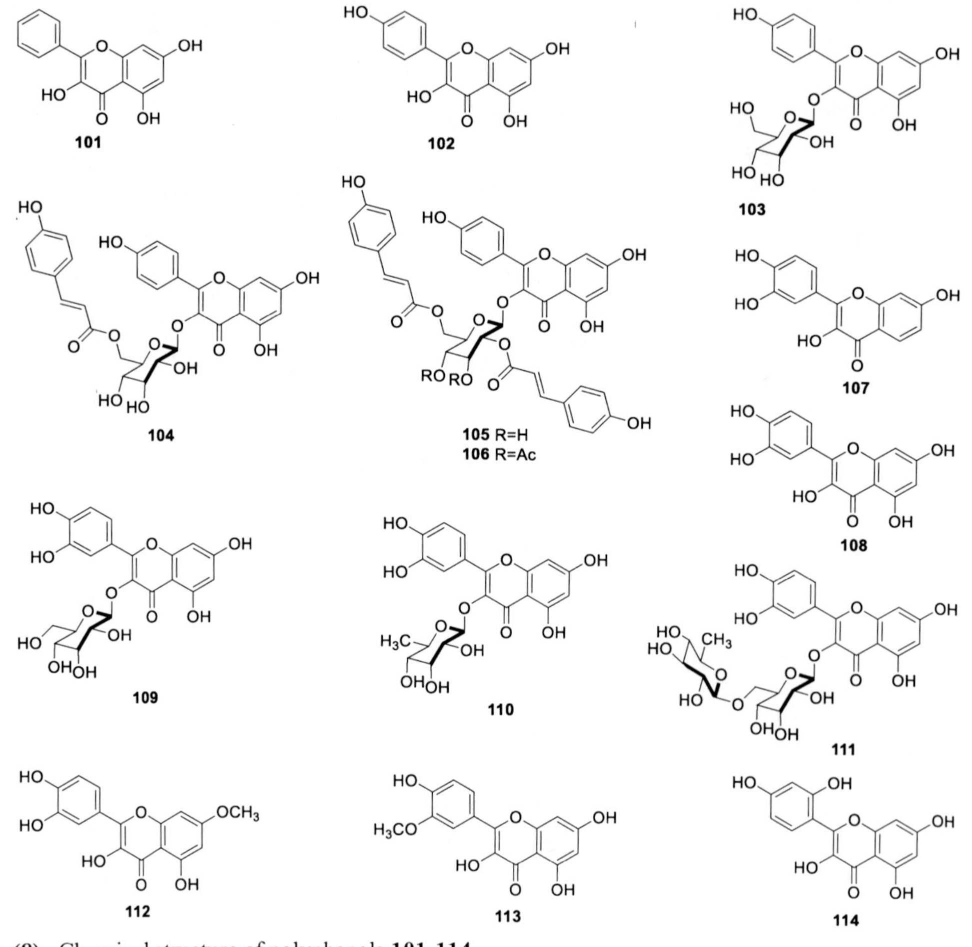

Fig. (8). Chemical structure of polyphenols **101-114**.

Table 4. Inhibition data of hCAs I-XIV with phenols 78-114, the reference phenol 1, and the standard sulfonamide inhibitor acetazolamide (AAZ) by a stopped-flow CO_2 hydrase assay [63].

cmpd	K_I[a] (μM)												Ref.
	hCA												
	I	II	III	IV	VA	VB	VI	VII	IX	XII	XIII	XIV	
1	10.2	5.5	2.7	9.5	218	543	208	710	8.8	9.2	697 (m)	11.5	[64 - 68]
78	2.42[c]	1.84[c]	3.58[c]	4.90[c]	4.21	4.02	4.91	0.45	5.03	4.72	10.51	11.55	[66 - 68, 79]
79	2.32	1.24	8.93[b]	3.98	-	-	4.36	-	-	.	-	-	[67, 73]
80	58.23	73.74	-	0.537	-	-	-	0.171	-	0.034	-	-	[76, 86]
81	4.10	2.70	2.21[b]	1.12	0.30	-	1.49	-	0.46	1.00	-	-	[67, 73, 89, 90]
82	>10	3.6	5.4[b]	4.4	-	-	-	0.004	-	0.060	-	-	[86, 89]
83	2.95	0.41	-	-	2.82	-	-	-	2.52	0.38	-	-	[90]
84	>10	>10	-	7.078	-	-	-	0.371	-	0.525	-	-	[86]
85	>10	>10	-	0.718	-	-	-	0.004	-	0.056	-	-	[86]
86	>10	>10	-	>10	-	-	-	0.452	-	0.515	-	-	[86]
87	87.2	83.1	-	-	-	-	-	-	-	-	-	-	[64]
88	471	235.7	-	-	-	-	-	-	-	-	-	-	[64]
89	3.66	0.34	-	9.09	4.24	-	-	0.49	0.43	0.19	-	-	[86, 90]
90	43.31	1.30	-	-	-	-	-	-	-	-	-	-	[91]
91	1.49	2.51	6.43	8.96	4.08	4.56	9.70	4.71	10.15	9.05	4.82	11.64	[66 - 68, 79]
92	>10	>10	-	0.079	-	-	-	0.004	-	0.044	-	-	[86]
93	20.51	37.50	-	-	2.10	-	-	-	3.39	0.24	-	-	[76, 90]
94	>10	>10	-	0.072	-	-	-	0.004	-	0.031	-	-	[86]
95	3.13	0.31	-	-	0.15	-	-	-	3.57	2.18	-	-	[90]
96	>10	>10	-	0.102	-	-	-	0.003	-	0.454	-	-	[86]
97	3.70[c,d]	2.98[c,d]	-	-	1.92	-	-	-	0.44	0.29	-	-	[76, 90]
98	46.2[c,d]	346.5[c,d]	-	-	-	-	-	-	-	-	-	-	[91]
99	18.73[c,d]	0.35[c,d]	-	-	-	-	-	-	-	-	-	-	[91]
100	115.5[c,d]	231.0[c,d]	-	-	-	-	-	-	-	-	-	-	[91]
101	>10	>10	-	0.568	-	-	-	0.024	-	0.041	-	-	[86]
102	>10	9.52	-	>10	-	-	-	0.025	-	142.9	-	-	[86]
103	>10	0.168	-	5.591	-	-	-	0.423	-	0.004	-	-	[86]

(Table 4) cont.....

cmpd	K_I[a] (μM)												Ref.
	hCA												
	I	II	III	IV	VA	VB	VI	VII	IX	XII	XIII	XIV	
104	>10	>10	-	5.468	-	-	-	0.004	-	0.134	-	-	[86]
105	>10	8.790	-	0.344	-	-	-	0.004	-	0.408	-	-	[86]
106	>10	6.863	-	0.062	-	-	-	0.026	-	0.399	-	-	[86]
107	0.83[d]	0.76[d]	-	-	-	-	-	-	-	-	-	-	[73]
108	2.68	2.54	8.10	7.89	6.81	11.9	6.17	4.84	7.00	9.39	9.03 (m)	5.41	[68]
109	>10	0.41	-	0.075	4.08	-	-	0.003	3.59	0.170	-	-	[86, 90]
110	>10	6.36	-	0.067	-	-	-	0.003	-	0.043	-	-	[86]
111	1.73	0.83	4.77[b]	3.76	-	-	7.82	-	-	-	-	-	[67, 73]
112	1.24[d]	0.87[d]	-	-	-	-	-	-	-	-	-	-	[73]
113	>10	>10	-	0.212	-	-	-	0.004	-	0.054	-	-	[73, 86]
114	12.8[c]	4.4[c]	21.3[b,c]	15.7[c]	-	-	-	-	-	-	-	-	[89]
AAZ	0.250	0.012	200	0.074	0.063	0.054	0.011	0.0025	0.025	0.0057	0.017 (m)	0.041	[18]

[a]Mean from 3 different assays, by a Stopped-Flow technique (errors were in the range of ± 5-10% of the reported values); [b]CA III from bovine. [c]Inhibition data measured by the 4-nitrophenylacetate esterase assay [83]. [d]Data reported as IC_{50} (μg/mL). m = murine; - = not available data.

Overall, approximately the half of phenol derivatives **1-114** resulted to be more active against hCA I (K_Is of 0.55–10.2 μM) and hCA II (K_Is of 0.090–5.5 μM) than phenol **1** (K_Is of 10.2 μM and 5.5 μM against hCA I and II, respectively). Among them, derivative **21** showed the lower K_I value against hCA I (K_I of 0.55 μM), whereas compounds **4**, **29** and **103** were the best hCA II inhibitors within this subset (K_Is of 0.090, 0.108 and 0.168 μM, respectively). All derivatives **1-114** showed to be more potent CA III inhibitors (K_Is of 0.71–63.73 μM) than the standard **AAZ** (K_I of 200 μM) with the exception of **3** and **8**. Only compounds **31** and **81** (K_Is of 0.71 and 2.21 μM) inhibit CA III more than phenol **1**.

Many derivatives reported with K_I values against hCA IV (K_Is of 0.062–9.09 μM), lower than that of phenol **1** (K_I of 9.5 μM). Among them, derivatives **72, 74, 95, 106** and **110** resulted as more potent inhibitors than **AAZ** (K_Is of 0.062-0.0072 μM *vs* 0.074 μM).

All compounds **1-114** were better hCA VA (K_Is of 0.085–65.0 μM) and VB (K_Is of 0.069–98.4 μM) than phenol **1** (K_Is of 0.063 and 0.054 μM against hCA VA and VB), except for derivatives **8**, **27-29**, **41** and **52**. Notably, phenols **36-38**, **56-58** and **60-69** exhibited low nanomolar K_I values against the two mitochondrial hCAs (K_Is of 0.085–0.110 μM and 0.069–0.125 μM against hCA VA and VB, respectively).

Most compounds produced a better inhibition of hCAs VI, VII, IX and XII than phenol **1** (hCA VI K_Is of 0.011, 0.0025, 0.025 and 0.0057 μM against hCA VI, VII, IX and XII respectively). Derivatives **5**, **71** and **77** (K_Is of 0.52, 0.59 and 0.34 μM) showed the lowest K_I values against hCA VI, whereas derivatives **82**, **85**, **92**, **94**, **96**, **104**, **105**, **109**, **110** and **113**, as aforementioned were the best hCA VII inhibitors within this subset (K_Is of 0.003–0.004 μM) and are comparable to **AAZ** (K_I of 0.0025 μM). Compounds **48**, **81**, **89** and **97** (K_Is of 0.81, 0.46, 0.43 and 0.49 μM, respectively) acted as the best hCA IX inhibitors of the subset. Among the several low nanomolar hCA XII inhibitors (K_Is of 0.004–0.060 μM), phenols **73** and **103** (both K_I of 0.004 μM) only inhibited this isoform with a K_I value slightly lower than that of **AAZ** (K_I of 0.0057 μM).

All derivatives were better CA XIII (K_Is of 4.09–657 μM) than phenol **1** (K_I of 697 μM), but none inhibited the isoform more than **AAZ** (K_I of 0.017 μM). Isoform hCA XIV was inhibited in the high nanomolar range only by compounds **14**, **21** and **48** (K_Is of 0.69, 0.65 and 0.83 μM), quite far from the K_I value of the standard **AAZ** (K_I of 0.041 μM).

Synthetic/Semisynthetic Phenolic Derivatives as Hcas Inhibitors

A vast research was done which developed synthetic/semisynthetic derivatives of natural phenols as hCAIs. Gul *et al.* produced several series of phenolic derivatives Table **5.** [92], which included Mannich bases of 1-[3,5-b-s-aminomethyl-4-hydroxyphenyl]-3-(4-halogenophenyl)-2-propen-1-ones (**115-117a–d**), mono and bis Mannich bases of 4-(1*H*-benzimidazol-2-yl)phenol (**118a-f, 119a–e**) [93] and 2–(4-hydroxybenzylidene)-2,3-dihydro-1*H*-inden-1-one (**120a-i, 121a–g**) [94], and mono Mannich bases of 2-(4-hydrox--3-((phenylpiperazin-1-yl)methyl)benzylidene)-2,3-di-hydro-1*H*-inden-1-one (**122a-e**) [95] as inhibitors of hCA I and II. Compounds from series **115-121** weakly inhibited hCA I and hCA II, with inhibition percentages of 18–43% and 6–45%, respectively at 1 μM inhibitor concentration. However, derivatives **115-117a–d** showed selectivity toward hCA I over II, as well as compounds **118a-f, 119a–e** at a minor extent. Compounds **120a-i, 121a–g** inhibited hCA II more efficiently than hCA I. Compounds of series **122** acted instead as low nanomolar inhibitors against both hCA I and II (K_Is of 29.6–58.4 and 38.1–69.7 nM against hCA I and II), being even more potent inhibitors than **AAZ** according to the adopted esterase assay.

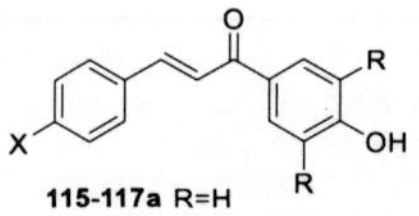

115a-d (X=F)
116a-d (X=Cl)
117a-d (X=Br)

115-117a R=H
115-117b R=$CH_2N(CH_2CH_2)_2CH_2$
115-117c R=$CH_2N(CH_2CH_2)_2O$
115-117d R=$CH_2N(CH_2CH_2)_2NCH_3$

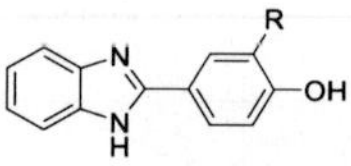

118a-f

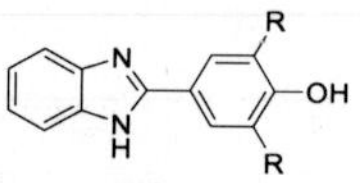

119a-e

118,119a R=$CH_2N(CH_3)_2$
118,119b R=$CH_2N(CH_2CH_2)_2$
118,119c R=$CH_2N(CH_2CH_2)_2CH_2$
118,119d R=$CH_2N(CH_2CH_2)_2NCH_3$
118,119e R=$CH_2N(CH_2CH_2)_2O$
118f R=H

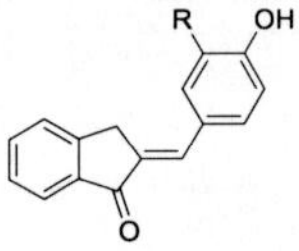

120a-i

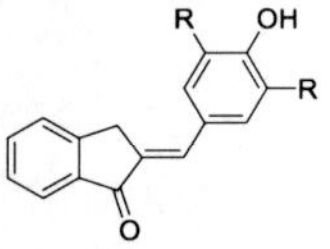

121a-g

120,121a R=$CH_2N(CH_2CH_2)_2NCH_3$
120,121b R=$CH_2N(CH_2CH_2)_2$
120,121c R=$CH_2N(CH_2CH_2)_2O$
120,121d R=$CH_2N(CH_2CH_2)_2CH_2$
120,121e R=$CH_2N(CH_3)_2$
120,121f R=$CH_2N(CH_2CH_2CH_3)_2$
120g R=$CH_2N(CH_2CH_3)_2$
120h R=$CH_2N(C_6H_5)_2$
120i R=H

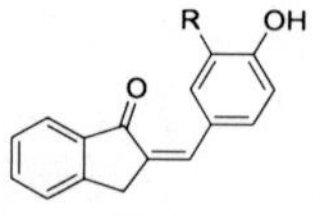

122a-e

122a R=$CH_2N(CH_2CH_2)_2NC_6H_5$
122b R=$CH_2N(CH_2CH_2)_2NCH_2C_6H_5$
122c R=$CH_2N(CH_2CH_2)_2N$-2-F-C_6H_5
122d R=$CH_2N(CH_2CH_2)_2N$-4-F-C_6H_5
122e R=$CH_2N(CH_2CH_2)_2N$-2-OCH_3-C_6H_5

Table 5. Inhibition % of hCAs I and II by the phenol series 115-121 at 1 μM concentration by a stopped-flow CO_2 hydrase assay [63] and inhibition data as K_Is of series 122 by a 4-nitrophenylacetate esterase assay [83], using AAZ as standard.

cmpd	% inhibition[a] hCA I	% inhibition[a] hCA II	Ref.
115a	34	17	[92]
115b	31	6	[92]
115c	26	16	[92]
115d	26	16	[92]
116a	30	11	[92]
116b	29	19	[92]
116c	30	20	[92]
116d	28	13	[92]
117a	43	9	[92]
117b	28	25	[92]
117c	29	17	[92]
117d	25	17	[92]
118a	26	21	[93]
118b	20	11	[93]
118c	23	20	[93]
118d	22	20	[93]

cmpd	% inhibition[a] hCA I	% inhibition[a] hCA II	Ref.
118e	18	24	[93]
118f	20	10	[93]
119a	20	7	[93]
119b	18	12	[93]
119c	21	13	[93]
119d	19	14	[93]
119e	18	25	[93]
120a	23	41	[94]
120b	24	41	[94]
120c	23	39	[94]
120d	31	42	[94]
120e	26	43	[94]
120f	25	45	[94]
120g	29	43	[94]
120h	23	44	[94]
120i	35	45	[94]

cmpd	% inhibition[a] hCA I	% inhibition[a] hCA II	Ref.
121a	25	38	[94]
121b	26	39	[94]
121c	31	42	[94]
121d	26	41	[94]
121e	26	36	[94]
121f	28	37	[94]
AAZ	79	95	[94]
cmpd	**K_I[b] (nM) hCA I**	**K_I[b] (nM) hCA II**	**Ref.**
122a	77.8	45.4	[95]
122b	63.8	40.7	[95]
122c	50.3	63.6	[95]
122d	29.7	71.4	[95]
122e	42.0	52.3	[95]
AAZ	183.4	104.6	[95]

[a]Mean from 3 different assays, by a Stopped-Flow assay. [b]Mean from 3 different assays, by the 4-nitrophenylacetate esterase assay. Errors were in the range of ± 5-10% of the reported values.

Riafrecha *et al.* appended different carbohydrate moieties to the phenol pharmacophore by a sulfonamide linker in *p*-position [96], demonstrating an improvement of the phenol CA inhibitory properties. The inhibition data of **123-125a,b** are reported in Table **6.** and showed a variably significant enhancement of the hCAs I and II inhibitory action (K_Is of 0.043–8.85 µM and 0.137–1.68 µM against hCA I and II) with respect to phenol **1**, up to the low nanomolar range. In contrast, the hCA IX and XII inhibition produced by **123-125a,b** dropped (K_Is >50 µM) with respect to lead **1**. Notably compound **123a**, the most potent hCAI inhibitor of the study, showed to be even more potent than **AAZ**.

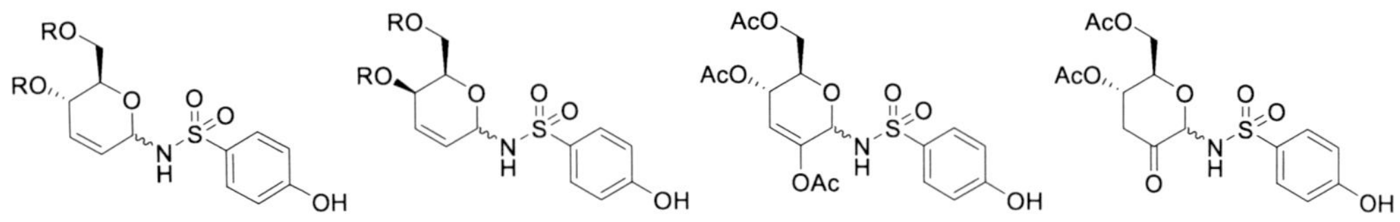

123a R=Ac
123b R=H
124a R=Ac
124b R=H
125a
125b

Table 6. Inhibition data of hCAs I, II, IX and XII with phenols 123-125a,b, the reference phenol 1, and the standard AAZ by a stopped-flow CO_2 hydrase assay [63].

cmpd	K_I[a] (µM)				Ref.
	hCA				
	I	II	IX	XII	
123a	0.043	0.139	>50	>50	[96]
123a	0.454	0.142	>50	>50	[96]
124a-α	6.63	0.695	>50	>50	[96]
124a-β	3.84	0.137	>50	>50	[96]
124b-α	8.85	0.34	>50	>50	[96]
124b-β	4.025	0.295	>50	>50	[96]
125a	6.69	0.36	>50	>50	[96]
125b	6.25	1.68	>50	>50	[96]
1	10.2	5.5	8.8	9.2	[64 - 68]
AAZ	0.250	0.012	0.025	0.0057	[18]

[a]Mean from 3 different assays, by a Stopped-Flow technique (errors were in the range of ± 5-10% of the reported values).

A series of antioxidant phenolic compounds (**126**, **127a-c**, **128a-c** and **129a,b**) were reported by Şentürk *et al.* [97] and tested against hCA I and II Table **7**. Generally, most such derivatives did not stand out for hCA inhibitory potency (K_Is 37.5–274.5 µM and 0.29–113.5 µM against hCA I and II). However, it was interesting to note that the bisphenol derivatives **128a-c** produced increased hCA

II inhibition than the corresponding phenol derivatives **127a-c**.

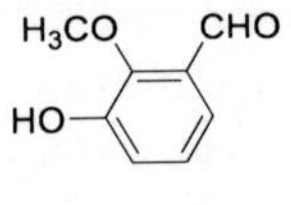

126

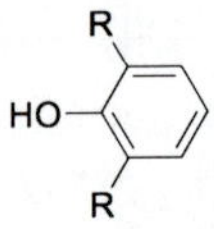

127a-c

127,128a R=CH_3
127,128b R=$CH(CH_3)_2$
127,128c R=$C(CH_3)_3$

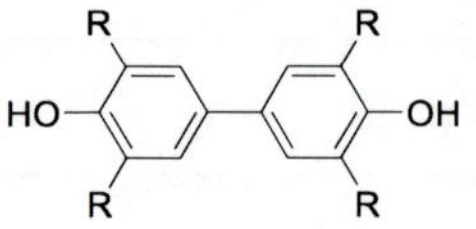

128a-c

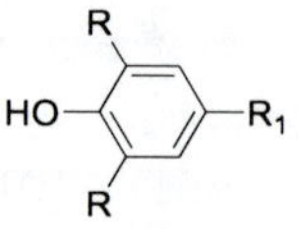

a R_1=CH_3
b R_1=OCH_3

129a,b (R=$C(CH_3)_3$)

Table 7. Inhibition data of hCAs I and II with phenols 126-129 and AAZ by a 4-nitrophenylacetate esterase assay [75].

cmpd	K_I[a] (μM) hCA		Ref.	cmpd	K_I[a] (μM) hCA		Ref.
	I	II			I	II	
126	55.6	1.25	[97]	**128b**	37.9	1.87	[97]
127a	198.3	113.5	[97]	**128c**	37.5	0.29	[97]
127b	98.9	18.5	[97]	**129a**	245.2	0.63	[97]
127c	274.5	0.51	[97]	**129b**	63.7	0.42	[97]
128a	92.8	4.05	[97]	**AAZ**	36.2	0.37	[97]

[a]Mean from 3 different assays, by the 4-nitrophenylacetate esterase method (errors were in the range of ± 5-10% of the reported values).

Two series of novel mono- and disubstituted phloroglucinol derivatives (**130, 131a-e**) were synthesized by Burmaoglu *et al.* [98, 99] and tested for their inhibitory activity against hCA I and II Table **8**. Except for compounds **130a** and **131a**, all derivatives resulted to act as low nanomolar inhibitors against the cytosolic isoforms with K_I values of 1.80–5.10 nM and 1.14–5.45 nM against hCA I and II, respectively.

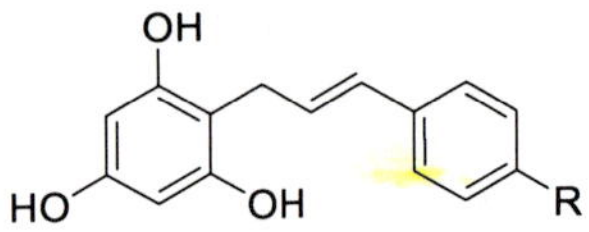

130a-e

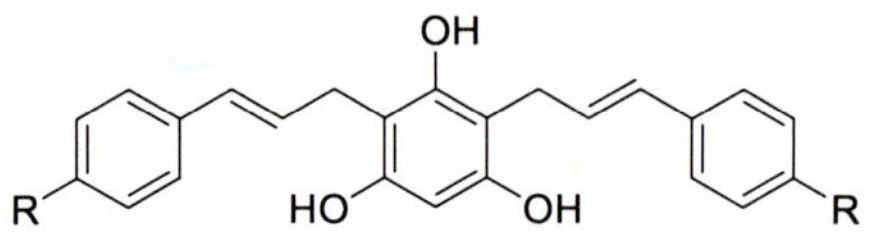

131a-e

130,131a R=OCH_3
130,131b R=F
130,131c R=Cl
130,131d R=Br
130,131e R=NO_2

Işik *et al.* reported a series of hydrazinecarbothioamides (**8a-f**) as semisynthetic derivatives of salicylic acid **8** [100]. Their inhibitory activity was tested against the cytosolic hCA I and hCA II and the transmembrane, tumor-associated hCA IX Table **9**. All derivatives **8a-f** produced greater inhibition of hCA I and IX and a weaker of hCA II with respect to the lead salicylic acid **8**. Specifically, **8c** and **8d** stood out in this study as low nanomolar hCA I inhibitors (K_Is of 0.086 and 0.043 μM, respectively).

Table 8. Inhibition data of hCAs I and II with phenols 130, 131a-e, and phenol 1 and AAZ as references by a 4-nitrophenylacetate esterase assay [83].

cmpd	K_I^a (nM) hCA I	K_I^a (nM) hCA II	Ref.	cmpd	K_I^a (nM) hCA I	K_I^a (nM) hCA II	Ref.
1	10200	5500	[64 - 68]	**131a**	n.d	83220	[98]
130a	77000	88920	[98]	**131b**	4.32	1.93	[99]
130b	5.10	1.77	[99]	**131c**	3.28	5.45	[99]
130c	4.35	1.48	[99]	**131d**	1.80	1.14	[99]
130d	5.08	1.86	[99]	**131e**	3.22	1.24	[99]
130e	3.17	2.84	[99]	**AAZ**	13.66	10.01	[99]

[a]Mean from 3 different assays, by the 4-nitrophenylacetate esterase method (errors were in the range of ± 5-10% of the reported values); n.d. = not detectable.

Table 9. Inhibition data of hCAs I, II and IX with phenols 8a-f, the lead salicylic acid 8, and the standard AAZ by a stopped-flow CO_2 hydrase assay [63].

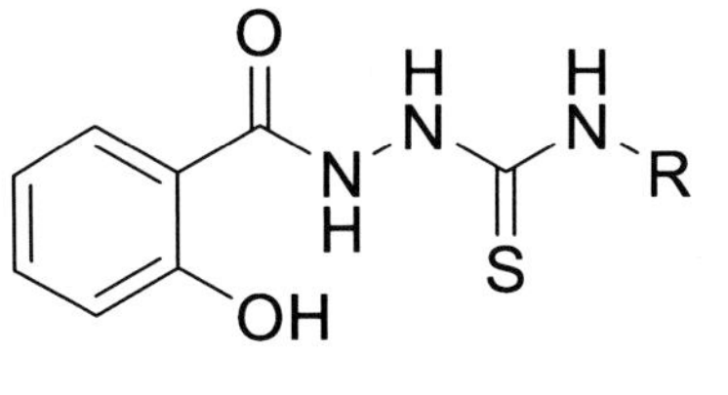

8a-f

8a R=H
8b R=CH_2CH_3
8c R=C_6H_5
8d R=4-CH_3-C_6H_4
8e R=$CH_2C_6H_5$
8f R=CH_2CHCH_2

cmpd	K_I^a (μM) hCA I	K_I^a (μM) hCA II	K_I^a (μM) hCA IX	Ref.	cmpd	K_I^a (μM) hCA I	K_I^a (μM) hCA II	K_I^a (μM) hCA IX	Ref.
8	9.9	7.1	78.7	[66]	**8d**	0.043	>10	1.245	[100]
8a	0.401	>10	1.005	[100]	**8e**	0.834	>10	0.980	[100]
8b	0.208	>10	0.878	[100]	**8f**	0.412	>10	0.760	[100]
8c	0.086	>10	1.220	[100]	**AAZ**	0.250	0.012	0.025	[18]

[a]Mean from 3 different assays, by a Stopped-Flow technique (errors were in the range of ± 5-10% of the reported values); n.d. = not detectable data.

Esters of natural phenols, such as *p*-hydroxybenzoic **10 (10a-c)**, protocatechuic **14 (14a-c)**, 2,4-dihydroxybenzoic **15 (15a-c)**, 2,5-dihydroxybenzoic **16 (16a-c)**, 2,6-dihydroxybenzoic **17 (17a-c)**, 3,5-dihydroxybenzoic **21 (21a-c)** and *p*-coumaric acid **40 (40a-c)** and amides of phenol **21 (21d,e)** were reported in two studies by Carta *et al.* and Arslan *et al.* These derivatives were evaluated by a stopped-flow CO_2 hydrase assay against the cytosolic CA I, II and VII, and the transmembrane CA IX, XII and XIV Table **10.** [75, 101]. Overall, the esterification of hydroxybenzoic acids **15, 16, 17, 21** and **40** variably increased the inhibitory action against all six tested CAs, except for **10a-c** and **16a**. In fact, esters **15a-c, 16a-c, 17a-c, 21a-e** and **40a-c** exhibited improved K_I values in a submicromolar range (K_Is *vs* hCA I of 0.32–0.97 µM; K_Is *vs* hCA II of 0.42–0.80 µM; K_Is *vs* hCA VII of 0.54–0.94 µM; K_Is *vs* hCA IX of 0.31–0.91 µM; K_Is *vs* hCA XII of 0.49–0.96 µM; K_Is *vs* hCA XIV of 0.33–0.89 µM). Amides **21d** and **21e** resulted to act as the worst hCA I and II inhibitors in this study.

Table 10. Inhibition data of hCAs I, II, VII, IX, XII and XIV with phenols 10a-c, 14a-c, 15a-c, 16a-c, 17a-c, 21a-e and 40a-c, phenol precursors 10, 14, 15, 16, 17, 21 and 40 as reference and the standard AAZ by a stopped-flow CO_2 hydrase assay [63].

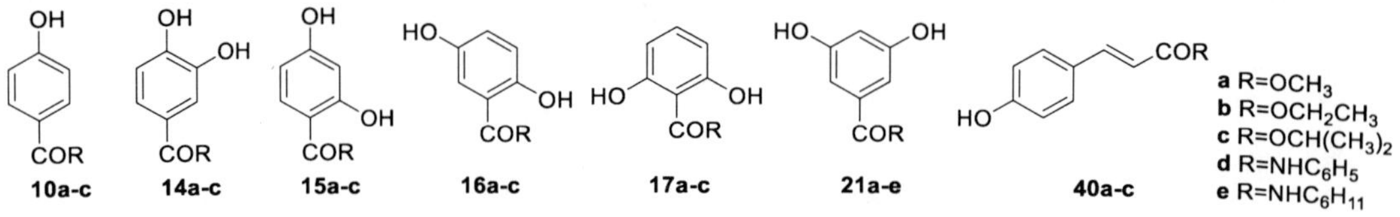

cmpd	K_I (µM)						Ref.
	hCA						
	I	II	VII	IX	XII	XIV	
10	9.8	10.6	4.08	3.73	6.27	6.16	[64, 65, 68, 69, 75]
10a	2.6	3.4	0.78	5.5	0.82	4.1	[75]
10b	7.9	4.8	8.7	8.2	8.6	7.7	[75]
10c	7.3	4.4	0.94	7.4	8.5	0.82	[75]
14	1.08	0.47	7.87	4.45	4.09	0.69	[69, 73 - 75]
14a	0.71	0.58	0.81	0.79	0.96	0.89	[75]
14b	0.65	0.61	0.75	0.78	0.83	0.86	[75]
14c	0.83	0.42	0.91	0.80	0.86	0.77	[75]
15	5.2	4.9	72	68	7.5	70	[69, 75]

(Table 10) cont.....

cmpd	**K_I (μM)**						**Ref.**
	hCA						
	I	**II**	**VII**	**IX**	**XII**	**XIV**	
15a	0.83	0.76	0.85	0.89	0.95	0.86	[75]
15b	0.63	0.52	0.81	0.82	0.77	0.74	[75]
15c	0.39	0.51	0.54	0.31	0.50	0.33	[75]
16	4.2	4.1	68	6.6	7.3	67	[75]
16a	0.82	0.77	8.3	0.84	0.83	0.80	[75]
16b	0.71	0.69	0.83	0.86	0.75	0.77	[75]
16c	0.97	0.58	0.84	0.81	0.82	0.84	[75]
17	5.7	5.2	6.6	5.9	7.2	6.5	[75]
17a	0.68	0.70	0.71	0.81	0.72	0.76	[75]
17b	0.67	0.56	0.76	0.78	0.84	0.82	[75]
17c	0.72	0.53	0.80	0.79	0.88	0.83	[75]
21	0.55	0.51	7.17	4.41	3.67	0.65	[69, 75]
21a	0.77	0.69	0.78	0.81	0.84	0.78	[75]
21b	0.69	0.66	0.90	0.91	0.85	0.83	[75]
21c	0.92	0.70	0.89	0.90	0.89	0.85	[75]
21d	441.5	10.76	-	-	-	-	[101]
21e	392.2	9.48	-	-	-	-	[101]
40	1.07	0.98	5.23	5.33	8.01	6.68	[64, 68, 75]
40a	0.78	0.80	0.82	0.85	0.81	0.83	[75]
40b	0.32	0.71	0.85	0.61	0.49	0.80	[75]
40c	0.54	0.52	0.69	0.68	0.76	0.73	[75]
AAZ	0.250	0.012	0.0025	0.025	0.0057	0.041	[18]

a. Mean from 3 different assays, by a Stopped-Flow technique (errors were in the range of ± 5-10% of the reported values); - = not available.

A thorough *in vitro* evaluation was conducted by Maresca *et al.* [102] with derivatives of *p*-coumaric **40 (40d-f)**, caffeic **42 (42a,b)**, ferulic acid **43 (43a-c)** esters bearing benzyl-, *m*/*p*-hydroxyphenethyl- and *p*-hydroxy-phenethoy-phenethyl moieties as hCAIs. The inhibitory profiles against hCA I-XIV are reported in Table **11**. The ubiquitous isoforms hCA I (K_I = 3.66– >50 μM) and II (K_I > 50 μM), as well as hCA III (K_I >50 μM), IV (K_I = 9.67–40.0 μM) and XII (K_I = 8.05–29.4 μM) were weakly inhibited by most such esters (*i.e.***40d-f**, **42a,b** and **43a-c**), though the precursors phenolic acids (**40**, **42** and **43**) were low micromolar inhibitors. Instead, the esters of series **40**, **42** and **43** showed increased inhibitory action against hCA VA (K_Is of 0.72–0.97 μM), VB (K_Is of 0.62–0.88 μM), VI (K_Is of 0.42–0.77 μM), VII (K_Is of 0.52–0.82 μM), IX (K_Is of 0.71–1.03 μM) and XIV (K_Is of 0.31–0.81 μM) with respect to the leads. Finally, **42a,b** and **43a-c** inhibited mCA XIII with intermediate K_I values in the range 0.84–0.94 μM, whereas compounds **40d-f** acted as low micromolar mCA XIII inhibitors (K_Is of 8.92–13.9 μM).

Table 11. Inhibition data of CAs I-XIV with phenols 40d-f, 42a,b and 43a-c, precursors phenols 40, 42 and 43 as references, and the standard AAZ by a stopped-flow CO_2 hydrase assay [63].

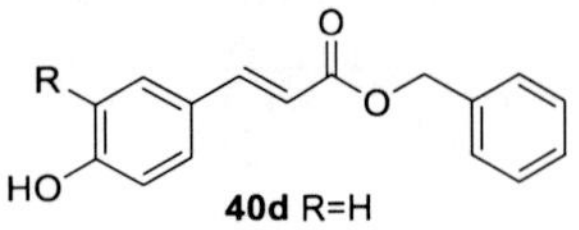

40d R=H
43a R=OCH_3

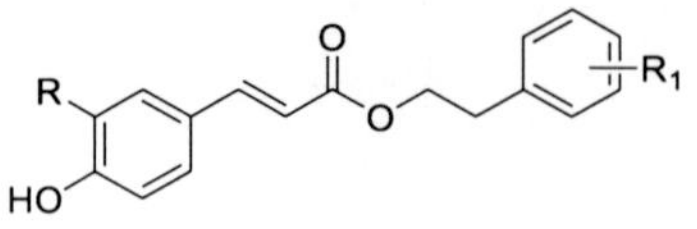

40e,f, 42a,b, 43b,c

40e R=H, R_1=*p*-OH
40f R=H, R_1=*m*-OH
42a R=OH, R_1=*p*-OCH_2CH_2-C_6H_4-*p*-OH
42b R=OH, R_1=*m*-OCH_2CH_2-C_6H_4-*m*-OH
43b R=OCH_3, R_1=*p*-OH
43c R=OCH_3, R_1=*m*-OH

cmpd	K_I[a] (μM)												Ref.
	hCA												
	I	II	III	IV	VA	VB	VI	VII	IX	XII	mXIII	XIV	
40	1.07	0.98	7.57	9.60	5.96	7.76	6.72	5.23	5.33	8.01	10.1	6.68	[64, 68, 75]
40d	>50	>50	>50	18.7	0.97	0.80	0.73	0.72	0.86	29.4	8.92	0.81	[102]
40e	3.87	>50	>50	9.67	0.85	0.62	0.51	0.73	0.71	12.7	13.9	0.37	[102]
40f	3.66	>50	>50	12.5	0.72	0.82	0.47	0.71	0.82	10.5	11.6	0.31	[102]
42	2.38	1.61	10.0	10.1	6.49	9.08	7.33	6.42	7.87	9.06	10.9	8.71	[102]
42a	5.23	>50	>50	24.1	0.79	0.74	0.56	0.73	0.93	8.05	0.84	0.64	[102]
42b	9.62	>50	>50	33.2	0.85	0.88	0.74	0.82	0.97	23.1	0.90	0.60	[102]
43	2.89	2.40	11.1	10.8	7.04	10.5	8.45	7.41	9.87	9.78	12.2	9.43	[64, 68]
43a	>50	>50	>50	39.5	0.88	0.66	0.42	0.63	1.03	8.89	0.94	0.78	[102]
43b	>50	>50	>50	44.0	0.81	0.67	0.77	0.62	0.81	8.47	0.93	0.72	[102]
43c	>50	>50	>50	40.5	0.93	0.76	0.54	0.52	0.99	29.2	0.91	0.75	[102]
AAZ	0.250	0.012	200	0.074	0.063	0.054	0.011	0.0025	0.025	0.0057	0.017	0.041	[18]

[a]Mean from 3 different assays, by a Stopped-Flow technique (errors were in the range of ± 5-10% of the reported values); m = murine.

In another study by Riafrecha *et al.* [103] synthetic derivatives of the *p/m*-coumaric acid **(132-135a,b)** were reported which include glycoside moieties. These derivatives were tested against the whole pattern of hCAs Table **12**. and showed to possess a rather flat CA inhibition profile against most isoforms. Indeed, mostly low micromolar K_I values were detected in the range 3.6–9.3 μM *vs* hCA I, K_I = 3.1–8.8 μM *vs* hCA II, 5.6–9.2 μM *vs* hCA IV, 3.4–9.8 μM *vs* hCA VA, 4.0– >100 μM *vs* hCA VB, 6.2– >100 μM *vs* hCA VI, 4.9–9.5 μM *vs* hCA VII, 2.9–9.2 μM *vs* hCA IX, 3.9–9.7 μM *vs* hCA XII, 4.9– >100 μM *vs* hCA XIII, 2.3– >100 μM *vs* hCA XIV. Most compounds, unlike the lead **1**, showed lack of action against hCA III (K_Is >100 μM). These results confirm that carbohydrate pendants applied to the phenol pharmacophore improve the hCA inhibitory activity. It should be stressed that the physicochemical properties of glycoside derivatives might physiologically orient CA inhibition towards the transmembrane isozymes such as the tumor-associated isoforms hCA IX and XII, according to a decreased membrane permeability. The authors claim that free C-cinnamoyl glycosides could be useful for intravenous chemotherapy, whereas the acetylated glycosides might be used as ester prodrugs.

Table 12. Inhibition data of hCAs I-XIV with phenols 132-135a,b, phenol 1 as reference and the standard AAZ by a stopped-flow CO_2 hydrase assay [63].

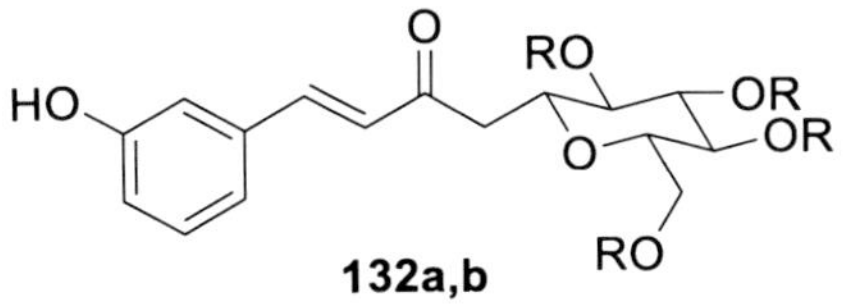

132a,b

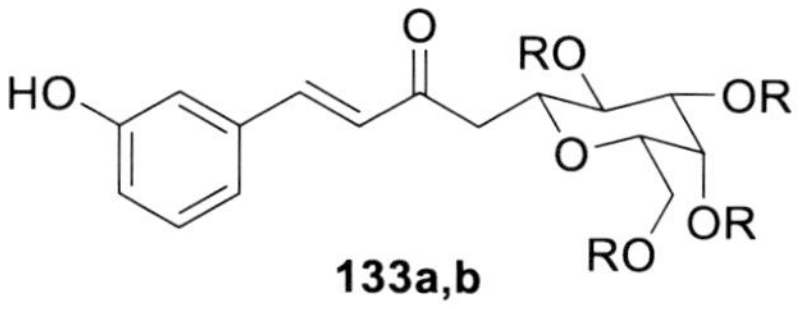

133a,b

a R=Ac
b R=H

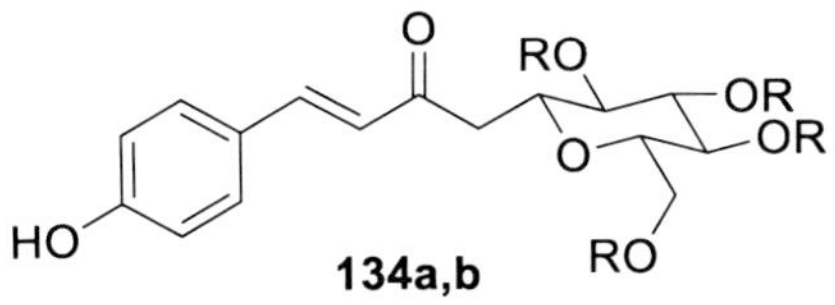

134a,b

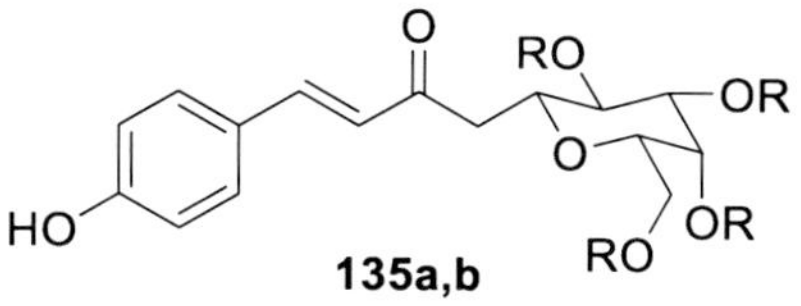

135a,b

Cmpd	K_I[a] (μM)												Ref.
	hCA												
	I	II	III	IV	VA	VB	VI	VII	IX	XII	XIII	XIV	
1	10.2	5.5	2.7	9.5	218	543	208	710	8.8	9.2	697(m)	11.5	[64 - 68]
132a	8.5	7.0	>100	5.6	9.8	6.0	8.8	9.5	5.2	6.7	5.1	5.9	[103]
132b	6.8	7.8	>100	8.3	7.4	>100	>100	4.9	4.5	7.4	8.8	4.3	[103]
133a	5.1	7.1	>100	7.8	9.5	6.9	7.7	7.1	3.3	3.9	7.2	4.6	[103]
133b	3.6	3.1	>100	9.2	3.4	>100	8.1	9.0	9.2	8.4	8.6	>100	[103]
134a	5.7	3.9	>100	4.9	8.4	4.0	6.2	6.3	5.9	6.2	4.9	5.6	[103]
134b	3.7	8.8	>100	7.1	4.4	>100	>100	8.5	8.2	8.7	8.6	7.1	[103]
135a	9.3	5.5	>100	6.7	9.3	5.2	7.9	5.8	2.9	4.2	6.7	2.3	[103]

(Table 12) cont.....

Cmpd	K_I^a (μM) hCA												Ref.
	I	II	III	IV	VA	VB	VI	VII	IX	XII	XIII	XIV	
135b	5.5	6.8	8.4	8.4	8.0	>100	>100	9.3	8.2	6.8	>100	>100	[103]
AAZ	0.250	0.012	200	0.074	0.063	0.054	0.011	0.0025	0.025	0.0057	0.017(m)	0.041	[18]

[a]Mean from 3 different assays, by a Stopped-Flow technique (errors were in the range of ± 5-10% of the reported values); m = murine.

Topal *et al.* [104] derived the lead eugenol **46** to yield novel semisynthetic phenol derivatives (**46a-e**) to be tested for their hCA I and II inhibitory action by a 4-nitrophenylacetate esterase assay Table **13**. These compounds demonstrated to inhibit hCA I and II in a low nanomolar range (K_Is of 0.113–0.738 μM and 0.092–0.530 μM, respectively), with an improved activity when compared to the lead **46**.

Table 13. Inhibition data of hCAs I and II with phenols 46a-e, eugenol 46 as the reference, and the standard AAZ by an esterase assay with 4-nitrophenylacetate as substrate [83].

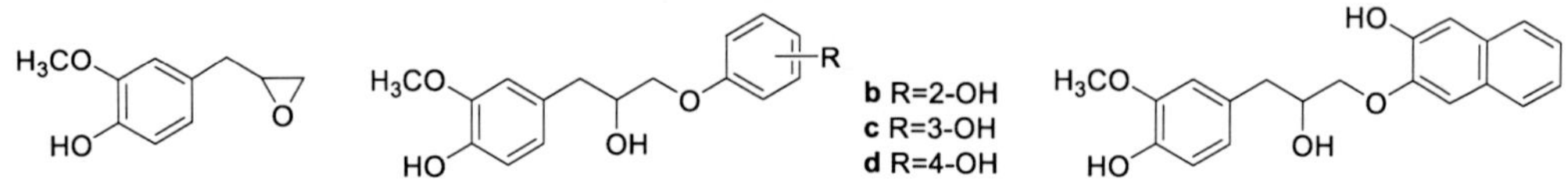

46a **46b-d** **46e**

cmpd	K_I^a (μM) hCA		Ref.	cmpd	K_I^a (μM) hCA		Ref.
	I	II			I	II	
46	0.738	0.530	[104]	**46c**	0.205	0.176	[104]
46a	0.568	0.470	[104]	**46d**	0.205	0.129	[104]
46b	0.224	0.092	[104]	**46e**	0.113	0.156	[104]
AAZ	0.594	0.120	[104]	**AAZ**	0.594	0.120	[104]

[a]Mean from 3 different assays, by the 4-nitrophenylacetate esterase method (errors were in the range of ± 5-10% of the reported values).

By using superacid chemistry, derivatives of the lactone phenolic hybrid dodoneine **52** (**52a-e**) were synthesized by Carreyre *et al.* [81] and tested as CAs I-XIV inhibitors Table **14**. Small chemical modifications of the basic scaffold revealed strong changes in the selectivity profile against different hCA isoforms. In fact, unlike the lead **52**, compounds **52a-e** selectively inhibited isoforms hCA I (K_Is of 0.13–0.76 μM), III (K_Is of 5.13–10.80 μM), XIV (K_Is of 2.44–7.24 μM), and mCA XIII (K_Is of 0.34–0.96 μM). Notably, derivatives **52d** and **52e** stood out as two new highly selective hCA III (K_Is of 10.80 and 5.13 µM, respectively) and mCA XIII (K_Is of 0.91 and 0.34 µM, respectively) inhibitors, being interesting targets of choice for further therapeutic evaluations.

Table 14. Inhibition data of CAs I-XIV with phenols 52a-e, dodoneine 52 as the reference, and the standard AAZ by a stopped-flow CO_2 hydrase assay [63].

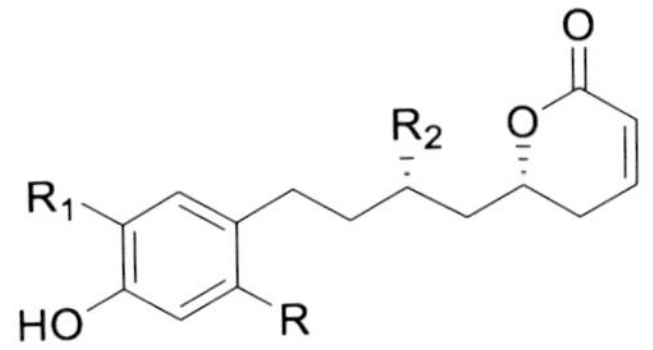

a R=R$_2$=OH, R$_1$=H
b R=R$_1$=Br, R$_2$=OH
c R=R$_1$=H, R$_2$=F

52a-c

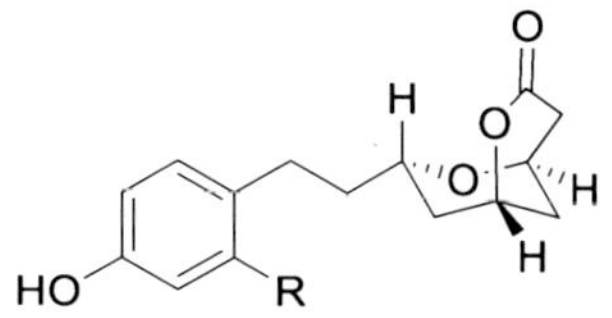

d R=H
e R=OH

52d,e

cmpd	K_I (µM)[a]												Ref.
	hCA												
	I	II	III	IV	VA	VB	VI	VII	IX	XII	mXIII	XIV	
52	5.48	>100	10.35	9.61	>100	>100	>100	>100	>100	>100	9.27	9.34	[81]
52a	0.38	>100	>100	4.12	21.6	13.7	>100	>100	32.6	24.5	8.13	7.24	[81]
52b	0.76	21.8	>100	13.7	8.55	6.32	>100	>100	15.7	10.8	7.89	12.5	[81]
52c	0.13	36.9	>100	5.36	7.13	1.36	>100	24.9	3.57	1.48	0.96	2.44	[81]
52d	>100	>100	10.80	>100	>100	>100	>100	>100	>100	>100	0.91	>100	[81]
52e	>100	>100	5.13	>100	>100	>100	>100	>100	>100	>100	0.34	>100	[81]
AAZ	0.250	0.012	200	0.074	0.063	0.054	0.011	0.0025	0.025	0.0057	0.017	0.041	[18]

[a]Mean from 3 different assays, by a Stopped-Flow technique (errors were in the range of ± 5-10% of the reported values); m = murine.

Davis *et al.* [78] studied the hCA I, II, VA and VB inhibition profiles with natural phenolic fungal metabolites **66-69** and their semisynthetic derivatives **67a-f** Table **15**. These compounds acted as low/medium micromolar inhibitors of the two cytosolic hCAs (K_I of 9.6–369 µM and 8.6–131 µM against hCA I and II, respectively). In contrast, a greater inhibition was interestingly measured against the mitochondrial hCAs VA and VB. The K_I values in a low/medium nanomolar range (0.094–0.110 µM and 0.079–0.125 µM, respectively) and a significant selectivity of action over the ubiquitous hCA I and II make these derivatives promising leads to develop new tools to target the mitochondrial hCAs.

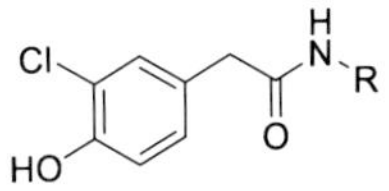

67a R=$CH_2CH_2OCH_3$
67b R=$C(CH_3)_3$
67c R=$CH_2CH_2CH_2CH_3$

67a-c

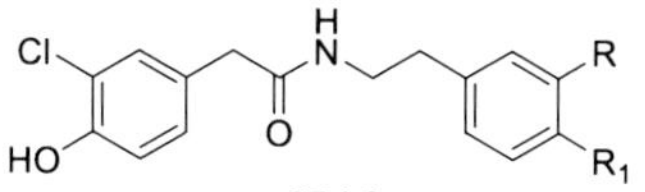

67d R=R$_1$=H
67e R=OCH_3, R$_1$=H
67f R=R$_1$=OCH_3

67d-f

Table 15. Inhibition data of hCA I, II, VA and VB with phenols 67a-f, phenols 66-69 as references and the standard AAZ by a stopped-flow CO_2 hydrase assay [43].

cmpd	K_I^a (μM)				Ref.
	hCA				
	I	II	VA	VB	
66	**10.5**	**11.4**	**0.096**	**0.085**	**[78]**
67	237	131	0.110	0.106	[78]
67a	158	10.4	0.102	0.084	[78]
67b	11.4	10.8	0.105	0.089	[78]
67c	10.7	9.4	0.108	0.081	[78]
67d	9.6	9.8	0.101	0.091	[78]
67e	11.2	10.8	0.103	0.087	[78]
67f	11.9	11.5	0.094	0.079	[78]
68	265	8.6	0.100	0.118	[78]
69	369	10.7	0.109	0.125	[78]
AAZ	0.250	0.012	0.063	0.054	[18]

[a]Mean from 3 different assays, by a Stopped-Flow technique (errors were in the range of ± 5-10% of the reported values).

Several series of bisphenol and bromophenol derivatives (compounds **71a-g**, **136a-c**, **137a-d** and **138a-j**) were developed from the natural compounds **70** (vidalol B) and **71** [84, 85, 105 - 108]. These derivatives were in part assayed as inhibitors of hCA I, II, IV and VI isoforms by the 4-nitrophenylacetate esterase assay Table **16**. Surprisingly, compounds from series **136**, **137** and **138** exhibited low nanomolar K_I values against hCAs I and II (K_Is of 1.85–93.48 nM and 2.01–67.05 nM).

Huyut *et al.* [91, 109] reported that the indole phenol derivatives **ID-8** can exert hCA I and II inhibitory actions with IC_{50} in a medium micromolar range Table **17**. Successively, Ekinci *et al.* investigated the CA inhibition profiles of other synthetic indole-based phenols (**139a-h**) against hCA I, II, IV, VI and bCA III Table **17**. Derivatives **139a-h** caused inhibition in the submicromolar range against hCA II (K_Is of 0.343–0.813 μM) and IV (K_Is of 0.435–1.032 μM), instead being low micromolar inhibitors against hCA I (K_Is of 2.14–3.48 μM), VI (K_Is of 1.92–9.21 μM) and bCAIII (K_Is of 2.13–9.62 μM).

Table 16. Inhibition data of hCAs I, II, IV and VI phenols 71a-g, 136a-c, 137a-d and 138a-j, phenols 70 and 71 as references and the standard AAZ by an esterase assay with 4-nitrophenylacetate as substrate [83].

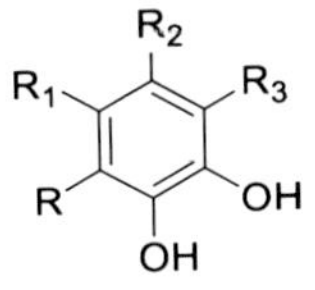

71a-g

a R=R_2=R_3=Br, R_1=CH_2OH
b R=R_2=R_3=Br, R_1=H
c R=R_1=R_2=R_3=Br
d R=H, R_1=$CH_2SO_2CH_3$, R_2=R_3=Br
e R=R_2=R_3=Br, R_1=$CH_2SO_2CH_3$
f R=R_2=H, R_1=$CH_2SO_2CH_3$, R_3=Br
g R=R_3=H, R_1=$CH_2SO_2CH_3$, R_2=Br

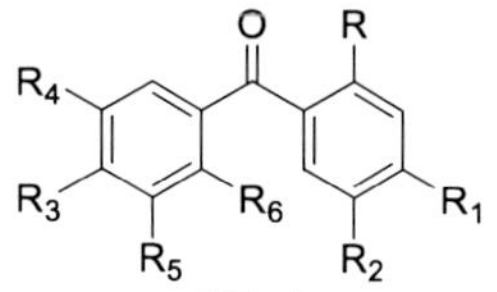

138a-j

a R=R_4=R_6=H, R_1=R_2=R_3=R_5=OH
b R=R_2=R_3=R_4=OH, R_1=Br, R_5=R_6=H
c R=R_2=R_3=R_4=R_5=OH, R_1=Br, R_6=H
d R=Br, R_1=OH, R_2=R_3=R_4=R_5=R_6=H
e R=Br, R_1=R_3=OH, R_2=R_4=R_5=R_6=H
f R=Br, R_1=R_3=R_4=OH, R_2=R_5=R_6=H
g R=Br, R_1=R_5=R_6=OH, R_2=R_3=R_4=H
h R=R_1=R_3=OH, R_2=Br, R_4=R_5=R_6=H
i R=R_2=R_3=OH, R_1=Br, R_4=R_5=R_6=H
j R=R_2=OH, R_1=Br, R_3=R_4=R_5=R_6=H

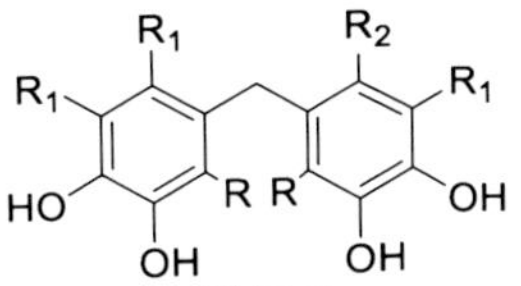

136a-c

a R=R_1=Br, R_2=H
b R=R_1=R_2=Br
c R=R_1=R_2=H

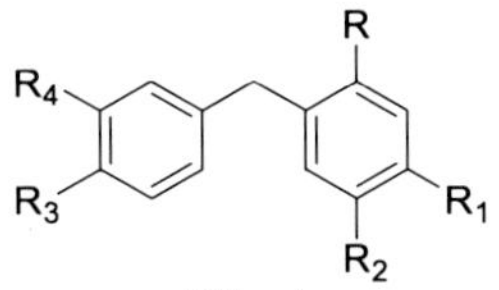

137a-d

a R=Br, R_1=OH, R_2=R_3=R_4=H
b R=R_2=OH, R_1=Br, R_3=R_4=H
c R=R_2=R_3=OH, R_1=Br, R_4=H
d R=Br, R_1=R_3=R_4=OH, R_2=H

cmpd	K_I[a] (nM)				Ref.	cmpd	K_I[a] (nM)				Ref.
	hCA						hCA				
	I	II	IV	VI			I	II	IV	VI	
70	12240	1130	1840	3410	[84]	**137b**	78.01	18.41	-	-	[107]
71	1670	560	1080	590	[85]	**137c**	67.30	27.44	-	-	[107]
71a	193240	34560	46350	158590	[84]	**137d**	40.92	22.84	-	-	[107]
71b	25340	26380	13120	11140	[84]	**138a**	18.03	1.437	-	11.42	[107]
71c	32150	29820	17480	29140	[84, 105]	**138b**	10.07	8.24	-	-	[107]
71d	89.37	67.05	-	-	[106]	**138c**	9.28	6.15	-	-	[107]
71e	64.12	54.76	-	-	[106]	**138d**	8.44	6.17	-	-	[107]
71f	53.75	42.84	-	-	[106]	**138e**	8.15	4.32	-	-	[107]
71g	57.43	53.75	-	-	[106]	**138f**	3.12	2.58	-	-	[107]
136a	34.41	21.16	27.48	17.43	[84]	**138g**	1.85	2.78	-	-	[107]
136b	35.12	21.47	28.04	17.83	[84]	**138h**	3.14	2.53	-	-	[107]
136c	18.36	5.64	7.64	13.69	[84]	**138i**	3.04	2.29	-	-	[107]
137a	93.48	57.30	-	-	[107]	**138j**	2.80	2.01	-	-	[107]
AAZ	36200	370	578	340	[105]	**AAZ**	36200	370	578	340	[105]

[a]Mean from 3 different assays, by the 4-nitrophenylacetate esterase method (errors were in the range of ± 5-10% of the reported values); - = not available data.

Table 17. Inhibition data of hCAs I-XIV with phenols ID-8 and 139a-h and the standard AAZ by an esterase assay with 4-nitrophenylacetate as substrate [83].

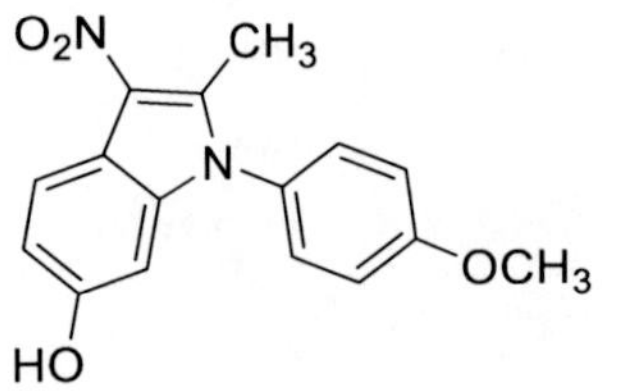

ID-8

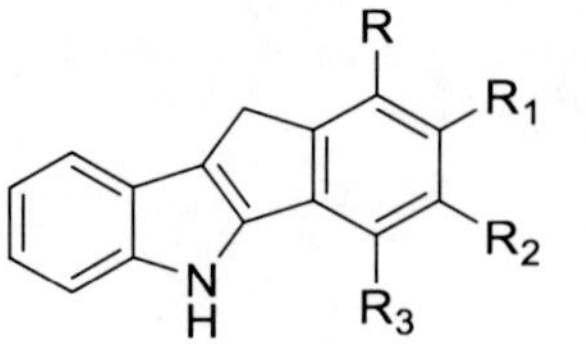

139a-h

a $R=OH, R_1=R_2=R_3=H$
b $R_1=OH, R=R_2=R_3=H$
c $R_2=OH, R=R_1=R_3=H$
d $R_3=OH, R=R_1=R_2=H$
e $R=R_1=OH, R_2=R_3=H$
f $R=R_3=OH, R_1=R_2=H$
g $R_1=R_2=OH, R=R_3=H$
h $R_1=R_3=OH, R=R_2=H$

Cmpd	K_I[a] (μM)					Ref.
	hCA					
	I	II	bIII	IV	VI	
ID-8	693.00[b]	53.30[b]	-	-	-	[91]
139a	2.14	0.648	8.84	0.875	8.31	[109]
139b	3.26	0.734	9.08	0.912	8.54	[109]
139c	3.29	0.785	9.42	0.943	8.98	[109]
139d	3.48	0.813	9.62	1.032	9.21	[109]
139e	2.47	0.447	2.13	0.543	1.92	[109]
139f	2.51	0.561	4.34	0.435	4.17	[109]
139g	2.59	0.343	5.17	0.842	4.95	[109]
139h	2.46	0.536	4.63	0.765	4.31	[109]
AAZ	36.20	0.370	83.40	0.578	0.34	[109]

[a]Mean from 3 different assays, by the 4-nitrophenylacetate esterase method (errors were in the range of ± 5-10% of the reported values); [b]Data reported as IC_{50} (μg/mL). b = bovine; - = not available data.

A new type of bis-chalcone (**140** and **141a-k** in Table **18.**) was reported by Arslan *et al.* and included a phenol moiety [110]. These compounds were thus tested for their CA inhibitory action against hCA I and II Table **18**. All such compounds inhibited both isoforms in a submicromolar range with K_Is in the range 0.111–325 μM and 0.154–0.645 μM, respectively.

Table 18. Inhibition data of hCA I and II with phenols 140 and 141a-k and the standard AAZ by a 4-nitrophenylacetate esterase assay [83].

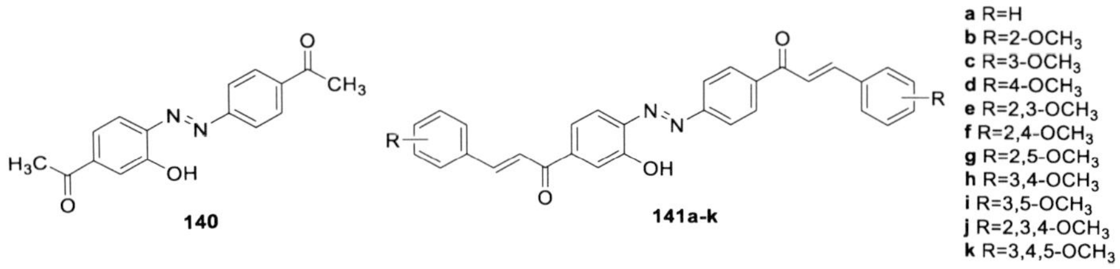

cmpd	K_I^a (μM)		Ref.	cmpd	K_I^a (μM)		Ref.
	hCA				hCA		
	I	II			I	II	
140	0.274	0.645	[110]	**141f**	0.177	0.446	[110]
141a	0.112	0.154	[110]	**141g**	0.188	0.208	[110]
141b	0.325	0.418	[110]	**141h**	0.323	0.182	[110]
141c	0.165	0.227	[110]	**141i**	0.072	0.166	[110]
141d	0.308	0.307	[110]	**141j**	0.179	0.268	[110]
141e	0.111	0.193	[110]	**AAZ**	36.20	0.370	[109]

[a]Mean from 3 different assays, by the 4-nitrophenylacetate esterase method (errors were in the range of ± 5-10% of the reported values).

Natural and Synthetic/Semisynthetic Phenols Inhibit Carbonic Anhydrases From Bacteria, Fungi, Protozoa, And Diatoms

Numerous phenolic derivatives, among which some mentioned above, were also tested as inhibitors of CA isoforms from bacteria (β- and γ-class CAs), fungal (β-CAs), protozoa (η-CAs) and diatoms (δ-CAs) searching for new promising anti-infective drugs with a novel mechanism of action.

Davis *et al.* [111] reported for the first time the inhibitory action of phenols against β-class CAs. In this study, the derivatives listed in Table **19.** (shown in above described Figures) were tested for the inhibition of hCAI and II, the three β-CAs from *Mycobacterium tuberculosis* (Rv1284, Rv3588c, Rv3273) and the β-CAs from *Candida albicans* (Nce103) and *Cryptococcus neoformans* (Can2).

The clinically used sulfonamide **AAZ** inhibits all these CAs in the submicromolar range up to low nanomolar K_Is with even single-digit values against hCA II Rv3588c and Can2 Table **19** [111]. Interestingly, most tested phenols provoked inhibition of the β-class enzymes in the submicromolar range, though with rather flat inhibition profiles. Notably, significant one to two orders of magnitude selectivity were detected for the β-class CAs over both hCAs. The two best performing phenolic CAIs, which are **58** and **67**, preferentially inhibited the fungal β-CAs Nce103 and Can2 over hCAs with a selective index (*SI*) of more than 2 orders of magnitude. Therefore, they represent promising leads for developing specific probes against β-CAs. These compounds provide the first non-canonical CA inhibitors with an important selectivity toward pathogen over host enzymes.

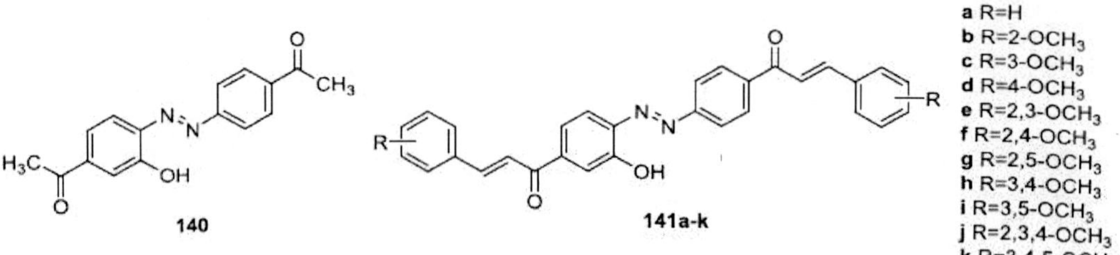

Table 19. Inhibition data of hCAs I, II, bacterial β-CAs from *Mycobacterium tuberculosis* (Rv1284, Rv3588c, Rv3273) and fungal β-CAs from *Candida albicans* (Nce103) and *Cryptococcus neoformans* (Can2) with phenols 36-68, phenol 1 and the AAZ as references by a stopped-flow CO_2 hydrase assay [63].

cmpd	K_I^a (μM)							Ref.
	hCA I	hCA II	Rv1284	Rv3588c	Rv3273	Nce103	Can2	
1	10.2	5.5	64.0	-	79.0	17.3	25.9	[111]
36	430	8.7	0.85	-	12.1	1.10	1.08	[111]
37	309	10.3	10.8	-	11.4	1.02	0.90	[111]
38	309	11.2	0.85	-	9.12	0.91	0.84	[111]
40	1.07	0.98	6.05	4.33	2.69	-	-	[111]
42	2.38	1.61	5.92	5.36	6.70	-	-	[111]
43	2.89	2.40	7.13	5.64	2.40	-	-	[111]
56	368	11.7	0.82	-	8.92	0.73	0.77	[111]
57	354	12.1	0.80	-	0.89	0.70	0.95	[111]
58	307	230	0.85	-	9.10	0.62	0.81	[111]
60	201	8.4	10.5	-	11.4	1.06	1.12	[111]
61	374	9.2	0.99	-	10.9	1.01	1.08	[111]
62	10.5	9.6	11.8	-	0.91	0.92	0.89	[111]
63	355	13.1	0.91	-	0.92	0.90	0.95	[111]
64	239	8.3	0.84	-	11.3	1.03	1.15	[111]

(Table 19) cont.....

cmpd	K_I[a] (μM)							Ref.
	hCA I	hCA II	Rv1284	Rv3588c	Rv3273	Nce103	Can2	
65	231	8.0	0.71	-	10.9	1.06	1.11	[111]
66	10.5	11.4	12.2	-	0.98	0.78	0.72	[111]
67	237	131	10.5	-	11.2	1.00	0.85	[111]
68	265	8.6	10.3	-	10.8	1.08	1.12	[111]
AAZ	0.250	0.012	0.480	0.0098	0.100	0.130	0.010	[111, 112]

[a]Mean from 3 different assays, by a Stopped-Flow technique (errors were in the range of ± 5-10% of the reported values).

The fungal metabolite **67** also represented the lead compound for the synthesis phenols **67a-f** that were thus assessed for the inhibition of the same pattern of CA isoforms Table **20** [78, 111]. Compounds **67d-f** showed improved inhibitory action than **67** against the β-CAs (K_Is of 0.80–1.78 μM against Rv1284; K_Is of 0.90–0.97 μM against Rv3273; K_Is of 0.72–0.93 μM against Nce103; K_Is of 0.81–0.94 μM against Can2). However, a loss of selectivity for β-CAs over hCAs occurred with respect to the lead **67**.

Table 20. Inhibition data of hCAs I, II, bacterial β-CAs from *M. tuberculosis* (Rv1284, Rv3273) and fungal β-CAs from *C. albicans* (Nce103) and *C. neoformans* (Can2) with phenols 67a-f, phenol 67 as a reference and the standard AAZ by a stopped-flow CO_2 hydrase assay [63].

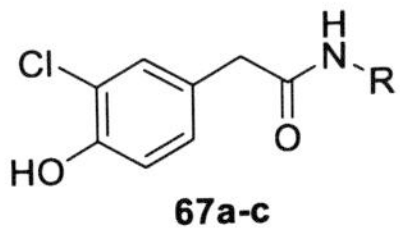

67a-c

67a R=$CH_2CH_2OCH_3$
67b R=$C(CH_3)_3$
67c R=$CH_2CH_2CH_2CH_3$

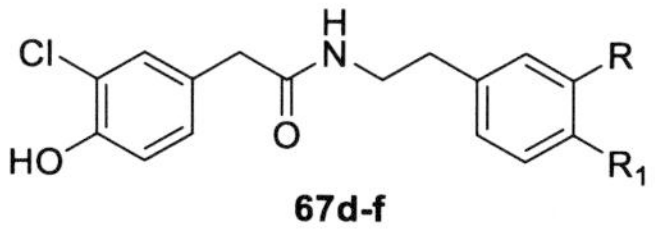

67d-f

67d R=R_1=H
67e R=OCH_3, R_1=H
67f R=R_1=OCH_3

cmpd	K_I (μM)[a]						Ref.
	hCA I	hCA II	Rv1284	Rv3273	Nce103	Can2	
67	237	131	10.5	11.2	1.00	0.85	[78, 111]
67a	158	10.4	11.0	1.14	0.99	0.95	[78, 111]
67b	11.4	10.8	12.3	10.2	0.96	0.91	[78, 111]
67c	10.7	9.4	11.6	10.4	0.81	0.73	[78, 111]
67d	9.6	9.8	0.80	0.97	0.93	0.81	[78, 111]
67e	11.2	10.8	1.27	0.91	0.72	0.94	[78, 111]
67f	11.9	11.5	1.78	0.90	0.75	0.86	[78, 111]
AAZ	0.250	0.012	0.480	0.100	0.130	0.010	[111, 112]

[a]Mean from 3 different assays, by a Stopped-Flow technique (errors were in the range of ± 5-10% of the reported values).

Cau *et al.* [113] studied the inhibitory activity of *p*-coumaric (**40**), caffeic (**42**) and ferulic acid (**43**) esters (**40d-f**, **42a,b** and **43a-c**) against the three β-CAs from *M. tuberculosis*. The K_I values collected in Table **21.** showed that all ester compounds were low micromolar inhibitors of the β-CAs (K_Is of 3.78–5.74 μM against Rv1284; K_Is of 4.33–8.03 μM against Rv3588c; K_Is of 1.84–6.83 μM against Rv3273) and notably did not show any inhibitory activity against the human widespread cytosolic isoforms hCA II (K_Is > 50 μM). Additionally, phenols **40d** and **43-c** showed a complete selectivity for the *M. tuberculosis* β-CAs over hCA I and II, as they did not inhibit hCA I also below a 50 μM concentration. Compounds **40d,f** and **42a,b** were instead low micromolar inhibitors of hCA I (K_Is of 3.66–9.62 μM).

Table 21. Inhibition data of hCAs I, II, and bacterial β-CAs from *Mycobacterium tuberculosis* (Rv1284, Rv3588c, Rv3273) with phenols 40d-f, 42a,b and 43a-c, phenols 40, 42 and 43 as references and the standard AAZ by a stopped-flow CO_2 hydrase assay [63].

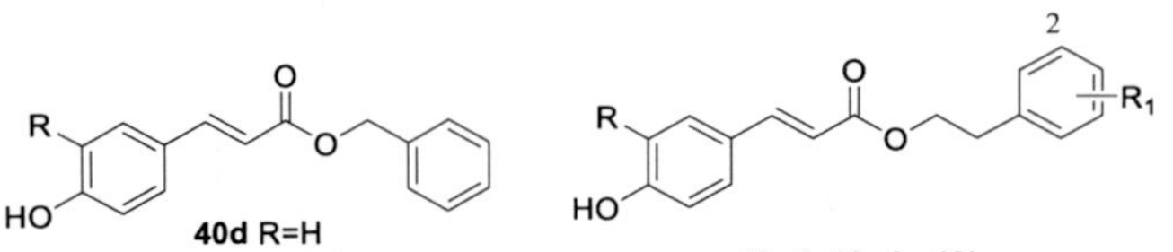

40d R=H
43a R=OCH_3

40e,f, 42a,b, 43b,c

40e R=H, R_1=*p*-OH
40f R=H, R_1=*m*-OH
42a R=OH, R_1=*p*-OCH_2CH_2-C_6H_4-*p*-OH
42b R=OH, R_1=*m*-OCH_2CH_2-C_6H_4-*m*-OH
43b R=OCH_3, R_1=*p*-OH
43c R=OCH_3, R_1=*m*-OH

cmpd	K_I[a] (μM)					Ref.
	hCA I	hCA II	Rv1248	Rv3588c	Rv3273	
40	1.07	0.98	6.05	4.33	2.69	[113]
40d	>50	>50	3.78	5.04	1.84	[113]
40e	3.87	>50	4.67	5.13	1.87	[113]
40f	3.66	>50	5.74	6.09	2.30	[113]
42	2.38	1.61	5.92	5.36	6.70	[113]
42a	5.23	>50	5.32	7.13	5.10	[113]
42b	9.62	>50	3.95	8.03	6.83	[113]
43	2.89	2.40	7.13	5.64	2.40	[113]
43a	>50	>50	4.51	7.05	3.19	[113]
43b	>50	>50	5.67	7.26	3.20	[113]
43c	>50	>50	4.69	5.40	2.32	[113]
AAZ	0.250	0.012	0.480	0.0098	0.100	[112]

[a]Mean from 3 different assays, by a stopped-flow technique (errors were in the range of ± 5-10% of the reported values).

The small series of C-cinnamoyl glycosides bearing a phenol moiety **132-135a,b** was also tested for the inhibition of the three β-CAs from *M. tuberculosis* and the two β-CAs from the bacterium *Brucella suis* (bsCA I and II) [114, 115]. The inhibition results are shown in Table **22**. The compounds resulted to act as low micromolar inhibitors against Rv1248 (K_Is of 0.14–4.5 μM), Rv3273 (K_Is of 3.25–19.0 μM), bsCA I (K_Is of 0.68–7.92 μM), and bsCA II (K_Is of 0.63–4.85 μM) showing instead a submicromolar activity against Rv3588c (K_Is of 0.13–1.5 μM). Specifically, the 3-hydroxyphenyl glycosides **132-133a,b** preferentially inhibited bsCAs over hCAs denoting such a scaffold as promising for the development of novel anti-infectives with a new mechanism of action. All compounds were also tested for the growth inhibition of a *M. tuberculosis* $H_{37}Rv$ strain, leading to the identification of **132a** that provoked a 99.9% reduction in the colony counts ($MIC_{99.9\%}$) at concentration values as low as 3.125–6.25μg/mL.

Table 22. Inhibition data of hCAs I, II, and bacterial β-CAs from *M. tuberculosis* (Rv1284, Rv3588c, Rv3273) and *Brucella suis* (BsCA I, BsCA II) with phenols 132-135a,b and the standard AAZ by a stopped-flow CO_2 hydrase assay [63].

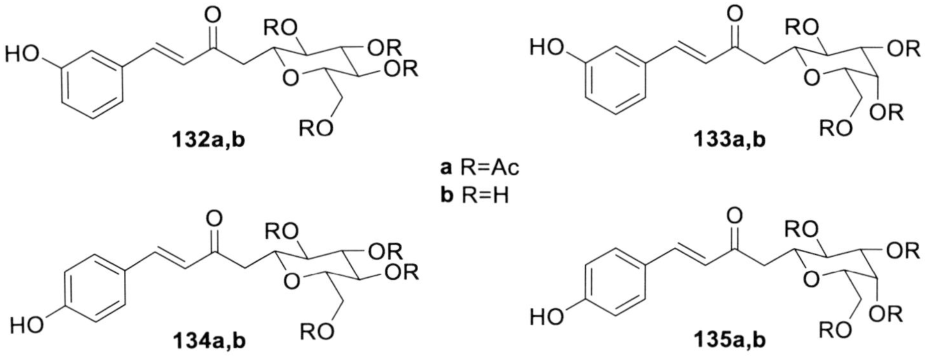

cmpd	K_I[a] (μM)							Ref.
	hCA I	hCA II	Rv1248	Rv3588c	Rv3273	bsCA I	bsCA II	
132a	8.5	7.0	2.1	0.64	19.0	0.92	0.71	[114, 115]
132b	6.8	7.8	0.14	0.24	6.21	3.45	0.78	[114, 115]
133a	5.1	7.1	3.8	0.87	15.6	0.68	0.63	[114, 115]
133b	3.6	3.1	1.16	0.51	3.25	6.54	0.83	[114, 115]
134a	5.7	3.9	2.9	0.35	13.1	5.65	2.68	[114, 115]
134b	3.7	8.8	0.93	0.13	4.13	7.92	4.75	[114, 115]
135a	9.3	5.5	4.5	1.15	12.0	7.18	4.85	[114, 115]
135b	5.5	6.8	4.5	0.64	4.13	5.43	2.80	[114, 115]
AAZ	0.250	0.012	0.480	0.104	0.0098	0.063	0.303	[112, 114, 115]

[a]Mean from 3 different assays, by a Stopped-Flow technique (errors were in the range of ± 5-10% of the reported values).

Two series of phenols incorporating tertiary amine and *trans*-2/3-pyridylethen-l-carbonyl moieties (**142a-g, 143a-f**) were reported by Bilginer *et al.* [116] and tested for the inhibition of hCA I and II isoforms and the β-CA from *Saccharomyces cerevisiae* (ScCA) Table **23**. The model organisms *S. cerevisiae* and ScCA are useful for detecting antifungals with a novel mechanism of action compared to the classical azole drugs to which significant drug resistance emerged. It should be also stressed that it was shown that some potent sulfonamide ScCA inhibitors inhibit the growth of the yeast *in vivo* [117].

All compounds resulted to be more active against ScCA (K_Is of 0.0049–0.0954 μM) than **AAZ** (K_I of 0.0826 μM), being instead worse hCA I and II inhibitors (K_Is of 0.78–23.5 μM and 10.8–52.4 μM, respectively). The best ScCA inhibitor **143d** even showed a nanomolar single-digit K_I of 4.9 nM.

Table 23. Inhibition data of hCAs I and II and β-CA of *Saccharomyces cerevisiae* (ScCA) with the synthetic phenols 142a-g and 143a-f and the standard AAZ by a stopped-flow CO_2 hydrase assay [63].

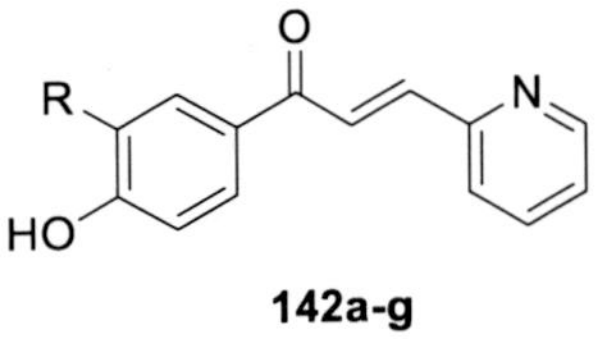

142a-g

a R=H
b R=$CH_2N(CH_3)_2$
c R=$CH_2N(CH_2CH_3)_2$
d R=$CH_2N(CH_2)_4$
e R=$CH_2N(CH_2)_5$
f R=$CH_2N(CH_2CH_2)_2NCH_3$
g R=$CH_2N(CH_2CH_2)_2O$

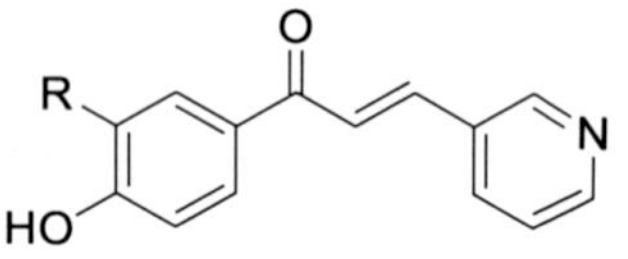

143a-f

cmpd	K_I[a] (μM)			Ref.	cmpd	K_I[a] (μM)			Ref.
	hCA I	hCA II	ScCA			hCA I	hCA II	ScCA	
142a	1.77	10.8	0.0658	[116]	**143a**	0.78	12.5	0.0765	[116]
142b	9.01	34.9	0.0901	[116]	**143b**	23.5	29.8	0.0235	[116]
142c	4.05	43.1	0.0819	[116]	**143c**	7.76	26.9	0.0771	[116]
142d	2.36	45.8	0.0858	[116]	**143d**	5.40	34.7	0.0049	[116]
142e	1.88	48.0	0.0791	[116]	**143e**	17.9	41.5	0.0650	[116]
142f	2.01	47.7	0.0795	[116]	**143f**	3.35	14.7	0.0765	[116]
142g	0.91	52.4	0.0954	[116]	**AAZ**	0.250	0.012	0.0826	[18, 116]

[a]Mean from 3 different assays, by a Stopped-Flow technique (errors were in the range of ± 5-10% of the reported values).

Entezari Heravi *et al.* [118] investigated for the first time the inhibitory activity of a panel of simple phenols, within the **1-40** subset, for the inhibition of the β-CA from the fungal parasite *Malassezia globosa* (MgCA), a validated anti-dandruff drug target. The inhibitory profiles displayed in Table **24.** were compared to those previously reported (in Tables **1** and **2**) against hCA I and II. All tested phenols showed to be better MgCA inhibitors (K_Is of 2.5–65.0 μM) than the clinically used sulfonamide **AAZ** (K_I of 74.0 μM). The effective MgCA inhibitory properties of simple phenols should be regarded with even greater interest in light of their poor inhibition against hCA I and II, making these compounds promising tools in the cosmetics field as potential anti-dandruff agents.

The inhibition profiles of these compounds were extended in a succeeding work by the same authors evaluating the inhibitory action of phenols against γ-class CAs from the pathogenic bacteria *Porphyromonas gingivalis* (PgiCA), *Vibrio cholerae* (VchCAγ) and *Burkholderia pseudomallei* (BpsCAγ), the antarctic/marine bacteria *Colwellia psychrerythraea* (CpsCAγ) and *Pseudoalteromonas haloplanktis* (PhaCAγ) Table **24** [71]. Many such compounds produced a submicromolar inhibition of BpsCAγ (K_Is of 0.45–8.6 μM), PgiCA (K_Is of 0.36–9.8 μM) and VchCAγ (K_Is of 0.47–9.6 μM). A subset of compounds, which are **6**, **10**, **27**, **30** and **32**, also demonstrated a significant selectivity for all γ-CAs over hCA I and II.

Another study by the same group reported the inhibitory profiles of these phenolic compounds against the poorly investigated η-CA from *Plasmodium falciparum* (PfCA), the protozoa responsible for malaria, and the δ-CA from the diatom *Thalassiosira weissflogii* (TweCA) Table **24**. Notably, some submicromolar inhibitors of these isoforms were also identified (K_Is of 0.62–78.7 μM against PfCA and 0.81–65.4 μM against TweCA) [119]. A subset of phenols, that are **6**, **8**, **10**, **16**, **27**, **30** and **32**, also demonstrated a significant selectivity for the η- and δ-CAs over the hCAs. This study promoted the identification of new potent and selective inhibitors of PfCA and TweCA, which could be considered as leads for finding drug candidates in the treatment of malaria or molecular probes in the study of carbon fixation processes, in which TweCA and orthologue enzymes are involved.

Table 24. Inhibition data of hCAs I, II, β-CA of *Malassezia globosa* (MgCA), γ-CAs of *Burkholderia pseudomallei* (BpsCAγ), *Colwellia psychrerythraea* (CpsCAγ), *Pseudoalteromonas haloplanktis* (PhaCAγ), *Porphyromonas gingivalis* (PgiCA), and *Vibrio cholerae* (VchCAγ), η-CA of *Plasmodium falciparum* (PfCA) and δ-CA of *Thalassiosira weissflogii* (TweCA) with 22 phenols 1-42 and the standard AAZ by a stopped-flow CO_2 hydrase assay [63].

cmpd	K_I (μM)[a]										Ref.
	hCA I (α)	hCA II (α)	MgCA (β)	BpsCA (γ)	CpsCA (γ)	PhaCA (γ)	PgiCA (γ)	VchCA (γ)	PfCA (η)	TweCA (δ)	
1	10.2	5.5	65.0	21.9	69.7	45.8	23.4	37.6	68.1	52.3	[71, 118, 119]
2	4003	9.91	7.0	2.6	23.4	18.7	3.8	1.2	1.4	4.5	[71, 118, 119]

(Table 24) cont.....

cmpd	K_I (µM)[a]										Ref.
	hCA I (α)	hCA II (α)	MgCA (β)	BpsCA (γ)	CpsCA (γ)	PhaCA (γ)	PgiCA (γ)	VchCA (γ)	PfCA (η)	TweCA (δ)	
3	795	7.7	6.1	16.8	38.9	68.2	22.6	11.2	26.9	48.2	[71, 118, 119]
4	10.7	0.090	6.3	2.2	10.6	24.8	5.1	4.2	21.0	34.9	[71, 118, 119]
6	>100	>100	7.4	0.69	5.1	2.9	1.3	0.47	0.83	2.0	[71, 118, 119]
8	9.9	7.1	6.6	15.6	37.5	30.5	19.2	14.8	0.72	0.95	[71, 118, 119]
10	9.8	10.6	4.9	0.45	2.3	3.9	0.86	0.69	0.90	1.4	[71, 118, 119]
15	5.2	4.9	6.5	0.55	4.8	4.8	0.36	0.89	1.6	4.9	[71, 118, 119]
16	4.2	4.1	4.5	18.1	26.9	26.9	12.5	18.7	0.62	0.81	[71, 118, 119]
17	5.7	5.2	5.9	23.5	36.5	36.5	9.8	17.4	2.5	2.7	[71, 118, 119]
26	4.9	4.7	3.9	10.3	15.7	29.1	4.7	7.9	78.7	65.4	[71, 118, 119]
27	159	752	32.0	14.5	43.6	10.8	19.5	15.7	33.8	17.6	[71, 118, 119]
28	10.0	6.2	2.5	8.6	20.7	18.2	5.6	7.3	26.4	7.9	[71, 118, 119]
29	131	0.108	0.7	30.5	46.5	66.5	39.6	28.7	36.9	56.9	[71, 118, 119]
30	134	870	29.7	2.8	18.5	18.5	3.4	7.2	41.3	30.7	[71, 118, 119]
31	38.8	33.9	8.8	3.6	20.3	20.3	4.8	9.6	32.7	21.0	[71, 118, 119]
32	>100	>100	36.4	1.3	13.6	13.6	5.8	2.6	22.8	13.8	[71, 118, 119]
33	6.3	4.9	44.9	0.72	14.3	18.9	0.85	2.8	>100	>100	[71, 118, 119]
34	57.8	57.5	>100	>100	>100	>100	>100	>100	>100	>100	[71, 118, 119]
35	68.9	95.3	6.1	5.6	31.1	44.0	10.5	8.6	47.1	35.9	[71, 118, 119]
40	1.07	0.98	3.3	0.85	2.9	2.9	1.3	1.9	5.7	14.5	[71, 118, 119]

(Table 24) cont.....

cmpd	K_I (μM)[a]										Ref.
	hCA I (α)	hCA II (α)	MgCA (β)	BpsCA (γ)	CpsCA (γ)	PhaCA (γ)	PgiCA (γ)	VchCA (γ)	PfCA (η)	TweCA (δ)	
42	2.38	1.61	0.6	6.3	15.4	15.4	5.4	2.9	11.2	5.9	[71, 118, 119]
AAZ	0.25	0.012	74.0	0.15	0.50	0.40	0.32	0.47	0.36	0.080	[71, 118, 119]

[a]Mean from 3 different assays, by a Stopped-Flow technique (errors were in the range of ± 5-10% of the reported values).

As simple phenols showed to preferentially inhibit MgCA over the off-target hCA I and II isoforms [118], the same authors evaluated a set of natural polyphenols, within the subset **72-113**, for MgCA inhibition Table **25** [120]. In fact, the antioxidant effects exerted by these compounds have considerable potential in cosmetics to enhance hair protection, correct the damage caused by neutralizing free radicals, and retard lipid oxidation. Relevantly, all tested compounds inhibited MgCA with K_I values in a narrow micromolar range (0.9–9.1 μM) showing a significant selectivity for the target CA over hCA I and II.

Table 25. Inhibition data of hCAs I, II, and β-CA of *M. globosa* (MgCA) with polyphenols of the 72-113 subset and the standard AAZ by a Stopped-Flow CO_2 hydrase assay [63].

cmpd	K_I (μM)[a]			Ref.	cmpd	K_I (μM)			Ref.
	hCA I	hCA II	MgCA			hCA I	hCA II	MgCA	
72	>10	9.594	0.9	[86, 120]	**96**	>10	>10	4.1	[86, 120]
73	>10	>10	2.6	[86, 120]	**101**	>10	>10	8.5	[86, 120]
74	>10	>10	3.3	[86, 120]	**102**	>10	9.52	8.6	[86, 120]
80	58.23	73.74	8.7	[76, 120]	**103**	>10	0.168	5.3	[86, 120]
82	>10	3.6	7.6	[86, 89, 120]	**104**	>10	>10	6.6	[86, 120]
84	>10	>10	8.9	[86, 120]	**105**	>10	8.790	4.3	[86, 120]
85	>10	>10	9.1	[86, 120]	**106**	>10	6.863	4.2	[86, 120]
86	>10	>10	3.7	[86, 120]	**109**	>10	0.41	3.7	[86, 90, 120]
89	3.66	0.34	4.8	[86, 90, 120]	**110**	>10	6.36	7.7	[86, 120]
92	>10	>10	8.6	[86, 120]	**113**	>10	>10	2.3	[73, 86, 120]
94	>10	>10	7.6	[86, 120]	**AAZ**	0.250	0.012	74.0	[119]

[a]Mean from 3 different assays, by a Stopped-Flow technique (errors were in the range of ± 5-10% of the reported values).

In Silico Studies of the Binding Mode of Phenolic Derivatives to CA Isoforms

The binding mode of phenolic compounds in the active site of CAs other than human ones was studied by means of *in silico* techniques. Also, computational procedures were used to evaluate the binding mode of α-estradiol **54** to hCA II (Fig. **9**) [82]. The phenolic OH of the estrogen is H-bonded to the zinc-bound hydroxide ion, which is in turn stabilized by two other H-bonds, acting as donors to the Thr199 side chain OH and as an acceptor with the Thr199 backbone NH. It should be noted that the phenolic portion of α-estradiol anchors to the nucleophile, locating more externally than cocrystallized simple ligands such as quinol **4** (pdb 4E3H) [60], because of the steric hindrance induced by the tetrahydrophenanthrenic core. The latter is involved in π-π and π-alkyl interactions with Leu198, Thr200, Phe131, Val121, His94, Gln92, Asn67, Asn62, and Leu60 side chain. Furthermore, the docked pose features an H-bond between the alcoholic moiety of **54** and the Asn67 side chain carbonyl group.

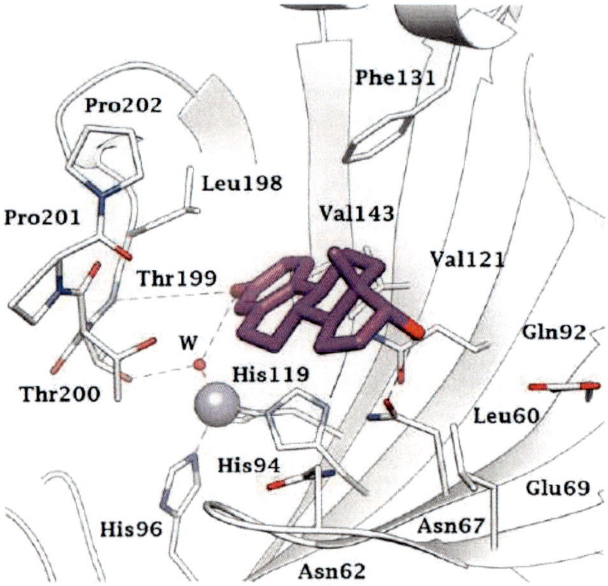

Fig. (9). Predicted binding mode of α-estradiol **54** to the hCA II active site [82].

Cau *et al.* [113] investigated *in silico* the binding mode of phenolic inhibitors **40**, **40d-f**, **42**, **42a,b**, **43** and **43a-c** to the active site of the β-CAs Rv1248 (crystal structure deposited as pdb 1YLK) [121] and Rv3588c (crystal structure deposited as pdb 2A5V) [122, 123]. The active site cleft of these enzymes is rather small in comparison to human CAs and is poorly accessible from the bulk solvent. The active site of β-CAs is at the interface between two distinct monomers (named here as A and B), whose dimerization is fundamental for the enzyme catalytic activity.

In the case of Rv1248, inhibitors **40d-f**, **42a,b** and **43b-c** were found to bind the Zn-coordinated water molecule by the phenolic moiety (Fig. **10A-B**). This interaction is reinforced by the H-bond with the backbone of Asp90(A) or the His54(B) or Arg39(A) side chain. Besides binding to the active site, **40d-f** and **43a,b** elongate at the dimer interface along the key loop Pro21(B)-Leu-Pro--et-Pro-Pro-Ser-Lys-His29(B), interacting with the Met24(B) backbone (**40f** and **43b,c**) or Arg39(A) side chain (inhibitor **40a,f**) (Fig. **10A-B**). In particular, for phenols **42a** and **42b**, which are rather long, their ester chain is docked in multiple conformations at the dimer interface.

Instead, as for Rv3588 β-CA, only inhibitors **40** (Fig. **10C**) and **42** were found to bind the water molecule by means of the phenolic moiety, while the carboxylic function is H-bonded and salt-bridged to the side chain of Lys43(B). Moreover, the phenolic OH also established H-bond interactions with the Ser106(A) backbone.

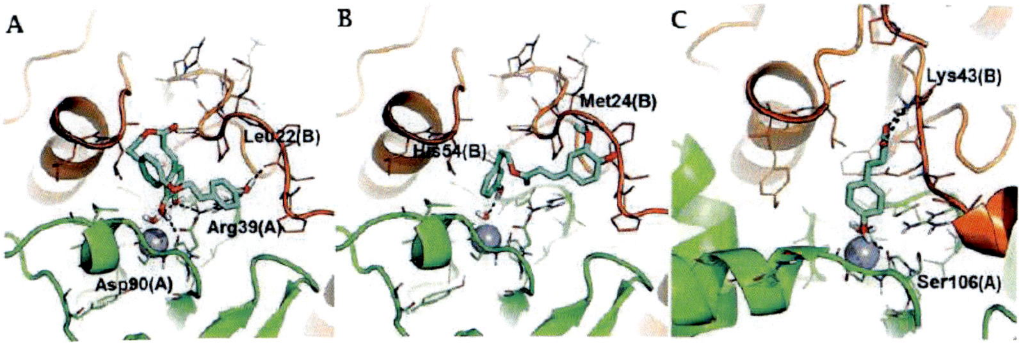

Fig. (10). Binding mode of A) **42a** and B) **43c** within the Rv1248 active site and C) **40** within Rv3588 active site. Reprinted with permission from ref [113]. Copyright 2016 Royal Society of Chemistry.

Because of the lack of the solved 3D structure of MgCA, our group built a model of it by homology using the deposited structure for Can2 as a template (pdb 2W3N) to assess the binding mode of the simple phenols **1-42** and polyphenols **72-113** set within MgCA active site [118, 120]. A wide network of H-bonds and hydrophobic interactions between the phenol and the active site residues were pointed out in the ligand-target adducts (Fig. **11**). The ligand OH function acts as an H-bond donor towards the Zn-bound hydroxide ion which, in turn, donates an additional hydrogen bond to Asp49(A) side chain. The ligand OH moiety also forms an H-bond with Ser48(A), which acts as a donor. The aromatic moiety is accommodated in a hydrophobic cavity formed by Phe66(B), Val71(A) and

Leu132(A). This positioning was strengthened by π-π (face to face) and π-alkyl interactions with the side chains of Phe88(B) and Val71(B), respectively, which sandwiched the aromatic portion. Substituted phenols, such as **26** in (Fig. **11**)., displayed some additional interactions, both within the hydrophobic cleft and the catalytic cavity, which improved the inhibitory effectiveness as clearly shown by the data in Table **24**. It is relevant that derivative **6**, hydroxyquinol, formed a three-center hydrogen bond involving the Zn-bound hydroxide group as an acceptor and the hydroxyl in positions 1 and 2 as donor groups (Fig. **11**).

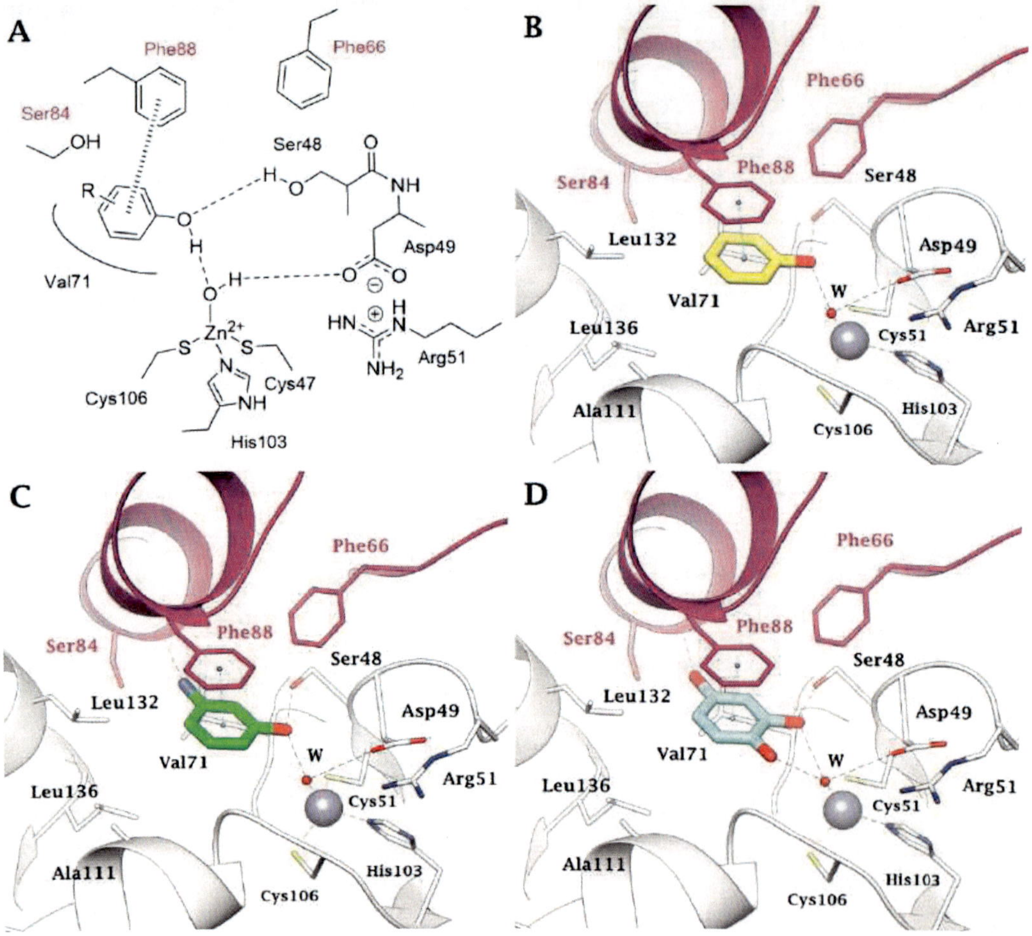

Fig. 11. A) 2D schematic representation of the binding mode of phenols within MgCA active site. Predicted binding mode of B) phenol **1**, C) *m*-aminophenol **26** and D) hydroxyquinol **6** to the MgCA active site [118]. Monomers A and B are colored white and magenta, respectively. Residues of monomers A and B are labeled black and magenta, respectively.

The authors also docked representative polyphenols of the **72-113** subset in the active site of MgCA and the *in silico* outcomes generally confirmed the interaction mode observed for simple phenols. Only luteolin **82** exhibited two isoenergetic docking solutions. They differ for the phenolic moiety that works as an anchoring group. In the first pose (Fig. **12A**), the 7-OH group acted both as an acceptor, for the side chain OH of S48(A), and as a donor anchoring the Zn-bound hydroxide ion. The 5-OH function instead donated an H-bond to the backbone carbonyl group of S84(B), the 1,4-benzopyrone system is stabilized by π-π (face to face) and π-alkyl interactions with the side chains of F88(B) and V71(A), respectively, and the two 3'- and 4'-OH functions of the flavone participate to a three-center H-bond set with K114(A). In the other luteolin docking solution (Fig. **12B**), the Zn^{2+}-bound hydroxide group acted as an acceptor in the three-center hydrogen bond that also involved the two 3'- and 4'-OH functions of the 2-phenyl-1,4-benzopyrone as donor groups. An analogue double anchoring was indeed reported for 1,2,4-benzenetriol (Fig. **11D**). Moreover, one of these two OH groups formed a hydrogen bond with the side chain hydroxyl group of S48(A), acting as a donor. The 3'-OH instead received an H-bond by the NH_2 of the Q38(B) side chain. The phenyl ring is accommodated in a hydrophobic cavity delimited by F66(B), V71(A) and L132(A), and was sandwiched by π-π (face to face) and π-alkyl interactions with the side chains of F88(B) and V71(A), respectively. The 1,4-benzopyrone moiety engaged π-alkyl interactions with A111(A) and G107(A), while the OH group in position 7 received an H-bond from the NH_3^+ of K114(A) side chain. All other polyphenols surprisingly provided a unique favoured docking orientation in the MgCA binding site that has the anchorage to the zinc-bound hydroxide made by the 7-OH group of the flavone. For instance, the binding mode of biochanin A **84** and taxifolin **89** is reported in Figs .**(12C-D)**. and included, as a matter of fact, the anchorage to the nucleophile by the OH at position 7 of the polyphenol scaffold.

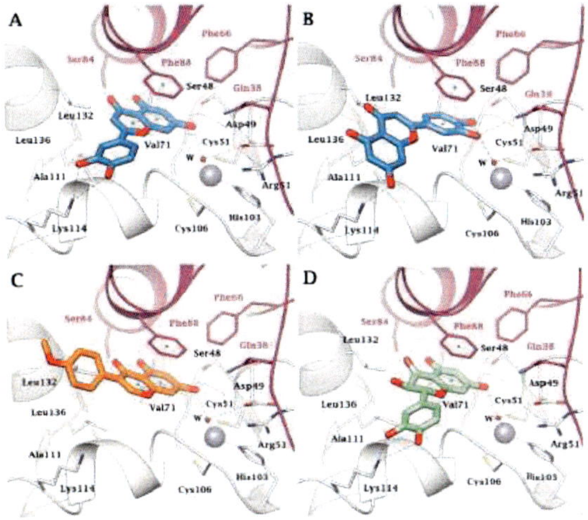

Fig. (12). Predicted binding mode of luteolin **82** A) pose 1 and B) pose 2, C) biochanin A **84** and D) taxifolin

89 to the MgCA active site [120]. Monomers A and B are colored white and magenta, respectively. Residues of monomers A and B are labeled black and magenta, respectively.

CONCLUSION

Thousands of phenolic derivatives have been extracted from plant sources. Many such derivatives were shown to produce pharmacological actions in humans which address their use in medicine as antiaging, anti-inflammatory, antioxidant, antidiabetic and antiproliferative agents among others. Numerous such pharmacological activities are likely to derive from the inhibition of human carbonic anhydrase (CAs, EC 4.2.1.1) isoforms. Phenols, in fact, are able to anchor to the zinc-bound nucleophile present in the enzyme active site, blocking the catalytic action of CAs in humans and/or encoded in various microorganisms. The inhibition potency of phenols against hCAs spans over a wide low nanomolar to high micromolar range, depending on the isoform and the substitution pattern of the phenolic scaffold. Hundreds of natural, semisynthetic and synthetic phenols were in fact evaluated as hCAIs by means of Stopped-Flow (chiefly) and 4-nitrophenylacetate esterase methods, which allowed to work out a thorough SAR. A more limited number of phenolic derivatives were evaluated as well for the inhibition of CAs from microorganisms, which include bacteria, fungi, protozoa and diatoms. In this context, potent CAIs were identified which exhibit selectivity against pathogen CAs over human isozymes. These derivatives represent valuable tools for the development of new anti-infective agents acting by an innovative mechanism of action.

CONSENT FOR PUBLICATION

Not applicable.

CONFLICT OF INTEREST

The authors declare no conflict of interest, financial or otherwise.

ACKNOWLEDGEMENT

Declared none.

REFERENCES

[1] Rajput, J.D.; Bagul, S.D.; Pete, U.D.; Zade, C.M.; Padhye, S.B.; Bendre, R.S. Perspectives on medicinal properties of natural phenolic monoterpenoids and their hybrids. *Mol. Divers.*, **2018**, *22*(1), 225-245.
[http://dx.doi.org/10.1007/s11030-017-9787-y] [PMID: 28988386]

[2] Durazzo, A.; Lucarini, M.; Souto, E.B.; Cicala, C.; Caiazzo, E.; Izzo, A.A.; Novellino, E.; Santini, A.

Polyphenols: A concise overview on the chemistry, occurrence, and human health. *Phytother. Res.*, **2019**, *33*(9), 2221-2243.
[http://dx.doi.org/10.1002/ptr.6419] [PMID: 31359516]

[3] Singla, R.K.; Dubey, A.K.; Garg, A.; Sharma, R.K.; Fiorino, M.; Ameen, S.M.; Haddad, M.A.; Al-Hiary, M. Natural polyphenols: chemical classification, definition of classes, subcategories, and structures. *J. AOAC Int.*, **2019**, *102*(5), 1397-1400.
[http://dx.doi.org/10.5740/jaoacint.19-0133] [PMID: 31200785]

[4] Lin, D.; Xiao, M.; Zhao, J. An overview of plant phenolic compounds and their importance in human nutrition and management of type 2 diabetes. *Molecules,* **2016**, *21*(10), 1374.
[http://dx.doi.org/10.3390/molecules21101374] [PMID: 27754463]

[5] Shukitt-Hale, B.; Lau, F.C.; Joseph, J.A. Berry fruit supplementation and the aging brain. *J. Agric. Food Chem.*, **2008**, *56*(3), 636-641.
[http://dx.doi.org/10.1021/jf072505f] [PMID: 18211020]

[6] Li, X.; Wang, T.; Zhou, B.; Gao, W.; Cao, J.; Huang, L. Chemical composition and antioxidant and anti-inflammatory potential of peels and flesh from 10 different pear varieties (Pyrus spp.). *Food Chem.,* **2014**, *152*, 531-538.
[http://dx.doi.org/10.1016/j.foodchem.2013.12.010] [PMID: 24444971]

[7] Moo-Huchin, V.M.; Moo-Huchin, M.I.; Estrada-León, R.J.; Cuevas-Glory, L.; Estrada-Mota, I.A.; Ortiz-Vázquez, E.; Betancur-Ancona, D.; Sauri-Duch, E. Antioxidant compounds, antioxidant activity and phenolic content in peel from three tropical fruits from Yucatan, Mexico. *Food Chem.,* **2015**, *166*, 17-22.
[http://dx.doi.org/10.1016/j.foodchem.2014.05.127] [PMID: 25053022]

[8] Sales, P.M.; Souza, P.M.; Simeoni, L.A.; Magalhães, P.O.; Silveira, D. α-Amylase inhibitors: a review of raw material and isolated compounds from plant source. *J. Pharm. Pharm. Sci.,* **2012**, *15*(1), 141-183.
[http://dx.doi.org/10.18433/J35S3K] [PMID: 22365095]

[9] Szkudelski, T.; Szkudelska, K. Anti-diabetic effects of resveratrol. *Ann. N. Y. Acad. Sci.,* **2011**, *1215*(1), 34-39.
[http://dx.doi.org/10.1111/j.1749-6632.2010.05844.x] [PMID: 21261639]

[10] Guo, W.; Kong, E.; Meydani, M. Dietary polyphenols, inflammation, and cancer. *Nutr. Cancer,* **2009**, *61*(6), 807-810.
[http://dx.doi.org/10.1080/01635580903285098] [PMID: 20155620]

[11] Franceschi, S.; Parpinel, M.; Vecchia, C.L.; Favero, A.; Talamini, R.; Negri, E. Role of different types of vegetables and fruit in the prevention of cancer of the colon, rectum, and breast. *Epidemiology,* **1998**, *9*(3), 338-341.
[http://dx.doi.org/10.1097/00001648-199805000-00020] [PMID: 9583427]

[12] Nöthlings, U.; Schulze, M.B.; Weikert, C. Intake of vegetables, legumes, and fruit, and risk for all-cause, cardiovascular, and cancer mortality in a European diabetic population. *J. Nutr.,* **2008**, *138*(4), 775-781.
[http://dx.doi.org/10.1093/jn/138.4.775] [PMID: 18356334]

[13] Grassi, D.; Mulder, T.P.J.; Draijer, R.; Desideri, G.; Molhuizen, H.O.F.; Ferri, C. Black tea consumption dose-dependently improves flow-mediated dilation in healthy males. *J. Hypertens.,* **2009**, *27*(4), 774-781.
[http://dx.doi.org/10.1097/HJH.0b013e328326066c] [PMID: 19516176]

[14] Heiss, C.; Finis, D.; Kleinbongard, P.; Hoffmann, A.; Rassaf, T.; Kelm, M.; Sies, H. Sustained increase in flow-mediated dilation after daily intake of high-flavanol cocoa drink over 1 week. *J. Cardiovasc. Pharmacol.,* **2007**, *49*(2), 74-80.
[http://dx.doi.org/10.1097/FJC.0b013e31802d0001] [PMID: 17312446]

[15] Keevil, J.G.; Osman, H.E.; Reed, J.D.; Folts, J.D. Grape juice, but not orange juice or grapefruit juice,

inhibits human platelet aggregation. *J. Nutr.*, **2000**, *130*(1), 53-56.
[http://dx.doi.org/10.1093/jn/130.1.53] [PMID: 10613766]

[16] Erlund, I.; Koli, R.; Alfthan, G.; Marniemi, J.; Puukka, P.; Mustonen, P.; Mattila, P.; Jula, A. Favorable effects of berry consumption on platelet function, blood pressure, and HDL cholesterol. *Am. J. Clin. Nutr.*, **2008**, *87*(2), 323-331.
[http://dx.doi.org/10.1093/ajcn/87.2.323] [PMID: 18258621]

[17] Ried, K.; Fakler, P.; Stocks, N.P. Effect of cocoa on blood pressure. *Cochrane Libr.*, **2017**, *2017*(5)CD008893
[http://dx.doi.org/10.1002/14651858.CD008893.pub3] [PMID: 28439881]

[18] Supuran, C.T. Carbonic anhydrases: novel therapeutic applications for inhibitors and activators. *Nat. Rev. Drug Discov.*, **2008**, *7*(2), 168-181.
[http://dx.doi.org/10.1038/nrd2467] [PMID: 18167490]

[19] Alterio, V.; Di Fiore, A.; D'Ambrosio, K.; Supuran, C.T.; De Simone, G. Multiple binding modes of inhibitors to carbonic anhydrases: how to design specific drugs targeting 15 different isoforms? *Chem. Rev.*, **2012**, *112*(8), 4421-4468.
[http://dx.doi.org/10.1021/cr200176r] [PMID: 22607219]

[20] Nocentini, A.; Supuran, C.T. Advances in the structural annotation of human carbonic anhydrases and impact on future drug discovery. *Expert Opin. Drug Discov.*, **2019**, *14*(11), 1175-1197.
[http://dx.doi.org/10.1080/17460441.2019.1651289] [PMID: 31436118]

[21] Xu, Y.; Feng, L.; Jeffrey, P.D.; Shi, Y.; Morel, F.M.M. Structure and metal exchange in the cadmium carbonic anhydrase of marine diatoms. *Nature,* **2008**, *452*(7183), 56-61.
[http://dx.doi.org/10.1038/nature06636] [PMID: 18322527]

[22] Jensen, E.L.; Clement, R.; Kosta, A.; Maberly, S.C.; Gontero, B. A new widespread subclass of carbonic anhydrase in marine phytoplankton. *ISME J.*, **2019**, *13*(8), 2094-2106.
[http://dx.doi.org/10.1038/s41396-019-0426-8] [PMID: 31024153]

[23] Maren, T.H. Carbonic anhydrase: chemistry, physiology, and inhibition. *Physiol. Rev.*, **1967**, *47*(4), 595-781.
[http://dx.doi.org/10.1152/physrev.1967.47.4.595] [PMID: 4964060]

[24] Del Prete, S.; Vullo, D.; Fisher, G.M.; Andrews, K.T.; Poulsen, S.A.; Capasso, C.; Supuran, C.T. Discovery of a new family of carbonic anhydrases in the malaria pathogen Plasmodium falciparum —The η-carbonic anhydrases. *Bioorg. Med. Chem. Lett.*, **2014**, *24*(18), 4389-4396.
[http://dx.doi.org/10.1016/j.bmcl.2014.08.015] [PMID: 25168745]

[25] Tripp, B.C.; Smith, K.; Ferry, J.G. Carbonic anhydrase: new insights for an ancient enzyme. *J. Biol. Chem.*, **2001**, *276*(52), 48615-48618.
[http://dx.doi.org/10.1074/jbc.R100045200] [PMID: 11696553]

[26] Ferry, J.G. The γ class of carbonic anhydrases. *Biochim. Biophys. Acta. Proteins Proteomics,* **2010**, *1804*(2), 374-381.
[http://dx.doi.org/10.1016/j.bbapap.2009.08.026] [PMID: 19747990]

[27] Smith, K.S.; Jakubzick, C.; Whittam, T.S.; Ferry, J.G. Carbonic anhydrase is an ancient enzyme widespread in prokaryotes. *Proc. Natl. Acad. Sci. USA,* **1999**, *96*(26), 15184-15189.
[http://dx.doi.org/10.1073/pnas.96.26.15184] [PMID: 10611359]

[28] Kikutani, S.; Nakajima, K.; Nagasato, C.; Tsuji, Y.; Miyatake, A.; Matsuda, Y. Thylakoid luminal θ-carbonic anhydrase critical for growth and photosynthesis in the marine diatom *Phaeodactylum tricornutum*. *Proc. Natl. Acad. Sci. USA,* **2016**, *113*(35), 9828-9833.
[http://dx.doi.org/10.1073/pnas.1603112113] [PMID: 27531955]

[29] Capasso, C.; Supuran, C.T. An overview of the alpha-, beta- and gamma-carbonic anhydrases from *Bacteria* : can bacterial carbonic anhydrases shed new light on evolution of bacteria? *J. Enzyme Inhib. Med. Chem.*, **2015**, *30*(2), 325-332.

[http://dx.doi.org/10.3109/14756366.2014.910202] [PMID: 24766661]

[30] Supuran, C.T.; Scozzafava, A.; Casini, A. Carbonic anhydrase inhibitors. *Med. Res. Rev.*, **2003**, *23*(2), 146-189.
[http://dx.doi.org/10.1002/med.10025] [PMID: 12500287]

[31] Supuran, C.T.; Scozzafava, A. Carbonic anhydrases as targets for medicinal chemistry. *Bioorg. Med. Chem.*, **2007**, *15*(13), 4336-4350.
[http://dx.doi.org/10.1016/j.bmc.2007.04.020] [PMID: 17475500]

[32] Temperini, C.; Scozzafava, A.; Supuran, C.T. Drug design of zinc-enzyme inhibitors: functional, structural, and disease applications Wiley, **2009**; p. Hoboken, NJ473.

[33] Gao, B.B.; Clermont, A.; Rook, S. Extracellular carbonic anhydrase mediates hemorrhagic retinal and cerebral vascular permeability through prekallikrein activation. *Nat. Med.*, **2007**, *13*(2), 181-188.
[http://dx.doi.org/10.1038/nm1534] [PMID: 17259996]

[34] Supuran, C.; Scozzafava, A.; Mincione, F. The development of topically acting carbonic anhydrase inhibitors as antiglaucoma agents. *Curr. Pharm. Des.*, **2008**, *14*(7), 649-654.
[http://dx.doi.org/10.2174/138161208783877866] [PMID: 18336310]

[35] Supuran, C. Diuretics: from classical carbonic anhydrase inhibitors to novel applications of the sulfonamides. *Curr. Pharm. Des.*, **2008**, *14*(7), 641-648.
[http://dx.doi.org/10.2174/138161208783877947] [PMID: 18336309]

[36] De Simone, G.; Scozzafava, A.; Supuran, C.T. Which carbonic anhydrases are targeted by the antiepileptic sulfonamides and sulfamates? *Chem. Biol. Drug Des.*, **2009**, *74*(3), 317-321.
[http://dx.doi.org/10.1111/j.1747-0285.2009.00857.x] [PMID: 19703035]

[37] Basnyat, B.; Gertsch, J.H.; Johnson, E.W.; Castro-Marin, F.; Inoue, Y.; Yeh, C. Efficacy of low-dose acetazolamide (125 mg BID) for the prophylaxis of acute mountain sickness: a prospective, double-blind, randomized, placebo-controlled trial. *High Alt. Med. Biol.*, **2003**, *4*(1), 45-52.
[http://dx.doi.org/10.1089/152702903321488979] [PMID: 12713711]

[38] Nocentini, A.; Supuran, C.T. Carbonic anhydrase inhibitors as antitumor/antimetastatic agents: a patent review (2008–2018). *Expert Opin. Ther. Pat.*, **2018**, *28*(10), 729-740.
[http://dx.doi.org/10.1080/13543776.2018.1508453] [PMID: 30074415]

[39] Barreiro, E.; Hussain, S.N.A. Protein carbonylation in skeletal muscles: impact on function. *Antioxid. Redox Signal.*, **2010**, *12*(3), 417-429.
[http://dx.doi.org/10.1089/ars.2009.2808] [PMID: 19686036]

[40] Capasso, C.; Supuran, C.T. Anti-infective carbonic anhydrase inhibitors: a patent and literature review. *Expert Opin. Ther. Pat.*, **2013**, *23*(6), 693-704.
[http://dx.doi.org/10.1517/13543776.2013.778245] [PMID: 23488877]

[41] Supuran, C.T. Structure and function of carbonic anhydrases. *Biochem. J.*, **2016**, *473*(14), 2023-2032.
[http://dx.doi.org/10.1042/BCJ20160115] [PMID: 27407171]

[42] Supuran, C.T. How many carbonic anhydrase inhibition mechanisms exist? *J. Enzyme Inhib. Med. Chem.*, **2016**, *31*(3), 345-360.
[http://dx.doi.org/10.3109/14756366.2015.1122001] [PMID: 26619898]

[43] Carta, F.; Aggarwal, M.; Maresca, A.; Scozzafava, A.; McKenna, R.; Masini, E.; Supuran, C.T. Dithiocarbamates strongly inhibit carbonic anhydrases and show antiglaucoma action *in vivo*. *J. Med. Chem.*, **2012**, *55*(4), 1721-1730.
[http://dx.doi.org/10.1021/jm300031j] [PMID: 22276570]

[44] Di Fiore, A.; Maresca, A.; Supuran, C.T.; De Simone, G. Hydroxamate represents a versatile zinc binding group for the development of new carbonic anhydrase inhibitors. *Chem. Commun. (Camb.)*, **2012**, *48*(70), 8838-8840.
[http://dx.doi.org/10.1039/c2cc34275h] [PMID: 22836518]

[45] Altcrio, V.; Cadoni, R.; Esposito, D.; Vullo, D.; Fiore, A.D.; Monti, S.M.; Caporale, A.; Ruvo, M.; Sechi, M.; Dumy, P.; Supuran, C.T.; Simone, G.D.; Winum, J.Y. Benzoxaborole as a new chemotype for carbonic anhydrase inhibition. *Chem. Commun. (Camb.),* **2016**, *52*(80), 11983-11986. [http://dx.doi.org/10.1039/C6CC06399C] [PMID: 27722534]

[46] Nocentini, A.; Gratteri, P.; Supuran, C.T. Phosphorus *versus* Sulfur: Discovery of benzenephosphonamidates as versatile sulfonamide-mimic chemotypes acting as carbonic anhydrase inhibitors. *Chemistry,* **2018**, *25*(5)chem.201805039 [http://dx.doi.org/10.1002/chem.201805039] [PMID: 30411821]

[47] Carta, F.; Akdemir, A.; Scozzafava, A.; Masini, E.; Supuran, C.T. Xanthates and trithiocarbonates strongly inhibit carbonic anhydrases and show antiglaucoma effects *in vivo. J. Med. Chem.,* **2013**, *56*(11), 4691-4700. [http://dx.doi.org/10.1021/jm400414j] [PMID: 23647428]

[48] Nocentini, A.; Ceruso, M.; Bua, S. Discovery of β-adrenergic receptors blocker-carbonic anhydrase inhibitor hybrids for multitargeted antiglaucoma therapy. *J. Med. Chem.,* **2018**, *61*(12), 5380-5394. [http://dx.doi.org/10.1021/acs.jmedchem.8b00625] [PMID: 29851481]

[49] Nocentini, A.; Moi, D.; Balboni, G.; Onnis, V.; Supuran, C.T. Discovery of thiazolin-4-one-based aromatic sulfamates as a new class of carbonic anhydrase isoforms I, II, IV, and IX inhibitors. *Bioorg. Chem.,* **2018**, *77*, 293-299. [http://dx.doi.org/10.1016/j.bioorg.2018.01.023] [PMID: 29421705]

[50] Nocentini, A.; Cadoni, R.; del Prete, S.; Capasso, C.; Dumy, P.; Gratteri, P.; Supuran, C.T.; Winum, J.Y. Benzoxaboroles as Efficient Inhibitors of the β-Carbonic Anhydrases from Pathogenic Fungi: Activity and Modeling Study. *ACS Med. Chem. Lett.,* **2017**, *8*(11), 1194-1198. [http://dx.doi.org/10.1021/acsmedchemlett.7b00369] [PMID: 29152053]

[51] Nair, S.K.; Ludwig, P.A.; Christianson, D.W. Two-site binding of phenol in the active site of human carbonic anhydrase II: structural implications for substrate association. *J. Am. Chem. Soc.,* **1994**, *116*(8), 3659-3660. [http://dx.doi.org/10.1021/ja00087a086]

[52] Carta, F.; Temperini, C.; Innocenti, A.; Scozzafava, A.; Kaila, K.; Supuran, C.T. Polyamines inhibit carbonic anhydrases by anchoring to the zinc-coordinated water molecule. *J. Med. Chem.,* **2010**, *53*(15), 5511-5522. [http://dx.doi.org/10.1021/jm1003667] [PMID: 20590092]

[53] Nocentini, A.; Carta, F.; Tanc, M.; Selleri, S.; Supuran, C.T.; Bazzicalupi, C.; Gratteri, P. Deciphering the mechanism of human carbonic anhydrases inhibition with sulfocoumarins: computational and experimental studies. *Chemistry,* **2018**, *24*(31), 7840-7844. [http://dx.doi.org/10.1002/chem.201800941] [PMID: 29603439]

[54] Tars, K.; Vullo, D.; Kazaks, A.; Leitans, J.; Lends, A.; Grandane, A.; Zalubovskis, R.; Scozzafava, A.; Supuran, C.T. Sulfocoumarins (1,2-benzoxathiine-2,2-dioxides): a class of potent and isoform-selective inhibitors of tumor-associated carbonic anhydrases. *J. Med. Chem.,* **2013**, *56*(1), 293-300. [http://dx.doi.org/10.1021/jm301625s] [PMID: 23241068]

[55] Maresca, A.; Temperini, C.; Vu, H.; Pham, N.B.; Poulsen, S.A.; Scozzafava, A.; Quinn, R.J.; Supuran, C.T. Non-zinc mediated inhibition of carbonic anhydrases: coumarins are a new class of suicide inhibitors. *J. Am. Chem. Soc.,* **2009**, *131*(8), 3057-3062. [http://dx.doi.org/10.1021/ja809683v] [PMID: 19206230]

[56] Maresca, A.; Temperini, C.; Pochet, L.; Masereel, B.; Scozzafava, A.; Supuran, C.T. Deciphering the mechanism of carbonic anhydrase inhibition with coumarins and thiocoumarins. *J. Med. Chem.,* **2010**, *53*(1), 335-344. [http://dx.doi.org/10.1021/jm901287j] [PMID: 19911821]

[57] Nocentini, A.; Carta, F.; Ceruso, M.; Bartolucci, G.; Supuran, C.T. Click-tailed coumarins with potent and selective inhibitory action against the tumor-associated carbonic anhydrases IX and XII. *Bioorg.*

Med. Chem., **2015**, *23*(21), 6955-6966.
[http://dx.doi.org/10.1016/j.bmc.2015.09.041] [PMID: 26432607]

[58] D'Ambrosio, K.; Carradori, S.; Monti, S.M.; Buonanno, M.; Secci, D.; Vullo, D.; Supuran, C.T.; De Simone, G. Out of the active site binding pocket for carbonic anhydrase inhibitors. *Chem. Commun. (Camb.)*, **2015**, *51*(2), 302-305.
[http://dx.doi.org/10.1039/C4CC07320G] [PMID: 25407638]

[59] Scozzafava, A.; Carta, F.; Supuran, C.T. Secondary and tertiary sulfonamides: a patent review (2008 – 2012). *Expert Opin. Ther. Pat.*, **2013**, *23*(2), 203-213.
[http://dx.doi.org/10.1517/13543776.2013.742065] [PMID: 23148584]

[60] Lomelino, C.; Supuran, C.; McKenna, R. Non-Classical Inhibition of Carbonic Anhydrase. *Int. J. Mol. Sci.*, **2016**, *17*(7), 1150.
[http://dx.doi.org/10.3390/ijms17071150] [PMID: 27438828]

[61] D'Ambrosio, K.; Carradori, S.; Cesa, S.; Angeli, A.; Monti, S.M.; Supuran, C.T.; De Simone, G. Catechols: a new class of carbonic anhydrase inhibitors. *Chem. Commun. (Camb.)*, **2020**, *56*(85), 13033-13036.
[http://dx.doi.org/10.1039/D0CC05172A] [PMID: 33000794]

[62] Temperini, C.; Innocenti, A.; Scozzafava, A.; Mastrolorenzo, A.; Supuran, C.T. Carbonic anhydrase activators: l-Adrenaline plugs the active site entrance of isozyme II, activating better isoforms I, IV, VA, VII, and XIV. *Bioorg. Med. Chem. Lett.*, **2007**, *17*(3), 628-635.
[http://dx.doi.org/10.1016/j.bmcl.2006.11.027] [PMID: 17127057]

[63] Khalifah, R.G. The carbon dioxide hydration activity of carbonic anhydrase. I. Stop-flow kinetic studies on the native human isoenzymes B and C. *J. Biol. Chem.*, **1971**, *246*(8), 2561-2573.
[http://dx.doi.org/10.1016/S0021-9258(18)62326-9] [PMID: 4994926]

[64] Innocenti, A.; Beyza Öztürk Sarıkaya, S.; Gülçin, İ.; Supuran, C.T. Carbonic anhydrase inhibitors. Inhibition of mammalian isoforms I–XIV with a series of natural product polyphenols and phenolic acids. *Bioorg. Med. Chem.*, **2010**, *18*(6), 2159-2164.
[http://dx.doi.org/10.1016/j.bmc.2010.01.076] [PMID: 20185318]

[65] Innocenti, A.; Vullo, D.; Scozzafava, A.; Supuran, C.T. Carbonic anhydrase inhibitors: Inhibition of mammalian isoforms I–XIV with a series of substituted phenols including paracetamol and salicylic acid. *Bioorg. Med. Chem.*, **2008**, *16*(15), 7424-7428.
[http://dx.doi.org/10.1016/j.bmc.2008.06.013] [PMID: 18579385]

[66] Innocenti, A.; Gülçin, I.; Scozzafava, A.; Supuran, C.T. Carbonic anhydrase inhibitors. Antioxidant polyphenols effectively inhibit mammalian isoforms I–XV. *Bioorg. Med. Chem. Lett.*, **2010**, *20*(17), 5050-5053.
[http://dx.doi.org/10.1016/j.bmcl.2010.07.038] [PMID: 20674354]

[67] Koz, Ö.; Ekinci, D.; Perrone, A.; Piacente, S.; Alankuş-Çalışkan, Ö.; Bedir, E.; Supuran, C.T. Analysis of saponins and phenolic compounds as inhibitors of α-carbonic anhydrase isoenzymes. *J. Enzyme Inhib. Med. Chem.*, **2013**, *28*(2), 412-417.
[http://dx.doi.org/10.3109/14756366.2011.651464] [PMID: 22299585]

[68] Supuran, C.T. Carbonic anhydrase inhibition with natural products: novel chemotypes and inhibition mechanisms. *Mol. Divers.*, **2011**, *15*(2), 305-316.
[http://dx.doi.org/10.1007/s11030-010-9271-4] [PMID: 20803169]

[69] Öztürk Sarikaya, S.B.; Topal, F.; Şentürk, M.; Gülçin, İ.; Supuran, C.T. *In vitro* inhibition of α-carbonic anhydrase isozymes by some phenolic compounds. *Bioorg. Med. Chem. Lett.*, **2011**, *21*(14), 4259-4262.
[http://dx.doi.org/10.1016/j.bmcl.2011.05.071] [PMID: 21669522]

[70] Ekinci, D.; Kurbanoglu, N.I.; Salamcı, E.; Şentürk, M.; Supuran, C.T. Carbonic anhydrase inhibitors: inhibition of human and bovine isoenzymes by benzenesulphonamides, cyclitols and phenolic compounds. *J. Enzyme Inhib. Med. Chem.*, **2012**, *27*(6), 845-848.

[http://dx.doi.org/10.3109/14756366.2011.621122] [PMID: 21999604]

[71] Nocentini, A.; Osman, S.M.; Del Prete, S.; Capasso, C.; ALOthman, Z.A.; Supuran, C.T. Extending the γ-class carbonic anhydrases inhibition profiles with phenolic compounds. *Bioorg. Chem.*, **2019**, *93*103336
[http://dx.doi.org/10.1016/j.bioorg.2019.103336] [PMID: 31604186]

[72] Scozzafava, A.; Passaponti, M.; Supuran, C.T.; Gülçin, İ. Carbonic anhydrase inhibitors: guaiacol and catechol derivatives effectively inhibit certain human carbonic anhydrase isoenzymes (hCA I, II, IX and XII). *J. Enzyme Inhib. Med. Chem.*, **2015**, *30*(4), 586-591.
[http://dx.doi.org/10.3109/14756366.2014.956310] [PMID: 25373500]

[73] Sahin, H.; Can, Z.; Yildiz, O.; Kolayli, S.; Innocenti, A.; Scozzafava, G.; Supuran, C.T. Inhibition of carbonic anhydrase isozymes I and II with natural products extracted from plants, mushrooms and honey. *J. Enzyme Inhib. Med. Chem.*, **2012**, *27*(3), 395-402.
[http://dx.doi.org/10.3109/14756366.2011.593176] [PMID: 21740099]

[74] Durdagi, S.; Şentürk, M.; Ekinci, D.; Balaydın, H.T.; Göksu, S.; Küfrevioğlu, Ö.İ.; Innocenti, A.; Scozzafava, A.; Supuran, C.T. Kinetic and docking studies of phenol-based inhibitors of carbonic anhydrase isoforms I, II, IX and XII evidence a new binding mode within the enzyme active site. *Bioorg. Med. Chem.*, **2011**, *19*(4), 1381-1389.
[http://dx.doi.org/10.1016/j.bmc.2011.01.016] [PMID: 21282059]

[75] Carta, F.; Vullo, D.; Maresca, A.; Scozzafava, A.; Supuran, C.T. Mono-/dihydroxybenzoic acid esters and phenol pyridinium derivatives as inhibitors of the mammalian carbonic anhydrase isoforms I, II, VII, IX, XII and XIV. *Bioorg. Med. Chem.*, **2013**, *21*(6), 1564-1569.
[http://dx.doi.org/10.1016/j.bmc.2012.05.019] [PMID: 22668600]

[76] Taslimi, P.; Caglayan, C.; Gulcin, İ. The impact of some natural phenolic compounds on carbonic anhydrase, acetylcholinesterase, butyrylcholinesterase, and α-glycosidase enzymes: An antidiabetic, anticholinergic, and antiepileptic study. *J. Biochem. Mol. Toxicol.*, **2017**, *31*(12)e21995
[http://dx.doi.org/10.1002/jbt.21995] [PMID: 28902458]

[77] Innocenti, A.; Vullo, D.; Scozzafava, A.; Supuran, C.T. Carbonic anhydrase inhibitors: Interactions of phenols with the 12 catalytically active mammalian isoforms (CA I–XIV). *Bioorg. Med. Chem. Lett.*, **2008**, *18*(5), 1583-1587.
[http://dx.doi.org/10.1016/j.bmcl.2008.01.077] [PMID: 18242985]

[78] Davis, R.A.; Innocenti, A.; Poulsen, S.A.; Supuran, C.T. Carbonic anhydrase inhibitors. Identification of selective inhibitors of the human mitochondrial isozymes VA and VB over the cytosolic isozymes I and II from a natural product-based phenolic library. *Bioorg. Med. Chem.*, **2010**, *18*(1), 14-18.
[http://dx.doi.org/10.1016/j.bmc.2009.11.021] [PMID: 19962903]

[79] Şentürk, M.; Gülçin, İ.; Beydemir, Ş.; Küfrevioğlu, Ö.İ.; Supuran, C.T. *In Vitro* inhibition of human carbonic anhydrase I and II isozymes with natural phenolic compounds. *Chem. Biol. Drug Des.*, **2011**, *77*(6), 494-499.
[http://dx.doi.org/10.1111/j.1747-0285.2011.01104.x] [PMID: 21332948]

[80] Arabaci, B.; Gulcin, I.; Alwasel, S. Capsaicin: a potent inhibitor of carbonic anhydrase isoenzymes. *Molecules,* **2014**, *19*(7), 10103-10114.
[http://dx.doi.org/10.3390/molecules190710103] [PMID: 25014536]

[81] Carreyre, H.; Coustard, J.M.; Carré, G. Natural product hybrid and its superacid synthesized analogues: Dodoneine and its derivatives show selective inhibition of carbonic anhydrase isoforms I, III, XIII and XIV. *Bioorg. Med. Chem.*, **2013**, *21*(13), 3790-3794.
[http://dx.doi.org/10.1016/j.bmc.2013.04.041] [PMID: 23685174]

[82] Nocentini, A.; Bonardi, A.; Gratteri, P.; Cerra, B.; Gioiello, A.; Supuran, C.T. Steroids interfere with human carbonic anhydrase activity by using alternative binding mechanisms. *J. Enzyme Inhib. Med. Chem.*, **2018**, *33*(1), 1453-1459.
[http://dx.doi.org/10.1080/14756366.2018.1512597] [PMID: 30221552]

[83] Verpoorte, J.A.; Mehta, S.; Edsall, J.T. Esterase activities of human carbonic anhydrases B and C. *J. Biol. Chem.*, **1967**, *242*(18), 4221-4229. [http://dx.doi.org/10.1016/S0021-9258(18)95800-X] [PMID: 4964830]

[84] Balaydın, H.T.; Şentürk, M.; Göksu, S.; Menzek, A. Synthesis and carbonic anhydrase inhibitory properties of novel bromophenols and their derivatives including natural products: Vidalol B. *Eur. J. Med. Chem.*, **2012**, *54*, 423-428. [http://dx.doi.org/10.1016/j.ejmech.2012.05.025] [PMID: 22687439]

[85] Balaydın, H.T.; Şentürk, M.; Menzek, A. Synthesis and carbonic anhydrase inhibitory properties of novel cyclohexanonyl bromophenol derivatives. *Bioorg. Med. Chem. Lett.*, **2012**, *22*(3), 1352-1357. [http://dx.doi.org/10.1016/j.bmcl.2011.12.069] [PMID: 22230050]

[86] Karioti, A.; Ceruso, M.; Carta, F.; Bilia, A.R.; Supuran, C.T. New natural product carbonic anhydrase inhibitors incorporating phenol moieties. *Bioorg. Med. Chem.*, **2015**, *23*(22), 7219-7225. [http://dx.doi.org/10.1016/j.bmc.2015.10.018] [PMID: 26498393]

[87] Gülçin, İ.; Scozzafava, A.; Supuran, C.T.; Koksal, Z.; Turkan, F.; Çetinkaya, S.; Bingöl, Z.; Huyut, Z.; Alwasel, S.H. Rosmarinic acid inhibits some metabolic enzymes including glutathione *S* -transferase, lactoperoxidase, acetylcholinesterase, butyrylcholinesterase and carbonic anhydrase isoenzymes. *J. Enzyme Inhib. Med. Chem.*, **2016**, *31*(6), 1698-1702. [http://dx.doi.org/10.3109/14756366.2015.1135914] [PMID: 26864149]

[88] Topal, M.; Gülçi̇n, İ. Rosmarinic acid: a potent carbonic anhydrase isoenzymes inhibitor. *Turk. J. Chem.*, **2014**, *38*, 894-902. [http://dx.doi.org/10.3906/kim-1403-5]

[89] Ekinci, D.; Karagoz, L.; Ekinci, D.; Senturk, M.; Supuran, C.T. Carbonic anhydrase inhibitors: *in vitro* inhibition of α isoforms (hCA I, hCA II, bCA III, hCA IV) by flavonoids. *J. Enzyme Inhib. Med. Chem.*, **2013**, *28*(2), 283-288. [http://dx.doi.org/10.3109/14756366.2011.643303] [PMID: 22168126]

[90] Gidaro, M.; Alcaro, F.; Carradori, S.; Costa, G.; Vullo, D.; Supuran, C.; Alcaro, S. Eriocitrin and Apigenin as New Carbonic Anhydrase VA Inhibitors from a Virtual Screening of Calabrian Natural Products. *Planta Med.*, **2015**, *81*(6), 533-540. [http://dx.doi.org/10.1055/s-0034-1396139] [PMID: 25590364]

[91] Huyut, Z.; Beydemir, Ş.; Gülçin, İ. Inhibition properties of some flavonoids on carbonic anhydrase I and II isoenzymes purified from human erythrocytes. *J. Biochem. Mol. Toxicol.*, **2017**, *31*(9)e21930 [http://dx.doi.org/10.1002/jbt.21930] [PMID: 28445001]

[92] Yamali, C.; Gul, H.I.; Sakagami, H.; Supuran, C.T. Synthesis and bioactivities of halogen bearing phenolic chalcones and their corresponding bis Mannich bases. *J. Enzyme Inhib. Med. Chem.*, **2016**, *31*(sup4), 125-131. [http://dx.doi.org/10.1080/14756366.2016.1221825] [PMID: 27594305]

[93] Gul, H.I.; Yazici, Z.; Tanc, M.; Supuran, C.T. Inhibitory effects of benzimidazole containing new phenolic Mannich bases on human carbonic anhydrase isoforms hCA I and II. *J. Enzyme Inhib. Med. Chem.*, **2016**, *31*(6), 1540-1544. [http://dx.doi.org/10.3109/14756366.2016.1156675] [PMID: 26985571]

[94] Yamali, C.; Tugrak, M.; Gul, H.I.; Tanc, M.; Supuran, C.T. The inhibitory effects of phenolic Mannich bases on carbonic anhydrase I and II isoenzymes. *J. Enzyme Inhib. Med. Chem.*, **2016**, *31*(6), 1678-1681. [http://dx.doi.org/10.3109/14756366.2015.1126715] [PMID: 26808123]

[95] Tugrak, M.; Gul, H.I.; Bandow, K.; Sakagami, H.; Gulcin, I.; Ozkay, Y.; Supuran, C.T. Synthesis and biological evaluation of some new mono Mannich bases with piperazines as possible anticancer agents and carbonic anhydrase inhibitors. *Bioorg. Chem.*, **2019**, *90*103095 [http://dx.doi.org/10.1016/j.bioorg.2019.103095] [PMID: 31288135]

[96] Riafrecha, L.E.; Bua, S.; Supuran, C.T.; Colinas, P.A. Synthesis and carbonic anhydrase inhibitory effects of new N-glycosylsulfonamides incorporating the phenol moiety. *Bioorg. Med. Chem. Lett.*, **2016**, *26*(16), 3892-3895.
[http://dx.doi.org/10.1016/j.bmcl.2016.07.015] [PMID: 27423482]

[97] Şentürk, M.; Gülçin, İ.; Daştan, A.; İrfan Küfrevioğlu, Ö.; Supuran, C.T. Carbonic anhydrase inhibitors. Inhibition of human erythrocyte isozymes I and II with a series of antioxidant phenols. *Bioorg. Med. Chem.*, **2009**, *17*(8), 3207-3211.
[http://dx.doi.org/10.1016/j.bmc.2009.01.067] [PMID: 19231207]

[98] Burmaoğlu, S.; Dilek, E.; Yılmaz, A.O.; Supuran, C.T. Synthesis of two phloroglucinol derivatives with cinnamyl moieties as inhibitors of the carbonic anhydrase isozymes I and II: an *in vitro* study. *J. Enzyme Inhib. Med. Chem.*, **2016**, *31*(sup2), 208-212.
[http://dx.doi.org/10.1080/14756366.2016.1181626] [PMID: 27173152]

[99] Burmaoglu, S.; Yilmaz, A.O.; Taslimi, P.; Algul, O.; Kilic, D.; Gulcin, I. Synthesis and biological evaluation of phloroglucinol derivatives possessing α-glycosidase, acetylcholinesterase, butyrylcholinesterase, carbonic anhydrase inhibitory activity. *Arch. Pharm. (Weinheim),* **2018**, *351*(2)1700314
[http://dx.doi.org/10.1002/ardp.201700314] [PMID: 29323749]

[100] Işık, S.; Vullo, D.; Durdagi, S.; Ekinci, D.; Şentürk, M.; Çetin, A.; Şentürk, E.; Supuran, C.T. Interaction of carbonic anhydrase isozymes I, II, and IX with some pyridine and phenol hydrazinecarbothioamide derivatives. *Bioorg. Med. Chem. Lett.,* **2015**, *25*(23), 5636-5641.
[http://dx.doi.org/10.1016/j.bmcl.2015.10.021] [PMID: 26520662]

[101] Arslan, M.; Şentürk, M.; Fidan, İ.; Talaz, O.; Ekinci, D.; Coşgun, S.; Supuran, C.T. Synthesis of 3,4-dihydroxypyrrolidine-2,5-dione and 3,5-dihydroxybenzoic acid derivatives and evaluation of the carbonic anhydrase I and II inhibition. *J. Enzyme Inhib. Med. Chem.*, **2015**, *30*(6), 896-900.
[http://dx.doi.org/10.3109/14756366.2014.983917] [PMID: 25744511]

[102] Maresca, A.; Akyuz, G.; Osman, S.M.; AlOthman, Z.; Supuran, C.T. Inhibition of mammalian carbonic anhydrase isoforms I–XIV with a series of phenolic acid esters. *Bioorg. Med. Chem.,* **2015**, *23*(22), 7181-7188.
[http://dx.doi.org/10.1016/j.bmc.2015.10.014] [PMID: 26498394]

[103] Riafrecha, L.E.; Rodríguez, O.M.; Vullo, D.; Supuran, C.T.; Colinas, P.A. Synthesis of C-cinnamoyl glycosides and their inhibitory activity against mammalian carbonic anhydrases. *Bioorg. Med. Chem.,* **2013**, *21*(6), 1489-1494.
[http://dx.doi.org/10.1016/j.bmc.2012.09.002] [PMID: 23010455]

[104] Topal, F.; Gulcin, I.; Dastan, A.; Guney, M. Novel eugenol derivatives: Potent acetylcholinesterase and carbonic anhydrase inhibitors. *Int. J. Biol. Macromol.*, **2017**, *94*(Pt B), 845-851.
[http://dx.doi.org/10.1016/j.ijbiomac.2016.10.096] [PMID: 27984137]

[105] Balaydin, H.T.; Durdaği, S.; Ekinci, D.; Şentürk, M.; Göksu, S.; Menzek, A. Inhibition of human carbonic anhydrase isozymes I, II and VI with a series of bisphenol, methoxy and bromophenol compounds. *J. Enzyme Inhib. Med. Chem.*, **2012**, *27*(4), 467-475.
[http://dx.doi.org/10.3109/14756366.2011.596836] [PMID: 21815772]

[106] Bayrak, C.; Taslimi, P.; Karaman, H.S.; Gulcin, I.; Menzek, A. The first synthesis, carbonic anhydrase inhibition and anticholinergic activities of some bromophenol derivatives with S including natural products. *Bioorg. Chem.*, **2019**, *85*, 128-139.
[http://dx.doi.org/10.1016/j.bioorg.2018.12.012] [PMID: 30605886]

[107] Öztaskın, N.; Taslimi, P.; Maraş, A.; Gülcin, İ.; Göksu, S. Novel antioxidant bromophenols with acetylcholinesterase, butyrylcholinesterase and carbonic anhydrase inhibitory actions. *Bioorg. Chem.*, **2017**, *74*, 104-114.
[http://dx.doi.org/10.1016/j.bioorg.2017.07.010] [PMID: 28772158]

[108] Taslimi, P.; Gülçin, İ.; Öztaşkın, N.; Çetinkaya, Y.; Göksu, S.; Alwasel, S.H.; Supuran, C.T. The

effects of some bromophenols on human carbonic anhydrase isoenzymes. *J. Enzyme Inhib. Med. Chem.*, **2016**, *31*(4), 603-607.
[http://dx.doi.org/10.3109/14756366.2015.1054820] [PMID: 26133541]

[109] Ekinci, D.; Çavdar, H.; Durdagi, S.; Talaz, O.; Şentürk, M.; Supuran, C.T. Structure–activity relationships for the interaction of 5,10-dihydroindeno[1,2-*b*]indole derivatives with human and bovine carbonic anhydrase isoforms I, II, III, IV and VI. *Eur. J. Med. Chem.*, **2012**, *49*, 68-73.
[http://dx.doi.org/10.1016/j.ejmech.2011.12.022] [PMID: 22245047]

[110] Arslan, T.; Çelik, G.; Çelik, H.; Şentürk, M.; Yaylı, N.; Ekinci, D. Synthesis and Biological Evaluation of Novel Bischalcone Derivatives as Carbonic Anhydrase Inhibitors. *Arch. Pharm. (Weinheim)*, **2016**, *349*(9), 741-748.
[http://dx.doi.org/10.1002/ardp.201600122] [PMID: 27435458]

[111] Davis, R.A.; Hofmann, A.; Osman, A.; Hall, R.A.; Mühlschlegel, F.A.; Vullo, D.; Innocenti, A.; Supuran, C.T.; Poulsen, S.A. Natural product-based phenols as novel probes for mycobacterial and fungal carbonic anhydrases. *J. Med. Chem.*, **2011**, *54*(6), 1682-1692.
[http://dx.doi.org/10.1021/jm1013242] [PMID: 21332115]

[112] Carta, F.; Maresca, A.; Covarrubias, A.S.; Mowbray, S.L.; Jones, T.A.; Supuran, C.T. Carbonic anhydrase inhibitors. Characterization and inhibition studies of the most active β-carbonic anhydrase from Mycobacterium tuberculosis, Rv3588c. *Bioorg. Med. Chem. Lett.*, **2009**, *19*(23), 6649-6654.
[http://dx.doi.org/10.1016/j.bmcl.2009.10.009] [PMID: 19846301]

[113] Cau, Y.; Mori, M.; Supuran, C.T.; Botta, M. Mycobacterial carbonic anhydrase inhibition with phenolic acids and esters: kinetic and computational investigations. *Org. Biomol. Chem.*, **2016**, *14*(35), 8322-8330.
[http://dx.doi.org/10.1039/C6OB01477A] [PMID: 27530867]

[114] Buchieri, M.V.; Riafrecha, L.E.; Rodríguez, O.M.; Vullo, D.; Morbidoni, H.R.; Supuran, C.T.; Colinas, P.A. Inhibition of the β-carbonic anhydrases from Mycobacterium tuberculosis with C-cinnamoyl glycosides: Identification of the first inhibitor with anti-mycobacterial activity. *Bioorg. Med. Chem. Lett.*, **2013**, *23*(3), 740-743.
[http://dx.doi.org/10.1016/j.bmcl.2012.11.085] [PMID: 23265903]

[115] Riafrecha, L.E.; Vullo, D.; Ouahrani-Bettache, S.; Köhler, S.; Dumy, P.; Winum, J.Y.; Supuran, C.T.; Colinas, P.A. Inhibition of **β** -carbonic anhydrases from *Brucella suis* with *C* -cinnamoyl glycosides incorporating the phenol moiety. *J. Enzyme Inhib. Med. Chem.*, **2015**, *30*(6), 1017-1020.
[http://dx.doi.org/10.3109/14756366.2014.986120] [PMID: 25676329]

[116] Bilginer, S.; Unluer, E.; Gul, H.I.; Mete, E.; Isik, S.; Vullo, D.; Ozensoy Guler, O.; Beyaztas, S.; Capasso, C.; Supuran, C.T. Carbonic anhydrase inhibitors. Phenols incorporating 2- or 3-pyridy--ethenylcarbonyl and tertiary amine moieties strongly inhibit *Saccharomyces cerevisiae* β-carbonic anhydrase. *J. Enzyme Inhib. Med. Chem.*, **2014**, *29*(4), 495-499.
[http://dx.doi.org/10.3109/14756366.2013.806497] [PMID: 23808805]

[117] Alafeefy, A.M.; Isik, S.; Al-Jaber, N.A.; Vullo, D.; Abdel-Aziz, H.A.; Ashour, A.E.; Awaad, A.S.; Capasso, C.; Supuran, C.T. Carbonic anhydrase inhibitors. Benzenesulfonamides incorporating cyanoacrylamide moieties strongly inhibit Saccharomyces cerevisiae β-carbonic anhydrase. *Bioorg. Med. Chem. Lett.*, **2013**, *23*(12), 3570-3575.
[http://dx.doi.org/10.1016/j.bmcl.2013.04.028] [PMID: 23642478]

[118] Entezari Heravi, Y.; Bua, S.; Nocentini, A.; Del Prete, S.; Saboury, A.A.; Sereshti, H.; Capasso, C.; Gratteri, P.; Supuran, C.T. Inhibition of Malassezia globosa carbonic anhydrase with phenols. *Bioorg. Med. Chem.*, **2017**, *25*(9), 2577-2582.
[http://dx.doi.org/10.1016/j.bmc.2017.03.026] [PMID: 28343756]

[119] Alissa, S.A.; Alghulikah, H.A.; ALOthman, Z.A.; Osman, S.M.; Del Prete, S.; Capasso, C.; Nocentini, A.; Supuran, C.T. Inhibition survey with phenolic compounds against the δ- and η-class carbonic anhydrases from the marine diatom *thalassiosira weissflogii* and protozoan *Plasmodium falciparum*. *J. Enzyme Inhib. Med. Chem.*, **2020**, *35*(1), 377-382.

[http://dx.doi.org/10.1080/14756366.2019.1706089] [PMID: 31856608]

[120] Nocentini, A.; Bua, S.; Del Prete, S.; Heravi, Y.E.; Saboury, A.A.; Karioti, A.; Bilia, A.R.; Capasso, C.; Gratteri, P.; Supuran, C.T. Natural polyphenols selectively inhibit β-carbonic anhydrase from the dandruff-producing fungus Malassezia globosa: activity and modeling studies. *ChemMedChem,* **2018**, *13*(8), 816-823.
[http://dx.doi.org/10.1002/cmdc.201800015] [PMID: 29575699]

[121] Covarrubias, A.S.; Larsson, A.M.; Högbom, M.; Lindberg, J.; Bergfors, T.; Björkelid, C.; Mowbray, S.L.; Unge, T.; Jones, T.A. Structure and function of carbonic anhydrases from *Mycobacterium tuberculosis. J. Biol. Chem.,* **2005**, *280*(19), 18782-18789.
[http://dx.doi.org/10.1074/jbc.M414348200] [PMID: 15753099]

[122] Covarrubias, A.S.; Bergfors, T.; Jones, T.A.; Högbom, M. Structural Mechanics of the pH-dependent Activity of β-Carbonic Anhydrase from Mycobacterium tuberculosis. *J. Biol. Chem.,* **2006**, *281*(8), 4993-4999.
[http://dx.doi.org/10.1074/jbc.M510756200] [PMID: 16321983]

[123] Berman, H.M.; Westbrook, J.; Feng, Z.; Gilliland, G.; Bhat, T.N.; Weissig, H.; Shindyalov, I.N.; Bourne, P.E. The Protein Data Bank. *Nucleic Acids Res.,* **2000**, *28*(1), 235-242.
[http://dx.doi.org/10.1093/nar/28.1.235] [PMID: 10592235]

CHAPTER 12

The Role of Flavonoids and other Selected (Poly) Phenols in Cancer Prevention and Therapy: A Focus on Epigenetics

Melissa D'Ascenzio[1,*]

[1] *D'Arcy Thompson Unit, Biological and Biomedical Sciences Education, School of Life Sciences, University of Dundee, DD1 4HN, Dundee, UK*

Abstract: The importance of diet in determining the incidence of chronic illnesses such as diabetes, cardiovascular disorders, neurodegenerative diseases, and cancer has inspired extensive research on the role of individual dietary components in chemoprevention. Flavonoids and (poly)phenols have often been identified as the ideal candidates for these types of studies, as they represent large classes of natural products that are widely available in fruit and vegetables. In this chapter, we will discuss the antiproliferative properties of flavonols, flavanols, flavones, isoflavones, anthocyanins, curcuminoids and resveratrol derivatives, with a particular focus on their ability to interfere with epigenetic processes and modulate gene expression. We will look at the challenges encountered during the optimisation of the pharmacokinetic and pharmacodynamic properties of these natural products and, where possible, we will define structure-activity relationships.

Keywords: Anthocyanins, Anticancer agents, Apigenin, Curcumin, Chemoprevention, Epigallocatechin-3-gallate, Epigenetics, Flavonoids, Flavonols, Flavones, Genistein, Isoflavones, Kaempferol, Polyphenols, Quercetin, Resveratrol.

INTRODUCTION

Chemoprevention and the Epigenetic Mechanisms Associated with Chronic Diseases

According to the latest World Population Prospect published in 2019 by the United Nations, the world's population is predicted to reach 9.7 billion by the year 2050 [1]. Thanks to the progress made by medicine and the implementation of

* **Corresponding author Melissa D'Ascenzio:** D'Arcy Thompson Unit, Biological and Biomedical Sciences Education, School of Life Sciences, University of Dundee, DD1 4HN, Dundee, UK; Tel.: +44 (0) 1382 384682; E-mail: m.dascenzio@dundee.ac.uk

public health measures aimed at improving the quality of care and raising awareness around healthy lifestyles, life expectancy is also expected to increase significantly over the next thirty years. As of today, the fastest-growing age group in terms of percentage of the overall population, is the one represented by persons aged 65 or over. Almost a fifth of the European and Northern American population is constituted by over 65s and this number is predicted to increase until it will reach 25% by 2050 [1]. Unfortunately, an extension in life expectancy does not necessarily translate into an increase in a healthy lifespan. In fact, ageing is one of the major contributing factors to the incidence of chronic diseases such as neurodegenerative disorders, cardiovascular diseases, chronic respiratory diseases, diabetes, obesity, and cancer [2]. In many instances, the decreased mortality associated with these pathologies leads to the development of comorbidities and the overall complication of the patient's clinical picture [3]. In 2002, the growing body of evidence linking dietary and lifestyle habits with the incidence of chronic diseases led the WHO and FAO to conduct a joint expert consultation aimed at producing evidence-based recommendations for the cost-effective prevention and control of chronic diseases [4]. In 2013, these recommendations were incorporated into a Global Action Plan for the prevention of non-communicable diseases (NCDs) and have since been translated into regional and national policies worldwide [5]. While WHO guidelines tend to focus mostly on limiting tobacco and alcohol consumption, reducing salt, sugar, and calorie intake, as well as promoting physical activity, scientific evidence demonstrates that the connection between diet and chronic diseases goes further than that. Recent studies report that the Mediterranean diet and the DASH (Dietary Approaches to Stop Hypertension) diet can slow down cognitive decline [6, 7], while high compliance to a hybrid Mediterranean-DASH diet reduces the incidence of Alzheimer's disease by more than 50% in patients aged 58-98 [8]. In a similar way, the regular consumption of fruits and vegetables has been associated with a significant reduction in the risk of developing several types of cancer, especially those involving the gastrointestinal tract and the respiratory system, but also including breast, bladder, prostate, kidney, cervix, ovary and endometrium cancer [9, 10]. These findings constitute the foundation upon which several dietary components, including micronutrients and phytochemicals, have been studied and adopted in clinical settings as adjuvants in cancer therapy and prevention [11]. This approach takes the name of chemoprevention.

Although there seems to be a general consensus around the fact that most dietary components show neuroprotective and anticancer behaviour thanks to their antioxidant properties, *i.e.* their ability to reduce the oxidative stress caused by the production of reactive oxygen and nitrogen species (ROS & RNS), there is a consolidated body of evidence suggesting that common phytochemicals found in vegetables and fruit can activate stress-response pathways that involve a large variety of effectors, including transcription factors, protein kinases, and epigenetic modifiers [12, 13].

The dramatic effect that dietary components can have on gene expression through the modulation of epigenetic mechanisms is beautifully captured in the honeybee (*Apis mellifera*) model, where the development of larvae with identical genetic material into queen or worker bees is determined by the food they receive [14]. While the queen bee is fed exclusively with royal jelly, worker bees receive royal jelly only for three days and then move onto a diet made of worker jelly, pollen, and beebread [15]. These dissimilar diets have been proven responsible for the physical and behavioural differences observed in the two honeybee phenotypes. At the cellular level, this phenomenon is caused by changes in DNA methylation levels, particularly at alternative splicing sites [14]. DNA methylation is an archaic mechanism that traces its origin back to bacteria and unicellular organisms and involves transferring a methyl group to the C-5 position of a cytosine base [16]. In humans, methylation usually happens at cytosine-rich regions known as CpG islands, which constitute over two-thirds of mammalian promoters [17]. Although humans do not exhibit the same developmental flexibility as honeybees, DNA methylation of gene promoters has a powerful silencing effect on downstream genes and it plays a fundamental role in embryonic development [18]. Changes in DNA methylation levels at this stage of development can dramatically increase the risk of chronic diseases later in life, as shown by studies conducted on individuals who were prenatally exposed to famine during the Dutch Hunger Winter in 1944-45 [19, 20]. Although these results would be difficult to confirm in humans due to ethical implications, it has been demonstrated in several animal studies that in the uterus and early life exposure to phytochemicals that are known for their ability to inhibit DNA methylation can reduce the incidence of cardiovascular diseases, obesity, and cancer [21 - 24]. In fact, maintaining a balanced DNA methylation status is particularly important to prevent cell transformation, as genome-wide demethylation associated with expression of oncogenes and hypermethylation of CpG islands promoters of onco-suppressor genes constitute a clear hallmark of cancer [17]. However, DNA methylation is not the only epigenetic process that has been found to be dysregulated in cancer development and progression. Epigenetic mechanisms associated with the onset of cancerous phenotypes include post-translational modification (PTM) of histone and non-histone proteins through acetylation, methylation, phosphorylation, ubiquitinylation, citrullination, ribosylation, and sumoylation, as well as non-coding RNA (ncRNA) mediated gene silencing [25]. In this chapter, we will discuss the antiproliferative activity of flavonoids and other selected (poly)phenols of plant origin, with particular reference to their ability to interfere with specific epigenetic mechanisms, such as DNA methylation and the methylation/acetylation of both histone and non-histone proteins.

Additionally, we will explore how some of the challenges related to potency, selectivity and ADME properties of these natural products led to the development of synthetic and semi-synthetic derivatives. For reasons of conciseness and space, we will leave the discussion on phytochemicals and miRNAs regulation out of the picture, although we recognise that this is an important topic exhaustively reviewed elsewhere [26].

EPIGENETIC MARKS AND EPIGENETIC PROTEINS

DNA Methyltransferases

The methylation status of the human genome is maintained by a class of enzymes called DNA methyltransferases (DNMTs) that catalyse the covalent addition of a methyl group to carbon 5 of cytosine bases. The DNA-methyltransferase family includes several enzymatic isoforms, such as DNMT1, DNMT3A, and DNMT3B. While DNMT3A and DNMT3B prefer binding to unmethylated DNA sequences and perform *de novo* methylation, DNMT1 is often recruited at partially methylated DNA *loci* and plays a fundamental role in maintaining physiological methylation levels. Moreover, DNMT1 is known to be involved in transferring the methylation pattern from mother to daughter cells during DNA replication [17].

Histone Acetyl Transferases (Hats) and Histone Deacetylases (Hdacs)

Inside the nucleus, DNA is tightly packed in structural units called nucleosomes. A nucleosome is constituted by a short strand of DNA wrapped around a set of basic proteins called histones. Each nucleosome contains two copies of each histone H2A, H2B, H3 and H4, to form an octamer core from which ten histone tails can be observed protruding, one N-terminal tail for each histone protein plus two additional C-terminal tails from histones H2A [27]. The interactions between the DNA backbone and the histone proteins in the nucleosome are mostly electrostatic in nature, as the negatively charged phosphate groups belonging to the DNA double helix interact with the protonated side chains of basic amino acids (Lys and Arg) belonging to the histone proteins. An extensive network of direct and water-mediated hydrogen bonds contributes to stabilise the binding [27]. As a consequence, a post-translational modification that reduces the accumulation of positive charge on the lateral chain of lysine residues like acetylation will result in the weakening of histones-DNA interactions and will increase chromatin accessibility to the transcriptional machinery [28]. Moreover, acetylated lysines constitute an anchoring point for proteins that recognise this epigenetic mark through a family of reader domains known as bromodomains (BRDs). These proteins are generally involved in chromatin remodelling and further histone modification [29]. Acetylation of the ε-amino group of lysine residues is often found at the *N*-terminal tails of histones, as they protrude from the nucleosome, and it is operated by a family of proteins called histone acetyl transferases (HATs), a class of enzymes that use Acetyl-CoA as a co-factor [30]. There are two main types of HATs: type A and type B. While type-B HATs specialise in acetylating newly synthesised histones, particularly H4K5 and H4K12, type-A HATs represent a more varied group divided into three main families (GNAT, MYST and p300/CBP) and they are involved in maintaining the acetylation status of both histone and non-histone proteins [31]. Like many other post-translational modifications, acetylation is a reversible process. The acetyl-lysine mark is removed by a class of enzymes known as histone deacetylases (HDACs). HDACs are divided into four major classes on the basis of sequence homology: HDAC1, HDAC2, HDAC3 and HDAC8 belong to class I; HDAC4, HDAC5, HDAC7, and HDAC9 belong to class IIa; HDAC6 and HDAC10 are classified as class IIb; there is only one class IV HDAC: HDAC11. Class I, II and IV HDACs are characterised by the presence of a catalytic zinc ion in the active site [32]. Histone deacetylases belonging to class III histone deacetylases are called sirtuins (SIRTs). There are seven known isoforms of SIRTs differing from each other in intracellular localisation: SIRT1, SIRT6, and SIRT7 are nuclear isoforms; SIRT3, SIRT4, and SIRT5 are localised in the mitochondria, while SIRT2 is mostly found in the cytosol. In contrast to other HDACs, SIRTs use NAD^+ as a co-factor. Given the high involvement of NAD^+ in several metabolic pathways, it is believed that these enzymes could constitute the link between gene transcription and cell metabolism, thus suggesting a potential involvement in mediating the effect of calories restriction on longevity [33, 34]. While acetylation promotes the activation of gene transcription and expression, lysine deacetylation has an opposite, silencing effect. Moreover, it exposes the side chain of lysine residues on histone tails to other post-translational modifications, such as methylation.

Histone Methyl Transferases (Hmts)

Histone methylation is an epigenetic mark commonly found on the side chain of basic amino acids, such as lysines and arginines. This post-translational modification is added to the *N*-terminal tails of histone proteins by histone methyltransferases (HMTs), a class of enzymes that uses S-adenosylmethionine (SAM) as a source of methyl groups. HMTs are grouped on the basis of their selectivity: lysine-specific isoforms are known as KMTs, while arginine specific isoforms take the name of PRMTs. Although it is estimated that the human genome could contain hundreds of KMTs, the methylation of highly conserved lysine residues on histone tails is operated by a small number of proteins, most of which possess a SET (Su(var)3-9, Enhancer of Zeste, and Trithorax) methyltransferase domain [35]. These enzymes are able to transfer one, two or three methyl substituents to the ε-amino group of lysine residues Fig. (**1**).

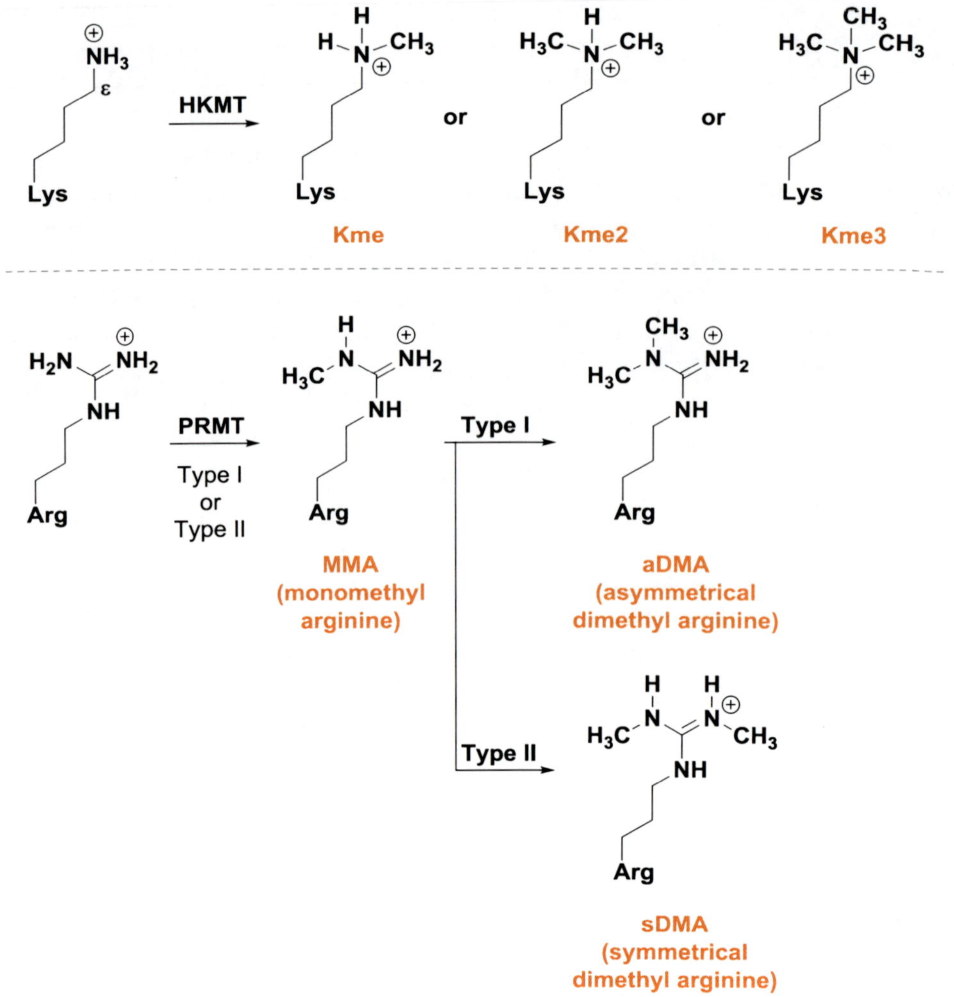

Fig. (1). Post-translational modification of lysine and arginine side chains operated by histone methyltransferases.

On the other end, only nine PRMTs have been identified in humans (PRMT1-9), with PRMT4 also taking the name of CARM1. PRMTs can be divided into two main classes: type I and type II methyl-arginine transferase. Although enzymes belonging to both classes are able to methylate the ω-guanidine group of arginine, only type I PRMTs (PRMT1-4, PRMT6 and PRMT8) can generate asymmetrical dimethyl arginine (aDMA), while type II PRMTs (PRMT5 and PRMT9) are responsible for the formation of symmetrical dimethyl arginine (sDMA) Fig. (**1**) [36]. PRMT7 is considered a unique type of arginine methyltransferase (type III), as it has been shown to produce only mono-methylated products [37].

Although methylation of lysine and arginine side chains reduces the ability of these residues to form hydrogen bonds and it increases their steric hindrance, this PTM does not affect their overall charge (Fig. **1**). In fact, these marks are believed to modulate the chromatin status by functioning as harbouring points for effector proteins that contain aromatic pockets capable of recognising methyl-lysine or methyl-arginine. These reader domains including chromodomains, ADD, ankyrin, PHD, tudor, MBT, PWWP, and WDR domains are found in proteins that tend to be a part of larger chromatin associating complexes inducing gene silencing, such as the Polycomb repressive complex, or transcription activation, like in the case of the basal transcription complex TFIID [38]. Moreover, these large multiprotein complexes can contain multiple reader subunits and display selectivity for specific combinations of post-translational modifications, a model that takes the name of "histone code" [39, 40]. Finally, the presence of specific marks on the histone tails can influence the further deposition of other epigenetic modifications, like in the case of H3K18 acetylation, which is known to facilitate the asymmetric methylation of the adjacent H3R17, or in the example provided by H3K9, whose acetylation prevents PRMT5 from methylating the vicinal H3R8 [41]. This phenomenon highlights the interdependence of epigenetic marks as well as the importance of the position of specific PTMs in determining which type of effector complex they are capable of recruiting. In particular, the methylation of H3K4, H3K36 and H3K79 has been associated with active chromatin and transcriptional activation, while the presence of the same mark on H3K9, H3K27 and H4K20 has been linked to reduced gene expression [42]. Similarly, the asymmetric methylation of H4R3 operated by PRMT1 has been reported to facilitate histone acetylation and the formation of active chromatin. On the other hand, the symmetric methylation of H4R3 and H3R8 by PRMT5 has been found to suppress gene expression [41 - 43]. Other arginine residues whose methylation status is involved in controlling chromatin activation include H3R2, H3R17, and H3R26. Although for a long time it was believed that methylation is an irreversible mark, it is now considered consolidated knowledge that most epigenetic marks, including methylation, are reversibly added and removed [36]. The enzymes responsible for the removal of methylation marks on histone tails take the name of histone demethylases and are characterised by the presence of a reader domain capable of recognising methylated amino acid side chains and a catalytic domain with oxidase activity [44, 45]. Lysine demethylases (KDMs) operate following two distinct mechanisms, both leading to the elimination of a methyl group in the form of formaldehyde. LSD demethylases (LSDs) use FAD^+ as a co-factor to induce oxidation of the methyl group following a mechanism that resembles the one operated by other monoamine oxidases Fig. (**2**). LSDs tend to be quite specific in their demethylating ability, with LSD1 showing preferential demethylation of H3K4me1/2 and H3K9m1/2, while LSD2 seems to prefer

H3K4me1 and H3K4me2 [46]. Jumonji C (JmJC) demethylases constitute the largest KDMs family, a group of metalloenzymes that utilise iron(II) ions to catalyse an α-ketoglutarate (2-oxoglutarate; 2-OG) dependent dioxygenase reaction that leads to the oxidation and elimination of the methyl group as formaldehyde (Fig. **2**) [46]. Like in the case of LSDs, distinct enzymes within the JmJC family present different selectivity against methylated lysines on histone H3, with the only difference that several isoforms can behave as trimethyl-lysine demethylases, especially against H3K9me3 and H3K36m3.

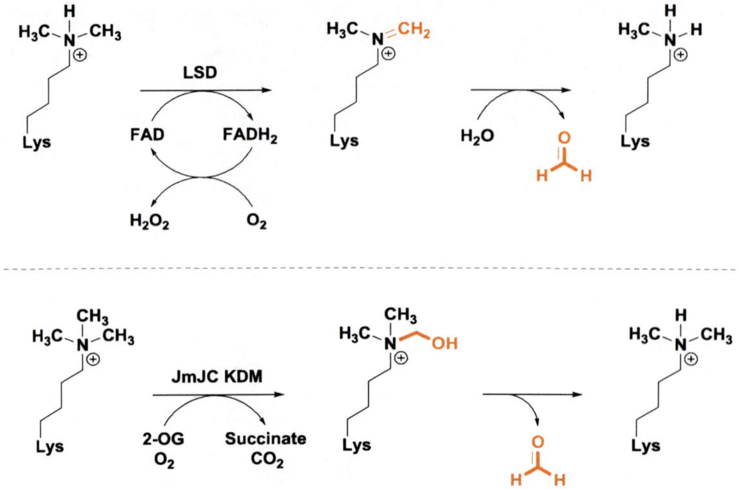

Fig. (2). Mechanism of demethylation operated by the two main classes of lysine demethylases: LSD and JmJC [46].

Although specific arginine demethylases have not been reported yet and the level to which arginine methylation constitutes a reversible modification is still a matter of debate, several lysine demethylases have been shown to possess the flexibility to act as arginine demethylases (RDMs). JMJD6, an enzyme belonging to the JmJC family of KDMs, is one of the first RDMs reported in the literature [47]. Moreover, a study conducted by Walport *et al.* [48] using purified isoforms of JmJC KDMs showed that this property is shared by other members of this family, including KDM3A, KDM4A, KDM4E, KDM5C, and KDM6B. Finally, the methyl mark on arginine lateral chains can be removed by deamination, a reaction catalysed by PAD4 (peptidyl arginine deaminase 4) that converts arginine into citrulline [49].

Other Post-Translational Modifications

Phosphorylation is a PTM (Post-Translational Modification) generally added to the side chains of amino acid residues such as threonine, tyrosine, and serine by a large family of protein kinases. However, this mark can also be found on less obvious amino acids such as histidine, lysine, aspartate, glutamate, and cysteine [50]. Histone phosphorylation is particularly important in regulating the process of DNA damage and repair, where the addition of a phosphate group to Ser139 and/or Tyr142 of histone H2A(X) initiates the recruitment of the DNA-repair machinery. Moreover, phosphorylation of histone H3 has been implicated in the expression of oncogenes such as *c-Fos*, *c-Jun*, and *c-Myc* [51]. Other histone modifications that will be discussed in less detail in this chapter include biotinylation, ubiquitylation, SUMOylation, citrullination, butyrylation, propionylation, and glycosylation.

FLAVONOIDS AS EPIGENETIC MODULATORS IN CHEMOPREVENTION AND CANCER THERAPY

Flavonoids are a large class of natural products extensively found in fruits and vegetables. They share a common three-ring system (A-C) characterised by a fused heterocyclic core. On the basis of their oxidation and hydroxylation state flavonoids can be divided into six different subclasses: flavonols, flavones, flavanones, isoflavones, flavanols and anthocyanins Fig. (**3**).

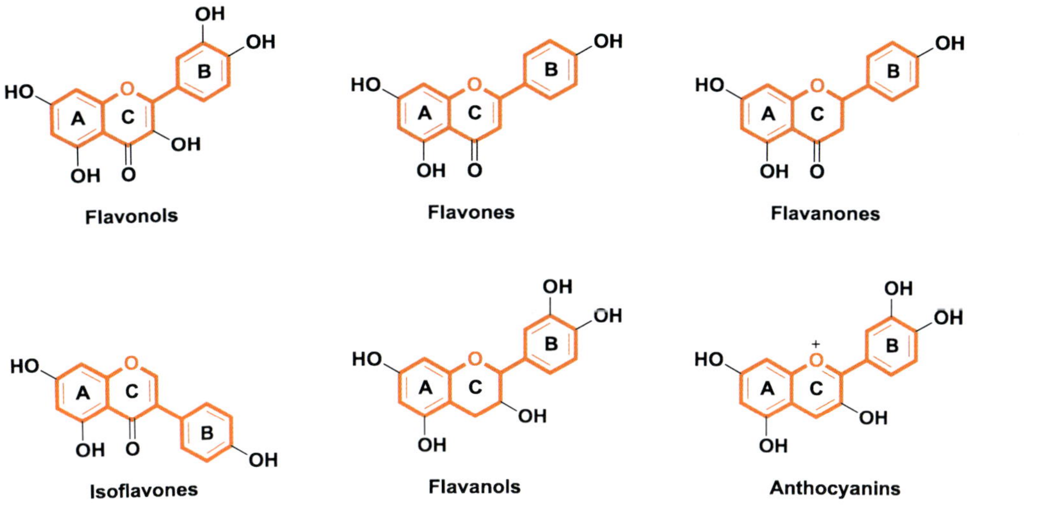

Fig. (3). Flavonoids classification. Structural differences between flavonoids subclasses: flavonols, flavones, flavanones, isoflavones, flavanols and anthocyanins.

These plant secondary metabolites are endowed with widespread biological activities and have been often associated with the health benefits derived from balanced diets. In several population and clinical studies, high flavonoids intake has been linked to a significant reduction or mitigation of cardiovascular and oncological diseases [52, 53]. The molecular mechanisms through which this heterogeneous class of compounds exert their protective action are varied and often rely on their anti-inflammatory, antioxidant, and radical scavenging properties [54]. Indeed, the chemopreventive and antiproliferative effect exerted by flavonoids on gastrointestinal, oral, hepatic, lung, and genitourinary cancers, as well as haematological malignancies, seems to be at least partially mediated by the inhibition of xanthine oxidases (XO), cyclooxygenases (COX) and lipoxygenases (LOX), alongside the reduction of highly reactive oxygen species (ROS) that are known to cause oxidative damage and promote cancer progression [55]. Amongst the non-specific mechanisms of action, flavonoids have been reported to inhibit several isoforms of CYP450, including CYP1A1 and CYP1A2, thus hindering the activation of procarcinogens that are often operated by these metabolic enzymes [56]. While this is a desirable effect, the inhibition of cytochrome P450 should always be considered a delicate matter, as it could cause pharmacokinetic interactions that interfere with the patient's exposure to life-saving drugs. Quercetin (**1**) and kaempferol's (**2**) inhibition of CYP3A has been associated with 43-51% reduction of exposure to orally administered cyclosporine, for example. On the other side, the co-administration of flavonoids and anti-cancer drugs metabolised by CYP3A such as tamoxifen, etoposide, doxorubicin and paclitaxel, resulted in increased bioavailability [57, 58]. Additionally, flavonoids are known to disrupt cancer growth thanks to their anti-angiogenetic properties. In particular, quercetin (**1**), kaempferol (**2**), genistein (**3**), and epigallocatechin-3-gallate (**4**) Fig. (**4**) have been reported to interfere with vascular endothelium grow factor (VEGF) signalling both at the receptor level, by reducing the expression of VEGFR2 and inhibiting its kinase activity, as well as acting directly on VEGF downstream signalling involving protein kinases such as MAPK, ERK 1/2 and AKT [59].

Other mechanisms that explain the anti-angiogenic effect of flavonoids have been proposed and include the downregulation of hypoxia induced factor HIF-α and fibroblast growth factor (FGF), as well as the inhibition of the activity and secretion of metalloproteinases MMP2 and MMP9 [59]. However, the most remarkable property of flavonoids with respect to cancer prevention and therapy is indeed their pro-apoptotic effect. Although members of the flavonol and flavone subclasses, like quercetin (**1**) and apigenin (**5**), have been shown to intercalate between DNA base pairs or bind to the minor groove of the double helix, DNA damage is not thought to constitute the main mechanism through which flavonoids induce cell death [60, 61]. In cancer cells, flavonoids have been reported to increase the levels of pro-apoptotic proteins such as p53, p16, p21, Bax and Fas, while reducing the expression of anti-apoptotic proteins like bcl-2, Fas, Bax, *N*- and *E*-cadherin, and cyclidins. At the same time, increased levels of cleaved caspases and the induced release of cytochrome C in the cytoplasm suggest the involvement of the intrinsic apoptosis pathway [60]. Recent studies have highlighted that the control that these natural products exert on intracellular levels of pro-apoptotic and anti-apoptotic factors could be ascribed, at least in part, to their ability to modulate epigenetic mechanisms involved in cell proliferation [62]. In particular, the inhibition of DNMTs activity and expression induced by this class of compounds has been correlated with the reactivation of onco-suppressor genes and consequential expression of proteins involved in DNA-damage repair, cell cycle arrest, and apoptosis [57]. Similarly, the ability that flavonoids have to interfere with the intracellular balance of acetylated/deacetylated histone and non-histone proteins has shown to be involved in mediating their antiproliferative effect [63].

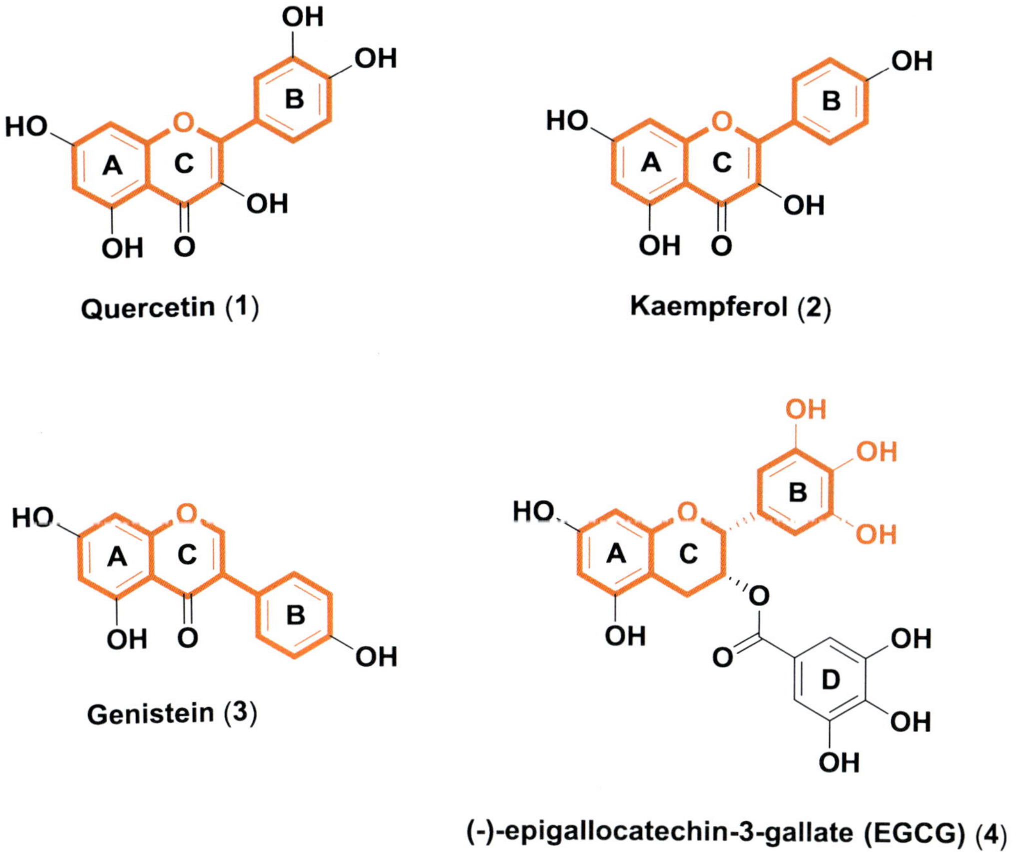

Fig. (4). Chemical structures of flavonoids that demonstrate antiangiogenetic activity through inhibition of VEGF and its downstream signalling.

FLAVONOLS, FLAVONES, ISOFLAVONES, AND ANTHOCYANINS

Flavonols: Quercetin and Kaempferol

Quercetin and Kaempferol are flavonoids extensively found in berries, grapes, apple peel and in a wide variety of plants and herbs including broccoli, tomatoes, capers, kale, onions, tea, *Ginkgo biloba*, *Hypericum perforatum* and *Sambucus canadensis*. Quercetin is also highly abundant in citrus fruits, red wine, and olive oil [64]. The two natural products belong to the class of flavonols and differ from each other only for the presence/absence of a hydroxyl group at the *meta*-position of the B ring. Similar to other members of the flavonoids family, quercetin (**1**) and kaempferol (**2**) have demonstrated high potential as preventive agents and/or co-adjuvants in the treatment of several forms of cancer. Although their chemopreventive properties have been often associated with their anti-inflammatory and antioxidant activity, these compounds have shown their antiproliferative effect through a variety of alternative mechanisms [60, 65, 66]. In oral cancer cell lines (SCC-1483, SCC-25, and SCC-QLL1), *Gingko biloba* extracts containing both flavonols induced apoptosis *via* a caspase-3-dependent pathway [67]. In acute lymphoblastic leukemia cells (MOLT-4), kaempferol-induced cell death seemed to be mediated by the involvement of the tumour necrosis factor-related apoptosis-inducing ligand TRAIL, through the activation of death receptors DR4 and DR5 [68]. In colon cancer models, kaempferol (**2**) was found to reduce the expression of several oncogenes like *K-Ras* and *c-Myc*, while inducing the expression of tumour suppressing genes (TSGs) such as AMPK and APC [69]. Interestingly, the combination of kaempferol (**2**) and quercetin (**1**) in a 1:2 ratio was reported to be more cytotoxic against HCT-116 colon cancer cells compared to individual treatment [70]. In a recent study involving HCT-116 colon cancer cells and human hepatoma cell lines (HepG2 and Hep3B), Berger *et al.* [71] demonstrated for the first time that kaempferol (**2**) could act as an *in vivo* pan-HDAC inhibitor and induce dose-dependent acetylation of histone H3. Treatment with 20-100 μM kaempferol (**2**) resulted in a significant reduction of cell proliferation and *via*bility in both cell lines, despite Hep3B being p53 deficient, while HDAC inhibition could be detected in nuclear extracts at concentrations as low as 5 μM. *In silico* docking of kaempferol and HDAC2, HDAC4, HDAC7 and HDAC8 confirmed that kaempferol (**2**) establishes constructive interactions with amino acid side chains and the catalytic zinc ion in the active site of these epigenetic enzymes Fig. (**5**) [71].

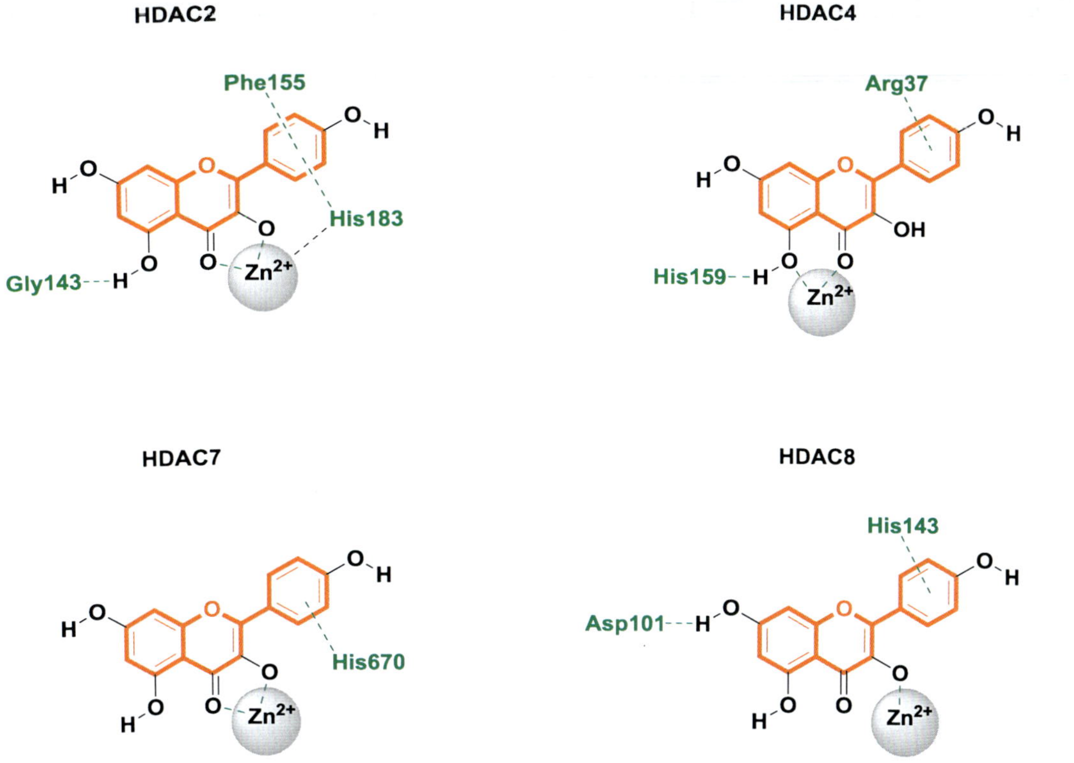

Fig. (5). Proposed interactions of kaempferol (**2**) within the active site of HDAC isoforms 2, 4, 7 and 8 [71].

Interestingly, kaempferol has also been reported to affect the expression and cellular localisation of SIRT3, a histone deacetylase belonging to the sirtuin family. In myelogenous leukemia K562 and promyelocytic leukemia U937 cell lines, the oxidative stress produced by treatment with 50 μM kaempferol for 24-72 hours caused an increment in SIRT3 mRNA expression and protein levels, while at the same time inhibiting the expression of Bcl-2 and Bcl-xL, inducing the expression of Bax and causing an increase of caspase activity [72]. Although the exact role that SIRT3 plays in mediating kaempferol's induced cell death has not been fully elucidated, SIRT3 has been previously reported to be essential in the apoptosis of HCT-116 colon cancer cells that follows Bcl-2 silencing under basal conditions [73]. Finally, kaempferol (150 mg/kg/day) has been shown to reduce the methylation levels of the *WRN* promoter, a region under the control of DNMT3B, in mice xenografts of bladder cancer (T24 cells) [74]. The analysis of expression levels of DNMTs after *in vitro* exposure to kaempferol (40 μM) showed that DNMT3B protein levels were, in fact, reduced in T24 and 5637 bladder cancer cells, despite its expression being significantly increased after 24 hours of treatment [74]. This discrepancy has led the authors to speculate that kaempferol exerts its control on DNMT3B levels by promoting its ubiquitination and proteasome degradation.

Similar to kaempferol (**2**), quercetin (**1**) has also been shown to possess antiproliferative properties in bladder cancer cell lines, particularly T24, EJ, and J82, although cell *via*bility was only halved at the highest tested concentration (100 μM) [75]. 72 hours treatment of T24 cells with 100 μM quercetin induced demethylation of the promoter region of genes that are usually hypermethylated in bladder cancer, such as *ER2* (gene encoding for the oestrogen receptor β), *p16*$^{INK\alpha}$, and *RASSF1A*. In the same cell line, quercetin (**1**) reduced the expression of survivin, a protein capable of inhibiting apoptosis and whose expression is considered a predictor of poor prognosis and high risk of recurrence in bladder cancer patients [75]. Moreover, quercetin was found to promote programmed cell death by preventing the translation and accumulation of mutated forms of p53 in both bladder (T24) and breast cancer cells (MDA-MB-468) [75, 76]. When quercetin was tested on cell lines expressing wild-type p53 (MCF-7), it seemed to have a much lower downregulating effect compared to the one reported in MDA-MB-468 cells [76]. Moreover, quercetin (**1**) was shown to induce Brca1 expression in ER(-) breast cancer cell lines like MDA-MB-468 and MDA-M--231 *via* a mechanism that implicates increased acetylation of the *BRCA1* promoter [77]. Since reduced levels of Brca1 have been correlated with activation of hypoxia induced factor HIF-1α and tumour progression, this result highlighted the potential benefits of using quercetin as a co-adjuvant in cancer therapy. Interestingly, the combination of quercetin (20 μM) and curcumin (10 μM) was more effective than single treatments against these two triple negative breast cancer cell lines, as it caused a 62-65% reduction in cell *via*bility and an even more apparent increase of Brca1 expression. Additionally, the combined treatment seemed to induce a genome-wide intensification of acetylation of lysine 9 on histone 3 (H3K9Ac) that was not observed when the same cell lines were treated with quercetin or curcumin alone [77]. Although the molecular mechanism through which quercetin can influence acetylation levels in breast cancer cells was not investigated in detail, there are reasons to believe it might involve direct modulation of epigenetic proteins. In a separate study involving MCF-7 and MDA-MB-231 breast cancer cells, Xiao *et al.* [78] used a luciferase assay to demonstrate that quercetin (25-300 μM) was capable of inducing a significant decrease of COX-2 expression by inhibiting the recruitment of transactivators such as CREB-2, c-Fos, C/EBPβ and NFκB to its promoter both *in vitro* and *in vivo*. This phenomenon was associated with direct inhibition of the histone acetyltransferase activity of p300, which was accompanied by diminished recruitment of this enzyme at the transcription site. Since the acetylase activity of p300 plays a pivotal role in enhancing chromatin access to the transcription machinery while stabilising the binding of transactivators - including NFκB - to gene promoters, its inhibition was directly correlated with COX-2 gene silencing [78]. This claim was supported by previous research conducted on a mouse model of chronic inflammation of the lower intestine, in which the treatment with 10 mg/kg/day of quercetin reduced the activation of proinflammatory genes (IP-10 and MIP-2) by inhibiting the recruitment of NFκB and CBP/p300, and decreasing histone 3 acetylation at the promoter regions [79]. It is important to note at this point that quercetin has also been found to induce apoptosis of colon and colorectal cancer cells in several studies, although the proposed mechanism of action varied significantly, from inhibition of EGF receptor kinase to interaction with type-II oestrogen binding sites [80, 81].

In vivo studies involving murine models of breast adenocarcinoma confirmed *in vitro* results, as the lifespan of tumour bearing mice receiving six doses of 1 mg/kg quercetin (**1**) every other third day increased five folds, while the volume of their tumours significantly decreased [60].

In human cervical cancer cells (HeLa), 25-50 μM quercetin (**1**) has been proven to cause a significant decrease in histone deacetylase (49-71%) and DNA-methyltransferase (32-63%) activity. This was accompanied by diminished expression of all the DNMT isoforms - DNMT1, DNMT3A, and DNMT3B - and histone deacetylases HDAC1-3, HDAC5-7 and HDAC11. Interestingly, quercetin (**1**) also seemed to induce reduced HAT1 and KDM5B expression, while inhibiting the activity of histone methyl transferase H3K9 (71% reported inhibition at 50 μM) [82]. This epigenetic unbalance resulted in the re-expression of a series of TSGs such as *DAPK1*, *RAR*-β, *PTEN*, *RASSF1*, *GSTP1*, *SOC51*, *MGMT*, *APC*, *CDH1*, *CDH13*, *FHIT*, *MLH1*, *TIMP3*, and *VHL* [82]. Molecular docking simulations of quercetin's binding mode within the active site of DNMTs and HDACs including HDAC2, HDAC4, HDAC7 and HDAC8 showed that quercetin (**1**) could act as a direct inhibitor of these enzymes. In fact, quercetin seems to fit the catalytic pocket of DNMT3A and DNMT3B, as well as the binding site of EZH2, a methyltransferase that plays an important role in DNMT1 recruitment and gene silencing. Similarly, quercetin places itself in the catalytic pocket of HDACs at a distance not higher than 5 Å from the zinc ion and it displays some overlap in the interactions it forms with those previously highlighted for kaempferol (**2**) Fig. (**5**)., such as for example the π-stacking interactions with Phe155 and His183 in HDAC2, or with His670 in HDAC7 [82]. Since inhibition of HDAC8 is thought to be particularly promising in the treatment of colon cancer [83], a series of quercetin derivatives have been synthesised (Fig. **6**) and tested for their ability to inhibit HDAC8 *in vitro* and prevent the proliferation of HCT116 cells Table **1** [84].

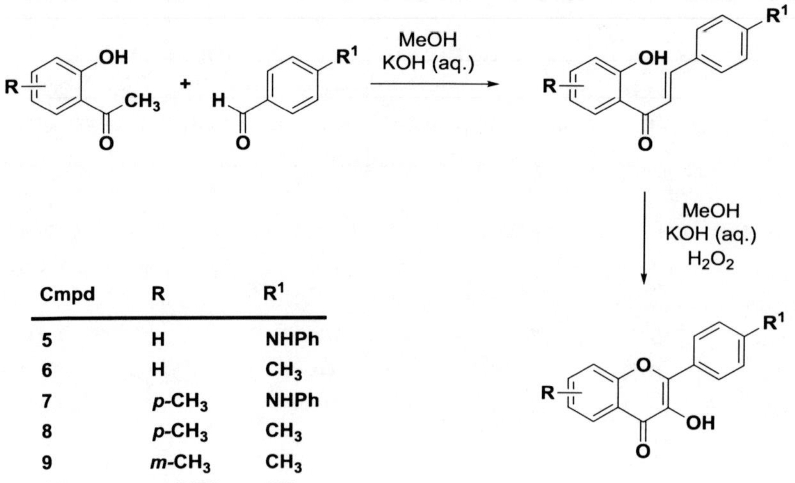

Cmpd	R	R^1
5	H	NHPh
6	H	CH_3
7	*p*-CH_3	NHPh
8	*p*-CH_3	CH_3
9	*m*-CH_3	CH_3
10	*m*-OCH_3	CH_3

Fig. (6). Synthesis of substituted quercetin derivatives as HDAC8 inhibitors [84].

Table 1. Cytotoxic activity of quercetin derivatives 6 and 9 against HCT116 colon cancer cells and Vero cells compared to quercetin (1) and SAHA (vorinostat). HDAC inhibition was measured both in whole cell assays and *in vitro* assays [84].

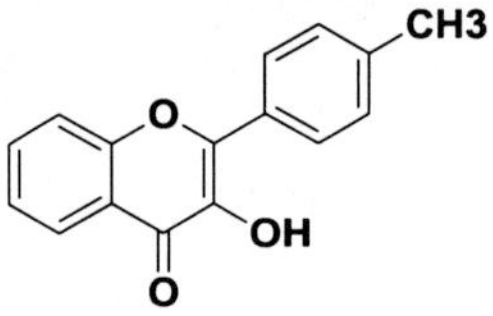

6

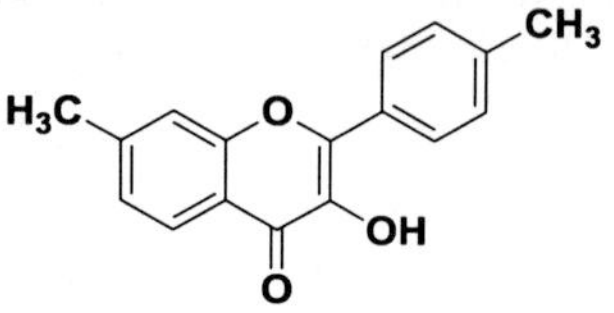

9

Cmpd	IC_{50} (μM)					
	HCT116	Vero	HDACs (whole cell)	HDAC8 (*in vitro*)	HDAC1 (*in vitro*)	HDAC6 (*in vitro*)
6	68 ± 2.3	140 ± 6.8	181.7 ± 22.04	36.03 ±4.17	34.11 ±3.83	165.1 ± 11.1
9	27.4 ± 1.8	55.6 ± 3.8	70.2 ± 4.3	24.00 ± 2.8	47.7 ± 6.3	163.35 ± 7.05
Quercetin	107.6 ± 1.2	201.5 ± 7.5	167.8 ± 6.9	15.4 ± 1.53	26.72 ± 3.77	43.39 ± 2.17
SAHA	3.1 ± 0.35	4.6 ± 1.6	1.2 ± 0.1	0.7 ± 0.025	0.026 ± 0.002	0.098 ± 0.012

This study showed that substitution of the B ring with a methyl group in the *para* position produced quercetin derivatives (**6** and **9**) with higher antiproliferative activity than quercetin (**1**), although especially in the case of compound **9**, this was associated with a general increase of cytotoxicity Table **1**. Although compounds **6** and **9** did not show higher HDAC inhibitory activity than quercetin (**1**) in *in vitro* studies, it is relevant to highlight that both compounds showed selectivity against class I HDACs (HDAC1 and 8) compared to class II HDACs, represented here by HDAC6 [84]. Hence, they could represent a good starting point for further development of selective HDAC inhibitors. Clearly, particular attention should be dedicated to the pharmacokinetic properties of future quercetin derivatives, as the addition of lipophilic groups to a scarcely water-soluble core could compromise further its bioavailability [85]. Multiple strategies have been attempted to improve quercetin's ADME properties, including the development of appropriate formulation and delivery systems, as well as the introduction of substituents that are able to modulate the compound's water solubility and logD, such as carboxylic acids and weak bases [86]. To achieve this task, Mukherjee *et al.* [86] developed a synthetic route for the regioselective substitution of positions C-3' and C-5 of quercetin Scheme (**1**).

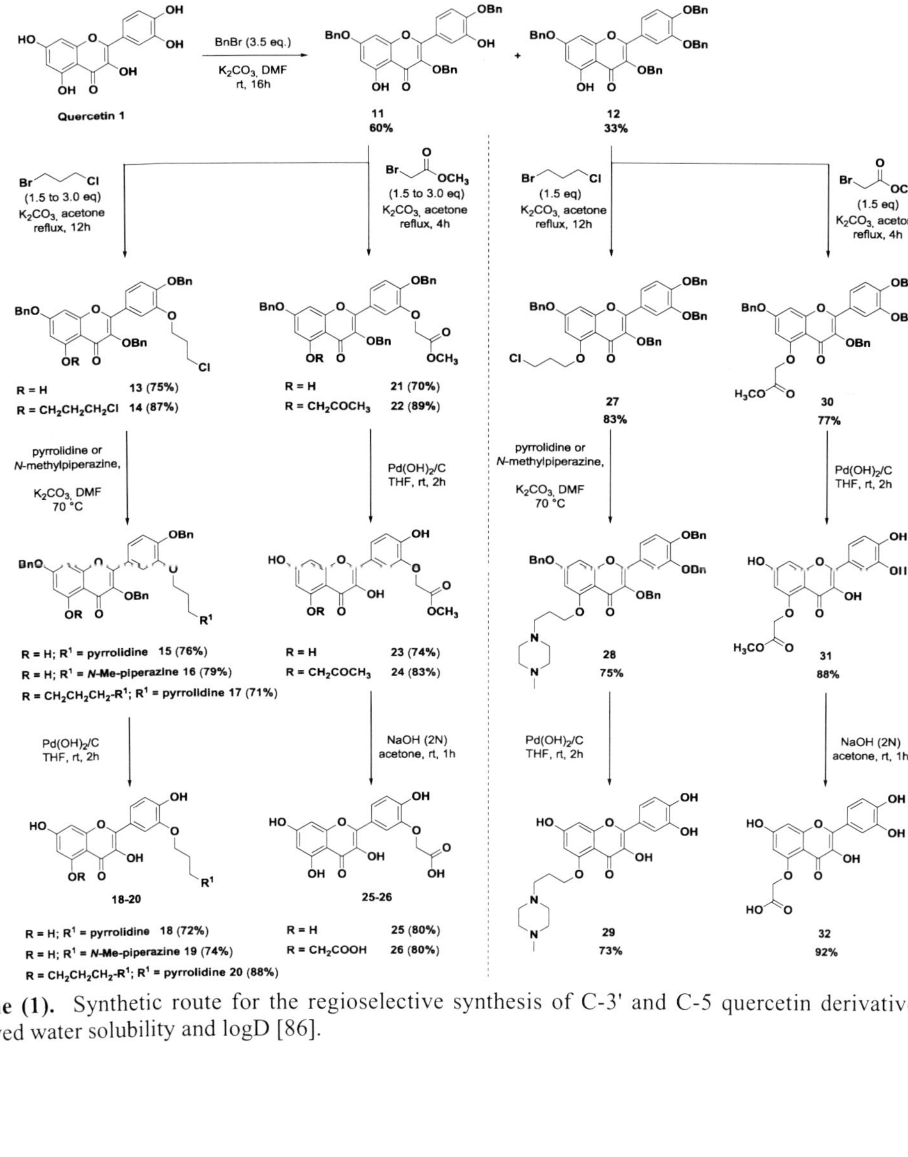

Scheme (1). Synthetic route for the regioselective synthesis of C-3' and C-5 quercetin derivatives with improved water solubility and logD [86].

Mono- and di-substitution of quercetin's core with carboxylic acid, pyrrolidine and *N*-methylpiperazine groups increased water solubility from 0.1 μg/mL up to 84.55 μg/mL in the case of pyrrolidine disubstituted compound **20**. Moreover, most derivatives showed an average ten-fold increase in antiproliferative activity against HCT116 colon cancer cells, with compounds **19**, **29** and **31** displaying sub-micromolar IC_{50} (Table **2**) [86].

Table 2. Solubility, dissociation and antiproliferative activity of semisynthetic quercetin derivatives (18-32) against HCT116 colon cancer cell lines and in CT-26 tumour carrying mice [86].

Cmpd	IC_{50} (μM)		LogD @ pH= 7.4	Water solubility μg/mL
	HCT116	CT 26		
18	1.98 ± 0.14	4.3 ± 0.08	2.15 ± 0.01	28.39 ± 0.40
19	0.47 ± 0.05	1.3 ± 0.06	2.53 ± 0.01	41.44 ± 0.58
20	2.04 ± 0.29	2.7 ± 0.09	0.65 ± 0.0	85.55 ± 2.32
29	0.55 ± 0.06	5.7 ± 0.20	ND	ND
31	0.34 ± 0.04	7.6 ± 0.16	1.81 ± 0.01	37.87 ± 0.48
32	1.74 ± 0.21	ND	0.98 ± 0.03	32.48 ± 0.21
Quercetin	45.32 ± 5.7	114	0.76 ± 0.09	0.1

When compounds were tested *in vivo* on mice carrying CT-26 tumours, they showed to be ten to a hundred times more potent than quercetin (**1**) and caused up to 60% reduction in tumour weight and increased mice lifespan. Finally, compound **29** was endowed with selective cytotoxic activity against cancer cells and high cell membrane permeability, as tested in Caco-2 assays [86].

A series of studies have proven that quercetin (**1**) has cytotoxic properties against leukemic cells. In a study involving CEM, K562 and Nalm6 leukaemia cell lines, Srivastava *et al.* [60] demonstrated that quercetin could induce apoptosis with estimated IC_{50} of 55, 44, and 20 μM, respectively. The molecular pathways involved included increased levels of phosphorylated and unphosphorylated p53, decreased levels of Bcl2 and Bcl-xL, mitochondrial release of cytochrome c, and activation of caspases [60]. However, when Alvarez *et al.* [87] looked at the pro-apoptotic effect of quercetin (**1**) in leukemic cell lines (HL60 and U937), they noticed that after 72 hours exposure to 50-75 μM quercetin the promoter methylation of TSGs such as *DAPK1* and *BCL2L11* was significantly reduced in HL60 cells, but not in U937 cells. However, DNMT1, DNMT3a, and STAT3 protein levels were found to be reduced in both cell lines [87]. At the same time, quercetin seemed to induce extensive acetylation of histones H3 and H4 across the genome, which resulted in the activation of a series of additional TSGs such as *APAF1*, *BAX*, *BNIP3*, and *BNIP3L*. These results were attributed at least in part to the ability of quercetin to induce protease degradation of class I HDACs, particularly HDAC1 and HDAC2, and they were validated in mice xenograft models of human leukaemia [87]. However, the epigenetic activity of quercetin is not limited to this class of HDACs, as this natural product has been shown to contrast the oxidative damage to the vascular endothelium caused by oxidised low-density lipoproteins (oxLDL) by increasing SIRT1 expression, even at doses as low as 2.5 μM [88]. On the other side, quercetin (**1**) and kaempferol (**2**) were reported to interact directly with enzymes belonging to the sirtuin family, particularly with SIRT6, a cytosolic isoform that is upregulated in hepatocellular carcinoma and multiple myeloma. The two flavonols seemed to behave as SIRT6 inhibitors at low concentrations (10 μM) and as activators at high concentrations (100 μM) [89]. These findings prompted the investigation of quercetin analogues as potential SIRT6 inhibitors for cancer therapy, as this enzyme is reported to play a fundamental role in DNA-damage/repair signalling and cell metabolism [90]. A study published in 2019 by Heger *et al.* [91] showed that two quercetin derivatives, diquercetin (**33**) and 2-chloro-1,4-naphthoquinone-quercetin (**34**), inhibited SIRT6 *in vitro* with IC_{50} values of 130 μM and 55 μM, respectively. Moreover, compound **34** was also able to inhibit SIRT2 with an IC_{50} value of 14 μM [91]. Docking simulations showed that diquercetin **33** forms productive hydrogen bonds and π-stacking interactions within the substrate binding site of SIRT6 and disrupts enzyme activity by interacting with the catalytic His131, while 2-chloro-1,4-naphthoquinone-quercetin **34** prefers to bind to the co-factor pocket (Fig. **7**) [91].

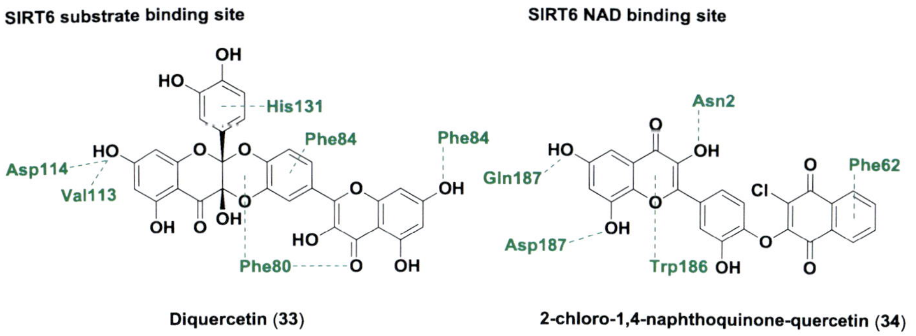

Fig. (7). Hydrogen bonding and π-stacking interactions identified by molecular docking of quercetin derivatives **33** and **34** in the substrate and co-factor pockets of histone deacetylase SIRT6 [91].

A broad *in silico* screening of a library containing thousands of flavonoids and flavonoid derivatives showed that this scaffold could be a promising starting point for the development of bromodomain inhibitors, particularly those belonging to the BET family, as it docks into the acetyl-lysine binding site that characterises these reader domains Fig. (**8A**) [92]. Interestingly, two of the derivatives that achieved the best docking scores, fisetin (**35**) and compound **36**, show structural similarity to RVX-208 (**37**), a known inhibitor of bromodomains belonging to the BET family (BRD2, BRD3, BRD4 and BRDTs) Fig. (**8B**)., and LY29002 (**39**), a dual kinase and BET bromodomain inhibitor Fig. (**8D**). Although the ability of fisetin (**35**) to act as an acetyl-lysine mimic has been reported in subsequent *in silico* studies, the best docking poses proposed for this natural compound in the binding site of the first bromodomain of BRD4 differ slightly (Fig. **8A** and **C**) [93]. In fact, one model focuses more on the hydrogen bonds formed between the inhibitor and the structural water molecules that are located at the back of the acetyl-lysine binding site Fig. (**8A**), while both studies confirm the interaction of **35** with Asn140, a highly conserved amino acid residue involved in the stabilisation of the acetyl-lysine moiety inside the pocket. As previously seen in the case of SIRT inhibitors, flavonoid dimers can imitate the behaviour of their corresponding monomers and sometimes even outperform them, thanks to their extended surface and ability to establish a higher number of weak interactions, as seen in Fig. (**8C**).

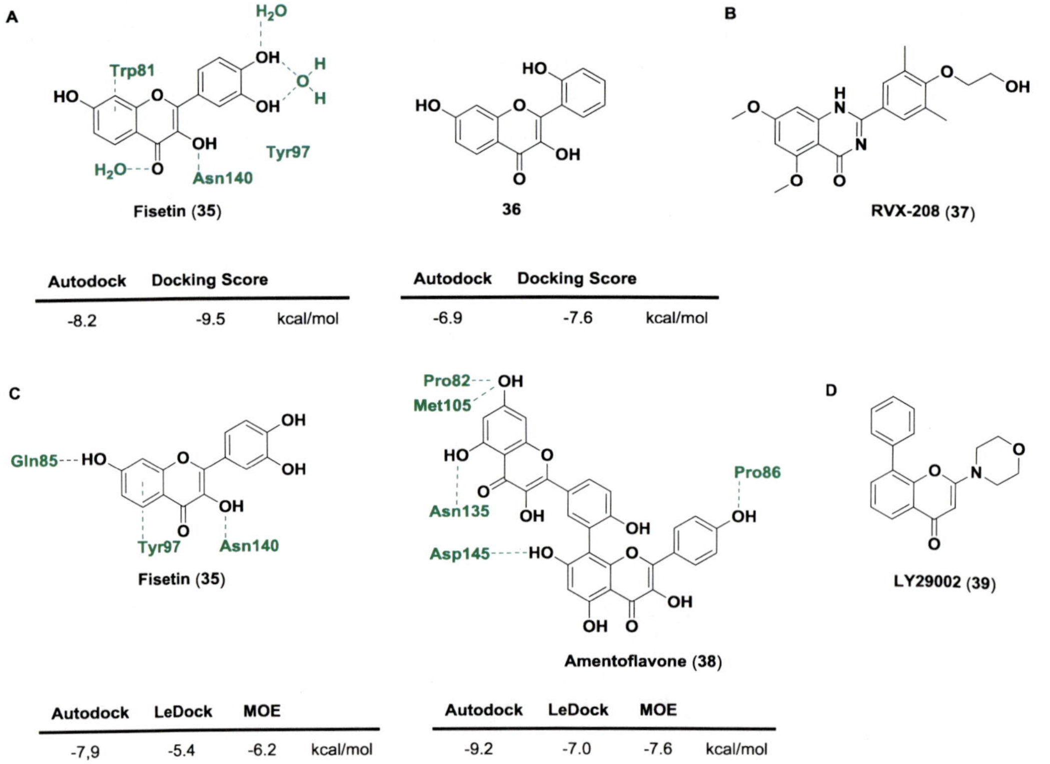

Fig. (8A and C). Flavonols identified by *in silico* screening as binders of the acetyl-lysine binding site of the first bromodomain (BD1) of BRD4. **B)** Chemical structure of RVX-28, a BET bromodomain inhibitor. **D)** Chemical structure of dual kinase and BET bromodomain inhibitor LY29002 [92, 93].

In all docking simulations involving flavonols and their derivatives, hydroxyl groups have been identified as pivotal in the formation of constructive hydrogen bonding interactions. It is therefore unsurprising that acetylation or methylation of these groups resulted in reduced interactions of the corresponding derivatives in the binding site of bromodomains. In fact, molecular modelling studies involving mono- or poly-acetylated and methylated flavonoid derivatives against the first bromodomain of BRD4 showed that the derivative forming the highest number of hydrogen bonds and showing the lowest docking score (-6.41 kcal/mol) was a monoacetylated compound **40** Fig. (**9**). However, it is important to remember that the acetyl-lysine binding side is lined with hydrophobic residues and that the ability of forming lipophilic interaction with the WPF (Trp, Pro, Phe) shelf, a highly conserved motif in the BET family situated at the entrance of the pocket, can greatly influence the activity and selectivity of bromodomain inhibitors. Given these considerations, it is possible to explain how poly-acetylated compounds were characterised by docking scores close to those recorded for a potent BRD4 inhibitor, (+)-JQ1 (-6.52 kcal/mol), despite forming a reduced number of hydrogen bonds, as shown in the case of compound **41** (Fig. **9**) [94].

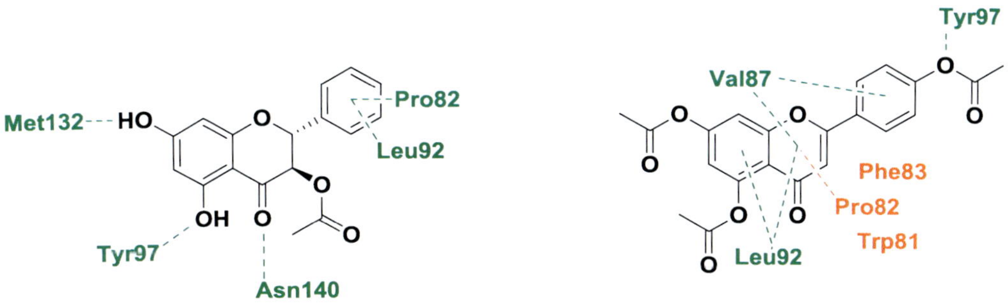

40

Docking Score -6.41 kcal/mol

41

Docking Score -6.29 kcal/mol

Fig. (9). Hydrogen bonding and steric interactions of mono- and poly-acetylated flavonoids in the binding pocket of the first bromodomain of BRD4 (PDB ID: 4CFK) [94].

Finally, flavonols have been found to be a promising starting point for the development of lysine demethylase (KDMs) inhibitors. In particular, quercetin (**1**) and its glycosylated derivatives, isoquercitrin (**42**) and rutin (**43**), showed low micromolar inhibitory activity against LSD1 (KMD1A) in *in vitro* assays (Fig. **10**) [95].

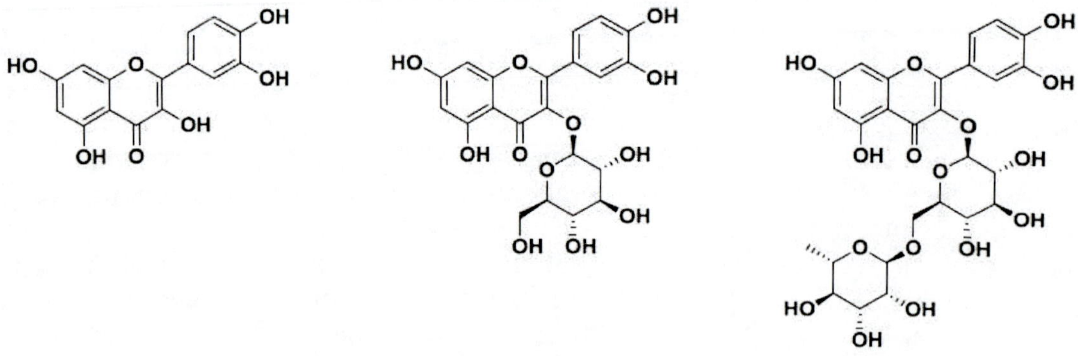

Quercetin (1) IC_{50} = 1.26 ± 0.04 μM

Isoquercitrin (42) IC_{50} = 0.95 ± 0.06 μM

Rutin (43) IC_{50} = 2.16 ± 0.33 μM

Fig. (10). Structures of quercetin (**1**) and its glycosylated analogues isoquercitrin (**42**) and rutin (**43**), and their *in vitro* inhibitory activity against histone demethylase LSD1 (KMD1A) [95].

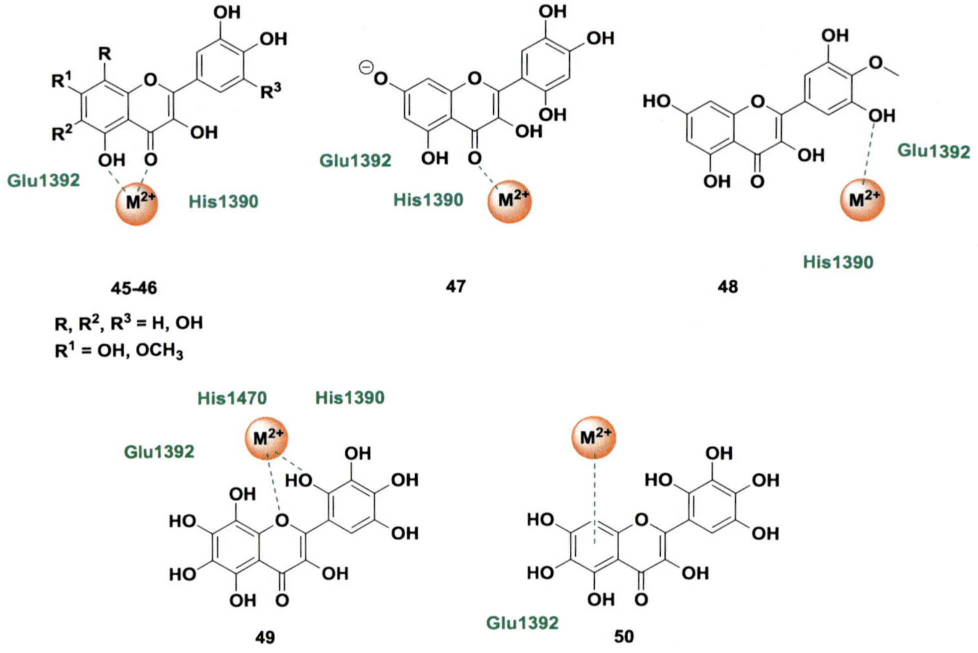

Fig. (11). Predicted mode of binding of flavonol derivatives in the active site of JMJD3 by molecular docking (PDB ID 4ASK). All reported derivatives have shown docking scores higher than 9 kcal/mol [97].

Isoquercitrin (**42**), the most active derivative, was confirmed to reduce methylation levels of H3K4 and H3K9 in MDA-MD-231 breast cancer cells in a dose-dependent manner. Moreover, Lineweaver-Burk analysis seemed to suggest that this compound behaves as a competitive inhibitor of LSD1 substrate H3K4me2 [95]. On the other hand, the flavonol myricetin (**44**) was identified as a low micromolar inhibitor (IC_{50} = 3.6 µM) of Jumonji histone demethylases JMJD2 in a high-throughput assay that screened a library of 1280 bioactive compounds (LOPAC^{1280}) [96]. This finding inspired the subsequent discovery of 65 myricetin derivatives as potential JMJD3 (KDM6B) inhibitors in *in silico* screenings based on the ZINC database. Some of these compounds (**45-50**) were capable of coordinating the central metal ion of KDMs, which in these enzymes is usually iron (II) but in the crystal structure (PDB ID: 4ASK) used in this study was replaced by cobalt(II). Moreover, they interacted with the catalytic triad constituted by two histidines (His1390 and His1470) and a glutamate residue (Glu1392) in the active site of JMJD3 (Fig. **11**) [97].

The promising antiproliferative activity showed by flavonol derivatives associated with their capacity to interact with different epigenetic proteins shows the versatility of this scaffold as a starting point for drug discovery programs on chemopreventive agents, although issues of bioavailability and metabolic stability remain to be solved.

Table 3. Summary of the epigenetic effects of flavonols in different types of cancer cells.

Cmpd	Pathology	Cell Model	Conc.	Time	Genes	Promoter Methylation		Promoter Acetylation	Histone Acetylation		Non Histone Proteins				Notes	Ref
											-	Expression	Activity			
Quercetin	Bladder Cancer	-	-	-	-	-		-	-	-	-	-	-	-	-	75
-	-	T24	100 µM	24-72 h	ESR2		⇩ 35%	-	-	-	-	-	-	-	-	-
-	-	-			$p16^{INK4a}$		⇩ 57%	-	-	-	-	-	-	-	-	-
-	-				RASSF1A		⇩ 73%			-	-	-	-	-	-	-
-	-	-			-	-	-	-	-	-	mutp53	⇩	-	-	-	-
-	-	-			-	-	-	-	-	-	survivin	⇩	-	-	-	-
Quercetin	Breast Cancer	-	-	-	-	-	-	-	-	-	-	-	-	-	-	77
-	-	MDA-MB-231	1-20 µM	48 h	-	-	-	-	H3K9	⇨	-	-	-	-	-	-
-	-				BRCA1	-	-	⇧	-	-	Brca1	⇧	-	-	-	-
-	-	MDA-MB-468					-			-				-	-	-
Curcumin	Breast Cancer	-	-	-	-	-	-	-	-	-	-	-	-	-	-	77
-	-	MDA-MB-231	1-20 µM	48 h	-	-	-	-	H3K9	⇨	-	-	-	-	-	-
-	-				BRCA1	-	-	⇧	-	-	Brca1	⇧	-	-	-	-
-	-	MDA-MB-468					-			-				-	-	-
Quercetin + Curcumin	Breast Cancer	-	-	-	-	-	-	-	-	-	-	-	-	-	-	77
-	-	MDA-MB-231	20 µM Q + 10 µM C	48 h	-	-	-	-	H3K9	⇨	-	-	-	-	Synergistic effect	
-	-				BRCA1	-	-	⇧	-	-	Brca1	⇧	-	-		
-	-	MDA-MB-468					-			-				-		

(Table 3) cont.....

Cmpd	Pathology	Cell Model	Conc.	Time	Genes	Promoter Methylation		Promoter Acetylation	Histone Acetylation		Non Histone Proteins				Notes	Ref
											-	Expression	Activity			
Quercetin	Cervical Cancer	-	-	-	-	-	-	-	-	-	-	-	-	-	-	82
-	-	HeLa	-	-	DAPK1	⇩	-	-	-	-	DNMT1	⇩		⇩ 49-71%		-
-	-	-	-	-	RARB	⇩	-	-	-	-	DNMT3A	⇩				-
-	-	-	-	-	PTEN	⇩	-	-	-	-	DNMT3b	⇩				-
-	-	-	-	-	RASSF1	⇩	-	-	-	-	HDAC1	⇩		⇩ 32-63%		-
-	-	-	-	-	GSTP1	⇩	-	-	-	-	HDAC2	⇩				-
-	-	-	-	-	SOC51	⇩	-	-	-	-	HDAC3	⇩				-
-	-	-	-	-	MGMT	⇩	-	-	-	-	HDAC5	⇩				-
-	-	-	-	-	APC	⇩	-	-	-	-	HDAC6	⇩				-
-	-	-	-	-	CDH1	⇩	-	-	-	-	HDAC7	⇩				-
-	-	-	-	-	CDH13	⇩	-	-	-	-	HDAC11	⇩				-
-	-	-	-	-	FHIT	⇩	-	-	-	-	KDM5B	⇩	-	-	-	-
-	-	-	-	-	MLH1	⇩	-	-	-	-	HAT1	⇩	-	-	-	-
-	-	-	-	-	TIMP3	⇩	-	-	-	-	HMT	-	-	-	-	-
-	-	-	-	-	VHL	⇩	-	-	-	-	-	-	-	-	-	-
Quercetin	Leukemia	-	-	-	-	-	-	-	-	-	-	-	-	-	-	87
-	-	HL60 & U937	50-75 µM	48-72 h	DAPK1	⇩	-	⇧	H3 and H4	⇧	DNMT1	⇩	-	-	-	-
-	-	-			BCL2L11	⇩	-	⇧			DNMT3a	⇩	-	-	-	-
-	-	-	-	-	BAX	-	-	⇧			STAT3	⇩	-	-	-	-
-	-	-	-	-	APAF1	-	-	⇧			HDAC1	-	-	-	-	-
-	-	-	-	-	BNIP3	-	-	⇧			HDAC2	-	⇩	-	increased proteasome degradation	
-	-	-	-	-	BNIP3L	-	-	⇧				-	⇩	-		
Kaempferol	Bladder Cancer	-	-	-	-	-	-	-	-	-	-	-	-	-	-	74
-	-	T24 xenografts	150 mg/Kg	-	WRN	⇩	-	-	-	-	DNMT3B	⇩	-	-		
-	-	T24 cell line	-	-	-	-	-	-	-	-	DNMT1	⇩	-	-		
-	-	5637 cell line	-	-	-	-	-	-	-	-	DNMT3A	⇩	-	-		
Kaempferol	Hepatoma	-	-	-	-	-	-	-	-	-	-	-	-	-	-	71
-	-	HepG2	5-100 µM	96 h	-	-	-	-	H3	⇧	HDACs	⇩	-	-		
-	-	Hep3B	5-100 µM	96 h	-	-	-	-	H3	⇧	-	-	-	-		
Kaempferol	Leukemia	-	-	-	-	-	-	-	-	-	-	-	-	-	-	72
-	-	K562 U937	50 µM	24-72 h	-	-	-	-	-	-	SIRT3	⇧	-	-		
-	-					-	-	-	-	-	Bax	⇧	-	-		
-	-					-	-	-	-	-	Bcl-2	⇩	-	-		
-	-					-	-	-	-	-	Bcl-xL	⇨	-	-		
-	-					-	-	-	-	-	Caspase3	-	⇧	-		
-	-					-	-	-	-	-	Caspase9	-	⇧	-		

Flavones: Apigenin, Luteolin and Chrysin

Flavones are a class of flavonoids characterised by a shared 4*H*-chromenone core variously substituted at the 2-, 5-, and 7- positions (Fig. **12**). The most abundant flavones in fruits and vegetables are apigenin (**51**) and luteolin (**52**), as they can be found in carrots, peppers, broccoli, herbs like celery, parsley, thyme, rosemary, oregano, peppermint, chamomile, and citrus fruits like grapefruits and oranges [98, 99]. In comparison, the dietary exposure to chrysin (**53**) is fairly limited, as although this flavone can be commonly found in plants and flowers, it finds its way in the diet through foods that are usually consumed in small amounts, such as honey and propolis [100].

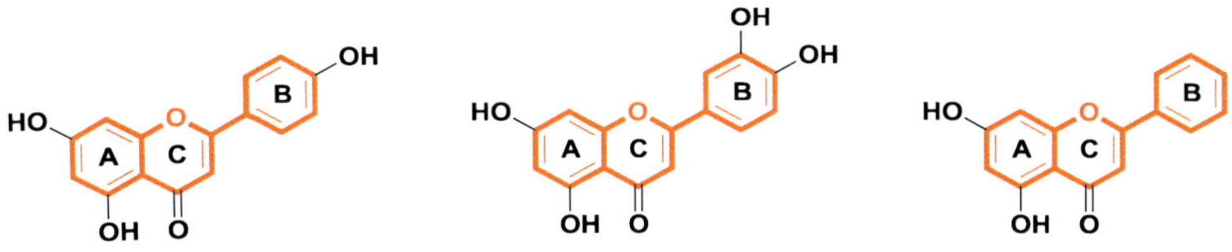

Fig. (12). Structure of the most abundant flavones Apigenin (**51**), Luteolin (**52**), and Chrysin (**53**).

Similarly to what has been observed for other members of the flavonoid family, flavones rich diets have been associated to reduced incidence of lung, ovarian, breast, prostate and colorectal cancer [98]. The antitumor activity of this class of phytochemicals has been ascribed to their ability to interfere with a wide range of pathways involved in cell proliferation, such as TNF-α induced activation of NFκB, as well as MAPK, PI3K/Akt, TRAIL, WNT/β-catenin, and JAK-STAT signalling [98, 99, 101, 102]. In the case of oestrogen-responsive cancers, such as breast and prostate cancer, flavones like apigenin have also been shown to induce apoptosis through a mechanism that involves selective activation of oestrogen receptor β (ER-β) [103]. However, further studies on breast and prostate cancer cell lines showed that the apoptotic process is often accompanied by significant inhibition of HDACs activity, resulting in genome-wide changes of acetylation levels. In triple negative breast cancer cells (MDA-MB-231), exposure to 40 μM apigenin for 1-4 days inhibited HDACs activity in a time-dependent manner and induced an increment in histone 3 acetylation that correlated with increased expression of cyclin dependent kinase inhibitor $p21^{WAF/CIP1}$ and cell cycle arrest in the G2/M phase. These *in vitro* results were reproduced *in vivo* using MDA-M--231 xenografts implanted on nude mice that received 5 or 25 mg kg^{-1} apigenin per day for a duration of 8 weeks [104]. Similarly, when prostate cancer cell lines (PC3 and 2 Rv1) were treated with 20-40 μM apigenin for 24 hours, an increase in $p21^{WAF/CIP1}$ and bax expression was observed as a consequence of dose-dependent HDAC inhibition and augmented promoter acetylation [105]. Although apigenin has been reported to inhibit class I HDACs *in vitro* (IC_{50} = 25 μM) and it is capable of binding the catalytic pocket of HDAC1 and 2 [106, 107], the reduced activity of HDAC1 and HDAC3 in these prostate cancer cell lines was clearly associated with a change in HDACs expression levels [105]. The treatment of mice carrying PC-3 xenografts with 20-50 μg/day apigenin confirmed the *in vivo* effectiveness of this flavone as an antiproliferative agent, as it caused 41.8-50.6% tumour shrinkage [105]. Interestingly, Kanwal *et al.* [61] recently reported that apigenin (**51**), luteolin (**52**) and chrysin (**53**) could also interfere with gene expression by acting as dual inhibitors of DNMT1 and histone methyltransferase EZH2. In fact, all three flavones were shown to bind *in silico* models of the catalytic pockets of DNMT1 (Fig. **13**) and EZH2 Fig. (**14**), while establishing effective hydrogen bonding and π-stacking interactions [61].

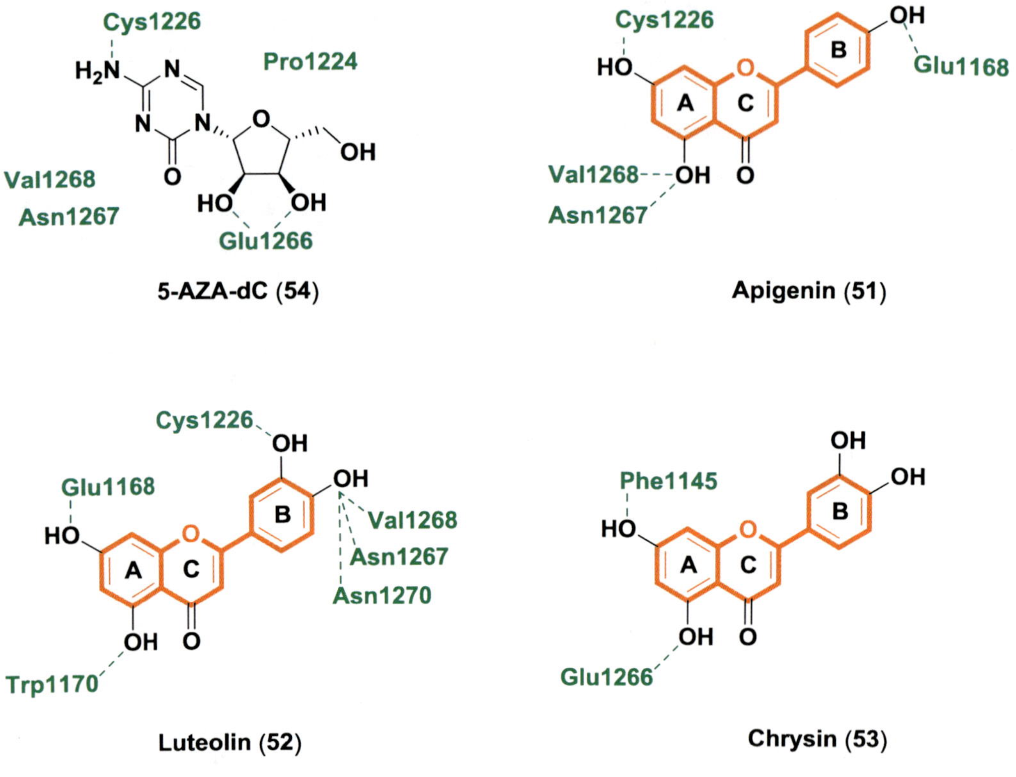

Fig. (13). Hydrogen bonding interactions identified by molecular docking of flavones apigenin, luteolin, and chrysin in the binding pocket of DNMT1, compared to the hydrogen bonding interactions formed by 5-az--2'deoxycitidine, a known DNMT1 inhibitor [61].

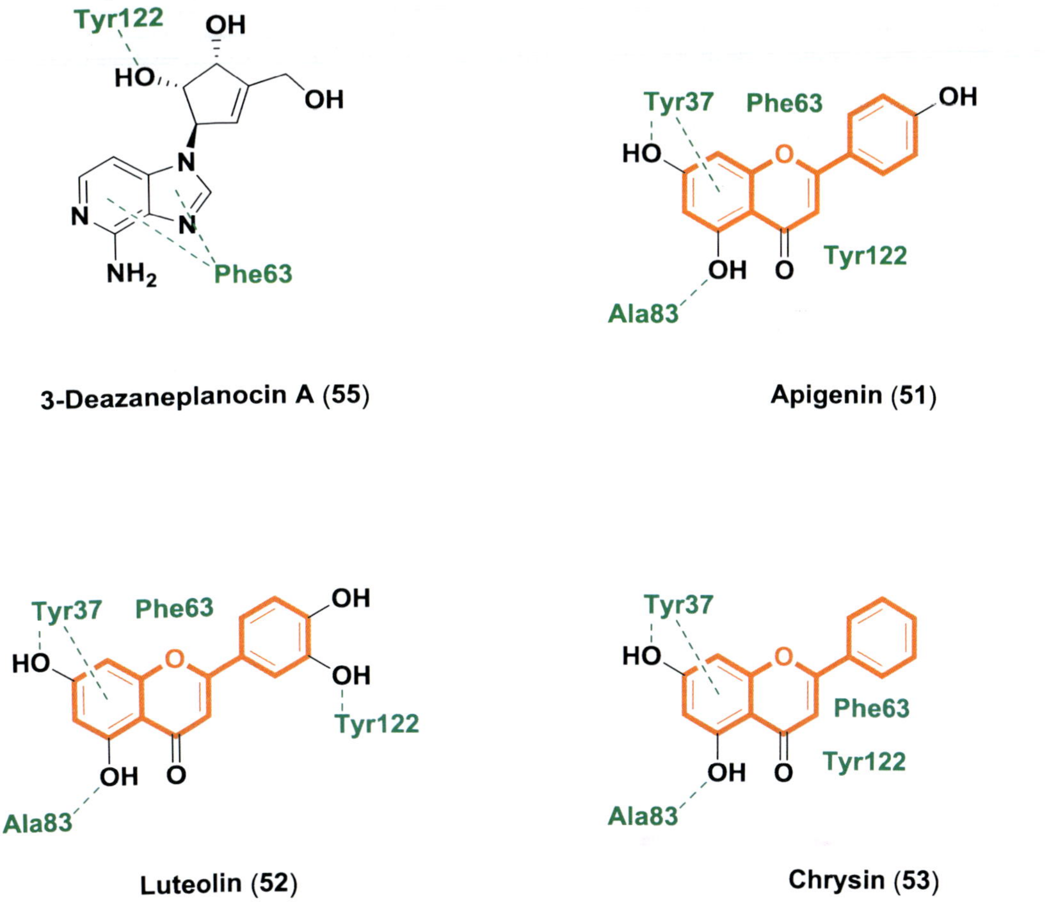

Fig. (14). Hydrogen bonding and π-stacking interactions identified by molecular docking of apigenin, luteolin, and chrysin in the binding pocket of methyl transferase EZH2, compared to the hydrogen bonding interactions formed by 3-deazaneplanocin A, a known EHZ2 inhibitor [61].

Both enzymes are known to possess a repressive effect on gene expression, as the enhancer of zeste 2 polycomb repressive complex 2 subunit (EZH2) induces trimethylation of H3K27, a known marker of transcriptional silencing, and the DNA methyltransferase 1 increases cytosine methylation at CpG sites. However, it has also been demonstrated that EZH2 plays an important role in the recruitment of DNMT1 at specific *loci* [108]. Therefore, the simultaneous inhibition of both enzymes could have a synergistic effect in promoting the activation of onco-suppressor genes. In fact, apigenin has been shown to reactivate the expression of Nrf2, a transcription factor that regulates the expression of enzymes involved in the cellular response to stress signals, in mouse

JBP6 P+ skin cancer cells [109]. This effect was directly correlated with a reduction in DNMT1, DNMT3A and DNMT3B expression, which resulted in decreased methylation of the Nrf2 promoter. At the same time, several HDACs were found to be downregulated, particularly HDAC3, HDAC4, HDAC6, HDAC7, and HDAC8, thus suggesting that this class of flavonoids can induce epigenetic changes and control cell-cycle progression simultaneously at multiple levels.

Table 4. Summary of the epigenetic effects of flavones in different types of cancer cells.

Cmpd	Pathology	Cell Model	Conc.	Time	Genes	Promoter Methylation		Promoter Acetylation	Histone Acetylation		Non Histone Proteins					Notes	Ref
											-	Expression		Activity			
Apigenin	Breast Cancer	-	-	-	-	-		-	-	-	-	-		-	-	-	104
-	-	MDA-MB-231	40 µM	24-96 h	p21		-	↑	H3	↑	$p21^{WAF1}$	↑		-	-	-	-
-	-	-			-		-	-	-	-	cyclidin A	↓		-	-	-	-
-	-	-			-		-	-	-	-	cyclidin B	↓		-	-	-	-
-	-	-				-	-	-	-	-	CDK1	↓		-	-	-	-
-	-	MDA-MB-231 xenografts	5-25 mg/Kg	8 weeks	p21		-	↑	H3	↑	$p21^{WAF1}$	↑		-	-	-	-
-	-					-	-	-	-	-	cyclidin A	↓		-	-	-	-
-	-	-				-	-	-	-	-	cyclidin B	↓		-	-	-	-
Apigenin	Prostate Cancer	-	-	-	-	-	-	-	-	-	-	-		-	-	-	104
-	-	PC-3	20 µM	24 h	-	-	-	-	H3	↑	HDAC1	↓	28%	HDACs	↓	-	-
-	-	-			-	-	-	-	H4	↑	HDAC3	↓	30%				-
-	-	-			p21	-	-	↑	-	-	$p21^{WAF1}$	↑	x 1.2	-	-	-	-
-	-	-				-	-	-	-	-	Bax	↑	x 3.9	-	-	-	-
-	-	-	40 µM			-	-	-	H3	↑	HDAC1	↓	46%	HDACs	↓	-	-
-	-	-			-	-	-	-	H4	↑	HDAC3	↓	48%				-
-	-	-			p21	-	-	-	-	-	$p21^{WAF1}$	↑	x 2.0	-	-	-	-
-	-	-				-	-	-	-	-	Bax	↑	x 11.2	-	-	-	-
-	-	22 Rv1	20 µM	24 h	-	-	-	-	H3	↑	HDAC1	↓	39%	HDACs	↓	-	-
-	-	-			-	-	-	-	H4	↑	HDAC3	↓	45%	-	-	-	-
-	-	-				-	-	-	-	-	$p21^{WAF1}$	↑	x 3.6	-	-	-	-
-	-	-				-	-	-	-	-	Bax	↑	x 1.7	-	-	-	-
-	-	-	40 µM			-	-	-	H3	↑	HDAC1	↓	52%	HDACs	-	-	-
-	-	-			-	-	-	-	H4	↑	HDAC3	↓	22%	-	-	-	-
-	-	-				-	-	-	-	-	$p2^{WAF1}$	↑	x 3.4	-	-	-	-
-	-	-				-	-	-	-	-	Bax	↑	x 1.8	-	-	-	-
-	-	-				-	-	-	-	-	p53	↑	-	-	-	-	-
-	-	PC- 3 xenografts	20-50 µg/day	8 weeks	-	-	-	-	-	-	HDAC1	↓	-	-	-	Tumour volume was reduced by 41.8% and 50.6%	
-	-					-	-	-	-	-	HDAC3	↓	-	-	-		
-	-	-				-	-	-	-	-	$p21^{WAF1}$	↑	-	-	-		
-	-	-				-	-	-	-	-	bax	↑	-	-	-		
-	-	-				-	-	-	-	-	bcl-2		-	-	-		

(Table 4) cont.....

Cmpd	Pathology	Cell Model	Conc.	Time	Genes	Promoter Methylation		Promoter Acetylation	Histone Acetylation		Non Histone Proteins				Notes	Ref
											-	Expression	Activity			
Apigenin	Prostate Cancer	-	-	-	-	-	-	-	-	-	-	-	-	-	-	61
-	-	LNCaP	10 μM	48 h	-	-	-	-	-	-	-		DNMTs	↓	-	-
-	-	-	20 μM		-	-	-	-	-	-	-					-
-	-	DU145	10 μM	48 h	-	-	-	-	H3K27		-	-	-	-	-	-
-	-	-	20 μM		-	-	-	-			-	-	-	-	-	-
-	-	-			-	-	-	-	-	-	EZH2	↓	-	-	-	-
Apigenin	Skin Cancer	-	-	-	-	-	-	-	-	-	-	-	-	-	-	109
-	-	JB6 P+	1.56 μM	120 h	NRF2	↓	-	-	-	-	Nrf2	↑	-	-	-	-
-	-	-	6.25 μM					-	-	-				-	-	-
-	-	-				-	-	-	-	-	DNMT1	↓	-	-	-	-
-	-	-				-	-	-	-	-	DNMT3A	↓	-	-	-	-
-	-	-				-	-	-	-	-	DNMT3b	↓	-	-	-	-
-	-	-				-	-	-	-	-	HDAC1	↓	-	-	-	-
-	-	-				-	-	-	-	-	HDAC2	↓	-	-	-	-
-	-	-				-	-	-	-	-	HDAC3	↓	-	-	-	-
-	-	-				-	-	-	-	-	HDAC4	↓	-	-	-	-
-	-	-				-	-	-	-	-	HDAC5	↓	-	-	-	-
-	-	-				-	-	-	-	-	HDAC6	↓	-	-	-	-
-	-	-				-	-	-	-	-	HDAC7	↓	-	-	-	-
-	-	-				-	-	-	-	-	HDAC8	↓	-	-	-	-

Isoflavones: Genistein and Daidzein

Thanks to their structural resemblance to sex hormones and their ability to bind the oestrogen receptors ER-α and ER-β, flavonoids are considered one of the most highly represented groups of phytoestrogens, xenobiotics of plant origin with oestrogenic properties [110]. In particular, isoflavones like genistein (**3**) are reported to behave as weak ER agonists, as they require concentrations 100-1000 times higher than the endogenous ligand 17β-estradiol (E2) to achieve the same receptor binding affinity. Other flavonoids like kaempferol (**2**) can act as very weak agonists or antagonists depending on the concentrations used [111]. Due to their capacity to mimic oestrogens mediated response, phytoestrogens have been considered for a long time potential adjuvants for the management of post-menopausal symptoms and the prevention of menopause associated diseases such as atherosclerosis and osteoporosis [112, 113]. On the other side, the oestrogenic activity of flavonoids like genistein (**3**) has been the cause of raising concerns regarding the safety of these natural remedies in patients at high risk of oestrogen-responsive malignancies [114, 115]. To complicate the matter, clinical studies in which pre- and post-menopausal women were administered elevated doses of isoflavones for a prolonged period of time (5 months to 2 years) returned contrasting results [116]. In some instances, isoflavones seemed to demonstrate weak oestrogenic activity, as they induced the secretion of breast fluid and the expression of cell proliferation markers [117, 118]. In others, despite low levels of oestrogenic stimulus, no changes could be detected in cell proliferation or expression of oestrogen receptors and breast cancer predictive markers [119 - 121]. Moreover, the prolonged exposure to phytoestrogens-rich diets has been correlated with reduced risk of developing cancer [122]. In particular, the low incidence of breast and prostate cancer in the Asian population, where the consumption of soy is tendentially very high, has prompted a wide number of investigations on the chemopreventive effects of soy isoflavones genistein (**3**) and daidzein (**56**) (Fig. **15**) [123].

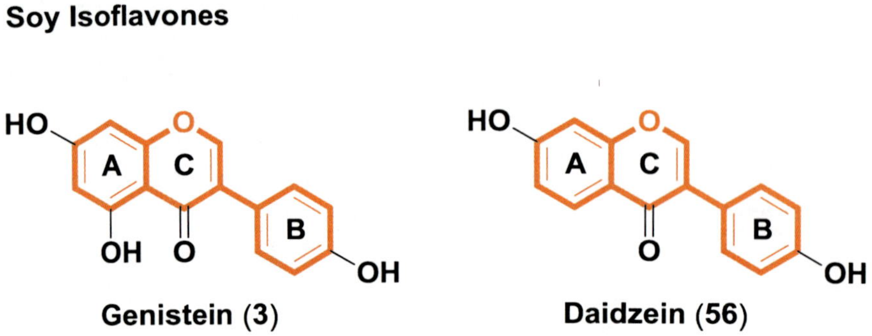

Fig. (15). Chemical structure of soy isoflavones Genistein (**3**) and Daidzein (**56**).

Several mechanisms have been proposed to explain genistein (**3**) and daidzein's (**56**) antiproliferative activity. In LNCaP prostate cancer cells, the treatment with doses lower than 20 μM of genistein (**3**) caused cell cycle block in the G_0/G_1 phase, while inducing the expression of p27^{KIP1} and p21^{WAF1}, two cyclin dependent kinase inhibitors whose genes are known to be downregulated in aggressive forms of prostate cancers [124]. However, genistein (**3**) induced cell apoptosis only at concentrations that are unlikely to be achieved following a soy-rich diet, thus confirming previous reports that placed its IC_{50} against different prostate cancer cell lines (LNCaP, DU145, and PC3) beyond 40 μM [125, 126]. Additional studies have shown that genistein can stop the cell cycle in the G_2/M phase by reducing the expression of cyclin B and inhibit cell growth by preventing the activation of several kinases (ERK1/2 and PI3K) involved in transmitting the proliferative signal of insulin-like and epidermal growth factors [127]. At the same time, genistein and daidzein are thought to induce apoptosis by inhibiting proteasome activity, potentiating the activity of TRAIL, a cytokine belonging to the tumour necrosis factor (TNF) family that selectively kills tumour cells, and activating necrosis factor NFκB and other cell-cycle inhibitors [128, 129].

A growing body of evidence suggests that these observed intracellular events could be the manifestation of a more profound control exerted by genistein and other flavonoids on genes regulation and expression through epigenetic mechanisms [116]. In a series of studies conducted in rats, the foetal and early-life exposure to genistein was associated with lifelong changes in DNA methylation at the promoter region of genes involved in haematopoiesis and proliferation of mammary epithelial cells, as well as down-regulation of oestrogen receptor mediated response [22, 24]. Two genes associated with increased survival chances in breast cancer patients, HPSE and RPS9, were found to be hypomethylated in rats subjected to early postnatal treatment with genistein [130]. Inhibition of DNMTs activity and expression have been proposed as one of the most plausible mechanisms through which genistein induces the re-expression of tumour suppressing genes (TSG), often silenced in cancer cells as a result of promoter hypermethylation. In a study that compared ER-α(+) and ER-α(-) breast cancer cells MCF-7 and MDA-MB-231, Xie *et al.* [131] showed that the treatment with 60-100 μM genistein for 48-72 hours caused significant reduction in both activity and expression of DNMT1, while DNMT3A and 3B did not seemed to be affected. ER-α(+) MCF-7 cells seemed to be more susceptible than ER-α(-) MDA-MB-231, as after treatment with 100 μM genistein (**3**) for 72 hours DNMT1 expression was reduced down to approximately 20% of its original level in MCF-7 cells, while it reached only 60% of its original levels in MDA-MB-231 cells. The authors conducted a molecular modelling study to explore the ability of this isoflavone to bind the catalytic pocket of DNMT1 and discovered that genistein is capable of forming effective hydrogen bonds with Phe1145 and Leu1153, two amino acid residues involved in the stabilisation of the flipped cytosine substrate. The direct interaction of genistein and DNMT1 was therefore proposed as one of the potential mechanisms responsible for the decrease in DNMT1 activity, which resulted in hypomethylation of a series of gene promoters often hypermethylated in breast cancer, such as *PTEN* and *APC* [131]. Most importantly, at physiologically achievable levels (1 μM) genistein can prevent the methylation of CpG islands at the promoter region of TSGs caused by the activation of the aryl hydrocarbon receptor (AhR), an environmental sensor that responds to xenobiotics such as polyaromatic hydrocarbons and other toxins [132]. It is interesting to note that activation of AhR in rodent models of breast cancer determines hypermethylation at the exon 1a of *BRCA1*, a tumour suppressor gene that is found to be responsible of 50% of familial forms of breast cancer and it is normally downregulated in sporadic forms [133]. Genistein (**3**) is reported to have a biphasic effect on *BRCA1* expression in ER-α(+) MCF-7 cells with activated AhR: at concentrations between 0.5-1.0 μM, genistein (**3**) restores *BRCA1* expression at levels normally induced by E2 stimulation, while at the same time increasing the expression of p53; at concentrations between 5-20 μM, way beyond the plasma levels achievable only by consuming a soy-rich diet, genistein can amplify the xenobiotic induced repression of *BRCA1* expression [131]. In ER-α(-) UACC-3199 cell lines, where AhR is constitutively expressed and does not require ligand-based activation, higher concentrations of genistein (10-20 μM) are required in order to witness similar levels of *BRCA1* promoter demethylation as seen in ER-α(+) MCF-7 cells [131]. Similarly, in triple negative breast cancer cell lines HCC38 where AhR is often overexpressed, 10 μM genistein reversed hypermethylation and caused a 74% reduction in AhR binding to the promoter of *BRCA1*, when compared to untreated cells [134]. Interestingly, pre-treatment with genistein seemed to sensitise HCC38 cells to the treatment with 4-hydroxytamoxifen. Since BRCA1 is required for the transactivation of *ESR1*, the gene encoding for ER-α, it has been suggested that genistein could induce sensitisation to antioestrogen drugs by restoring, at least in part, the ER-α mediated response in triple negative breast cancer cells. Moreover, mice being fed a genistein-rich diet since conception showed a decrease of basal *BRCA1* promoter methylation levels in the mammary gland [134].

DNA-methylation is not the exclusive epigenetic mechanism affected by exposure to genistein. In MCF-7 cells treated with 1 μM genistein for 48 hours, researchers reported an increase in HDACs activity, which was associated with enhanced HDAC6 expression, while registering a simultaneous decrease in HATs activity [135]. Increased deacetylase activity associated with diminished binding of HAT/p300 at the distal promoter of catechol-*O*-methyl transferase (COMT) resulted in decreased levels of H3K4 and H3K9 acetylation in this region and consequent repression of COMT transcription. Interestingly, this study found a simultaneous increase of DNA methylation at the same *loci*. In fact, E2 induced expression of COMT in the same cell line could be reversed by treatment with a DNMT inhibitor such as 5-azacytidine (5-AZA), or a HDAC inhibitor like trichostatin A (TSA) [135]. Since the inhibition of COMT has been linked to increased susceptibility of breast epithelial cells to oxidative DNA damage and has been implicated in the pathogenesis of breast cancer, it would be important to assess the extent to which genistein-induced COMT inhibition impacts on the safety of this chemopreventive agent. Dietary combination of natural epigenetic modulators might provide a response to some of these concerns. For example, when genistein (**3**) was combined with sulforaphanes (SFN), a class of highly abundant compounds in cruciferous vegetables renowned for their HDAC inhibitory activity, the mixture (5 μM SFN and 15 μM GEN) seemed to exert synergistic effect against MCF-7 and MDA-MB-231 cells but did not reduce cell *via*bility of non-cancerous cells (MCF10A) [136]. Treated cells showed a decrease in HDACs activity and expression, especially in the case of HDAC2 and HDAC3. The combination of sulforaphanes and genistein was confirmed to produce a synergistic chemopreventive and chemotherapeutic effect in a transgenic mouse model for breast cancer (C(3)1-SV40), as both tumour incidence and growth were significantly reduced in comparison to the control cohort, as well as the two cohorts subjected to single interventions. In adult humans, the doses administered would correspond roughly to the equivalent of two cups of broccoli sprouts and two grams of genistein (**3**) per day [136].

Of course, the ability of genistein to modulate epigenetic mechanisms is not restricted to breast cancer cells. When human cervical cancer cells (HeLa) were treated with 15 μM genistein for 24-96 hours, a reduction was observed in both expression and activity of DNMTs, including DNMT1, DNMT3A and DNMT3B, as well as HDACs, particularly HDAC1, HDAC3, HDAC6, and HDAC7 [137]. Unsurprisingly, DNMTs inhibition led to extensive demethylation of CpG islands in the promoter region of TSGs such as MGMT, RARβ, p21, *E*-cadherin, and DAPK1. HDAC inhibition can also have significant impact on cancer progression. Specifically, the overexpression of HDACs in cervical cancer represents a known predictor of poor prognosis and lowered chances of patient survival, especially with reference to HDAC6, a cytoplasmic isoform that plays a fundamental role in regulating the acetylation state of Hsp90 chaperone and the maturation of oncoproteins, such as Bcr-Abl and Her2 [138]. A molecular modelling study confirmed that genistein (**3**) can dock in the substrate binding pocket of both DNMTs and HDACs, and that its interactions with amino acid residues within these pockets largely overlap with those described for known DNMT and HDAC inhibitors 5-AZA-2'-deoxycytidine (**54**) and TSA, respectively [137].

The incidence and progression of prostate cancer is similarly thought to be affected by exposure to isoflavones in the diet [127]. An investigation on how genome-wide methylation levels vary after exposure to soy isoflavones showed that genistein **3** (40 μM) induced demethylation of 37.5% of regions in androgen insensitive (DU-145) prostate cancer cells and 61.1% in androgen sensitive (LNCaP) cells. In the same way, exposure to 110 μM daidzein for 48 hours caused demethylation of 32.9% and 84.9% of methylated regions in DU-145 and LNCaP cells, respectively. The registered changes in methylation patterns were reported to implicate 58 genes, amongst which we find proteins involved in the control of the mitotic checkpoint (*MAD1L1*), an E3 ubiquitin ligase involved in the downregulation of NFκB activity (tumour necrosis factor associated protein 7, *TNF7*), a lysine demethylase (*KDM4B*) known to play a pivotal role in ubiquitination and degradation of AhR, and *hTERT*, the telomerase reverse transcriptase unit of the human telomerase complex [139]. However, when ARCap-E prostate cancer cells were treated with a much lower concentration of genistein **3** (20 μM), this natural product did not seem to have any effect on the methylation state of CpG islands across the genome. On the contrary, an increment of *HAT1* expression was recorded, together with an increase in promoter acetylation and consequent expression of tumour suppressing genes such *APC* and *WIF1* [140]. In the case of KYSE 510 oesophageal squamous cell carcinoma, the treatment with genistein **3** (2-20 μM) reversed hypermethylation at the promoter region of TSGs such as retinoic acid receptor β (RARβ), MGMT, and p16$^{INK\alpha}$ and increased their mRNA levels. However, much higher concentrations (50-100 μM) were required to see substantial (40-70%) inhibition of DNMTs activity [141]. The activity of histone deacetylases was also inhibited by the exposure of KYSE 510 cells to 20-100 μM genistein, although the decrement was significantly lower (10-30%) than the one observed in the case of DNMTs [141].

Table 5. Summary of the epigenetic effects of isoflavones in different types of cancer cells.

Cmpd	Pathology	Cell Model	Conc.	Time	Genes	Promoter Methylation		Promoter Acetylation	Histone Acetylation		Non Histone Proteins				Notes	Ref
											-	Expression	Activity			
Genistein	Breast Cancer	-	-	-	-	-		-	-	-	-	-	-	-	-	132
-	-	MCF-7	1 μM	24-48 h	BRCA1	↓	-	-	-	-	Brca1	↑	-	-	-	-
-	-	-	-	-	-		-	-	-	-	Cyclidin D1	↓	-	-	-	-
-	-	-	-	-	-		-	-	-	-	DNMT1	↓	-	-	-	-
-	-	-	-	-	-	-	-	-	-	-	p53	↑	-	-	-	-
Genistein	Breast Cancer	-	-	-	-	-	-	-	-	-	-	-	-	-	-	132
-	-	UACC-3199	1 μM	-	BRCA1	→	-	-	-	-	Brca1	→	-	-	-	-
-	-	-			-	-	-	-	-	-	CYP1A1	↑	-	-	-	-
-	-	-	5 μM	-	BRCA1	→	-	-	-	-	Brca1	-	-	-	-	-
-	-	-			ESR1	↓	-	-	-	-	-	-	-	-	-	-
-	-	-		-				-	-	-	-	-	-	-	-	-
-	-	-	10 μM		-	-	-	-	-	-	Cyclidin D1	-	-	-	-	-
-	-	-			BRCA1	↓	-	-	-	-	Brca1		-	-	-	-
-	-	-	20 μM	-				-	-	-				-	-	-
Genistein	Breast Cancer	-	-	-	-	-	-	-	-	-	-	-	-	-	-	134
-	-	HCC38	10 μM	-	BRCA1	↓	-	-	-	-	Brca1	-	-	-	-	-
-	-	-	-	-	-	-	-	-	-	-	ERα	-	-	-	-	-
Genistein	Breast Cancer	-	-	-	-	-	-	-	-	-	-	-	-	-	-	135
-	-	MCF-7	1 μM	-	COMT	↓	-	-	H3K4	↓	COMT	↓	-	-	-	-
-	-	-	-	-	-	-	-	-	H3K9	↓	-	-	-	-	-	-
-	-	-	-	-	-	-	-	-	-	-	DNMT1	↑	DNMTs	↑	-	-
-	-	-	-	-	-	-	-	-	-	-	DNMT3A	→				-
-	-	-	-	-	-	-	-	-	-	-	DNMT3B	→				-
-	-	-	-	-	-	-	-	-	-	-	HDAC1	→	HDACs	↑	-	-
-	-	-	-	-	-	-	-	-	-	-	HDAC6	↑				-
-	-	-	-	-	-	-	-	-	-	-	HAT/p300	↓	HATs	↓	-	-

(Table 5) cont.....

Cmpd	Pathology	Cell Model	Conc.	Time	Genes	Promoter Methylation		Promoter Acetylation	Histone Acetylation		Non Histone Proteins				Notes	Ref
											-	Expression	Activity			
Genistein	Breast Cancer	-	-	-	-	-	-	-	-	-	-	↑	-	-	-	131
-	-	MCF-7	60 μM	48 h	-	-	-	-	-	-	DNMT1	↓ 10%	-	-	-	-
-	-	-		72 h	-	-	-	-	-	-		↓ 60%	-	-	-	-
-	-	-	60 μM	72 h	-	-	-	-	-	-	ATM	↑	-	-	-	-
-	-	-				-	-	-	-	-	APC	↑	-	-	-	-
-	-	-				-	-	-	-	-	PTEN	↑	-	-	-	-
-	-	-	100 μM	48 h	-	-	-	-	-	-	DNMT1	↓ 40%	-	-	-	-
-	-	-		72 h	-	-	-	-	-	-	-	↓ 80%	-	-	-	-
-	-	-			ATM	-	-	-	-	-	ATM	↑	-	-	-	-
-	-	-			APC	-	-	-	-	-	APC	↑	-	-	-	-
-	-	-			PTEN	-	-	-	-	-	PTEN	↑	-	-	-	-
-	-	-			SERPINB5	-	-	-	-	-	SERPINB5	↑	-	-	-	-
-	-	MDA-MB-231	60 μM	48 h	-	-	-	-	-	-	DNMT1	↓ 10%	-	-	-	-
-	-	-		72 h	-	-	-	-	-	-		↓ 20%	-	-	-	-
-	-	-				-	-	-	-	-	ATM	↑	-	-	-	-
-	-	-				-	-	-	-	-	APC	↑	-	-	-	-
-	-	-	100 μM	48 h	-	-	-	-	-	-	DNMT1	↓ 20%	-	-	-	-
-	-	-		72 h	-	-	-	-	-	-	-	↓ 40%	-	-	-	-
-	-	-			ATM	-	-	-	-	-	ATM	↑	-	-	-	-
-	-	-			APC	-	-	-	-	-	APC	↑	-	-	-	-
-	-	-			PTEN	-	-	-	-	-	PTEN	↑	-	-	-	-
Genistein	Cervical Cancer	-	-	-	-	-	-	-	-	-	-	-	-	-	-	137
-	-	-	15 μM	24-96 h		-	-	-	-	-	DNMT1	↓	DNMTs	↓	-	-
-	-	-	-			-	-	-	-	-	DNMT3A	↓				-
-	-	-	-			-	-	-	-	-	DNMT3B	↓				-
-	-	-	-			-	-	-	-	-	HDAC1	↓	HDACs	↓	-	-
-	-	-	-			-	-	-	-	-	HDAC3	↓				-
-	-	-	-			-	-	-	-	-	HDAC6	↓				-
-	-	-	-			-	-	-	-	-	HDAC7	↓				-
-	-	-	-		RARβ	↓	-	-	-	-	RARβ	↑	-	-	-	-
-	-	-	-		p21	↓	-	-	-	-	p21	↑	-	-	-	-
-	-	-	-		E-cad.	↓	-	-	-	-	E-cadherin	↑	-	-	-	-
-	-	-	-		DAPK1	↓	-	-	-	-	DAPK1	↑	-	-	-	-
-	-	-	-		MGMT	↓	-	-	-	-	-	-	-	-	-	-
Genistein	Prostate Cancer	-	-	-	-	-	-	-	-	-	-	-	-	-	-	139
-	-	DU-145	40 μM	48 h	MAD1L1	↓	-	-	-	-	-	-	-	-	androgen insensitive	
-	-	-			TRAF7	↓	-	-	-	-	-	-	-	-		
Daidzein	Prostate Cancer	-	-	-	-	-	-	-	-	-	-	-	-	-	-	139
-	-	DU-145	110 μM	-	MAD1L1	↓	-	-	-	-	-	-	-	-	-	-
-	-	-			KDM4B	↑	-	-	-	-	-	-	-	-	-	-
-	-	LNCaP			*h*TERT	↑	-	-	-	-	-	-	-	-	androgen sensitive	
	-	-	-	-	-	-	-	-	-	-	-	-	-	-		

(Table 5) cont.....

Cmpd	Pathology	Cell Model	Conc.	Time	Genes	Promoter Methylation		Promoter Acetylation	Histone Acetylation		Non Histone Proteins				Notes	Ref
											-	Expression	Activity			
Genistein	Prostate Cancer	-	-	-	-	-	-	-	-	-	-	-	-	-	-	140
-	-	ARCaP-E	20 µM	-	SOX7	-	-	⇧	-	-	-	-	-	-	-	-
-	-	-			APC	-	-	⇧	-	-	-	-	-	-	-	-
-	-	-			DKK3	-	-	⇧	-	-	-	-	-	-	-	-
-	-	-			WIF1	-	-	⇧	-	-	-	-	-	-	-	-
-	-	-			SFRP1	-	-	⇧	-	-	-	-	-	-	-	-
-	-	-			SFRP2	-	-	⇧	-	-	-	-	-	-	-	-
-	-	-				-	-	-	-	-	HAT1	⇧	-	-	-	-
Genistein	Oesophageal Cancer	-	-	-	-	-	-	-	-	-	-	-	-	-	-	141
-	-	KYSE 510	20 - 100 µM	-		-	-	-	-	-	-	-	DNMTs	⇩	DNMT1 IC_{50}=30 µM	
-	-	-				-	-	-	-	-	-	-	HDACs	⇩	-	-
-	-	-	5-20 µM	24-144 h	MGMT	-	-	-	-	-	MGMT	⇧	-	-	-	-
-	-	-			RARβ	-	-	-	-	-	RARβ	⇧	-	-	-	-
-	-	-	-	-	$P16^{INK\alpha}$	-	-	-	-	-	$P16^{INK\alpha}$	⇧	-	-	-	-

Anthocyanins

Anthocyanins are a subclass of flavonoids highly abundant in apples, grapes, purple cabbage, and various types of berries, such as strawberries, raspberries, and blackberries. Their highly conjugated structure allows them to absorb visible light in the green/blue wavelength and confer fruits and vegetable their characteristic red, purple, and blue colours. Although conclusive results on the effectiveness of anthocyanins as chemopreventive agents in human tumorigenesis have not been produced yet, it is important to note that the consumption of anthocyanin-rich berry extracts has shown beneficial effects in mice models of oesophageal, skin, breast, and colon cancer [142]. The analysis of *in vitro* effects of anthocyanins on cell proliferation has led to the conclusion that these natural compounds can reduce oxidative cell damage, limit the production of pro-inflammatory mediators, inhibit angiogenesis, and control invasiveness of cancer cells by affecting the expression of matrix metalloproteases (MMPs). Moreover, anthocyanins have been shown to cause cell cycle arrest and apoptosis in different type of cancers by interfering with MAPK signalling and by activating the intrinsic and extrinsic apoptosis pathway [142]. Interestingly, amongst the few successful human trials involving anthocyanins, those concerning colon cancer patients and patients with familial adenomatous polyposis seemed particularly promising, as regular consumption of black raspberries determined changes in the methylation status of tumour suppressor and marker genes such as *WIF1*, $p16^{INK\alpha}$ and *SFRP2* (secreted frizzled-related protein 2) [143]. In fact, the exposure of HCT-116, Caco2 and SW480 colon cancer cells to 0.5-25 µg/ml anthocyanins derived from black raspberries showed to induce promoter demethylation of *SFRP2* and *WIF1* in all cell lines, while the promoter of *CDKN2A* was demethylated in HCT116 and SW480, and the one of *SFRP5* only in Caco2 cells. This change seemed to be closely correlated with strong inhibition of DNMT1 and DNMT3B activity in all tested cell-lines [144]. However, promoter demethylation was not a good predictor of increased mRNA levels and protein expression. In fact, only SFRP2 mRNA levels were increased in all three cell lines, while WIF1 expression was enhanced in HCT116 and SW480 cells. Moreover, SFRP5 mRNA levels were amplified only in HCT-116 cells [144]. The strong inhibitory effect on DNMTs associated with the exposure to anthocyanins was found in JB6 P+ skin cancer cells as well. When these cells were treated with 5-20 μM delphinidin (**57**) Fig. (**16**)., one of the most abundant anthocyanins in berries and black currants, a decrease in DNMT1 and DNMT3A expression was recorded [145].

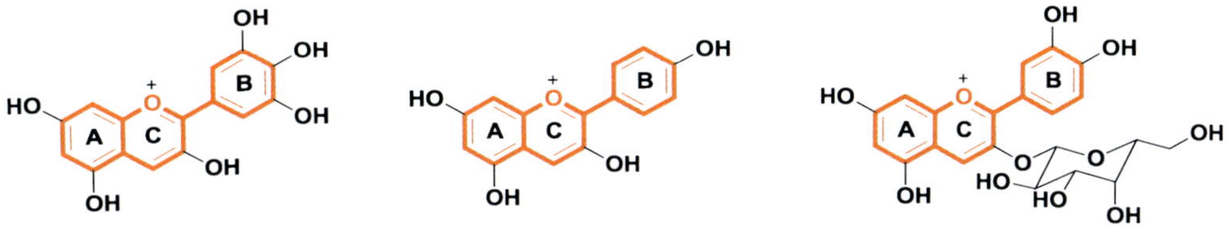

Delphinidin (57) Pelargonidin (58) Idaein (59)

Fig. (16). Chemical structure of anthocyanins delphinidin (**57**), pelargonidin (**58**) and idaein (**59**).

This effect was associated with reduced methylation at the promoter of *NRF2*, a gene involved in modulating the cellular response to oxidative stress, and consequent upregulated expression of Nrf2 and its target genes *Nqo1*, *Sod-1*, and *Ho-1*. At the same time, the expression of histone deacetylases HDAC1-5 and HDAC7 was found to be reduced by delphinidin (**57**) in a dose-dependent manner [145]. The involvement of HDACs in mediating delphinidin's anti-proliferative activity was further demonstrated in a separate study on LNCaP, CP-3 and DU145 prostate cancer cells lines, where HDACs activity was reported to be reduced after 24 hours treatment with 100-150 μM delphinidin (**57**) in both LNCaP and CP-3 cells [146]. The most sensitive cells to delphinidin were LNCaP cells, the only cell line of the three that expresses normal levels of functional p53. This finding led the authors to speculate that delphinidin-induced apoptosis in LNCaP cells could be promoted by the stabilisation of p53 resulting from the loss of HDAC3 activity, which was highly pronounced after 100-150 μM treatment when compared to other HDAC isoforms in the same cell line [146]. The loss of HDAC3 activity was not only associated with its reduced expression but also with the upregulation and activation of caspase-7, an enzyme responsible for HDAC3 proteolytic cleavage, a crucial step in cell programmed death [147]. A very similar mechanism of action seemed to be enacted by the galactosylated anthocyanin derivative idaein (**59**) (Fig. **16**) when inducing p53 mediated apoptosis in HPV positive ovarian cancer cells (HeLa), although in this case reduced expression of DNMTs was reported as well [148]. In a molecular modelling study, Karthi *et al.* [149] investigated the mechanism through which the anthocyanin pelargonidin (**58**) Fig. (**16**) caused changes in DNA methylation in cancer cells and they highlighted that these natural compounds have the potential of binding directly to the catalytic pocket of DNMT1 and DNMT3A Fig. (**17**).

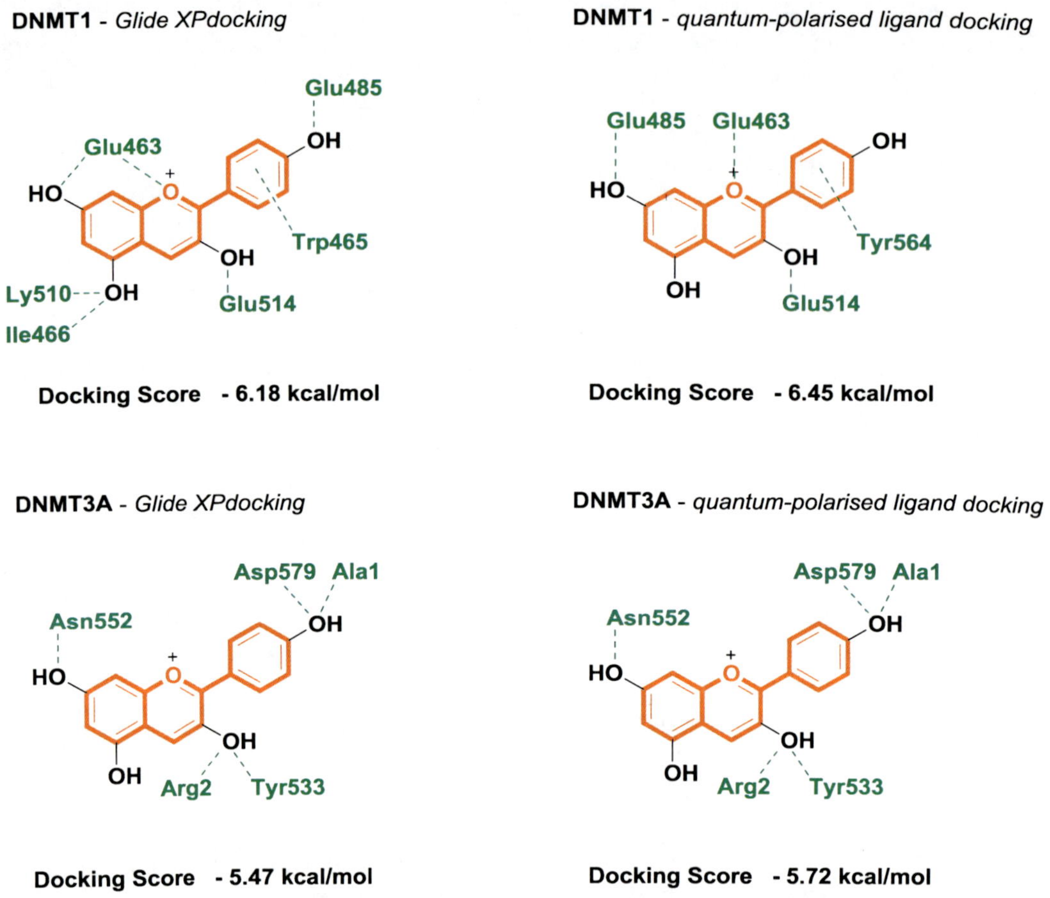

Fig. (17). A comparison between hydrogen bonding and π-stacking interactions identified by docking pelargonidin (**58**) in DNMT1 (PDB ID: 3EPZ) and DNMT3A (PDB ID: 4QBQ) using two different docking and scoring methods available in the Schrödinger software package [149].

Finally, anthocyanins have been reported to possess HAT inhibitory activity as well. Screening increasing concentrations (10-100 μM) of delphinidin against HeLa nuclear extracts showed that this compound could cause up to 70%

reduction in HAT activity, while not significantly affecting the activity of other epigenetic modulators such as SIRT1, HDACs or HMTs. Moreover, delphinidin (**57**) inhibited the acetylation of synthetic histone H4 from recombinant p300 and CBP in a dose-dependent manner [150]. Suppression of p300/CBP activity has also been correlated to reduced acetylation of the nuclear factor NFκB, which prevented its nuclear translocation and stopped TNF-α induced activation of the inflammatory response in human rheumatoid arthritis syno*via*l cells (MH7A) [150].

Table 6. Summary of the epigenetic effects of anthocyanins in different types of cancer cells.

Anthocyanin	Pathology	Cell model	Cell *via* bility	Conc.	Duration	Genes	Promoter Methylation	Non histone proteins					Notes	Ref
									Expression	Acetylation	Activity			
Black raspberry	Colon Cancer	**HCT116**	-	-	-		-	-	-	-	-	-	-	144
-	-	-	-	25 µg/mL	72 h	-	-	DNMT1	⇩	-	DNMTs	⇩	-	-
-	-	-	-			-	-	DNMT3B	⇩	-			-	-
-	-	-	-			CDKN2A	⇩	CDKN2A	⇨	-	-	-	-	-
-	-	-	-			SFRP5	⇨	SFRP5	⇧	-	-	-	-	-
-	-	-	-			SFRP2	⇩	SFRP2	⇧	-	-	-	-	-
-	-	-	-			WIF1	⇩	WIF1	⇧	-	-	-	-	-
-	-	**Caco2**	-	-	-	-	-	-	-	-	-	-	-	144
-	-	-	-	25 µg/mL	72 h	-	-	DNMT1	⇩	-	DNMTs	⇩	-	-
-	-	-	-			-	-	DNMT3B	⇩	-			-	-
-	-	-	-			CDKN2A	⇨	CDKN2A	⇨	-	-	-	-	-
-	-	-	-			SFRP5	⇩	SFRP5	⇨	-	-	-	-	-
-	-	-	-			SFRP2	⇩	SFRP2	⇧	-	-	-	-	-
-	-	-	-			WIF1	⇩	WIF1	⇨	-	-	-	-	-
-	-	**SW480**	-	-	-	-	-	-	-	-	-	-	-	144
-	-	-	-	25 µg/mL	72 h	-	-	DNMT1	⇩	-	DNMTs	⇩		
-	-	-	-			-	-	DNMT3B	⇩	-			-	-
-	-	-	-			CDKN2A	⇩	CDKN2A	⇨	-	-	-	-	-
-	-	-	-			SFRP5	⇨	SFRP5	⇨	-	-	-	-	-
-	-	-	-			SFRP2	⇩	SFRP2	⇧	-	-	-	-	-
-	-	-	-			WIF1	⇩	WIF1	⇨	-	-	-	-	-
Delphinidin	Skin Cancer	**JB6 P+**	-	-	-	-	-	-	-	-	-	-	-	145
-	-	-	-	-	120 h	-	-	DNMT1	⇩	-	-	-	-	-
-	-	-	-	-			-	DNMT3A	⇩	-	-	-	-	-
-	-	-	-	-			-	HDAC1	⇩	-	-	-	-	-
-	-	-	-	5 µM			-	HDAC2	⇩	-	-	-	-	-
-	-	-	-	10 µM			-	HDAC3	⇩	-	-	-	-	-
-	-	-	-25%	20 µM			-	HDAC4	⇩	-	-	-	-	-
-	-	-	-	-			-	HDAC5	⇩	-	-	-	-	-
-	-	-	-	-			-	HDAC7	⇩	-	-	-	-	-

(Table 6) cont.....

Anthocyanin	Pathology	Cell model	Cell *via* bility	Conc.	Duration	Genes	Promoter Methylation	Non histone proteins					Notes	Ref
									Expression	Acetylation	Activity			
-	-	-	-	-	-	NRF2	↓	Nrf2	↑	-	-	-	-	-
-	-	-	-	5 µM 10 µM 20 µM	120 h	-	-	Nqo1	↑	-	-	-	Nrf2 target genes	
-	-	-	-				-	HP-1	↑	-	-	-		
-	-	-	-				-	Sod-1	↑	-	-	-		
-	-	-	-				-	HO-1	↑	-	-	-		
Delphinidin	Prostate Cancer	**LNCaP**	-	-	-	-	-	-	-	-	-	-	-	146
-	-	-	-30%	50 µM	12 h	-	-	HDAC3	→	-	HDACs	↓	-	-
-	-	-					-	cleaved PARP-1	→	-	-	-	-	-
-	-	-					-	Caspase 3	→	-	Caspases	→	-	-
-	-	-					-	Caspase 7	→	-			-	-
-	-	-					-	Caspase 8	→	-			-	-
-	-	-	-40 to -50%	100 µM	12 h	-	-	HDAC3	↑	-	HDACs	↓	-	-
-	-	-					-	cleaved PARP-1	↑	-	-	-	-	-
-	-	-					-	Caspase 3	↑	-	Caspases	-	-	-
-	-	-					-	Caspase 7	↑	-			-	-
-	-	-					-	Caspase 8	↑	-			-	-
-	-	-			24 h	-	-	p53	-	↑	-	-	-	-
-	-	-	-60%	150 µM	12 h	-	-	HDAC3	↑	-	HDACs	↓	-	-
-	-	-					-	cleaved PARP-1	↑	-	-	-	-	-
-	-	-					-	Caspase 3	↑	-	Caspases	-	-	-
-	-	-					-	Caspase 7	↑	-			-	-
-	-	-					-	Caspase 8	↑	-			-	-
-	-	-			24 h	-	-	p53	-	↑	-	-	-	-
Idaein	Cervical Cancer	HeLa HPV+	-	-	-	-	-	-	-	-	-	-	-	148
-	-	-	-	0.97 µg/mL	6 h	-	-	DNMT1	↓	-	-	-	-	-
-	-	-	-	1.95 µg/mL			-	DNMT3A	↓	-	-	-	-	-
-	-	-	-	2.59 µg/mL			-	DNMT3B	↓	-	-	-	-	-
	-	-	-	-	-	-	-	-	-	-	-	-	-	-
	-	-	-	-	-	-	-	-	-	-	-	-	-	-
	-	-	-	-	-	-	-	-	-	-	-	-	-	-
	-	-	-	-	-	-	-	-	-	-	-	-	-	-
Anthocyanin	**Pathology**	**Cell Model**	**Cell *via* bility**	**Conc.**	**Duration**	**Genes**	**Promoter Methylation**	**Non histone proteins**					**Notes**	**Refs.**
									Expression	Acetylation	Activity			
-	-	-	-	2.59 µg/mL	6-12 h	-	-	DAPK1	-	-	-	-	-	-
-	-	-	-				-	$p16^{INKa}$	-	-	-	-	-	-
-	-	-	-				-	Bax	-	-	-	-	-	-

(Table 6) cont.....

Anthocyanin	Pathology	Cell model	Cell via bility	Conc.	Duration	Genes	Promoter Methylation	Non histone proteins					Notes	Ref
									Expression	Acetylation	Activity			
-	-	-	-			-	-	Bcl-2	-	-	-	-	-	-
-	-	-	-				-	Cyt-c	-	-	-	-	-	-
-	-	-	-	2.59 µg/mL	6-12 h		-	Caspase3	-	-	-	-	-	-
-	-	-	-				-	Caspase9	-	-	-	-	-	-
-	-	-	-				-	PARP	-	-	-	-	-	-
-	-	-	-				-	p53	-	-	-	-	-	-
-	-	-	-				-	$p21^{WAF1}$	-	-	-	-	-	-

Flavanols: Catechins from Green Tea

Green tea is a popular beverage obtained from the unfermented leaves of *Camellia sinensis*. The alleged health benefits associated with the consumption of green tea have been often attributed to its abundance in natural polyphenols, including catechins, theaflavins, thearubigens, and other flavonoids [151]. Although the composition of tea leaves and their extracts can change depending on cultivation, climate, and brewing conditions, catechins tend to constitute between 30-42% of the dry weight of green tea. In particular, the four most abundant catechins are: (-)-epicatechin (EC) **60**, (-)-epigallocatechin (EGC) **61**, (-)-epicatechin-3-*O*-gallate (ECG) **62**, and (-)-epigallocatechin-3-*O*-gallate (EGCG) **63**, with EGCG accounting for 50-80% of the whole catechin content in green tea Fig. (**18**).

Over the past thirty years, there have been a growing number of studies reporting on the potential therapeutic effects of tea polyphenols and despite promising *in vitro* results, the association between the consumption of green tea and cancer chemoprevention remains to be demonstrated. Similar to other flavonoids, catechins are characterised by poor bioavailability and undergo extensive metabolism *in vivo* [152]. The HPLC-DAD/MS analysis of plasma and urine samples after the ingestion of green tea has revealed the presence of ECG (**62**) and EGCG (**63**) together with a series of methyl, sulfate, and glucuronide derivatives (Table **7**) [153].

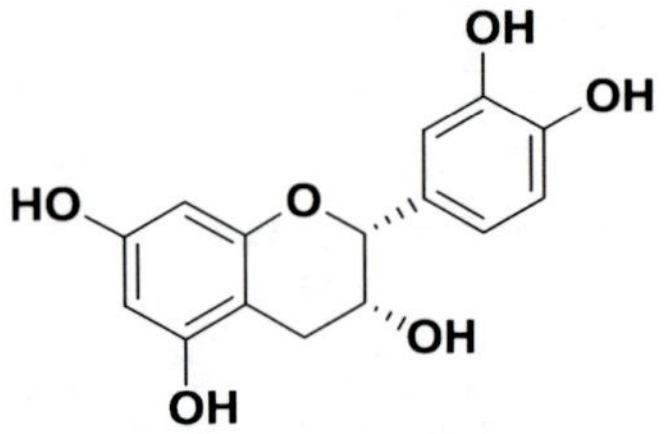

(-)-epicatechin (EC)

(60)

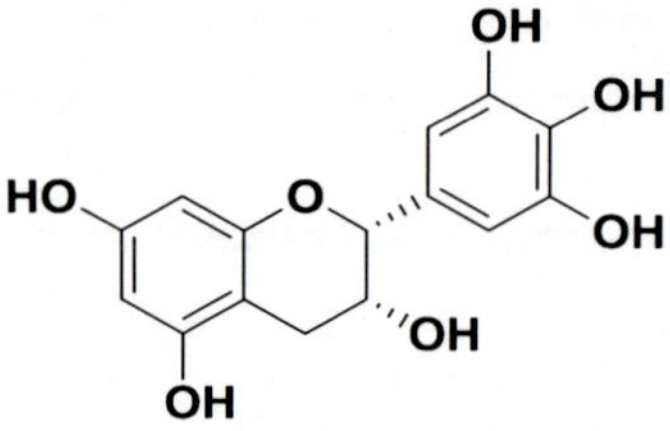

(-)-epigallocatechin (EGC)

(61)

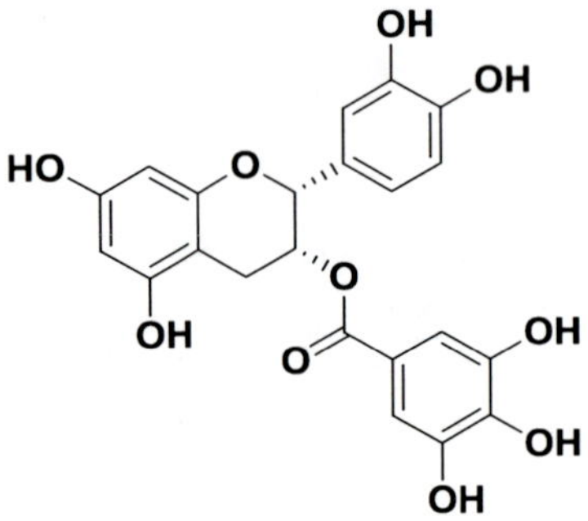

(-)-epicatechin-3-gallate (ECG)

(62)

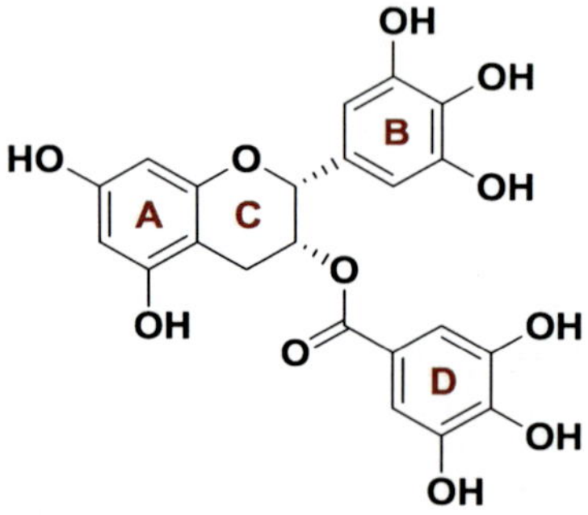

(-)-epigallocatechin-3-gallate (EGCG)

(63)

Fig. (18). Chemical structure of the major polyphenol components of green tea.

Table 7. Levels of catechins and their metabolites detected in the plasma samples of volunteers (n = 10) after the ingestion of 500 mL of green tea [153].

Catechin	C_{max} (nM)	T_{max} (h)	$T_{1/2}$ (h)
(-)-Epigallocatechin-3-*O*-gallate	55 ± 12	1.9 ± 0.1	1.0
EGC-*O*-Glucuronide	126 ± 19	2.2 ± 0.2	1.6
4'-*O*-Methyl-EGC-*O*-Glucuronide	46 ± 6.3	2.3 ± 0.3	3.1
4'-*O*-Methyl-EGC-*O*-Sulfate	79 ± 12	2.2 ± 0.2	2.2
(-)-Epicatechin-3-*O*-gallate	25 ± 3.0	1.6 ± 0.2	1.5
O-Methyl-epicatechin-*O*-sulfate	90 ± 15	1.7 ± 0.2	1.5
EC-3-*O*-Glucuronide	29 ± 4.7	1.7 ± 0.2	1.6
EC-*O*-Sulfate	89 ± 15	1.6 ± 0.2	1.9

Catechins are both substrates and inhibitors of catechol-*O*-methyltransferase, the most potent inhibitor being EGCG (**63**), with IC_{50} = 0.07 µM. EGCG metabolites, 4"-*O*-methyl- and 4',4"-di-*O*-methyl-EGCG derivatives **64-65**, can also inhibit COMT, despite their lower IC_{50} of 0.10 µM and 0.15 µM, respectively Fig. (**19**) [154]. The presence of the D-ring was proposed to be fundamental for the inhibition of COMT, as catechins that did not bear the gallate substituent, such as EGC (**61**), showed 100-1000-fold decrease in potency.

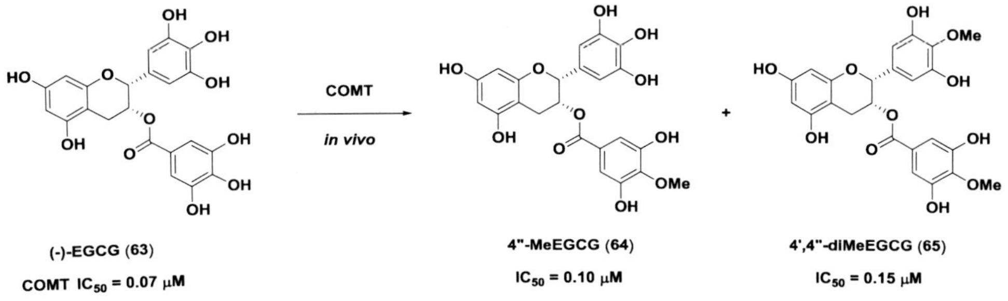

Fig. (19). EGCG is methylated *in vivo* by catechol-*O*-methyltransferase to form methyl- and dimethyl-EGCG.

The methylation reaction catalysed by COMT is believed to affect the therapeutic potential of catechins *in vivo,* as an inverse association was established between the risk to develop breast cancer and women carrying a low activity allele for COMT if they were tea drinkers compared to non-tea drinkers. No significant difference was found in women that were homozygous for the high-activity allele [155]. Catechol-*O*-methyltransferase (COMT) and DNA *N*-methyltransferases (DNMT) belong to the same superfamily of *S*-adenosyl methyltransferases that use the same cofactor, *S*-adenosyl-L-methionine (SAM) as the methyl donor. For this reason, it has been proposed that the mechanism through which EGCG (**63**) could induce DNA hypomethylation is mediated by the depletion of cellular SAM and the subsequent production of *S*-adenosyl-L-homocysteine (SAH) resulting from the extensive metabolism of catechins operated by COMT [156]. However, when EGCG (**63**) was tested for its ability to inhibit DNMT1-mediated DNA methylation *in vitro*, it demonstrated to be a dose-dependent, potent inhibitor (IC_{50} = 0.47 µM) of DNA methylation both in the presence and in the absence of COMT. In contrast, the DNMT1 inhibitory activity of (-)-epicatechin (EC) **60** increased significantly when COMT was added to the assay, from 40% inhibition at 20 µM in the absence of COMT, to IC_{50} = 4.6 µM in the presence of COMT. The impact of EGCG (**63**) on the methylation status of treated cells was confirmed by incubating MCF-7 and MDA-MB-231 breast cancer cells with EGCG (**63**) at 0, 0.2, 1, 5, 25 and 50 µM. Although cell growth was not substantially inhibited after 6 days of treatment, the unmethylation-specific PCR bands related to the promoter of retinoic acid receptor α (*RAR*α) were shown to be increased, while methylation-specific bands appeared to be decreased in a dose-dependent manner [156]. In a previous study, EGCG (**63**) had already been reported as capable of inhibiting DNMT activity in a competitive fashion (K_i = 6.89 μM). In particular, treatment of human oesophageal cancer cell line KYSE 510 with 5, 10, 20 or 50 μM EGCG (**63**) for 12-144 hours reactivated a series of methylation-silenced genes including *RAR*α, the tumor suppressor $p16^{INK4a}$, *O6*-methylguanine methyltransferase (*MGMT*), and mismatch repair human *mutL* homologue 1 (*hMLH1*) in a time- and dose-dependent manner (IC_{50} = 20 μM) [157]. Re-expression of the genetic products of *RAR*α and *hMLH1* after treatment with EGCG was confirmed by Western blot in oesophageal cancer cells (KYSE 510), human colon cancer cells (HT-29), and prostate cancer cells (PC3). These findings led Fang *et al.* [157] to conduct a molecular modelling simulation to propose a binding mode for EGCG (**63**) in the cytosine binding site of DNMT1. Their results highlighted the importance of the hydrogen bonds formed by the D-ring of EGCG (**63**) with the backbone of Pro^{1225} and the lateral chain of Glu^{1223}, which are the residues involved in the stabilisation of the flipped-out cytosine substrate inside the pocket Fig. (**20**). In fact, catechin derivatives that do not carry the gallate substituent (ring D), such as EC (**60**) and EGC (**61**), or in which the hydroxyl-groups of the gallate moiety have ben alkylated, like in the case of 4”-MeEGCG (**64**) and 4’,4”-diMeEGCG (**65**), show lower binding affinity scores to DNMT1 and reduced inhibitory activity in *in vitro* DNA methylation assays [157].

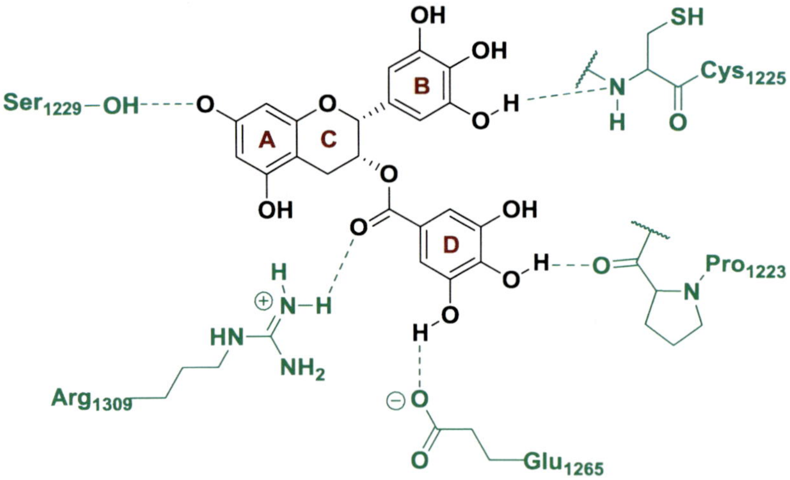

Fig. (20). Modelled interactions of EGCG (**63**) into the putative cytosine pocket of DNMT1. Insight II Homology Module was used to construct a structural model of the binding site of DNMT1 using the crystal structure of HhaI Mtase (PDB 5MHT) and DNMT1 protein sequence (accession number NP_00137) [157].

In their study, Fang *et al.* [157] focused on DNMT1, as the most abundant DNA-*N*-methyltransferase in nuclear extracts. However, they could not exclude that DNMT3a and 3b could also be present in small amounts in their *in vitro* assay and therefore contribute to the observed results. In fact, a later study by Khan *et al.* [158] reported that, according to molecular modelling predictions, EGCG (**63**) can bind to the cytosine pocket of DNMT3b, which, for the purpose of this study, was modelled from the crystal structure of DNMT3a (PDB: 2QRV). The relevance of the interactions established by the D-ring of EGCG with key residues in the modelled substrate binding site of DNMT3b (Arg^{832}, Arg^{823}, Ser^{778} and Asn^{652}) were highlighted in this occasion as well. Moreover, the treatment of human cervical cancer cells (HeLa) with 25 μM EGCG (**63**) for 3 days showed a time-dependent decrease in the expression of DNM3b mRNA at levels comparable with those induced by subjecting the same cells to 1 μM 5-aza--'-deoxycytidine (**54**), a known modulator of the DNMT1 and DNMT3b mediated DNA damage response in cancer cells [159]. In the same study, Khan *et al.* [158] investigated the ability of EGCG (**63**) to inhibit the deacetylase activity of HDAC1. Although docking simulations predicted that EGCG (**63**) could bind the same acetyl lysine pocket occupied by trichostatin A (TSA), a broad spectrum inhibitor of class I and II HDACs, ECGC (**63**) showed to be significantly less effective than TSA in modulating histone deacetylase activity in HeLa cells. However, when the epigenetic modulation initiated by EGCG (**63**) in prostate cancer cell lines (LNCaP) was compared to the one promoted by a quantified extract of *Camellia sinensis* leaves (Polyphenon E®), Pandey *et al.* [160] found that green tea polyphenols (GTP) were able to inhibit DNMT activity in LNCaP cells at higher levels (36%, 62% and 78% after a 7 days treatment with 5, 10, and 20 μM GTP, respectively) than EGCG (**63**) at the same dosages (16%, 28% and 56%). At the same time, GTP induced a dose- and time-dependent re-expression of glutathione-*S*-transferase *pi* (GSTP1) in the same cell lines *via* demethylation of the promoter region [160]. Interestingly, the treatment with GTP did not cause extensive and aspecific DNA demethylation, which is known to cause DNA instability and promote the expression of pro-metastatic genes [161]. Moreover, GTP seemed to be able to inhibit the expression of HDAC1 (38%) and HDAC3 (51%) in LNCaP cells after a 7 days treatment with 10 μg/mL extract, while the expression of HDAC2 was increased 120%. This induced an overall reduction of HDAC activity in treated cells, with a consequent 22-fold increase in acetylation levels of histones H3 and a 2.2-fold increase in acetylation of histone H4 [160]. The ability of green tea polyphenols to down-regulate the expression of DNMT1 and HDAC1 in cancer cells was further demonstrated by subjecting colorectal cancer cells (RKO, HCT-116, and HT-29) to a combined treatment with 10 μM EGCG (**63**) and 5 mM sodium butyrate, a short chain fatty acid commonly released in the intestine as a result of the degradation of dietary fibres by the gut microbiota [162]. EGCG (**63**) and sodium butyrate showed synergistic effect as the levels of DNMT1 and HDAC1 were significantly lower when the two compounds were co-administered compared to individual treatments. Moreover, the authors reported a decrease in DNMT3a and DNMT3b levels as well. Although no influence on histone acetyl transferases (HATs) could be found in colorectal cancer cells, a separate study from Choi *et al.* [163] revealed that EGCG (**63**) is capable of regulating the acetylation state of p65 (RelA), a subunit of the nuclear factor NFkB, *via* the inhibition of histone acetyl transferases (HATs) p300 (IC_{50} = 30 μM) and CBP (IC_{50} = 50 μM), both *in vitro* and *in vivo*. The reduction in acetyltransferase activity after treatment with EGCG (**63**) was observed in human embryonic kidney cells (HEK293) and leukemic monocyte cells (THP-1), and it was correlated with a decreased binding of NFkB to the promoter of the *IL-6* gene, a proinflammatory cytokine. Given that IL-6 and IL-2 are overexpressed in EBV-associated B cell lymphoma and that EGCG (**63**) demonstrated to reverse the aberrant expression of these inflammatory markers in EBV-infected cells, it was proposed that EGCG (**63**) could act as a chemopreventive agent in population groups at high risk of developing lymphoma. Moreover, the ability of EGCG (**63**) to behave as a dual DNA-methyltransferase and histone acetyltransferase inhibitor had already been reported by Meeran *et al.* [164] while studying *h*TERT, a human telomerase reverse transcriptase known to be overexpressed in a high percentage of cancers. According to this study, ECGC **63** (40 μM) and pro-EGCG **66** (20 μM), a prodrug obtained by modifying the hydroxyl groups of EGCG (**63**) with acetate groups Fig. (**21**). in order to improve its stability and cell permeability, can inhibit *h*TERT expression in breast cancer cell lines (MCF-7 and MDA-MB-231) and induce apoptosis. ChiP-qPCR experiments demonstrated that the downregulation of *h*TERT levels was associated with hypomethylation and hypoacetylation of its promoter region, as well as reduced acetylation of specific markers of chromatin activation, such as histone 3 (ac-H3), lysine 9 of histone 3 (ac-H3K9), and histone 4 (ac-H4).

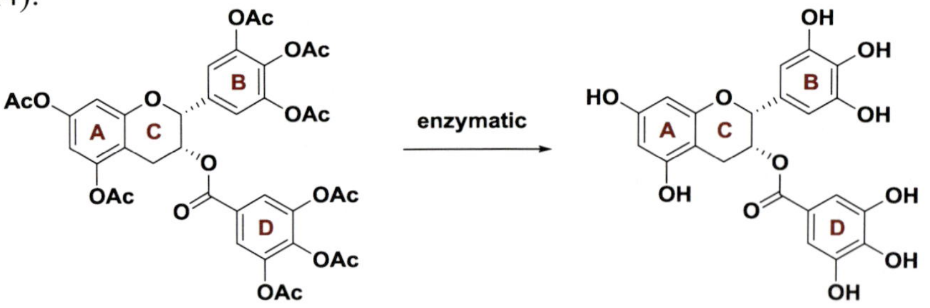

pro-EGCG (66) **EGCG (63)**

Fig. (21). Structure and enzymatic conversion of pro-EGCG (**66**) into EGCG (**63**) [165].

It is important to note that most studies reporting on the effect of EGCG (**63**) on the methylation/acetylation status of cancer cells have relied on indirect PCR analysis and that defining the mode of inhibition of epigenetic proteins has mostly relied on *in silico* simulations. In fact, these results have sometimes proven difficult to reproduce in enzymatic essays. For example, when EGCG (**63**) was subjected to a more systematic investigation alongside other known DNMT inhibitors, it did not seem to inhibit purified recombinant DNA methyltransferase and it performed its cytotoxic activity without affecting the overall levels of genomic DNA-methylation [166]. At the same time, EGCG (**63**) was reported to produce highly reactive radical species and inhibit several restriction enzymes, which could suggest an indirect, non-specific mechanism. In a similar way, the inhibitory activity exerted by EGCG (**63**) on recombinant SIRT1, a NAD^+ dependent histone deacetylase, has been demonstrated to be reduced by the co-administration of Vitamin C as a stabilising agent [167]. Despite these contrasting results, the virtual screening of a library containing 14,000 lead-like natural products against a validated model of the catalytic domain of DNMT1 primarily returned compounds characterised by a benzopyran-2-one (chromen-2-one or coumarin), 2-phenyl-4H-chromen-4-one, or 2-phenyl-1,4-benzopyrone (flavone) core [168]. These findings reinforce the idea that epigenetic modulators can indeed be found amongst polyphenolic structures of natural origin, while at the same time calling for more rigorous biochemical and cellular characterisation. Over the years, the search for synthetic flavan-3-ols analogues with improved pharmacokinetic properties, higher metabolic stability, and increased antiproliferative activity, has prompted the development of several SAR studies aimed at evaluating the contribution of the A, B, C, and D ring to the biological activity of catechins. Moreover, synthetic derivatives could play a pivotal role in elucidating the mechanism of action of catechin derivatives. In 2001, Zaveri [169] reported on the synthesis of 2,3-*syn* and 2,3-*anti* D-ring analogues of EGCG (**75** and **77**), where the hydroxyl groups of the gallate substituent previously reported to be involved in the formation of hydrogen bonds in the active site of DNMT1 and HDAC1 were methylated (Scheme 2).

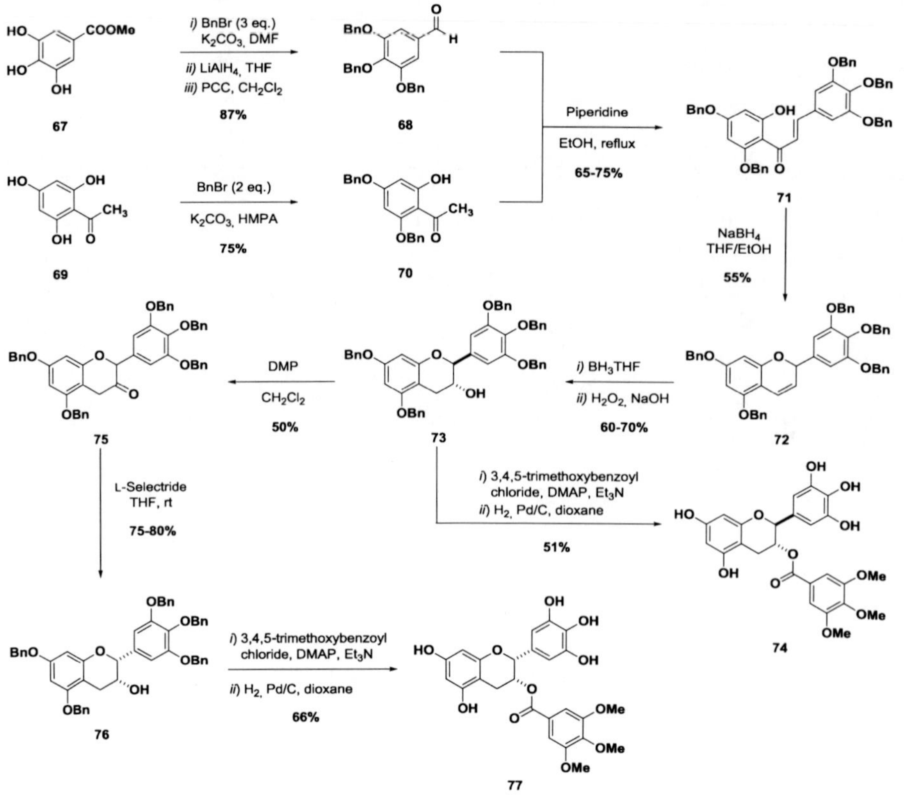

Scheme (2). Synthetic strategy for the development of 2,3-*syn* and 2,3-*trans* isomers of methylated D-ring derivatives of EGCG [169].

Interestingly, both *syn*- and *anti*-isomer inhibited the growth of breast cancer cells *in vitro*, with the 2,3-*syn* isomer **77** being slightly less potent than the 2,3-*anti* isomer **74**. In particular, the latter was demonstrated to inhibit the proliferation of MCF-7 and MDA-MB-231 cancer cells with IC_{50} values (11.4 ± 1.1 μM in MCF-7 and 8.8 ± 0.56 μM in MDA-MB-231) that were comparable to the IC_{50} measured for EGCG (**63**) when tested on the same cell lines, *i.e.* 12.5 ± 0.79 μM and 7.8 ± 1.6 μM, respectively [170]. The fact that modifications of the D-ring seemed to have little to no influence on the activity of EGCG derivatives **74** and **77** seemed to validate the theory according to which the B-ring and not the D-ring is responsible for the antiproliferative effect of catechins, as it has been demonstrated to take part in antioxidant reactions with peroxyl radicals [171]. Flavan-3-ols like EGCG (**63**) and other catechins can be distinguished from other flavonoids by the presence of two vicinal chiral centres. Therefore, the synthesis proposed by Zaveri [169] in 2001 yields racemic mixtures of *syn*- and *anti*-isomers. Over the past twenty years, a series of asymmetric strategies have been employed to achieve the enantioselective synthesis of the flavan-3-ol framework, including Sharpless asymmetric dihydroxylation [172, 173], Sharpless epoxidation [174], Shi epoxidation, and chiral resolution of enantiomeric mixtures Scheme (**3**) [175].

These strategies have been widely applied to evaluate the influence of B- and/or D-ring substitution on the pro-apoptotic activity of ECG and EGCG derivatives [176], they have been used to study the *in vivo* conversion of acetylated precursors into their corresponding active metabolites and have allowed the production of UPLC-MS/MS standards for the identification of plasma, bile and urine metabolites [177]. At the same time, the direct modification of the catechin core was also considered a valid strategy for the production of flavan-3-ol derivatives. In particular, this strategy was utilised for the synthesis of C4 and C8-modified derivatives of both (+)-catechin and (-)-epicatechin-3-gallate that were subsequently tested for their potential anticancer activity against several human cancer cell lines Scheme (**4**). and Table **8** [178].

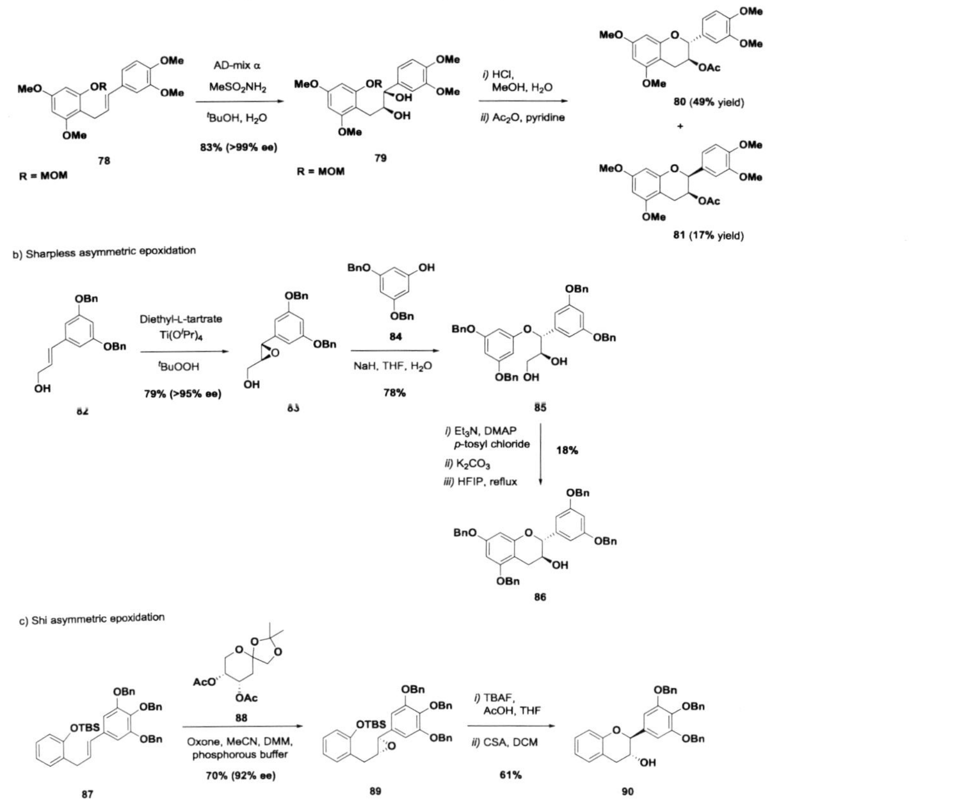

Scheme (3). Generic synthetic strategies for the construction of the C2 and C3 chiral centers of flavan-3-ols [175].

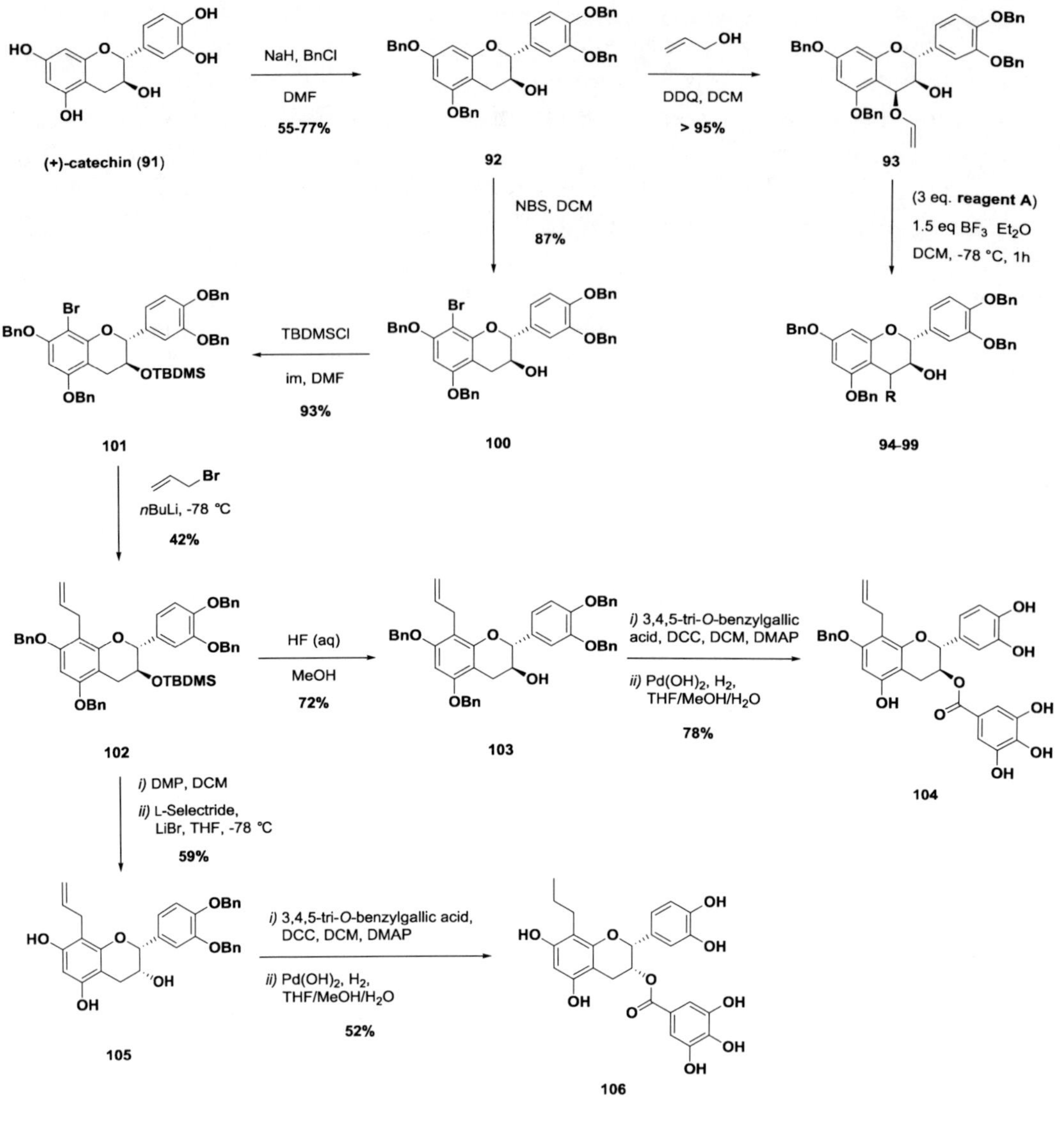

Scheme (4). General synthesis of C4 and C8-modified derivatives of (+)-catechin and (-)-epicatechi--3-gallate [178].

Table 8. Reagents used for the synthesis of C4 derivatives of (+)-catechin [178].

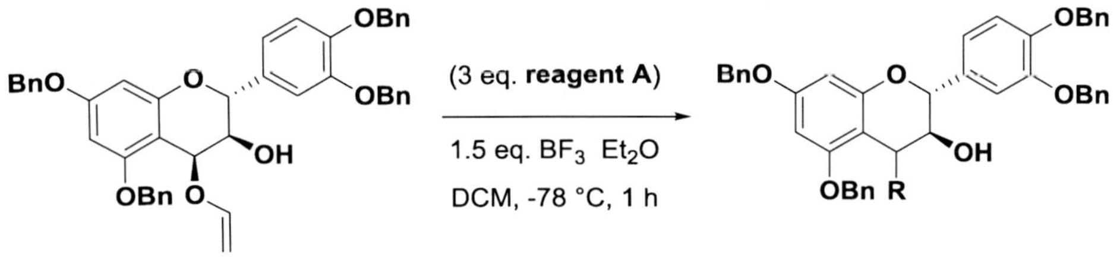

93 **94-99**

Reagent A	R	Yield%	Comp.
$TMSN_3$	$-N_3$	60%	94
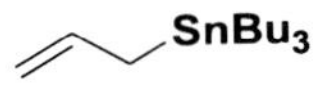	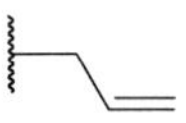	45%	95
PhSH	–SH	75%	96
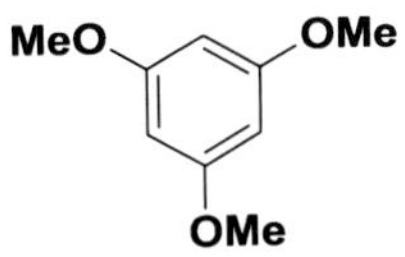	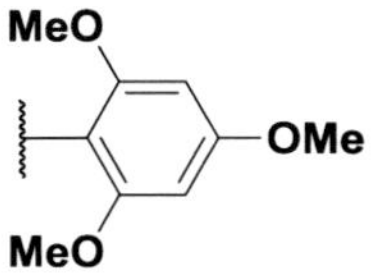	80%	97
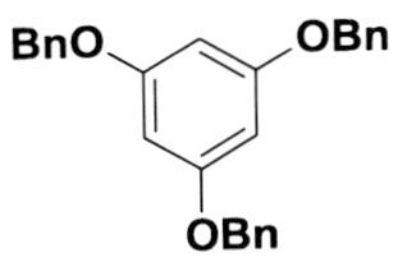	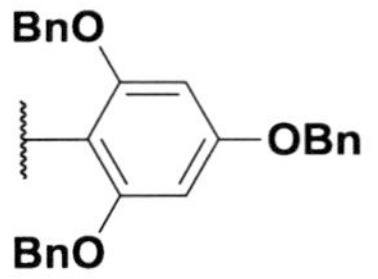	68%	98
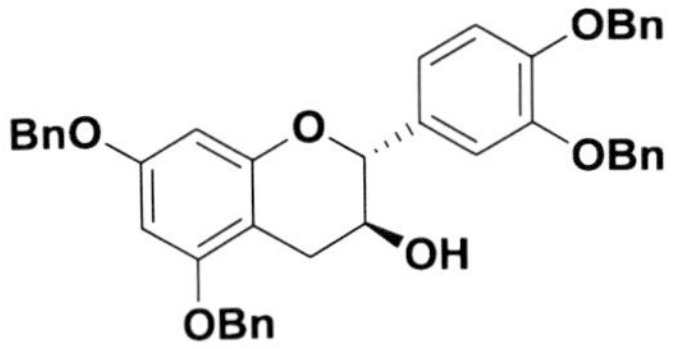	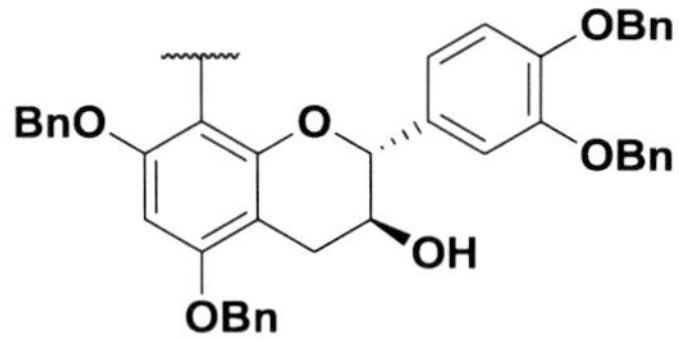	52%	99

Amongst these derivatives, 8-propyl-(+)-catechin gallate **106** displayed higher inhibitory activity (IC_{50} = 31 μM) on the *in vitro* proliferation of colorectal adenocarcinoma cell lines (HCT116) than (+)-catechin-3-gallate **107** (IC_{50} = 53 μM) and (-)-epicatechin-3-gallate **61** (IC_{50} = 76 μM). Bladder (RT112), stomach (MGLVA1), and liver (HepG2) cancer cells also showed to be sensitive to the treatment with **106** at levels comparable to colorectal cancer cell lines [178]. More recently, the substitution at C-3 of the flavan-3-ol ring has been proposed to modulate the binding affinity of catechins to bovine serum albumin (BSA) and human serum albumin (HSA) [179]. When a series of catechin derivatives was tested in a tryptophan fluorescence quenching assay against BSA, it was revealed that acylation at the C-3 position increased the quenching constant (Kq). In particular, the gallate moiety was proposed to induce fluorescence quenching by interacting with two tryptophan residues on the enzyme surface (Trp134) and in the binding site (Trp213) assuming two different binding poses. Replacing the gallate substituent with long carbon chains (C6-C18) improved the lipophilicity of these derivatives and, at the same time, enhanced the binding affinity towards BSA and HAS of both (+)-catechins and (-)-epicatechins, with the ideal length of the carbon chain being 10 carbon atoms [179]. When 3-*O*-acyl and -alkyl (-- -epicatechin derivatives were tested for their ability to inhibit the growth of prostate (PC3), ovarian (SKOV5), and human glioblastoma astrocytoma (U-373 MG) cancer cells, derivatives carrying carbon chains of 10-12 carbon atoms showed the greatest activity Table **9** [180]. In particular, C-3 alkyl derivatives substituted with 10-12 carbon atom chains had lower IC_{50} than their corresponding C-3 acyl derivatives and the naturally occurring catechins EC (**60**) and ECG (**61**). Interestingly, the replacement of the gallate moiety with substituted aromatic rings also had a positive effect on the *in vitro* anticancer activity of these derivatives.

Table 9. Structure and antiproliferative activity of 3-*O*-acyl and alkyl (-)-epicatechin derivatives 108-114 against prostate (PC3), ovarian (SKOV3), and human glioblastoma astrocytoma (U-373 MG) cell lines [180].

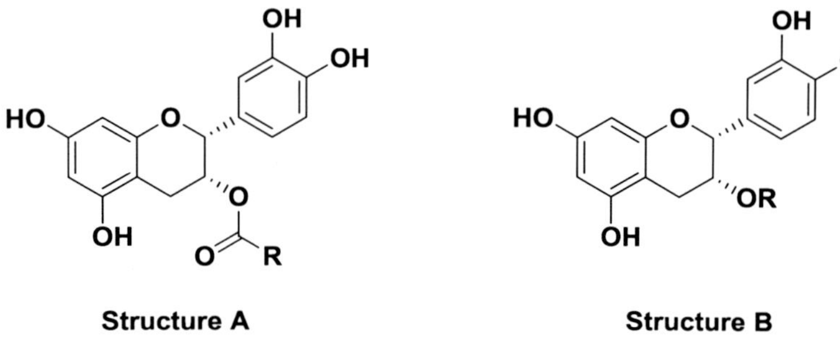

Cmpd	R	Structure	IC_{50} (μM)		
			PC3	SKOV3	U373MG
108	3,4,5-trihydroxyphenyl	A	168.2	185.4	157
109	-H	B	>500	>500	>500
110	$-CH_2(CH_2)_7CH_3$	A	14.6	20.8	19.2
111	$-CH_2(CH_2)_9CH_3$	A	23.1	22.4	24.3
112	$-CH_2(CH_2)_7CH_3$	B	8.9	7.9	6.4
113	$-CH_2(CH_2)_9CH_3$	B	9.3	8.6	7.1

(Table 9) cont.....

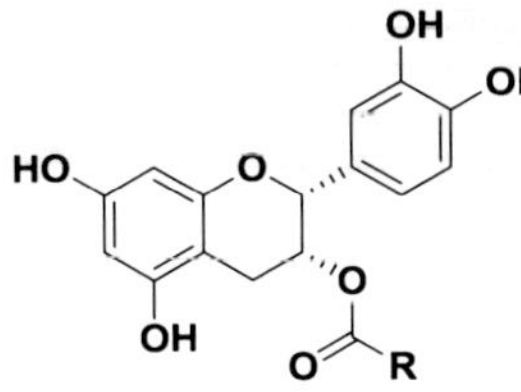

Structure A

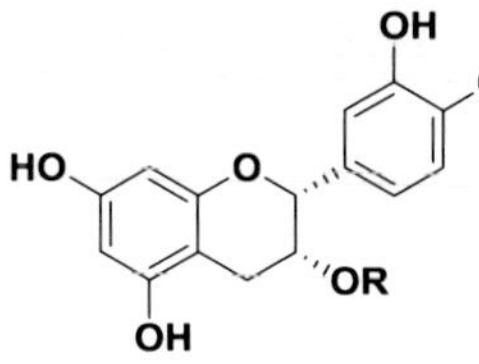

Structure B

Cmpd	R	Structure	IC_{50} (μM)		
			PC3	SKOV3	U373MG
114	4-trifluoromethoxyphenyl	B	14.	19.1	11.2

Metabolically stable 3-*O*-alkyl derivatives that resist the cleavage from esterases and possess increased cell permeability properties have attracted some attention as antiproliferative agents, as confirmed in a later publication from Kumar *et al.* [181], where a series of (-)-catechin C-3 derivatives **115-118** were tested for their antiproliferative activity against breast (MDA-MB-231), prostate (DU145), liver (HepG2) and lung (A549) cancer cell lines Table **10**.

Table 10. Structure and antiproliferative activity of C-3 alkyl substituted derivatives of (-)-catechin [181].

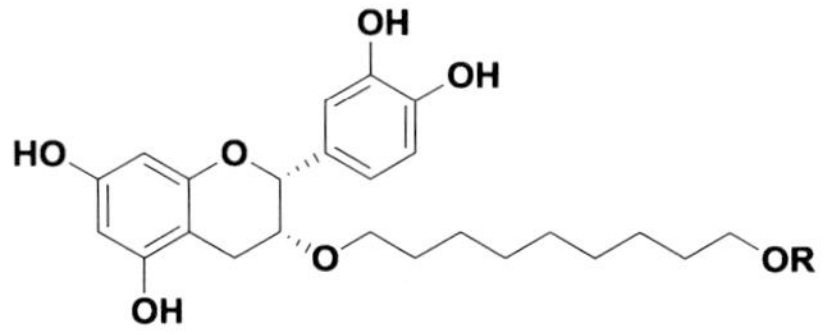

Cmpd	R	IC_{50} (μM)				
		A549	MDMB-231	DUI451	HepG2	cLogP
115	-H	9.4 ± 0.32	23.4 ± 0.21	22.4 ± 0.22	10.4 ± 0.34	3.39
116	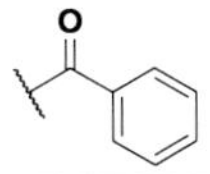	4.8 ± 0.22	7.8 ± 0.12	5.4 ± 0.14	2.5 ± 0.22	6.27
117	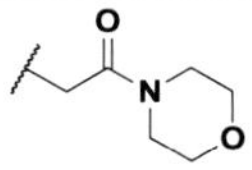	9.5 ± 0.24	8.9 ± 0.32	9.1 ± 0.16	7.4 ± 0.18	3.67

(Table 10) cont.....

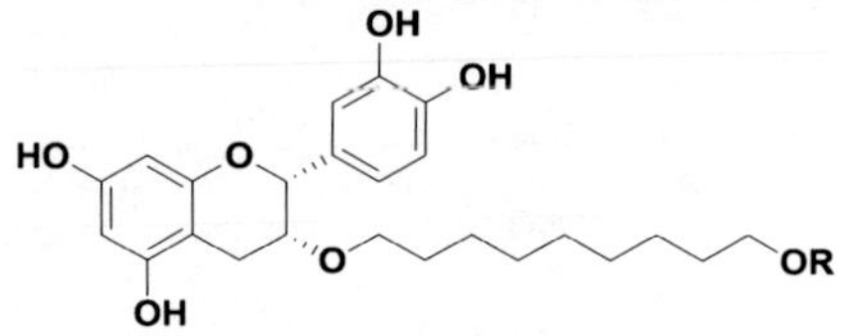

Cmpd	R	IC_{50} (μM)				
		A549	MDMB-231	DUI451	HepG2	cLogP
118	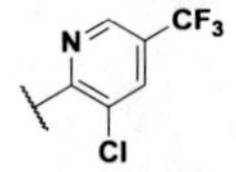	7.9 ± 0.09	6.6 ± 0.11	8.2 ± 0.18	5.5 ± 0.08	7.10
119	Doxorubicin	0.7 ± 0.12	0.9 ± 0.11	0.9 ± 0.08	0.6 ± 0.18	-

Provided the promising antiproliferative activity of catechin derivatives and the availability of efficient routes for the asymmetric synthesis and selective derivatisation of positions C-3, C-4, and C-8 of both the (+)-catechin and (---epicatechin core, further investigation should be conducted to assess the full potential of this class of polyphenols as anticancer agents and the development of accurate SAR analysis. Although the direct engagement with epigenetic proteins has not been demonstrated yet, *in silico* studies have indicated the possibility for this scaffold to be employed in future drug discovery programs focused on epigenetics and chemoprevention.

CURCUMIN AND CURCUMINOIDS

Curcumin (**120**) is the major bioactive component of turmeric, a spice obtained from the rhizome of *Curcuma longa*. It is commonly found in Asian cuisine, where turmeric-based dishes are extremely popular. Moreover, *Curcuma longa* finds extensive use in traditional Chinese and Ayurvedic medicine for the treatment of joint pain and inflammation [182]. Investigations into the therapeutic properties of curcumin (**120**) showed that this natural product, together with its most abundant analogues and metabolites such as demethoxycurcumin (**121**), bisdemethoxycurcumin (**122**), dihydrocurcumin (**123**) and tetrahydrocurcumin (**124**) Fig. (**22**)., is characterised by a variety of biological properties, including anti-inflammatory, anti-oxidant, anti-bacterial, anti-angiogenic and anti-proliferative activity [183].

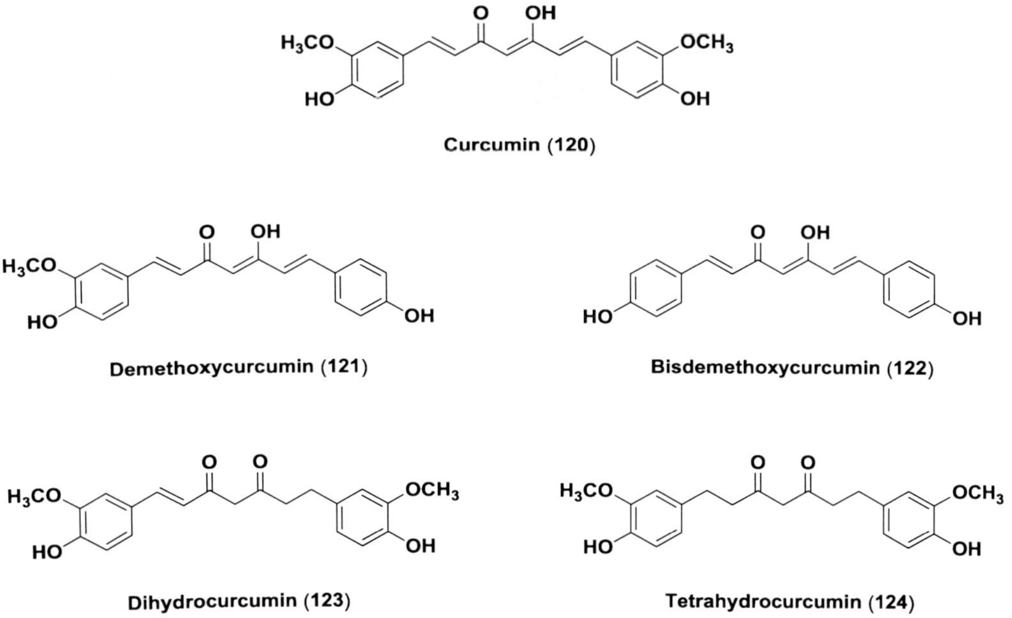

Fig. (22). Curcumin and curcuminoids found in the rhizome of *Curcuma longa*..

The chemotherapeutic and chemopreventive properties of curcumin have been mostly ascribed to its ability to interrupt the cell cycle at the G1/S or G2/M phase and induce apoptosis *via* a multiplicity of mechanisms [184]. In fact, curcumin has been proposed to interfere with the cell cycle directly, by influencing the activity of several cyclin dependent kinases (CDK 1, 2 and 4), or indirectly, by inducing the expression of CDK inhibitors such as p16^{INKa}, p21$^{WAF1/CIP1}$, and p27^{KIP1} [185]. The involvement of the Ras/ERK1 and 2 pathway has also been proposed in specific cancer cell lines, like human adenocarcinoma cells [186]. On the other side, curcumin (**120**) can induce apoptosis by producing highly reactive ROS species that cause direct DNA damage [187]. However, a series of alternative paths have been involved in curcumin-induced apoptosis, including proteasome inhibition [188], modulation of the Wnt/β-catenin pathway [189], upregulation of pro-apoptotic effectors such as Fas and FasL, and interference with the TNF-α induced expression of anti-apoptotic proteins such as Bcl-2 and Bcl-xL [190, 191]. In some cases, kinases (EGFR, MAPK, and AKT) and nuclear factors (NFκB, STATs, AP1, and PPR-γ) have been shown to behave as mediators of curcumin's antiproliferative activity. However, a growing body of evidence seems to implicate that curcumin-induced cell cycle arrest and apoptosis could involve a significant contribution from specific epigenetic mechanisms. In fact, curcumin (**120**) has been found to control gene expression by inhibiting DNA methylation, interfering with the acetylation state of histones and other intracellular proteins, and regulating the expression of miRNAs [192]. Although the molecular mechanisms behind curcumin's influence on epigenetic pathways remain elusive and in need of further validation, it is undoubtable that curcumin can have a significant impact on both the function and the expression level of epigenetic proteins. Firstly, curcumin (**120**) is a well-known inhibitor of the histone acetyltransferase activity of the transcriptional co-activators p300/CBP [193]. The treatment of purified histones extracted from HeLa cells with [H^3]acetyl CoA and recombinant p300/CBP in the presence of 20, 40, 60, 80 μM curcumin (**120**), showed a dose-dependent reduction in acetylated histones H3 and H4, with reported IC_{50} = 25 μM. When intact HeLa cells were exposed to 75-100 μM curcumin (**120**) for 24 hours, they underwent extensive apoptosis; when histones acetylation levels were enhanced by pre-treating cells with deacetylase inhibitors such TSA and sodium butyrate, significant changes in H3 and H4 acetylation levels were recorded after exposure to 100 μM curcumin (**120**) [193]. Interestingly, p300/CBP is not only involved in the acetylation of the *N*-terminal tails of histones, but also in the acetylation of non-histone proteins such as p53 and RelA. In fact, it is through these secondary effectors that some of the chemopreventive effects of curcumin (**120**) are achieved [190]. Acetylation of p53 leads to increased protein stability and consequent increase in activity, which usually results in an arrest of the cell cycle to allow DNA repair, or cell death by apoptosis [194]. In 2006, Shankar and Srivastava [195] reported that curcumin could induce extensive apoptosis in LNCaP prostate cancer cells. When they treated LNCaP cells with 10-30 μM curcumin (**120**), they noticed a significant increment of acetylated and phosphorylated p53 after 4 h of exposure, with no changes in expression levels. At the same time, increased acetylation of histones H3 and H4 was registered [195]. In Burkitt lymphoma (Raji) and leukemia (THP-1) cell lines, the inhibition of p300/CBP HAT was correlated to reduced activity of the transcription factor NFκB as a result of the acetylation of RelA (p65), a protein involved in the formation of the most abundant forms of NFκB, the p65/p50 heterodimer and the p65/p65 homodimer, and in the IκBα-mediated attenuation of NFκB [192, 196]. In a few instances, it has been theorised that the α,β-unsaturated ketone of curcumin (**120**) could facilitate the formation of a covalent adduct with p300 [197]. As the acetylation and deacetylation of histone and non-histone proteins is a dynamic equilibrium under the control of both histone acetyltransferases (HATs) and histone deacetylases (HDACs), it is not surprising that curcumin (**120**) exerts its antiproliferative activity by influencing both systems. In Rajii cells, curcumin **120** (12.5 μM) was found to reduce intracellular levels of p300 together with HDAC1 and HDAC3 [198]. In a similar way, HDAC4 expression and activity were demonstrated to be reduced in curcumin (**120**) treated medulloblastoma cells (DAOY) [199]. Interestingly, the reduction in HDAC3 expression levels was confirmed in LNCaP prostate cancer cells, while the expression of HDAC1, HDAC4, HDAC5 and HDAC8 seemed to increase after treatment with 5 μM curcumin (**120**). Moreover, when curcumin was tested in an *in vitro* assay performed using HeLa nuclear extracts, it caused dose-dependent inhibition of HDAC activity, with IC_{50} = 115 μM [200]. Docking curcumin in the active site of HDAC8 showed that this natural compound could assume a stable pose inside the channel connecting the surface of the protein to the acetyl-lysine pocket, despite not reaching far enough to interact with the catalytic zinc ion [200]. More recently, the inhibition of DNA-methyltransferases has been proposed as an alternative epigenetic mechanism subject to curcumin's control. The treatment of a variety of cancer cell lines with curcumin (**120**) has been largely associated with hypomethylation of the promoter region of several oncosuppressor genes. Since methylation of CpG islands in the promoter region is associated with gene silencing, demethylation is expected to cause an increase in gene expression. In fact, the expression of Neurog1, a cancer-related CpG-methylation marker, was reactivated by treatment of LNCaP prostate cancer cells with 5 μM curcumin (**120**) for 7 days [201]. Although no changes in the expression of DNMTs was observed, chromatin immunoprecipitation assays showed a reduction in methylated lysine 27 on histone 3 (H3K27me3), a validated marker of transcriptional activity [202]. In a similar way, curcumin **120** (5 or 10 μM for 5 days) reversed the hypermethylation of the promoter region of *Nrf2*, the gene encoding for nuclear factor erythroid-1 related factor-2, a regulator of the cell antioxidant response system, in prostate cancer cells from TRAMP mice [203]. Again, no transcriptional activation of *DNMT1*, *DNMT3a* or *DNMT3b* was observed. These findings suggest that, although the mechanism of curcumin-induced DNA hypomethylation has not been fully elucidated yet, it would be unlikely to result from the direct control of intracellular levels of DNMTs. However, this claim has been contrasted by two separate studies on MCF-7 breast cancer cells and multidrug resistant melanoma cells, in which curcumin (**120**) has been reported to reactivate the expression of methylation-silenced genes (*FANCF* in MCF-7 and cyclin-dependent kinase inhibitor genes in melanoma cells) by reducing the expression of DNMT1 at both the mRNA and protein level [204, 205]. At the same time, several *in vitro* methylation assays confirmed that curcumin (**120**) is capable of inhibiting bacterial CpG-specific DNA-methyltransferase *M. SssI*, an enzyme characterised by high similarity to the catalytic domain of DNMT1, in a dose-dependent manner [203, 206]. According to Liu *et al.* [207], the apparent IC_{50} of curcumin (**120**) against *M. SssI* is in the low nanomolar range (30 nM). Moreover, virtual docking of curcumin (**120**) in the active site of human DNMT1, obtained by homology modelling, returned a binding pose suggesting that curcumin could inhibit DNMT1 by blocking the access to its catalytic cysteine, C1226 [207]. However, with the only exception of a study where curcumin (**120**) was demonstrated to reduce the growth of human prostate cancer cell xenografts in mice [208], clinical trials in which curcumin was added to the diet of cancer patients have not produced consistent results [209]. In part, this discrepancy could be justified by the fact that curcumin (**120**) is characterised by low bioavailability and high instability at physiological pH. Moreover, it undergoes extensive first passage metabolism to generate sulfate, glucuronide, dihydro and tetrahydrocurcumin derivatives that are excreted in the bile and in the urines. In fact, only patients treated with high doses of curcumin (**120**) showed plasma concentration in the therapeutic range: when patients were administered 8 g of curcumin (**120**) per day, the registered plasma concentration was 1.75 ± 0.80 μM; when the patients received roughly half of the dose, 3.6 g of curcumin per day, the plasma concentration fell as low as 11.1 nM, while maintaining micromolar concentration in colorectal tissue [210]. In the search to improve its pharmacokinetic properties, several attempts have been made at modifying the structure of curcumin (**120**) in order to identify its pharmacophore and remove any metabolic liability. Most studies have focused on protecting or removing the hydroxyl groups at position four of the aromatic rings, which is known to constitute an anchor for phase II type metabolic reactions. Several isosteric substitutions and simplification operations have been proposed to replace the β-hydroxyketone moiety as although it was deemed essential for biological activity, it is responsible for curcumin's instability and susceptibility to aldo-ketoreductase enzymes. In 2009, Fuchs *et al.* [211] published a comprehensive study on the effect of chemical modifications on the anti-proliferative activity of curcumin derivatives. The synthesised analogues were tested on four panels of breast cancer (MCF-7 and MDA-MD-231) and prostate cancer (LNCaP and PC-3) cell lines (selected results are reported in Table **11**).

Table 11. Structure and antiproliferative activity of curcumin derivatives 125-130 against breast (MCF-7 and MDA-MD-231) and prostate cancer (LNCaP and PC-3) cell lines [211].

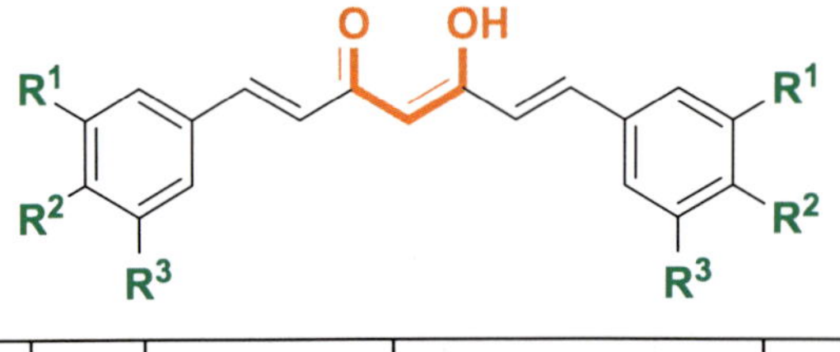

Cmpd	R^1	R^2	R^3	MCF-7 (IC_{50})	MDA-MD-231 (IC_{50})	LNCaP (IC_{50})	PC-3 (IC_{50})
120	OCH_3	OH	H	21.5 ± 4.7 μM	25.6 ± 4.8 μM	19.6 ± 3.7 μM	19.8 ± 2.1 μM
125	OCH_3	OSO_2NH_2	H	5.5 ± 1.2 μM	3.1 ± 1.3 μM	5.9 ± 1.7 μM	7.5 ± 1.8 μM
126	OCH_3	OCH_3	H	5.4 ± 0.8 μM	4.9 ± 0.9 μM	3.9 ± 0.6 μM	5.9 ± 1.3 μM
127	OCH_3	OSO_2NH_2	OCH_3	4.7 ± 0.7 μM	5.5 ± 0.1 μM	10.4 ± 1.6 μM	13.1 ± 2.1 μM
128	OCH_3	H	H	25.9 ± 9.5 μM	31.9 ± 11.1 μM	34.7 ± 6.6 μM	40 ± 4.9 μM

(Table 11) cont.....

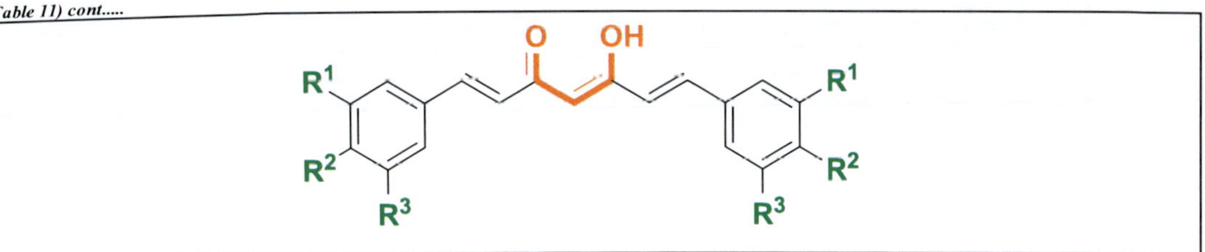

Cmpd	R^1	R^2	R^3	MCF-7 (IC_{50})	MDA-MD-231 (IC_{50})	LNCaP (IC_{50})	PC-3 (IC_{50})
129	H	OCH_3	H	> 40 μM	> 40 μM	> 40 μM	> 40 μM

Table 12. Curcumin derivatives as HDAC inhibitors [212].

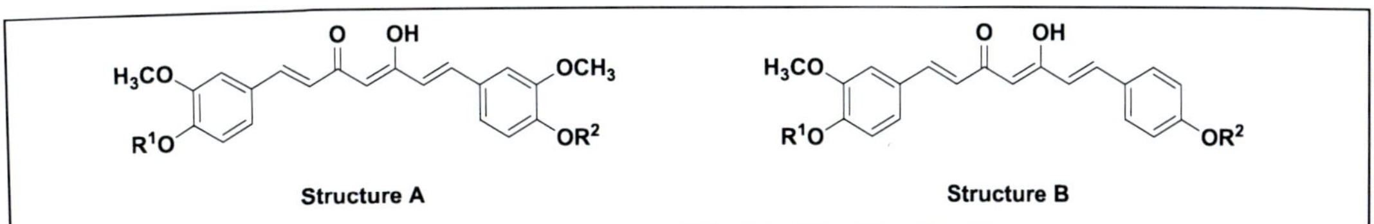

Cmpd	Structure	R^1	R^2	Remaining HDAC activity	HDAC1 binding activity	HDAC2 binding activity	HDAC8 binding activity	HeLa cells	HCT116 cells	MCF-7 cells
				%	K_i (μM)	K_i (μM)	K_i (μM)	72h	72h	72h
120	curcumin	-	-	33 ± 0.25	50.79	97.67	64.90	3.56 ± 0.47	2.40 ± 0.15	2.03 ± 0.16
130	A	*sec*-C_4H_9	*sec*-C_4H_9	7 ± 0.17	20.71	7.47	10.22	10.20 ± 0.20	7.89 ± 0.19	13.89 ± 0.67
131	A	CH_2COOH	CH_2COOH	5 ± 0.02	1.96	3.99	14.24	> 100	> 100	>100
132	A	$CH(CH_3)CONH_2$	$CH(CH_3)CONH_2$	7 ± 0.04	0.936	0.55	0.88	19.56 ± 1.14	14.60 ± 1.19	30.71 ± 1.10
133	B	H	*sec*-C_4H_9	6 ± 0.06	2.50	1.06	3.60	9.33 ± 0.38	7.33 ± 0.98	18.08 ± 1.44

Interestingly, the protection of hydroxyl groups at positions R^1 and R^2 in β-hydroxyketone derivatives **125-127** with a range of functional groups, including methyl and sulfamate, led to an average four folds increase in anti-proliferative activity compared to curcumin (**120**). On the contrary, the removal of substituent R^1 or R^2 caused a significant loss of activity, with R^1 seemingly being necessary for biological activity Table **11**. Although the molecular mechanism through which these compounds exerted their cytotoxic activity was not investigated in this study, a recent publication from Somsakeesit *et al.* [212] seems to suggest that they could behave as HDAC inhibitors. When three series of curcumin, demethoxycurcumin and bisdimethoxycurcumin derivatives were tested for their ability to inhibit histone deacetylase activity in three human cancer cell lines (HeLA, HCT-116 and MCF-7), most compounds induced more than 80% inhibition of HDAC activity at 100 µM. These derivatives included substituents at the R group such as methyl, ethyl, butyl, *sec*-butyl, allyl, propargyl, benzyl, 4-fluorobenzyl, 4-*tert*-butyl benzyl, TBDSM, linear and branched methyl esters, their carboxylic acids and amide derivatives [212]. The four most potent derivatives (**130-133**) showed higher HDAC inhibitory activity than curcumin (**120**) as well as higher binding affinity to the active sites of HDAC1, HDAC2 and HDAC8. However, none of these compounds had cytotoxic activity comparable to curcumin (**120**) when tested against cervical (HeLa), colon (HCT116), and breast (MCF-7) cancer cell lines (Table **12**).

When compound **132** was docked in the active site of HDAC2, it was predicted to bind the catalytic Zn^{2+} ion with its amide substituent and engage in at least four hydrogen bonding interactions with the backbone of Gly32 and Leu276 and the lateral chains of Glu103, and Tyr209. Unfortunately, modifications of the β-hydroxyketone functional group involving the addition of an alkyl or aryl substituent at the α-carbon (**134-136**) or the reduction to a 1,3-diol (**137**) caused a significant reduction in HDAC inhibition. The activity was rescued only when the α-carbon was doubly substituted with two methyl-ester moieties (**138**) Table **13**

Table 13. Effects of the modification of the β-hydroxyketone on the HDAC inhibitory activity of curcumin derivatives (100 µM) [212].

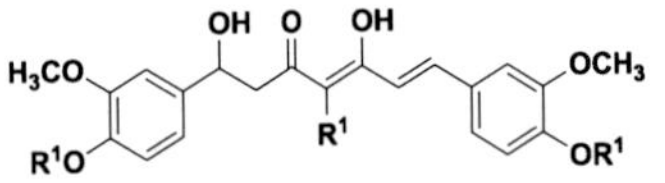

Structure A

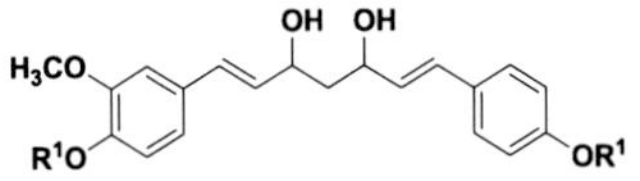

Structure B

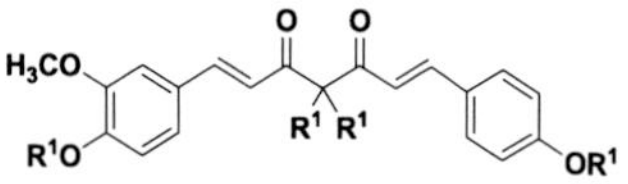

Structure C

	R^1	Remaining HDAC activity %			R^1	Remaining HDAC activity %			R^1	Remaining HDAC activity %
134	CH_3	51 ± 0.83	-	137	H	85 ± 0.62	-	138	$CH_2CO_2CH_3$	18 ± 0.46
135	benzyl	31 ± 0.33	-							
136	$CH_2CO_2CH_3$	28 ± 0.30	-							

However, when the derivatisation of the α-carbon of curcumin (**120**) was performed using prenyl and geranyl groups, a remarkable loss of HDAC inhibitory activity of the corresponding derivatives (**139-143**) was recorded when they were tested on HeLa cell nuclear extracts [213]. On the other side, the introduction of a farnesyl appendix to one of the aromatic rings led to a more active derivative (**142**, IC_{50} = 84.2 μM) than coumarin (**120**, IC_{50} = 187 μM) Fig. (**23**).

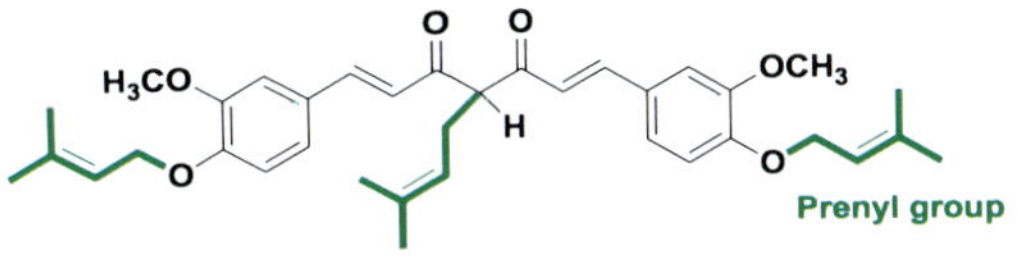

139

No inhibition

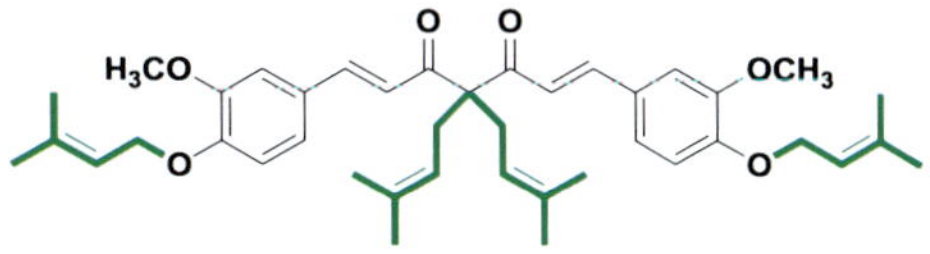

140

No inhibition

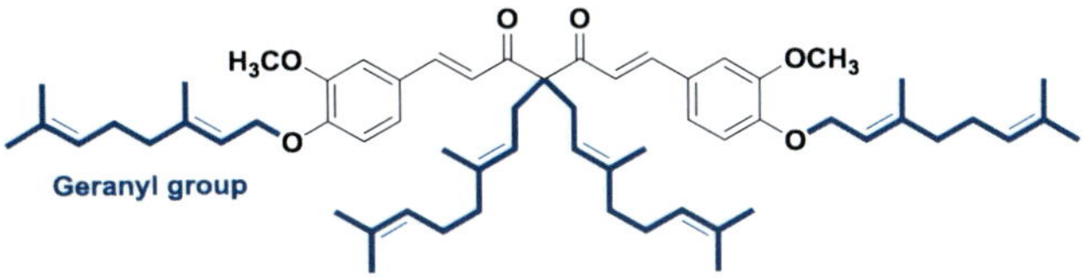

141

IC_{50} = 217 μM

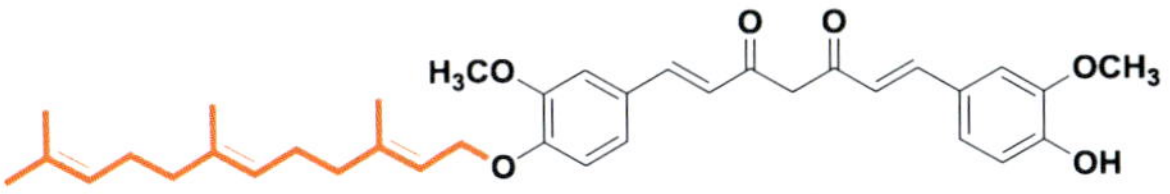

Farnesyl group

142

IC_{50} = 84.2 μM

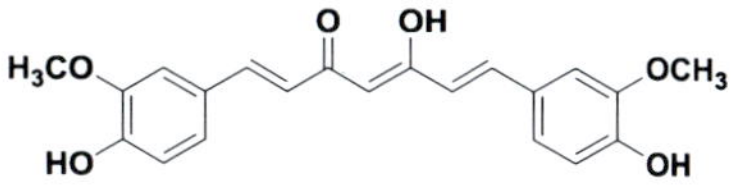

143

IC_{50} = 187 μM

Fig. (23). Prenyl, geranyl, and farnesyl derivatives of curcumin and their inhibitory activity against HDAC in HeLa cell nuclear extracts [213].

The predicted binding mode of compound **142** in the active site of HDAC2 showed that this compound can bind the Zn^{2+} ion in a bidentate fashion and, at the same time, establish extensive hydrophobic contacts with the surface of the protein using its farnesyl group [213]. Beyond the substitution/alkylation of the α-carbon, an appealing strategy adopted to generate metabolically stable derivatives involves replacing the β-hydroxyketone functional group with heterocyclic structures. In fact, five membered ring heteroaromatic structures could mimic the monodentate chelation of the catalytic Zn^{2+} ion while optimising the interaction with aromatic residues within the active sites of HDACs. Despite these premises, none of the oxazole or imidazole derivatives (**144-148**) recently reported by Kumboonma *et al.* [214] showed significantly higher HDAC inhibitory activity compared to curcumin (**120**), which was found to reduce 62% of HDAC activity in HeLa nuclear extracts at a concentration of 100 μM Table **14**.

Table 14. Heterocyclic curcumin derivatives as HDAC inhibitors in HeLa nuclear extracts [214].

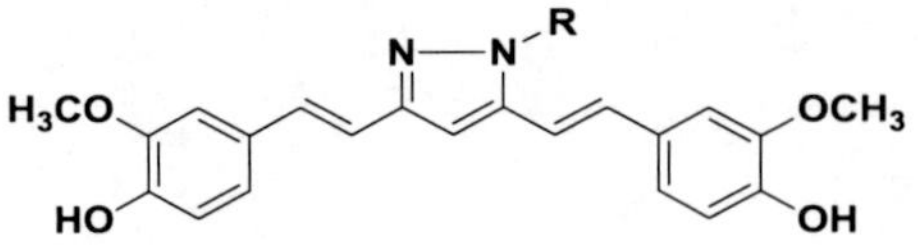

Structure A

Cmpd	R	Remaining HDAC activity
144	H	49%
145	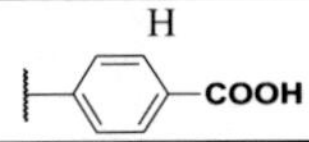	36%
146	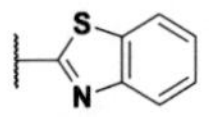	33%
147	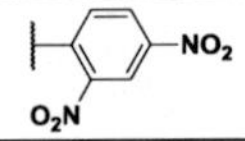	35%

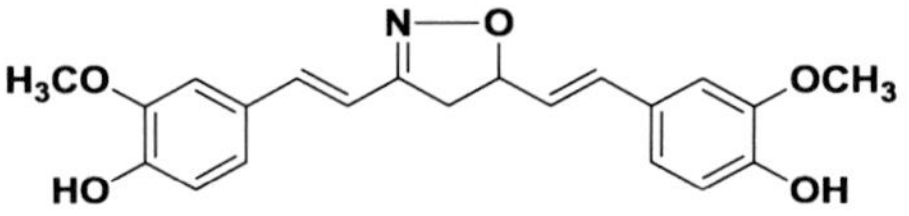

Structure B

Cmpd	R	Remaining HDAC activity
144	H	49%

When compound **148** was tested against breast carcinoma cell lines (MCF-7) and their multi-drug resistant variant (MCF-7R), it showed promising cytotoxic activity (IC_{50} values of 13.1 ± 1.6 μM and 12.0 ± 2.0 μM, respectively) despite its molecular mechanism not being confirmed.[215] On the contrary, hydroxycurcumin **149** and its substituted amine and methoxy-amino equivalents **150-151** showed a slight increase in HDAC inhibitory activity compared to curcumin Table **15** [214].

Table 15. HDAC inhibitory activity and antiproliferative effect of hydroxy (149), arylamine (150) and methoxyamino (151) derivatives of curcumin (120) [214].

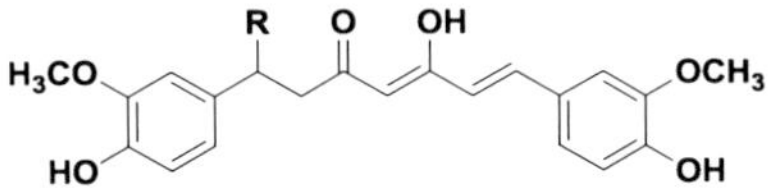

Cmpd	R	Remaining HDAC activity	HDAC2 binding activity	HDAC4 binding activity	HDAC7 binding activity	HDAC8 binding activity	HeLa cells	HCT116 cells	MCF-7 cells
		%	K_i (μM)	K_i (μM)	K_i (μM)	K_i (μM)	72 h	72 h	72 h
120	curcumin	38	9.54	1.91	10.63	18.38	3.57 ± 0.50	2.67 ± 0.20	2.08 ± 0.12
149	OH	24	0.98	13.99	2.64	8.01	-*	-*	-*
150	aniline	18	20.23	2.11	8.26	3.97	12.81 ± 0.31	2.97 ± 0.06	13.27 ± 1.49
151	$NHOCH_3$	27	-*	-*	-*	-*	4.69 ± 0.14	4.69 ± 0.14	5.23 ± 0.21

[1]Data not reported.

In particular, mapping the interactions of compound **150** in the active site of HDAC4, it was proposed that this compound could bind the Zn^{2+} ion *via* the hydroxyl group, while forming hydrogen bonds with three amino acids within the catalytic pocket (Lys20, Gly331, and His198) using both its hydroxyl and amino groups. Moreover, the benzene ring of aniline was reported to establish π-π interactions with the lateral chain of His198, a residue involved in the coordination of the catalytic zinc. Although this evidence seemed to suggest that substituting the hydroxyl group in curcumin with an amino groups could be beneficial, the replacement of the β-hydroxyketone group with variedly substituted β-aminoketones (**152-156**) caused a significant loss in cytotoxic activity against breast cancer cells, with IC_{50} values against MCF-7 and MCF-7R in the range of 49-100 μM Table **16** [215]. On the contrary, the di-oxime derivative **157** showed to be two to four folds more potent than curcumin (**120**) against the same cell lines Table **16**.

Table 16. Cytotoxic activity of amine and hydroxylamine derivatives of curcumin on breast cancer cell lines (MCF-7 and MCF-7R) [215].

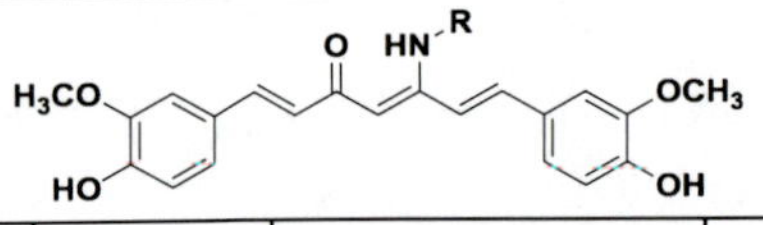

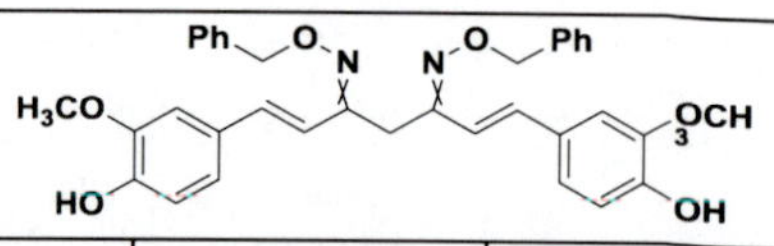

Cmpd	R	MCF-7 (IC_{50})	MCF-7R (IC_{50})		Cmpd	MCF-7 (IC_{50})	MCF-7R (IC_{50})
		μM	μM			μM	μM
120	curcumin	29.3 ± 1.7	26.2 ± 1.6	-	**157**	7.1 ± 0.2	9.3 ± 1.7
152	H	49.9 ± 4.6	54.7 ± 4.6	-	-	-	-
153	CH_2Ph	>100	>100	-	-	-	-
154	$CH(CH_3)_2$	70.3 ± 8.0	49.8 ± 6.6	-	-	-	-
155	$CHCH_3)Ph$	>100	>100	-	-	-	-
156	CH_2CH_3	93.0 ± 6.7	67.6 ± 7.4	-	-	-	-

The replacement of the β-hydroxyketone group with a dienone moiety (**158-161**) showed to be a successful strategy to increase the stability of the corresponding derivatives and, at the same time, improve their cytotoxicity against breast and prostate cancer cell lines Table **17** [211].

Table 17. Antiproliferative activity of dienone curcumin analogues (158-163) against breast (MCT-7 and MDA-MD-231) and prostate (LNCaP and PC3) cancer cell lines [211].

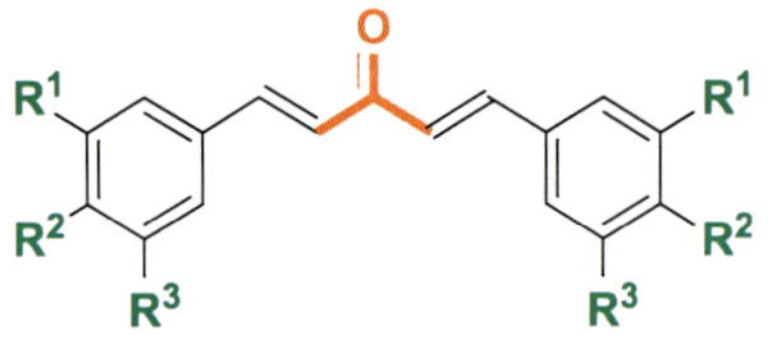

Cmpd	R^1	R^2	R^3	MCF-7 (IC_{50})	MDA-MD-231 (IC_{50})	LNCaP (IC_{50})	PC-3 (IC_{50})
158	OCH_3	OH	H	2.4 ± 0.4 μM	2.8 ± 1.0 μM	2.7 ± 0.4 μM	3.9 ± 1.1 μM
159	OCH_3	OSO_2NH_2	H	6.6 ± 1.1 μM	1.7 ± 0.1 μM	2.4 ± 0.6 μM	6.1 ± 0.3 μM
160	OCH_3	OCH_3	H	2.5 ± 0.4 μM	1.6 ± 0.4 μM	2.2 ± 0.5 μM	2.9 ± 0.6 μM
161	OCH_3	OSO_2NH_2	OCH_3	1.5 ± 0.1 μM	0.6 ± 0.2 μM	1.9 ± 0.4 μM	2.4 ± 0.2 μM

(Table 17) cont.....

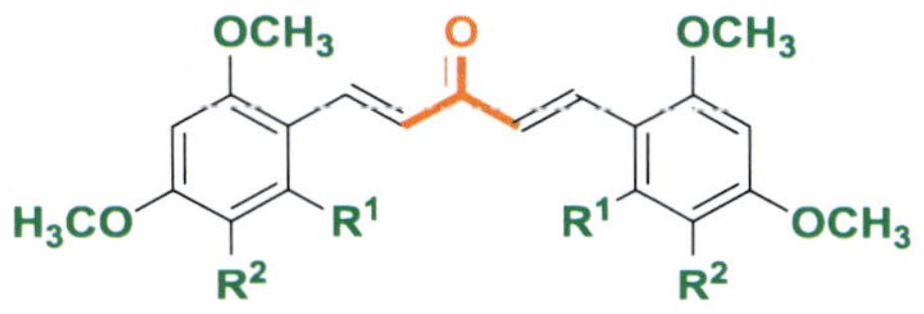

Cmpd	R^1	R^2	MCF-7 (IC_{50})	MDA-MD-231 (IC_{50})	LNCaP (IC_{50})	PC-3 (IC_{50})
162	OCH_3	H	0.4 ± 0.1 μM	0.6 ± 0.1 μM	0.5 ± 0.1 μM	2.1 ± 1.1 μM
163	H	OCH_3	2.4 ± 1.0 μM	2.4 ± 0.4 μM	1.7 ± 0.6 μM	4.6 ± 0.2 μM

Table 18. Antiproliferative activity of non-conformationally restrained (164-171) and conformationally restrained (172-179) dienone curcumin analogues against a panel of gastric (BGC-823), nasopharyngeal (CNE), leukemia (HL-60), epidermal (KB), colorectal (LS174T), prostate (PC3), and cervical (HeLa) cancer cell lines [216].

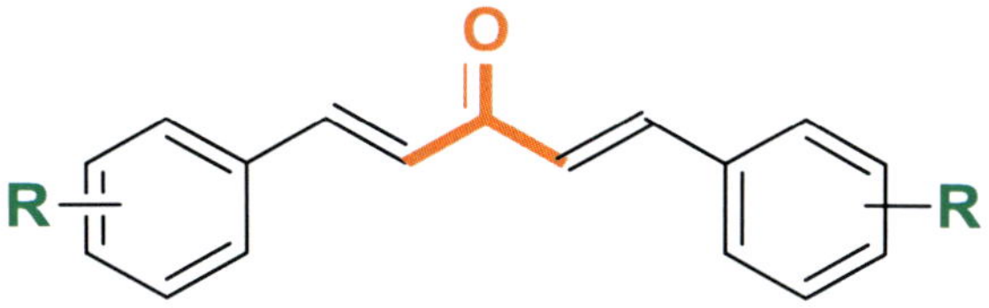

Comp	R	IC_{50} (μM)						
		BGC-823	CNE	HL-60	KB	LS174T	PC3	HeLa
164	3'-OCH_3, -4'OH	-	6.8 ± 1.6	-	-	3.7 ± 0.7	-	-
165	2'-OCH_3, 3'-OCH_3	24.4 ± 2.6	-	4.5 ± 3.6	24.3 ± 3.9	48.0 ± 10.7	-	-
166	2'-CH_3, 5'-CH_3	-	17.7 ± 2.6	-	-	103 ± 19.3	5.2 ± 2.1	6.1 ± 1.0
167	4'-$C(CH_3)_3$	-	89.8 ± 24.0	-	-	-	12.0 ± 2.9	21.8 ± 6.3
168	4'-F	-	-	-	94.6 ± 14.3	98.8 ± 19.1	15.2 ± 2.9	-
169	2'-Br	16.1 ± 2.6	-	-	-	4.0 ± 0.6	15.4 ± 6.0	34.2 ± 7.8
170	2'-Cl	-	-	8.6 ± 2.6	59.0 ± 12.0	-	-	-
171	2'-CF_3	-	-	<10	<3.70	-	0.35 ± 0.1	-
120	Curcumin	16.7 ± 2.3	32.8 ±6.7	11.6 ± 0.9	35.9 ± 21.0	6.4 ± 1.0	15.0 ± 2.9	17.5 ±2.2

(Table 18) cont.....

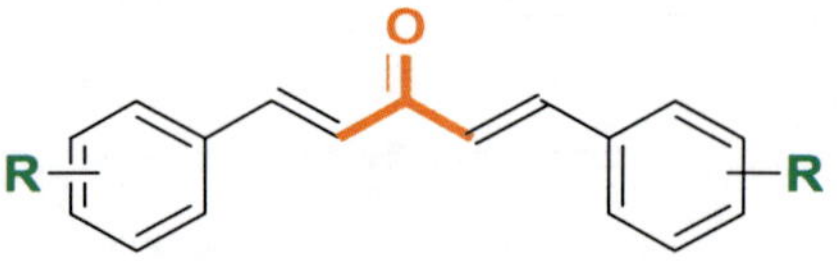

Comp	R	IC$_{50}$ (μM)						
		BGC 823	**CNE**	**HL-60**	**KB**	**LS174T**	**PC3**	**HeLa**
172	3'-OCH_3, -4'OH	-	17.6 ± 6.9	-	<10.10	4.6 ± 2.5	-	
173	2'-OCH_3, 3'-OCH_3	55.3 ± 16.5	-	-	179 ± 67.0	84.5 ± 23.1	-	
174	2'-CH_3, 5'-CH_3	-	-	-	35.3 ± 10.8	-	-	
175	4'-$C(CH_3)_3$	-	-	-	78.9 ± 25.6	-	-	
176	4'-F	87.3 ± 26.9	77.9 ± 20.7	58.1 ± 15.4	150 ± 41.3	7.4 ± 2.4	-	
177	2'-Br	-	-	-	55.3 ± 14.6	-	-	
178	2'-Cl	4.4 ± 0.9	-	98.3 ± 17.8	6.7 ± 1.5	4.2 ± 2.1	13.8 ± 3.2	
179	2'-CF_3	-	-	-	54.0 ± 19.9	-	-	46.3 ± 15.9
120	Curcumin	16.7 ± 2.3	32.8 ±6.7	11.6 ± 0.9	35.9 ± 21.0	6.4 ± 1.0	15.0 ± 2.9	17.5 ±2.2

These findings were confirmed in a contemporary study conducted by Liang *et al.* [216] on the bioavailability and cytotoxicity of curcumin derivatives. In this study, the authors reported that the oral administration of 500 mg/Kg of derivative **164**, a compound that differs from curcumin only for the presence of a dienone functional group instead of a β-hydroxyketone, to healthy rats showed a nine folds increase in plasma concentration (C_{max} = 0.82 μg/mL) compared to curcumin **120** (C_{max} = 0.091 μg/mL), while its clearance (125.4 L/Kg h) was significantly lower than the parent compound **120** (835.2 L/Kg h). Compound **169** showed the most promising pharmacokinetic properties, as it reached a plasma concentration of 4.1 μg/mL and its clearance was as low as 38.98 L/Kg h. When these derivatives were tested on seven different cancer cell lines, non-conformationally restrained compounds (**164-171**) displayed higher cytotoxicity than the corresponding cyclic compounds (**172-179**) Table **18**. The dimension of the ring was deemed essential to maintain biological activity. In particular, when the 6-membered ring was replaced by a 5-membered ring, most derivatives lost activity [216].

When the aromatic ring was replaced by isosteric heteroaromatic rings, the cytotoxic effect of the corresponding derivatives was detectable only at high micromolar concentrations, with the notable exception of pyrrole (**182-183**), thiophene (**180**) and 2-bromo-thiophene (**181**) derivatives Table **19** [216].

Table 19. Antiproliferative effect of heterocyclic isosteres of curcumin (180-183) against prostate (PC3), cervical (HeLa), colorectal (LS147T), and epidermal (KB) cancer cells [216].

Compd	Structure	Cell type	IC_{50} (μM)*
180	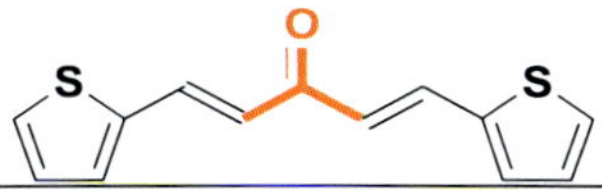	PC3	10.3 ± 2.8
		HeLa	6.2 ± 2.2
181	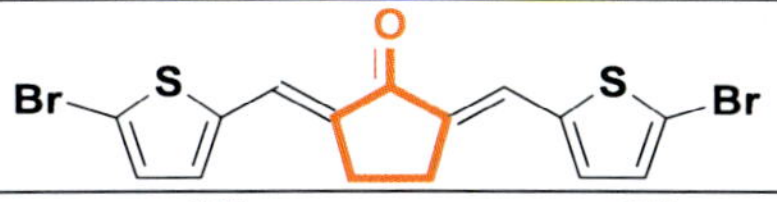	LS147T	9.0 ± 2.5
182	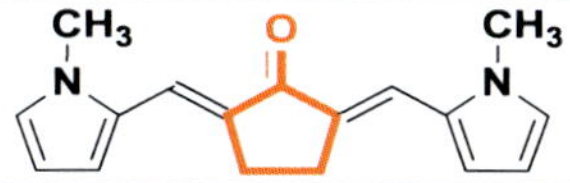	LS147T	9.2 ± 2.9
183	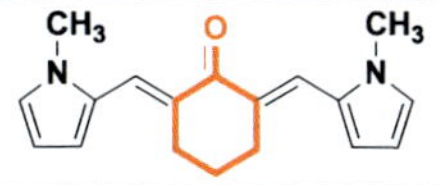	KB	2.3 ± 0.6

An analogous approach was taken by Yadav *et al.* [217] when they synthesised a series of cyclopentanone and cyclohexanone derivatives of curcumin, alongside heterocyclic and bicyclic compounds, to evaluate their cytotoxicity against MDA-MB-231 breast cancer cells and their ability to inhibit the nuclear factor NFκB in K563 leukemia cells. Similarly to the work conducted by Liang *et al.* [216], heterocyclic structures such as pyridine, thiophene, imidazole, pyrrole and indole were considered isosteric replacements for the substituted benzene rings of curcumin. Of the eighteen compounds tested, only five of them showed cytotoxic activity in the low micromolar range (≈ 1 μM), usually associated with potent inhibition of NFκB (Table **20**) [217].

Although the cellular mechanisms involved in controlling NFκB activity could be diverse, it cannot be excluded that these compounds act through the modulation of epigenetic pathways. Similar compounds, in which the tetrahydropyridine ring has been replaced with a tetrahydropyran (**190**) or tetrahydrothiopyran (**191**) were shown to inhibit the proliferation of humane prostate cancer cell lines CWR-22Rv1 and LNCaP Table **21**. while, at the same time, reactivating the methylation silenced gene Nrf2 in TRAMP-C1 prostate cancer cells when tested with a luciferase activity essay [203, 218].

Table 20. Cytotoxicity and NFκB inhibitory activity of conformationally-restrained heterocyclic analogues of curcumin [217].

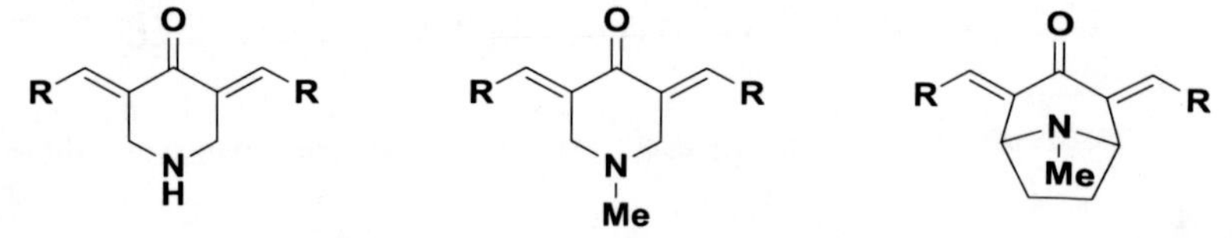

Cmpd	Series	R	MDA-MB-231	NFkB
			EC_{50} (μM)	IC_{50} (μM)
120	curcumin	-	7.6	15 ± 5
184	A	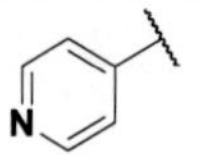	1.1	2.5 ± 0.2
185	B	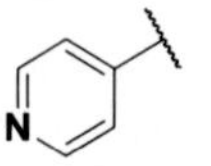	0.8	1.0 ± 0.3
186	B	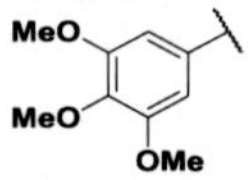	0.3	0.9 ± 0.1
187	B	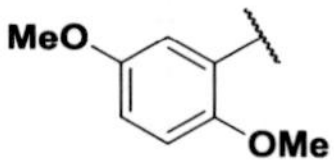	1.1	6.3 ± 0.3
188	C	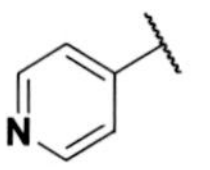	1.1	1.5 ± 0.2

Table 21. Antiproliferative activity of heterocyclic conformationally restrained coumarin analogues 189-191 against two prostate cancer cell lines [218].

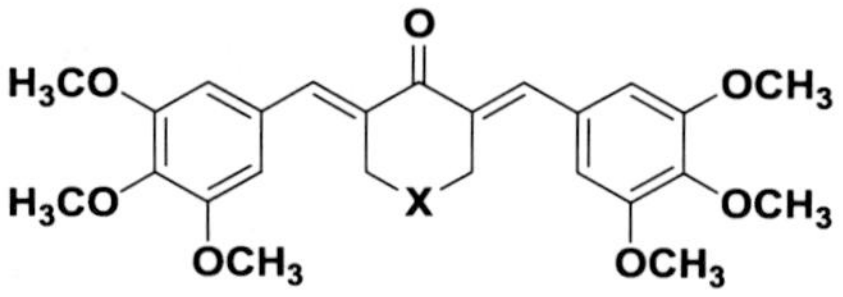

Cmpd	X	CWR-22Rv1 (IC_{50}) μM	LNCaP μM
120	curcumin	16.99 ± 3.0	13.59 ± 1.8
189	CH_2	8.76 ± 0.5	9.8 ± 1.2
190	O	0.82 ± 0.1	0.65 ± 0.2

(Table 21) cont.....

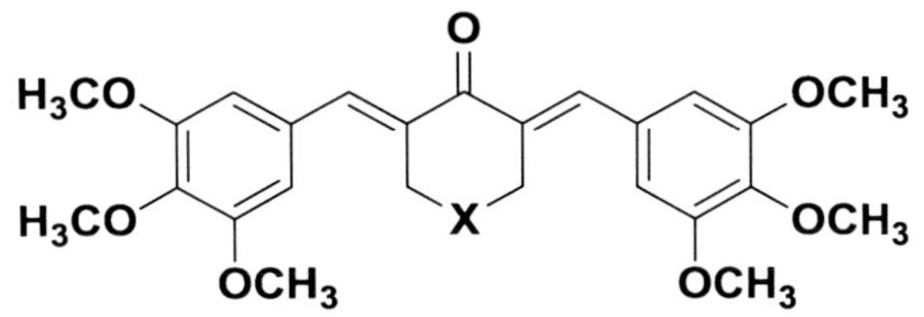

Cmpd	X	CWR-22Rv1 (IC_{50}) µM	LNCaP µM
191	S	0.96 ± 0.1	0.81 ± 0.2

In accordance with the proposed reactivation of Nerf2 *via* demethylation of its promoter, the expression and activity levels of DNMT1, DNMT3a and DNMT3b were found to be reduced in TRAMP-C1 cells after treatment with both 50 nM and 100 nM compound **191**. In contrast, compound **190** did not seem to induce a similar change in DNMTs levels: treating TRAMP-C1 cells with 100 nM **190** caused an increase of DNMT1 expression and did not affect DNTM3a and DNMT3b. At the same time, both compounds **190** and **191** caused a reduction in HDACs expression, although compound **191** inhibited total HDAC activity, while compound **190** increased it. Interestingly, when a series of this kind of exocyclic dienone derivatives were tested against a panel of HATs (p300 and PCAF), sirtuins (SIRT1 and 2), KMT (EZH2) and PRMT (CARM1), they showed to be dual and selective p300/CARM1 inhibitors Table **22** [219]. In fact, the treatment of several cancer cell lines including leukaemia (NB4), lymphoma (U937), neuroblastoma (SH-SY5Y), and breast cancer (MCF-7) with derivatives **186**, **189-190**, and **192-202** showed that most compounds were able to arrest the cell cycle at the G2/M or G1/S phase and decrease the levels of acetyl-H3, acetyl-H4, acetyl-H3K9/14 and H3R17me2.

These results are particularly promising as they address some of the major concerns around the chemopreventive and therapeutic use of curcumin derivatives, which include metabolic susceptibility and instability under physiological conditions. Although these compounds have shown promising activity against HDACs, HATs, and even PRMTs, their bioavailability and *in vivo* efficacy remains to be demonstrated.

Table 22. ***In vitro*** **inhibition of HAT, SIRT, KMT and PRMT enzymatic activity by exocyclic dienone compounds 186, 189-190, 192-202 [219].**

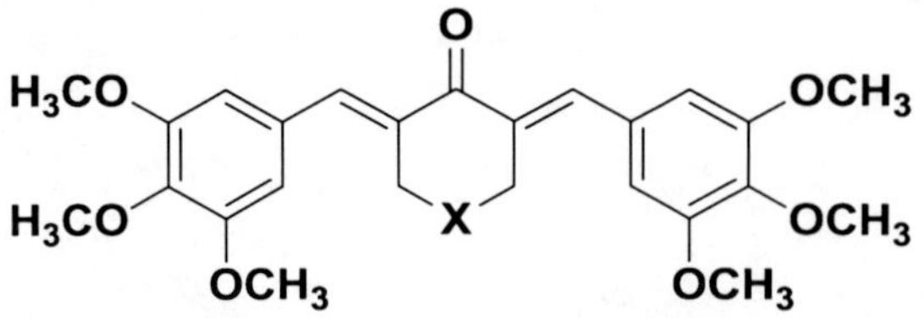

Cmpd	X	IC$_{50}$ (μM)					
		p300	PCAF	SIRT1	SIRT2	PRC2/EZH2	CARM1
189	CH_2	1.38 ± 0.24	>200	>200	>200	117 ± 6	16.8 ± 3.4
190	O	2.56 ± 0.23	>200	>200	>200	>200	23.3 ± 0.5
192	NH	23.2 ± 0.51	>200	>200	>200	>200	44.8 ± 6.0
186	N-CH_3	2.66 ± 0.15	>200	>200	>200	46.7 ± 1.1	3.24 ± 1.22
193	CH_2Ph	2.19 ± 0.77	>200	>200	>200	44.2 ± 0.2	6.50 ± 0.86
194	CH_2CH_2Ph	30.17 ± 2.71	>200	>200	>200	>200	18.5 ± 0.9
195	$CH_2(CH_2)_2$Ph	40.7 ± 2.39	>200	>200	>200	>200	12.6 ± 2.6
196	CH_2COPh	1.03 ± 0.22	>200	>200	>200	46.0 ± 8.1	5.52 ± 0.78
197	CH_2CH_2COPh	1.57 ±0.72	>200	>200	>200	60.6 ± 10.5	6.96 ± 0.9
198	$CH_2(CH_2)_2$COPh	2.13 ± 1.35	>200	>200	>200	68.5 ± 6.2	4.80 ± 1.72
199	COPh	2.09 ± 0.79	>200	>200	>200	40.7 ± 15.3	1.33 ± 0.14
200	COCH_2Ph	0.45 ± 0.03	>200	>200	>200	15.2 ± 2.2	0.43 ± 0.12
201	COCH_2CH_2COPh	0.46 ± 0.10	>200	>200	>200	11.3 ± 0.08	0.79 ± 0.06
202	COCH=CHPh	1.23 ± 0.29	>200	>200	>200	13.9 ± 1.8	7.14 2.54

RESVERATROL AND OTHER STILBENE DERIVATIVES

Resveratrol (**203**), pterostilbene (**204**) and piceatannol (**204**) are polyphenols characterised by a *trans*-stilbene core and are produced by plants as a defensive mechanism in response to physical stressors, parasites, and other pathogens [220]. They are abundantly found in grapes, berries, and red wine, often in association with other polyphenols and flavonoids, such as anthocyanins and quercetin [221]. Their significant presence in red wine and not in white wine has been mostly ascribed to differences in the fermentation process that, in the latter case, requires the removal of the skin.

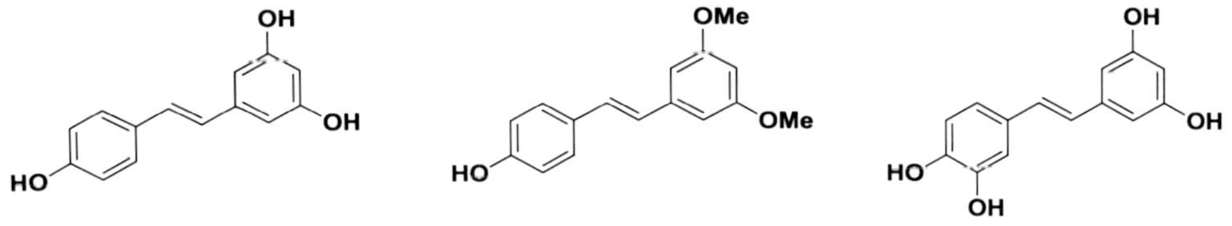

Resveratrol
203

Pterostilbene
204

Piceatannol
205

Fig. (24). Structure of trans-stilbene derivatives resveratrol (**203**), pterostilbene (**204**), and piceatannol (**205**).

The alleged role of red wine in reducing the incidence of cardiovascular diseases in the French population, despite them following a diet involving high alcohol and fat intake together with widespread tobacco consumption, gave origin to the so called "French paradox", which has prompted numerous investigations into the potential chemopreventive effects of its components [222, 223]. These studies have shown that stilbene derivatives, like other polyphenols, possess anti-oxidant and anti-inflammatory properties that involve a wide variety of molecular targets and cellular pathways. In fact, the activity of resveratrol (**203**) and its analogues spans from preventing the formation of oxygen reactive species (ROS) and acting as radical scavengers to inhibiting low-density lipoprotein (LDL) peroxidation and protecting the vascular endothelium from lipid damage [224]. They have also been found to inhibit cyclooxygenase isoforms 1 and 2, and induce the expression of antioxidant enzymes such as Heme Oxygenase 1 (HO-1), glutathione reductase (GR), and quinone reductase (QR) [225, 226]. In fact, some of the cardiovascular protective effects exerted by this class of polyphenols have ben ascribed to their ability to interact with epigenetic modulators and affect gene expression. In particular, resveratrol (**203**) has been reported to be an activator of SIRT1, a (NAD^+)-dependent histone deacetylase highly expressed in the vascular endothelium, where it regulates the expression of genes involved in angiogenic activity and vascular remodelling [227, 228]. The resveratrol induced activity of SIRT1 has been associated with a reduction in angiotensin II receptor mediated hypertension and cardiac fibroblast proliferation, while at the same time having a preventive effect on cardiomyocytes cell death [227, 229]. While originally presented as a SIRT1 activator, resveratrol was subsequently proposed to be a weak inhibitor of SIRT2 and SIRT3, and an activator of SIRT5 [230]. However, studies aimed at defining the binding mode of resveratrol in SIRT1 have concluded that this polyphenol is not a direct SIRT1 activator. In fact, resveratrol seems to induce deacetylation of different fluorophore-tagged peptides but not of unmodified SIRT1 peptide substrates [231, 232]. The direct interaction of resveratrol with the coumarin-based fluorophore attached to a p53 derived peptide was confirmed by X-Ray crystallography [233]. Despite the controversy surrounding their exact mechanisms of action and epigenetic targets, it has been repeatedly demonstrated that resveratrol and its derivatives can induce epigenetic changes and modulate gene expression in several types of cancers, both *in vitro* and *in vivo* [234]. Studies conducted on hepatocellular carcinoma cell lines (HepG2) showed that resveratrol (50-100 μM) acts as a pan-HDAC inhibitor and promotes histone hyperacetylation [235]. When similar dosages were tested in prostate cancer cell lines (DU145 and LNCaP), it was reported that resveratrol could modulate the acetylation state and consequently the activity of tumour suppressor proteins such as p53 and PTEN. This effect was associated with resveratrol's ability to destabilise the nucleosome remodelling and deacetylation (NuRD) corepressor complex including metastasis-associated protein 1 (MTA1), an epigenetic reader overexpressed in aggressive prostate cancer, and HDAC1/2 [236, 237]. A preclinical study using mice models of prostate cancer showed that the upregulation of MTA1 associated with increased tumorigenesis and cancer progression could be contrasted by the administration of resveratrol's more metabolically stable and bioavailable derivative pterostilbene (**204**) [238]. When PTEN heterozygous mice were fed a pterostilbene (**204**) supplemented diet (100 mg/Kg of AIN-76A diet) for 8-10 months, the authors observed a significant reduction in prostatic intraepithelial neoplasia (PIN), thus suggesting a chemopreventive effect of this polyphenol. At the same time, daily intraperitoneal injections of 10 mg/kg of pterostilbene (**204**) in PTEN-null mice led to a 5-fold reduction of the incidence of pre-invasive or invasive prostatic adenocarcinoma [238]. When a series of natural and synthetic stilbenoids were tested against (AR^-) DUP145, (AR^+) LNCaP, and highly metastatic PC3M prostate cancer cells, Li *et al.* [239] found that although resveratrol **203**, pterostilbene **204** and piceatannol **205** (5-100 μM) were all able to inhibit MTA1 expression in a dose-dependent manner, pterostilbene was the compound with the highest pro-apoptotic activity. Moreover, the daily administration of resveratrol (**203**) or pterostilbene (**204**) (50 mg/kg/day) to mice carrying DU145 prostate cancer xenografts led to a significant slowdown of tumour growth, progression and metastasis [239]. Given the proposed mode of action, it should not surprise that the combination of both resveratrol (**203**) and pterostilbene (**204**) with clinically approved HDAC inhibitors, such as SAHA (suberoylanilide hydroxamic acid), revealed a synergistic effect and led researchers to postulate that stilbenoids could be included in the future as sensitisers in well-established therapeutic protocols [236, 240]. However, the epigenetic role of stilbenoids is not limited to modulating histone acetylation: a wide variety of studies has demonstrated that resveratrol and pterostilbene can also influence the methylation state of oncogenes and tumour suppressor genes [241]. With this respect, resveratrol (**203**) and pterostilbene (**204**) have shown promising therapeutic potential for breast cancer, despite their phytoestrogen properties would suggest that their use could be problematic in oestrogen responsive cancers [234]. Genome-wide analysis of methylation patterns recorded in MCF10CA1a and MCF10CA1h breast cancer cell lines treated with resveratrol (**203**) and pterostilbene (**204**) (0-20 μM) showed that these compounds can induce DNMT3b mediated silencing of oncogenes involved in the NOTCH pathway, such as *MAML2* [242]. Similarly, Kala *et al.* [243] reported that a combined treatment of 15 μM resveratrol (**203**) and 5 μM pterostilbene (**204**) selectively reduced the *via*bility of HCC1806 and MDA-MB-157 triple negative breast cancer cells with respect to MCF10A control cells [243]. The synergistic inhibition of cancer cells growth was associated with downregulation of SIRT1, DNMT1, DNMT3a and DNMT3B expression and activity. In fact, while SIRT1 plays an important role in protecting healthy cells from potential stressors, in cancerous cells this histone deacetylase seems to contribute to maintain the malignant phenotype by preventing apoptosis, promoting angiogenesis, and inducing the deacetylation of tumour suppression proteins [244]. Similarly, the combined treatment of MDA-MB-321 and MCF-7 breast cancer cells with resveratrol (**203**) (10-20 μM) and proanthocyanidins extracted from grape seeds (20-40 μg/mL) for 48 hours showed a marked inhibition of DNMTs and HDACs activity associated with reduction in cell *via*bility that reached 91% when the highest dosage was used [245]. Moreover, resveratrol (**203**) was shown to have a preventive effect on the epigenetic silencing of *BRCA-1* in MCF-7 cell lines and in mice exposed to xenobiotics that are known to activate the aromatic hydrocarbon receptor (AhR) such as TCDD (2,3,7,8-tetrachlorodibenzo-p-dioxin), with consecutive recruitment of DNMTs and hypermethylation of CpG islands at the *BRCA-1* promoter [246, 247]. The chemopreventive effect of this polyphenol was also reported in a small clinical study in which thirty-nine women at high risk of breast cancer were treated with placebo or 5-50 mg of resveratrol (**203**) twice a day [248]. Interestingly, a marginally significant correlation was found between the concentration of resveratrol (**203**) in the plasma (p=0.047), the nipple aspirate fluid concentration of prostaglandin E_2 (p=0045), and the methylation state of tumour suppressor gene *RASSF-1α* [248]. However, the doses used in this study largely exceed the amount of resveratrol that could be taken up by diet only, especially since its content varies between different types of grapes, with the highest recorded concentrations being in the range of 50-100 μg/g, and wines (0.1-15 mg/L) [225]. Moreover, resveratrol (**203**) is characterised by low water solubility and high susceptibility to phase I and phase II metabolism, as it is converted into its corresponding glucuronide and sulfate derivatives. The need for more potent and selective resveratrol analogues with enhanced pharmacokinetic properties led to a plethora of synthetic studies aimed at exploring the effect of structural changes to the stilbenoid scaffold on the pro-apoptotic, anticancer activity of the resulting compounds. Two of these studies focused on epigenetic targets: DNMT3 and

LSD1. In the first study, *in vitro* analysis of methylated, acylated and carboxylated *trans*-resveratrol derivatives led to the discovery of two low micromolar DNMT3a and DNMT3b selective inhibitors **206-207** Fig. (**25**) [249].

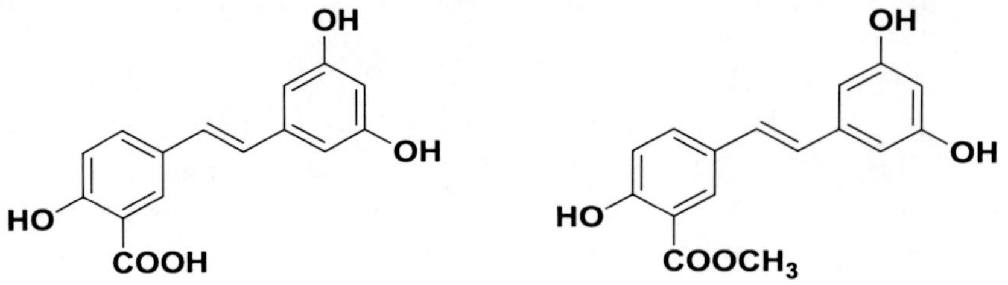

206

DNMT3a: IC_{50} = 40 μM

DNMT3b: IC_{50} = 52 μM

DNMT1: IC_{50} = NI

207

DNMT3a: IC_{50} = 25 μM

DNMT3b: IC_{50} = 62 μM

DNMT1: IC_{50} = NI

Fig. (25). *In vitro* inhibitory activity of trans-resveratrol derivatives **206-207** against inducible (DNMT3a and DNMT3b) and constitutive (DNMT1) isoforms of DNA methyltransferase. (NI = no inhibition at the highest tested concentration > 300 μM) [249].

In the second study, the authors combined the structure of resveratrol (**203**), a low-micromolar LSD1 inhibitor (IC_{50} = 10.20 μM), with the one of a previously reported amidoxime inhibitor **208** (IC_{50} = 10.20 μM) to generate a new series of compounds with nanomolar activity against this epigenetic modulator Fig. (**26**) [250].

Since *cis*-resveratrol isomers are not found in grape skin and they scarcely appear in wine, where their presence is thought to be the result of light-induced isomerisation during production and conservation processes, these compounds have been considered less appealing as chemopreventive agents. Hence, most synthetic studies have been focused on *trans*-stilbenoid derivatives instead, with a few notable exceptions [251 - 253]. An interesting study aimed at comparing the relative antiproliferative effect of various substituted *cis*- and *trans*-stilbenes against HL60 leukaemia cell lines showed that *cis*-compounds (**211**, **213**, **215**) can be more cytotoxic than their corresponding *trans*-isomers (**212**, **214**, **216**) Table **23** [254].

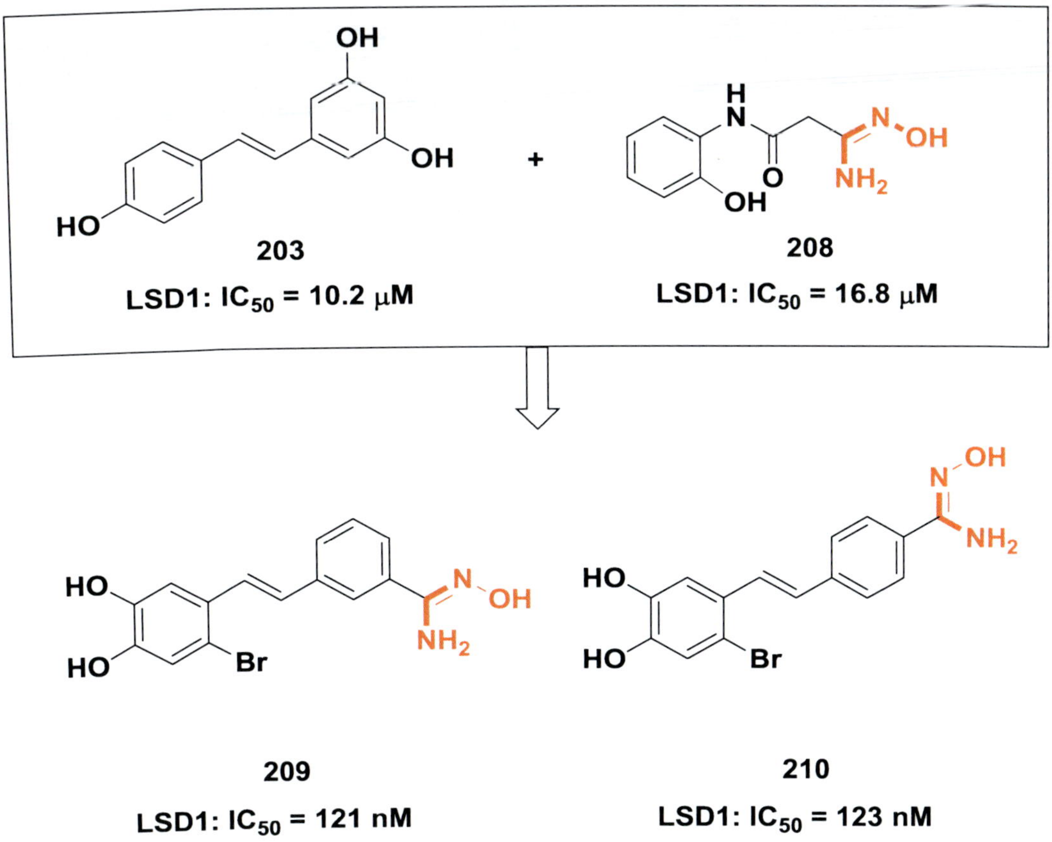

Fig. (26). Rational design of resveratrol-inspired nanomolar LSD1 inhibitors (**209-210**) [250].

Table 23. Comparing the apoptotic activity of *cis*- and *trans*-stilbenoids against HL60 leukaemia cells [254].

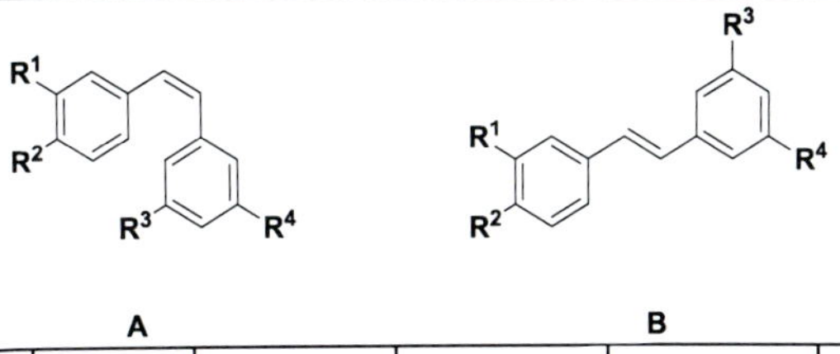

Cmpd	Scaffold	R^1	R^2	R^3	R^4	HL60 (IC_{50} μM)
211	A	NH_2	OCH_3	OCH_3	OCH_3	0.03 ± 0.005 μM
212	B	NH_2	OCH_3	OCH_3	OCH_3	4 ± 0.8 μM
213	A	OH	OCH_3	OCH_3	OCH_3	0.03 ± 0.0012 μM
214	B	OH	OCH_3	OCH_3	OCH_3	0.7 ± 0.09 μM
215	A	OH	OH	OCH_3	OCH_3	0.05 ± 0.008 μM

(Table 23) cont.....

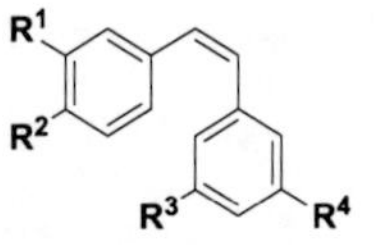

A

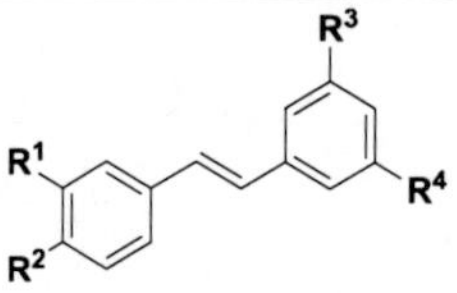

B

Cmpd	Scaffold	R[1]	R[2]	R[3]	R[4]	HL60 (IC_{50} μM)
216	**B**	OH	OH	OCH_3	OCH_3	0.8 ± 0.1 μM

Inspired by the higher metabolic stability and cell permeability of alkylated resveratrol derivatives like pterostilbene (**204**), the antiproliferative activity of methoxy and thiomethyl substituted *cis*-analogues was further tested against a wide range of cancer cell lines, showing promising sub-micromolar activity against SW480 human colorectal cancer Table **24**. and MCF-7 breast cancer cells Table **25** [251, 253].

Table 24. Antiproliferative activity of *cis*-resveratrol derivatives (217-223) against SW480 human colorectal cancer cells [251].

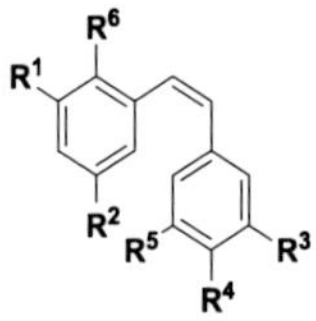

217-223

Cmpd	R[1]	R[2]	R[3]	R[4]	R[5]	R[6]	SW480 (IC_{50} μM)
(*E*)-Resv. 203	-	-	-	-	-	-	20 ± 3 μM
(*Z*)-Resv. 217	OH	OH	H	OH	H	H	90 ± 12 μM
218	OCH_3	OCH_3	H	OCH_3	H	H	0.3 ± 0.04 μM
219	OCH_3	OCH_3	H	OCH_3	H	OH	18 ± 2 μM
220	OCH_3	OCH_3	OCH_3	H	OCH_3	H	13 ± 2 μM
221	OCH_3	OCH_3	OCH_3	H	OCH_3	OH	7 ± 2 μM
222	OCH_3	OCH_3	OCH_3	OCH_3	H	H	9.5 ± 2 μM
223	OCH_3	OCH_3	OCH_3	OCH_3	H	OH	10 ± 2 μM

Table 25. Cytotoxicity of *cis*-stilbenoid derivatives (224-225) on a wide panel of cancer cell lines using MTT assay [253].

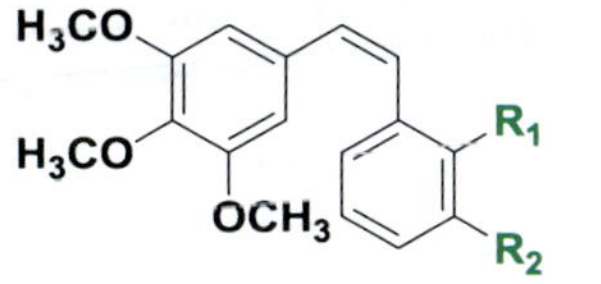

224-225

Cmpd	R^1	R^2	IC_{50} (μM)					
			A431	HeLa	MCF-7	MDA-MB-231	SKOV3	HaCaT
224	SCH_3	OCH_3	3.61 ± 2.44	6.18 ± 0.46	0.65 ± 0.19	11.73 ± 0.85	14.47 ± 1.25	9.56 ± 3.03
225	SCH_3	H	8.22 ± 2.66	11.68 ± 2.54	2.35 ± 1.04	14.20 ± 0.54	14.08 ± 0.61	12.82 ± 1.83

The structural similarity of these compounds to combretastatin A-4, a known tubulin inhibitor, has driven speculations that the antiproliferative activity of *cis*-resveratrol analogues could be derived by the interaction with to the same colchicine binding site on β-tubulin subunits [251]. Interestingly, the most promising results in terms of cytotoxicity and tubulin polymerisation inhibition were obtained when the *cis*-alkene was replaced by a heterocyclic structure, especially isoxazole Table **26** [253].

Table 26. Antiproliferative and tubulin inhibitory activity of isoxazole analogues of *cis*-resveratrol (226-228) [253].

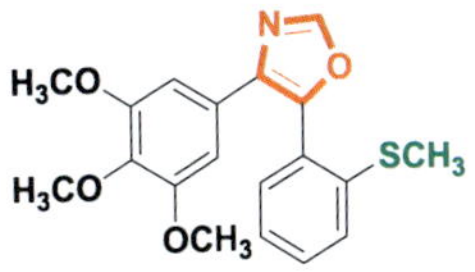

226

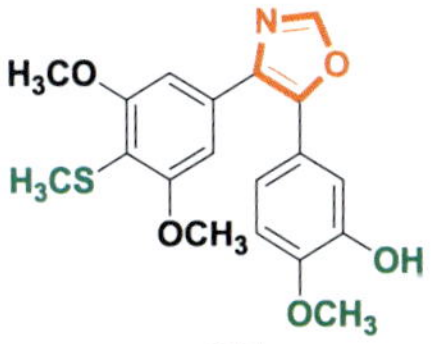

227

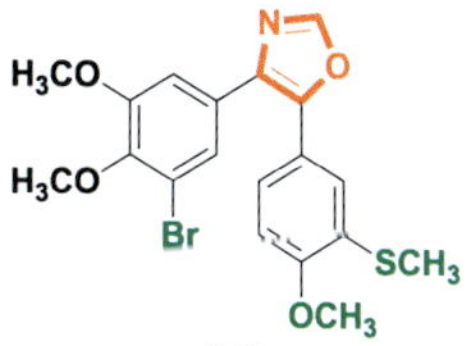

228

Cmpd	IC_{50} (μM)						
	A431	HeLa	MCF-7	MDA-MB-231	SKOV3	HaCaT	Tubulin polymerisation
226	>20	7.33 ± 0.19	1.43 ± 0.37	>20	>20	>20	0.86
227	0.25 ± 0.20	0.009 ± 0.002	0.45 ± 0.14	0.71 ± 0.16	0.25 ± 0.12	0.32 ± 0.09	1.05
228	0.43 ± 0.11	0.63 ± 0.04	2.78 ± 0.77	0.92 ± 0.14	1.16 ± 0.13	0.52 ± 0.08	0.85

Since embedding the alkene inside a heterocyclic ring prevents the light-induced interconversion of *cis/trans*-isomers and eliminates a source of metabolic instability, this strategy has also been applied to the development of *trans*-resveratrol derivatives. In particular, Mayhoub *et al.* [255] reported that thiadiazole and thiazole containing derivatives had promising aromatase and quinone reductase inhibitory activity (Fig. **27**). Modulating the substitution pattern and electronic properties of the phenyl substituents, the authors managed to increase the potency and selectivity of these compounds, an effect that was exacerbated by the isosteric substitution of the thiadiazole moiety in compounds **229-232** with a thiazole ring in derivatives **233-234** Fig. (**27**) [256, 257].

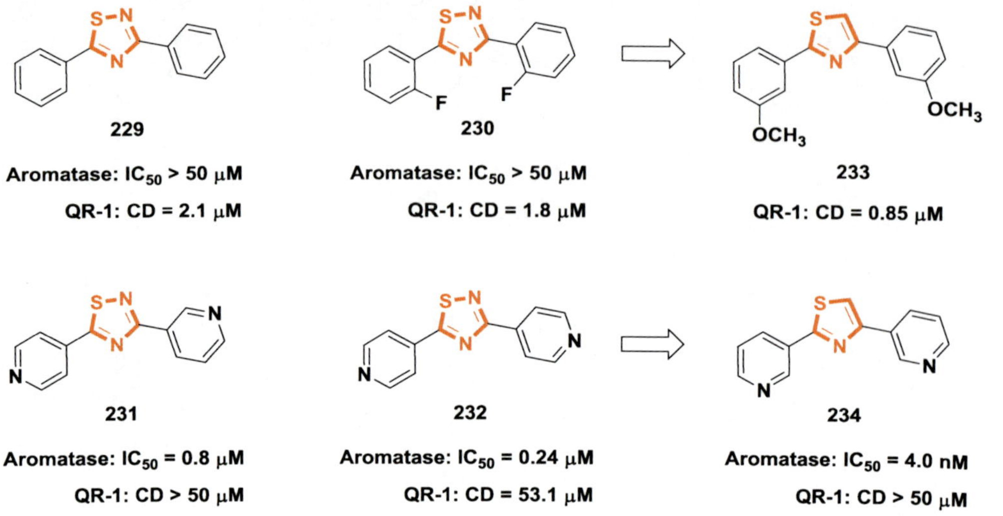

Fig. (27). Optimisation of di-benzothiadiazole and thiazole inhibitors of aromatase and quinone reductase as potential anticancer agents [255 - 257].

Further studies by Ertas *et al.* [258] showed that these types of derivatives have indeed the capacity of inhibiting aromatase at sub-micromolar concentrations Fig. (**28**). However, their *in vitro* antiproliferative activity against hormone responsive cancer cell lines (MCF-7) remained quite low [258].

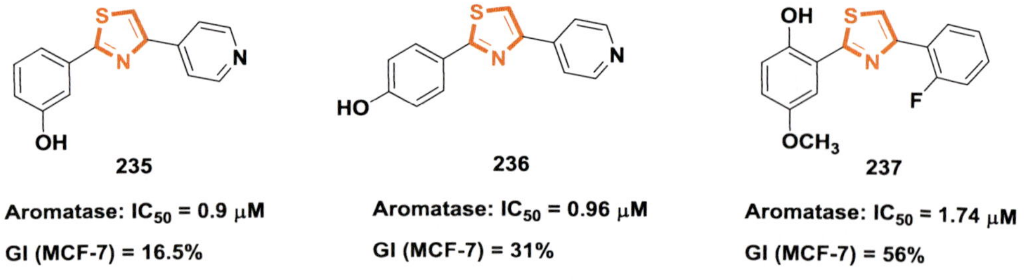

Fig. (28). Aromatase inhibition and antiproliferative activity of di-phenylthiazole derivatives **235-237** [258].

On the contrary, the replacement of one of the aryl rings of *trans*-resveratrol with variously substituted heteroaromatic structures resulted in promising pro-apoptotic activity. A clear example is provided by styrylcoumarin derivatives **238-239**, which were reported to induce p21 mediated cell cycle arrest and apoptosis at sub-micromolar concentrations in lung carcinoma cell lines (H460), and derivatives **240-242** that are endowed with low-micromolar, selective antiproliferative activity against SW480 colon cancer cells (Fig. **29**) [259, 260].

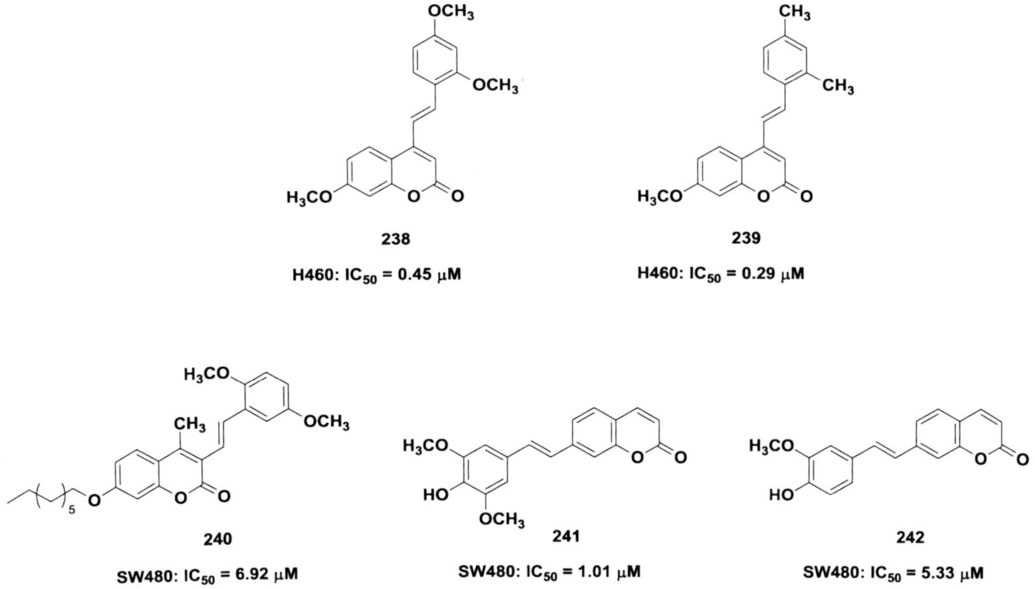

Fig. (29). *In vitro* antiproliferative activity of *trans*-stilbenoid and coumarin hybrids on lung carcinoma (H460) and colon cancer (SW480) cell lines [259, 260].

Alternatives to the coumarin scaffold include pyridine, thiophene Table **27**., haloquinolines (Table **28**) and naphtho[2,3-*d*]imidazolium halides Table **29**. Pyridine and thiophene derivatives were tested against three prostate cancer cell lines and showed promising micromolar activity, with compound **243** inducing a reduction in cell *via*bility higher than 50% in PC-1 and PC-3 cells [261].

Quinolino-stilbene derivatives were reported to be very active against a panel of breast cancer cell lines, with compound **245** showing sub-micromolar activity against the highly metastatic MDA-MB-468 cell line while retaining high selectivity against healthy mammary tissue. These compounds were proposed to inhibit microtubule polymerisation by interacting the podophyllotoxin-binding site on tubulin [262].

Table 27. Antiproliferative activity of heterocyclic derivatives of resveratrol 243-244 against three prostate cancer cell lines [261].

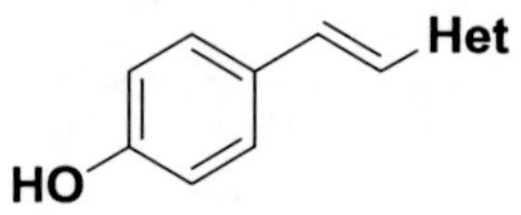

243-244

Cmpd	Het	IC_{50} (μM) AsPC-1	BxPC-3	Capan-2
243	2-thiophenyl	20.39 ± 0.04	20.64 ± 0.71	19.29 ± 0.37
244	4-pyridinyl	18.18 ± 0.33	18.38 ± 0.43	18.05 ± 0.33

Table 28. Antiproliferative activity of quinoline-stilbene derivatives 245-246 against a panel of cancerous and non-cancerous cell lines [262].

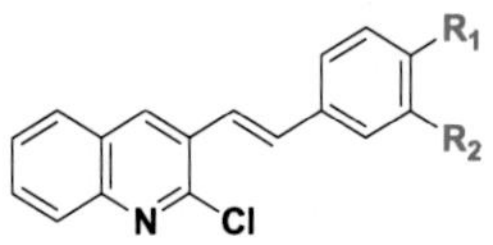

245-246

Cmpd	R^1	R^2	IC_{50} (μM)				
			HeLa	MCF-7	MDA-MB-231	MDA-MB-468	184B5
245	F	H	>50	15.13 ± 5.79	>50	0.12 ± 0.02	38.45 ± 9.5
246	H	CF_3	2.85 ± 0.02	3.53 ± 0.74	3.75 ± 0.29	3.70 ± 0.37	6.15 ± 0.40

Similarly, a series of substituted imidazolium compounds derived by fusing the *trans*-stilbenoid scaffold with the structure of sepantronium bromide (YM155), a known inhibitor of survivin (IC_{50} 0.54 nM), led to the discovery of potent cytotoxic agents against prostate (PC-3), melanoma (A375), and cervical cancer (HeLa) cell lines Table **29** [263, 264].

In general, *trans*-stilbenoid analogues have been proposed to exert their antitumour activity through a wide variety of mechanisms and molecular effectors. Multiple studies have reported on the ability of stilbene derivatives to inhibit angiogenesis by affecting the expression and secretion of VEFG and to restore cell senescence by inhibiting the expression of oncogenes such as *hTERT* and *c-Myc* [265 - 267]. Unfortunately, most of these compounds showed low selectivity against the screened cancer cell lines and were found to be cytotoxic against non-cancerous HEK-293 cells, with the exception of derivatives **249-254** Table **30** [266, 267].

Table 29. Antiproliferative activity of two naphtho[2,3-*d*]imidazolium halides derivatives 247-248 inspired by the surviving inhibitor sepantronium bromide (YM155) on prostate, melanoma, and cervical cancer cell lines [263].

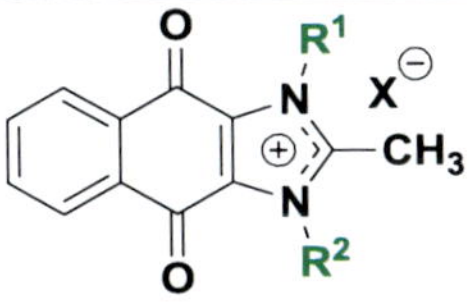

YM155

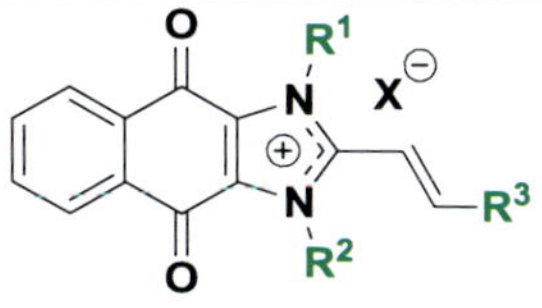

247-248

Cmpd	R^1	R^2	R^3	X	IC$_{50}$ (μM) PC-3	A375	HeLa
247	CH_2CH_3	*i*Pr	4-CH_3-C_6H_4	I	0.022 ± 0.001	1.068 ± 0.069	1.120 ± 0.270
248	CH_2-C_6H_5	CH_2-C_6H_5	3-indolyl	Br	0.128 ± 0.017	0.212 ± 0.029	0.059 ± 0.011
YM155	$(CH_2)_2$-OCH_3	CH_2-pyrazine	-	Br	0.005 ± 0.001	0.015 ± 0.003	0.137 ± 0.013

Both compounds **247-248** were found to inhibit the expression of survivin and Bcl-2, thus promoting cell apoptosis.

Table 30. Antiproliferative activity (IC$_{50}$) and selectivity (α, β) of imine analogues of *trans*-resveratrol against human colorectal (HT-29) and breast (MCF-7) cancer cell lines; α = IC$_{50}$ (HEK-293)/IC$_{50}$ (HT-29), β = IC$_{50}$ (HEK-293)/IC$_{50}$ (MCF-7) [267].

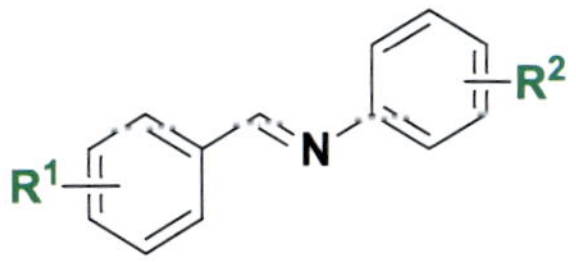

249-254

Cmpd	R^1	R^2	IC$_{50}$ (μM)				
			HT-29	MCF-7	HEK-293	α	β
249	H	3-Br	>350	9 ± 3	>350	-	>40
250	H	4-OCH_3	15 ± 4	14 ± 3	>450	>30	>30
251	2-OH	4-Br	18.8 ±2.3	>350	25.7 ± 1.5	1.4	<0.1
252	3-OH	4-Br	35 ± 8	51 ± 18	>350	>10	>7
253	4-OH	H	31.8 ± 1	96 ± 46	>500	>15	>5
254	4-OH	4-OCH_3	123 ± 40	>400	>400	>3.6	-

Compound **254** was also capable of lowering VEGF secretion (-35%) and expression (-42%) in HT-29 cells with respect to control. A more marked effect was registered on the expression levels of *h*TERT, which was reduced up to 70% in HT-29 cells treated with 110 μM compound **254**. Low micromolar (12-32 μM) concentrations of compounds **249-253** were also demonstrated to significantly inhibit *h*TERT expression [267]. The regulation of oncogenes observed after the treatment of cancer cells with resveratrol and pterostilbene could also be ascribed to upstream inhibition of the Wnt pathway. These two natural stilbenoids are able to inhibit the expression of Wnt-target genes such as *c-Myc* and *Cyclin-D1* in colorectal cancer cells (LS174) at 100 μM concentration [268]. The search for more potent inhibitor of this regulatory pathway led to the development of a series of fluorinated aminostilbenes **255-260** with antiproliferative activity in the low micromolar range Table **31** [268]. In particular, compound **260** was found to repress the expression of Axin2 and c-Myc at concentrations as low as 0.5 μM and to inhibit the growth of LS174 xenografts *in vivo*.

Table 31. Concentrations at which fluorinated aminostilbenes 255-260 inhibit the expression of WNT-target genes in LS174 colorectal cancer cell line [268].

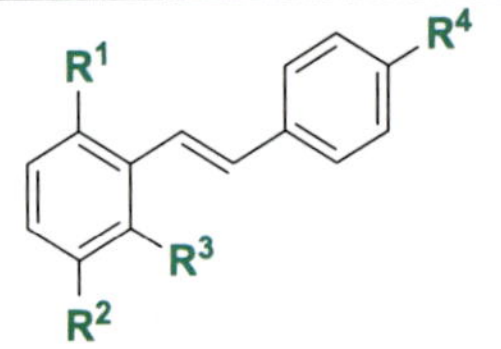

255-260

Cmpd	R¹	R²	R³	R⁴	Active Concentration (μM)
255	H	H	H	NH_2	30
256	H	H	F	$N(CH_3)_2$	10
257	H	F	H	$N(CH_3)_2$	10
258	H	F	F	$N(CH_3)_2$	10
259	F	F	H	$N(CH_3)_2$	10
260	F	H	F	$N(CH_3)_2$	0.5

Modification of the alkene linker between the two aromatic groups of stilbene derivatives, as seen in compounds **249-254**, has also revealed to be a successful strategy for the development of potent antiproliferative agents. In 2006, a study from Yoo *et al.* [269] reported a series of imine and amide analogues of resveratrol with nanomolar inhibitory activity against PC-3 and LNCaP prostate cancer cell lines Fig. (**30**).

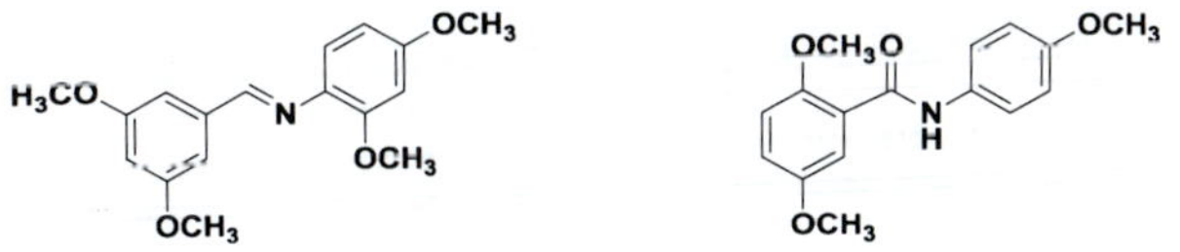

261 PC-3: IC_{50} = 0.07 ± 0.01 µM LNCaP: IC_{50} = 0.03 ± 0.01 µM

262 PC-3: IC_{50} = 0.09 ± 0.04 µM LNCaP: IC_{50} = 0.04 ± 0.01 µM

Fig. (30). Antiproliferative activity of imine and amide analogues **261-262** of alkylated *trans*-resveratrol and pterostilbene against two prostate cancer cell lines (PC-3 and LNCaP) [269].

In several studies the *trans*-alkene has been substituted by an acrylonitrile moiety. Compounds carrying this functional group were shown to possess cytotoxic activity against a wide variety of cancer cell lines including colon, lung, cervical, ovarian, breast, skin cancer and leukemia Table **32** [270 - 272].

Table 32. Cytotoxic activity of acrylonitrile derivatives 263-268 against colon (HCT116 and HCT15), cervical (HeLa), ovarian (SK-OV-3), lung (A549), and skin (SK-MEL-2) cancer cell lines [270, 271].

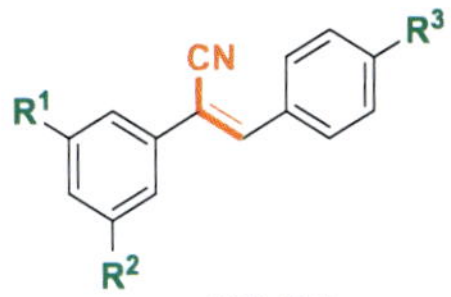

263-268

				IC_{50} (µM)			
Cmpd	**R¹**	**R²**	**R³**	**HCT116**	**HeLa**	-	-
263	OCH_3	OCH_3	Br	11.37 ± 1.85	4.20 ± 0.23	-	-
264	OCH_3	OCH_3	$N(CH_3)_2$	0.59 ± 0.29	>100	-	-
265	OCH_3	OCH_3	OCH_2CH_3	1.30 ± 0.22	>100	-	-
-	-	-	-	IC_{50} (µg mL^{-1})			
-	-	-	-	**HCT15**	**SK-OV-3**	**A549**	**SK-MEL-2**
266	H	H	$N(CH_3)_2$	0.34	0.14	0.57	0.65
267	H	H	Cl	1.22	0.20	1.81	1.53
268	H	H	CH_3	1.54	0.58	1.82	1.63

When a series of naphthalene analogues of compounds **263-268** were tested against a panel of 54 different cancer cell lines, they showed antiproliferative activity at nanomolar concentrations Table **33**. Compounds **269-271** were able to reduce tubulin polymerisation by more than 50% in MV4-11 acute myeloid leukemia cells and *in silico* studies indicated that this effect might be mediated by their binding to the colchicine pocket [272]. Moreover, these compounds showed much higher antitumour activity then DMU-212 (**271**), a widely studied resveratrol derivative with broad antiproliferative activity and high chemopreventive potential in colorectal cancer, due to its preferential pharmacokinetic properties (Table **33**) [273]. In fact, this compound tends to accumulate in the intestine and colon and, differently from resveratrol, its metabolism involves mainly hydroxylation and demethylation.

Table 33. Naphthalene acrylonitrile derivatives 269-270 inhibit the growth of a wide variety of cancer cell lines at nanomolar concentrations while showing a potency two orders of magnitude higher than the widely studies resveratrol derivative DMU-212 (271) [272].

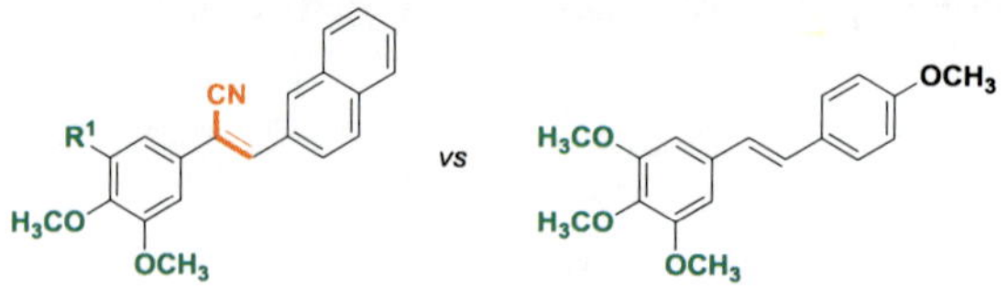

269-270 vs 271 DMU-212

		IG_{50} (µM)							
		Leukemia		Non-Small-Cell Lung Cancer		Colon Cancer			
Cmpd	R[1]	HL-60	SR	HOP-62	NCI-H552	HCT116	HCT-15	KM12	SW-620
269	H	0.060	0.068	0.095	0.067	0.045	0.057	0.080	0.054
270	OCH_3	0.031	0.032	0.044	0.027	0.030	0.031	0.039	0.038
271	-	3.90	3.93	3.14	3.70	3.23	2.82	2.32	3.63
-	-	CNS Cancer			Melanoma				
Cmpd	R[1]	SF-295	SF-539	SNB-75	MDA-MB-435	M14	SK-MEL-5	UACC-62	
269	H	0.041	0.048	0.091	0.025	0.048	0.066	0.035	
270	OCH_3	0.028	0.025	0.044	0.021	0.026	0.023	0.039	
271	-	2.18	2.18	1.88	1.04	2.81	2.50	2.37	
-	-	Ovarian	Renal Cancer				Breast		
Cmpd	R[1]	OVCAR-3	786-0	A498	CAKI-1	RXF 393	T-47D	MDA-MB-468	
269	H	0.051	0.062	0.049	0.091	0.077	0.064	0.094	
270	OCH_3	0.036	0.035	0.033	0.051	0.054	0.048	0.027	
271	-	3.45	5.42	0.74	3.00	2.36	3.55	2.22	

It is important to remember that acrylonitrile groups are electrophilic and, in specific circumstances, they could engage in reversible covalent inhibition [274]. While this could explain, at least in part, their potency and cytotoxicity, a full investigation of their mechanism of action should be conducted to assess potential off-targets.

In conclusion, while preclinical studies have shown that low doses of resveratrol (**203**) supplementation (200 µg–2 mg/kg/day) in the diet would allow to reach plasma concentrations that justify its use as a chemopreventive agent [275], the search for potent *trans*-stilbene derivatives with adequate pharmacokinetic properties and high selectivity against cancerous *vs* non-cancerous cells is still very much open. Several approaches have been attempted, including the substitution of the aryl rings with isosteric heterocycles, the embedment of the double bond inside heterocyclic structures, and the replacement of the *trans*-double bond with imines, amides and, possibly the most promising of all, acrylonitrile groups. The resulting compounds have shown increased anticancer activity compared to the parent compounds, although in most cases their mechanism of action remained elusive. Preliminary *in vitro* studies exploring the inhibitory effect of resveratrol derivatives (**206-207** and **209-210**) on epigenetic modulators, such as DNA-methyltransferases and lysine demetylases, constitute a foundation for the further exploration of this scaffold for cancer therapy.

CONCLUDING REMARKS

Flavonoids and (poly)phenols are highly abundant natural products found in fruit and vegetables that have always attracted a lot of attention because of their potential chemopreventive properties. A large number of *in vitro* studies have demonstrated that these compounds possess promising antiproliferative activity against different cancer cell lines, although, with the only exception of a few preclinical studies, their *in vivo* efficacy remains to be demonstrated. Regardless, these relatively safe scaffolds continue to be of high interest in drug discovery programs, as flavonoids and (poly)phenols have been shown to exert their pro-apoptotic activity through a wide variety of mechanisms involving molecular effectors that regulate processes such as inflammation, angiogenesis, and cell cycle progression. In many cases, epigenetic modulators have been identified as potential targets of both natural and synthetic derivatives of flavonoids and (poly)phenols. However, promiscuity, low bioavailability, and metabolic stability remain major challenges in the development of synthetic flavonoids and (poly)phenols analogues. In this chapter we presented a selection of the most common and successful drug discovery strategies that have been applied to study and improve the pharmacokinetic and pharmacodynamic properties of these naturally occurring compounds.

CONSENT FOR PUBLICATION

Not applicable.

CONFLICT OF INTEREST

The author declares no conflict of interest, financial or otherwise.

ACKNOWLEDGEMENTS

Declared none.

REFERENCES

[1] United Nations; Department of Economic and Social Affairs; Population Division. World population prospects highlights, 2019 Revision highlights, 2019 Revision; **2019**.

[2] Kennedy, B.K.; Berger, S.L.; Brunet, A. Aging: a common driver of chronic diseases and a target for novel interventions. *Cell,* **2014**, *159*(4), 709-713. [http://dx.doi.org/10.1016/j.cell.2014.10.039] [PMID: 25417146]

[3] Divo, M.J.; Martinez, C.H.; Mannino, D.M. Ageing and the epidemiology of multimorbidity. *Eur. Respir. J.,* **2014**, *44*(4), 1055-1068. [http://dx.doi.org/10.1183/09031936.00059814] [PMID: 25142482]

[4] WHO | Diet, nutrition and the prevention of chronic diseases. Report of the joint WHO/FAO expert consultation https://www.who.int/dietphysicalactivity/publications/trs916/summary/en/ (accessed Nov 7, 2020)

[5] Noncommunicable diseases progress monitoring - Background paper (Moscow, Russian Federation, 8–9 June **2017**.https://www.euro.who.int/en/health-topics/noncommunicable-diseases/pages/w-o-european-office-for-the-prevention-and-control-of-noncommunicable-diseases-ncd-office/data-publications-and-tools/latest-reports/noncommunicable-diseases-pr-gress-monitoring-background-paper-moscow,-russian-federation,-89-june-2017

[6] Martínez-Lapiscina, E.H.; Clavero, P.; Toledo, E. Mediterranean diet improves cognition: the PREDIMED-NAVARRA randomised trial. *J. Neurol. Neurosurg. Psychiatry,* **2013**, *84*(12), 1318-1325. [http://dx.doi.org/10.1136/jnnp-2012-304792] [PMID: 23670794]

[7] Smith, P. J.; Blumenthal, J. A.; Babyak, M. A.; Craighead, L.; Welsh-Bohmer, K. A.; Browndyke, J. N.; Strauman, T. A.; Sherwood, A. *Effects of the dietary approaches to stop hypertension.,* **2010**.

[8] Morris, M.C.; Tangney, C.C.; Wang, Y.; Sacks, F.M.; Bennett, D.A.; Aggarwal, N.T. MIND diet associated with reduced incidence of Alzheimer's disease. *Alzheimers Dement.,* **2015**, *11*(9), 1007-1014. [http://dx.doi.org/10.1016/j.jalz.2014.11.009] [PMID: 25681666]

[9] Surh, Y.J. Cancer chemoprevention with dietary phytochemicals. *Nat. Rev. Cancer,* **2003**, *3*(10), 768-780. [http://dx.doi.org/10.1038/nrc1189] [PMID: 14570043]

[10] Willett, W.C. Diet and Cancer. *Oncologist,* **2000**, *5*(5), 393-404. [http://dx.doi.org/10.1634/theoncologist.5-5-393] [PMID: 11040276]

[11] Aly, M.S.; Mahmoud, A.A.E. Cancer chemoprevention by dietary polyphenols. *Carcinogenesis,* **2013**.

[12] Calabrese, V.; Cornelius, C.; Mancuso, C. Cellular stress response: a novel target for chemoprevention and nutritional neuroprotection in aging, neurodegenerative disorders and longevity. *Neurochem. Res.,* **2008**, *33*(12), 2444-2471. [http://dx.doi.org/10.1007/s11064-008-9775-9] [PMID: 18629638]

[13] Ullah, M.F.; Usmani, S.; Shah, A.; Abuduhier, F.M. Dietary molecules and experimental evidence of epigenetic influence in cancer chemoprevention: an insight. *Semin. Cancer Biol.,* **2020**.

[PMID: 33152485]

[14] Lyko, F.; Foret, S.; Kucharski, R.; Wolf, S.; Falckenhayn, C.; Maleszka, R. The honey bee epigenomes: differential methylation of brain DNA in queens and workers. *PLoS Biol.,* **2010**, *8*(11)e1000506 [http://dx.doi.org/10.1371/journal.pbio.1000506] [PMID: 21072239]

[15] Mao, W.; Schuler, M.A.; Berenbaum, M.R. A dietary phytochemical alters caste-associated gene expression in honey bees. *Sci. Adv.,* **2015**, *1*(7)e1500795 [http://dx.doi.org/10.1126/sciadv.1500795] [PMID: 26601244]

[16] Zemach, A.; McDaniel, I.E.; Silva, P.; Zilberman, D. Genome-wide evolutionary analysis of eukaryotic DNA methylation. *Science,* **2010**, *328*(5980), 916-919. [http://dx.doi.org/10.1126/science.1186366] [PMID: 20395474]

[17] Jin, B.; Li, Y.; Robertson, K.D. DNA methylation: superior or subordinate in the epigenetic hierarchy? *Genes Cancer,* **2011**, *2*(6), 607-617. [http://dx.doi.org/10.1177/1947601910393957] [PMID: 21941617]

[18] Greenberg, M.V.C.; Bourc'his, D. The diverse roles of DNA methylation in mammalian development and disease. *Nat. Rev. Mol. Cell Biol.,* **2019**, *20*(10), 590-607. [http://dx.doi.org/10.1038/s41580-019-0159-6] [PMID: 31399642]

[19] Heijmans, B.T.; Tobi, E.W.; Stein, A.D.; Putter, H.; Blauw, G.J.; Susser, E.S.; Slagboom, P.E.; Lumey, L.H. Persistent epigenetic differences associated with prenatal exposure to famine in humans. *Proc. Natl. Acad. Sci. USA,* **2008**, *105*(44), 17046-17049. [http://dx.doi.org/10.1073/pnas.0806560105] [PMID: 18955703]

[20] Schulz, L.C. The Dutch Hunger Winter and the developmental origins of health and disease. *Proc. Natl. Acad. Sci. USA,* **2010**, *107*(39), 16757-16758. [http://dx.doi.org/10.1073/pnas.1012911107] [PMID: 20855592]

[21] Bonacasa, B.; Siow, R.C.M.; Mann, G. Impact of dietary soy isoflavones in pregnancy on fetal programming of endothelial function in offspring. *Microcirculation,* **2011**, *18*(4), 270-285. [http://dx.doi.org/10.1111/j.1549-8719.2011.00088.x] [PMID: 21418378]

[22] Vanhees, K.; Coort, S.; Ruijters, E.J.B.; Godschalk, R.W.L.; Schooten, F.J.; Doorn-Khosrovani, S.B.W. Epigenetics: prenatal exposure to genistein leaves a permanent signature on the hematopoietic lineage. *FASEB J.,* **2011**, *25*(2), 797-807. [http://dx.doi.org/10.1096/fj.10-172155] [PMID: 21048042]

[23] Dolinoy, D.C.; Weidman, J.R.; Waterland, R.A.; Jirtle, R.L. Maternal genistein alters coat color and protects Avy mouse offspring from obesity by modifying the fetal epigenome. *Environ. Health Perspect.,* **2006**, *114*(4), 567-572. [http://dx.doi.org/10.1289/ehp.8700] [PMID: 16581547]

[24] Blei, T.; Soukup, S.T.; Schmalbach, K. Dose-dependent effects of isoflavone exposure during early lifetime on the rat mammary gland: Studies on estrogen sensitivity, isoflavone metabolism, and DNA methylation. *Mol. Nutr. Food Res.,* **2015**, *59*(2), 270-283. [http://dx.doi.org/10.1002/mnfr.201400480] [PMID: 25410811]

[25] Shanmugam, M.K.; Arfuso, F.; Arumugam, S. Role of novel histone modifications in cancer. *Oncotarget,* **2018**, *9*(13), 11414-11426. [http://dx.doi.org/10.18632/oncotarget.23356] [PMID: 29541423]

[26] Babashah, S.; Bakhshinejad, B.; Birgani, M.T.; Pakravan, K.; Cho, W.C. Regulation of microRNAs by phytochemicals: a promising strategy for cancer chemoprevention. *Curr. Cancer Drug Targets,* **2018**, *18*(7), 640-651. [http://dx.doi.org/10.2174/1568009617666170623124710] [PMID: 28669335]

[27] McGinty, R.K.; Tan, S. Nucleosome structure and function. *Chem. Rev.,* **2015**, *115*(6), 2255-2273. [http://dx.doi.org/10.1021/cr500373h] [PMID: 25495456]

[28] Verdone, L.; Agricola, E.; Caserta, M.; Di Mauro, E. Histone acetylation in gene regulation. *Brief. Funct. Genomics Proteomics,* **2006**, *5*(3), 209-221.
[http://dx.doi.org/10.1093/bfgp/ell028] [PMID: 16877467]

[29] Fujisawa, T.; Filippakopoulos, P. Functions of bromodomain-containing proteins and their roles in homeostasis and cancer. *Nat. Rev. Mol. Cell Biol.,* **2017**, *18*(4), 246-262.
[http://dx.doi.org/10.1038/nrm.2016.143] [PMID: 28053347]

[30] Bannister, A.J.; Kouzarides, T. Regulation of chromatin by histone modifications. *Cell Res.,* **2011**, *21*(3), 381-395.
[http://dx.doi.org/10.1038/cr.2011.22] [PMID: 21321607]

[31] Hodawadekar, S.C.; Marmorstein, R. Chemistry of acetyl transfer by histone modifying enzymes: structure, mechanism and implications for effector design. *Oncogene,* **2007**, *26*(37), 5528-5540.
[http://dx.doi.org/10.1038/sj.onc.1210619] [PMID: 17694092]

[32] Gallinari, P.; Marco, S.D.; Jones, P.; Pallaoro, M.; Steinkühler, C. HDACs, histone deacetylation and gene transcription: from molecular biology to cancer therapeutics. *Cell Res.,* **2007**, *17*(3), 195-211.
[http://dx.doi.org/10.1038/sj.cr.7310149] [PMID: 17325692]

[33] Nakagawa, T.; Guarente, L. Sirtuins at a glance. *J. Cell Sci.,* **2011**, *124*(6), 833-838.
[http://dx.doi.org/10.1242/jcs.081067] [PMID: 21378304]

[34] Lee, S.H.; Lee, J.H.; Lee, H.Y.; Min, K.J. Sirtuin signaling in cellular senescence and aging. *BMB Rep.,* **2019**, *52*(1), 24-34.
[http://dx.doi.org/10.5483/BMBRep.2019.52.1.290] [PMID: 30526767]

[35] Husmann, D.; Gozani, O. Histone lysine methyltransferases in biology and disease. *Nat. Struct. Mol. Biol.,* **2019**, *26*(10), 880-889.
[http://dx.doi.org/10.1038/s41594-019-0298-7] [PMID: 31582846]

[36] Greer, E.L.; Shi, Y. Histone methylation: a dynamic mark in health, disease and inheritance. *Nat. Rev. Genet.,* **2012**, *13*(5), 343-357.
[http://dx.doi.org/10.1038/nrg3173] [PMID: 22473383]

[37] Zurita-Lopez, C.I.; Sandberg, T.; Kelly, R.; Clarke, S.G. Human protein arginine methyltransferase 7 (PRMT7) is a type III enzyme forming ω-NG-monomethylated arginine residues. *J. Biol. Chem.,* **2012**, *287*(11), 7859-7870.
[http://dx.doi.org/10.1074/jbc.M111.336271] [PMID: 22241471]

[38] Musselman, C.A.; Lalonde, M.E.; Côté, J.; Kutateladze, T.G. Perceiving the epigenetic landscape through histone readers. *Nat. Struct. Mol. Biol.,* **2012**, *19*(12), 1218-1227.
[http://dx.doi.org/10.1038/nsmb.2436] [PMID: 23211769]

[39] Strahl, B.D.; Allis, C.D. The language of covalent histone modifications. *Nature,* **2000**, *403*(6765), 41-45.
[http://dx.doi.org/10.1038/47412] [PMID: 10638745]

[40] Margueron, R.; Trojer, P.; Reinberg, D. The key to development: interpreting the histone code? *Curr. Opin. Genet. Dev.,* **2005**, *15*(2), 163-176.
[http://dx.doi.org/10.1016/j.gde.2005.01.005] [PMID: 15797199]

[41] Yang, Y.; Bedford, M.T. Protein arginine methyltransferases and cancer. *Nat. Rev. Cancer,* **2013**, *13*(1), 37-50.
[http://dx.doi.org/10.1038/nrc3409] [PMID: 23235912]

[42] Ng, S.S.; Yue, W.W.; Oppermann, U.; Klose, R.J. Dynamic protein methylation in chromatin biology. *Cell. Mol. Life Sci.,* **2009**, *66*(3), 407-422.
[http://dx.doi.org/10.1007/s00018-008-8303-z] [PMID: 18923809]

[43] Litt, M.; Qiu, Y.; Huang, S. Histone arginine methylations: their roles in chromatin dynamics and transcriptional regulation. *Biosci. Rep.,* **2009**, *29*(2), 131-141.

[http://dx.doi.org/10.1042/BSR20080176] [PMID: 19220199]

[44] Tian, X.; Fang, J. Current perspectives on histone demethylases. *Acta Biochim. Biophys. Sin. (Shanghai),* **2007**, *39*(2), 81-88.
[http://dx.doi.org/10.1111/j.1745-7270.2007.00272.x] [PMID: 17277881]

[45] D'Oto, A.; Tian, Q.; Davidoff, A.M.; Yang, J. Histone demethylases and their roles in cancer epigenetics. *Journal of Medical Oncology and Therapeutics,* **2016**, *1*(2), 34-40.
[http://dx.doi.org/10.35841/medical-oncology.1.2.34-40] [PMID: 28149961]

[46] Kooistra, S.M.; Helin, K. Molecular mechanisms and potential functions of histone demethylases. *Nat. Rev. Mol. Cell Biol.,* **2012**, *13*(5), 297-311.
[http://dx.doi.org/10.1038/nrm3327] [PMID: 22473470]

[47] Chang, B.; Chen, Y.; Zhao, Y.; Bruick, R.K. JMJD6 is a histone arginine demethylase. *Science,* **2007**, *318*(5849), 444-447.
[http://dx.doi.org/10.1126/science.1145801] [PMID: 17947579]

[48] Walport, L.J.; Hopkinson, R.J.; Chowdhury, R.; Schiller, R.; Ge, W.; Kawamura, A.; Schofield, C.J. Arginine demethylation is catalysed by a subset of JmjC histone lysine demethylases. *Nat. Commun.,* **2016**, *7*(1), 11974.
[http://dx.doi.org/10.1038/ncomms11974] [PMID: 27337104]

[49] Zhang, J.; Jing, L.; Li, M.; He, L.; Guo, Z. Regulation of histone arginine methylation/demethylation by methylase and demethylase (Review). *Mol. Med. Rep.,* **2019**, *19*(5), 3963-3971.
[http://dx.doi.org/10.3892/mmr.2019.10111] [PMID: 30942418]

[50] Makwana, M.V.; Muimo, R.; Jackson, R.F.W. Advances in development of new tools for the study of phosphohistidine. *Lab. Invest.,* **2018**, *98*(3), 291-303.
[http://dx.doi.org/10.1038/labinvest.2017.126] [PMID: 29200202]

[51] Rossetto, D.; Avvakumov, N.; Côté, J. Histone phosphorylation. *Epigenetics,* **2012**, *7*(10), 1098-1108.
[http://dx.doi.org/10.4161/epi.21975] [PMID: 22948226]

[52] Bisol, Â.; Campos, P.S.; Lamers, M.L. Flavonoids as anticancer therapies: A systematic review of clinical trials. *Phytother. Res.,* **2020**, *34*(3), 568-582.
[http://dx.doi.org/10.1002/ptr.6551] [PMID: 31752046]

[53] McCullough, M.L.; Peterson, J.J.; Patel, R.; Jacques, P.F.; Shah, R.; Dwyer, J.T. Flavonoid intake and cardiovascular disease mortality in a prospective cohort of US adults. *Am. J. Clin. Nutr.,* **2012**, *95*(2), 454-464.
[http://dx.doi.org/10.3945/ajcn.111.016634] [PMID: 22218162]

[54] Panche, A.N.; Diwan, A.D.; Chandra, S.R. Flavonoids: an overview. *J. Nutr. Sci.,* **2016**, *5*e47
[http://dx.doi.org/10.1017/jns.2016.41] [PMID: 28620474]

[55] Sharma, N.; Dobhal, M.P.; Joshi, Y.C.; Chahar, M.K. Flavonoids: A versatile source of anticancer drugs. *Pharmacogn. Rev.,* **2011**, *5*(9), 1-12.
[http://dx.doi.org/10.4103/0973-7847.79093] [PMID: 22096313]

[56] Tsyrlov, I.B.; Mikhailenko, V.M.; Gelboin, H.V. Isozyme- and species-specific susceptibility of cDNA-expressed CYP1A P-450s to different flavonoids. *Biochim. Biophys. Acta Protein Struct. Mol. Enzymol.,* **1994**, *1205*(2), 325-335.
[http://dx.doi.org/10.1016/0167-4838(94)90252-6] [PMID: 8155716]

[57] Gilbert, E.R.; Liu, D. Flavonoids influence epigenetic-modifying enzyme activity: structure - function relationships and the therapeutic potential for cancer. *Curr. Med. Chem.,* **2010**, *17*(17), 1756-1768.
[http://dx.doi.org/10.2174/092986710791111161] [PMID: 20345345]

[58] Srinivas, N.R. Recent trends in preclinical drug-drug interaction studies of flavonoids - Review of case studies, issues and perspectives. *Phytother. Res.,* **2015**, *29*(11), 1679-1691.
[http://dx.doi.org/10.1002/ptr.5447] [PMID: 26343418]

[59] Mirossay, L.; Varinská, L.; Mojžiš, J. Antiangiogenic effect of flavonoids and chalcones: an update. *Int. J. Mol. Sci.*, **2017**, *19*(1), 27.
[http://dx.doi.org/10.3390/ijms19010027] [PMID: 29271940]

[60] Srivastava, S.; Somasagara, R.R.; Hegde, M.; Nishana, M.; Tadi, S.K.; Srivastava, M.; Choudhary, B.; Raghavan, S.C. Quercetin, a natural flavonoid interacts with DNA, arrests cell cycle and causes tumor regression by activating mitochondrial pathway of apoptosis. *Sci. Rep.*, **2016**, *6*(1), 24049.
[http://dx.doi.org/10.1038/srep24049] [PMID: 27068577]

[61] Kanwal, R.; Datt, M.; Liu, X.; Gupta, S. Dietary flavones as dual inhibitors of DNA methyltransferases and histone methyltransferases. *PLoS One*, **2016**, *11*(9)e0162956
[http://dx.doi.org/10.1371/journal.pone.0162956] [PMID: 27658199]

[62] Busch, C.; Burkard, M.; Leischner, C.; Lauer, U.M.; Frank, J.; Venturelli, S. Epigenetic activities of flavonoids in the prevention and treatment of cancer. *Clin. Epigenetics*, **2015**, *7*(1), 64.
[http://dx.doi.org/10.1186/s13148-015-0095-z] [PMID: 26161152]

[63] Vahid, F.; Zand, H.; Nosrat-Mirshekarlou, E.; Najafi, R.; Hekmatdoost, A. The role dietary of bioactive compounds on the regulation of histone acetylases and deacetylases: A review. *Gene*, **2015**, *562*(1), 8-15.
[http://dx.doi.org/10.1016/j.gene.2015.02.045] [PMID: 25701602]

[64] Kumari, A.; Bhawal, S.; Kapila, S.; Yadav, H.; Kapila, R. Health-promoting role of dietary bioactive compounds through epigenetic modulations: a novel prophylactic and therapeutic approach. *Crit. Rev. Food Sci. Nutr.*, **2020**, 1-21.
[PMID: 33081489]

[65] Sezer, E.D.; Oktay, L.M.; Karadadaş, E.; Memmedov, H.; Selvi Gunel, N.; Sözmen, E. Assessing anticancer potential of blueberry flavonoids, quercetin, kaempferol, and gentisic acid, through oxidative stress and apoptosis parameters on HCT-116 cells. *J. Med. Food*, **2019**, *22*(11), 1118-1126.
[http://dx.doi.org/10.1089/jmf.2019.0098] [PMID: 31241392]

[66] Imran, M.; Rauf, A.; Shah, Z.A. Chemo-preventive and therapeutic effect of the dietary flavonoid kaempferol: A comprehensive review. *Phytother. Res.*, **2019**, *33*(2), 263-275.
[http://dx.doi.org/10.1002/ptr.6227] [PMID: 30402931]

[67] Kang, J.W.; Kim, J.H.; Song, K.; Kim, S.H.; Yoon, J.H.; Kim, K.S. Kaempferol and quercetin, components of *Ginkgo biloba* extract (EGb 761), induce caspase-3-dependent apoptosis in oral cavity cancer cells. *Phytother. Res.*, **2010**, *24*(S1) Suppl. 1, S77-S82.
[http://dx.doi.org/10.1002/ptr.2913] [PMID: 19585476]

[68] Hassanzadeh, A.; Naimi, A.; Hagh, M.F.; Saraei, R.; Marofi, F.; Solali, S. Kaempferol improves TRAIL-mediated apoptosis in leukemia MOLT-4 cells by the inhibition of anti-apoptotic proteins and promotion of death receptors expression. *Anticancer. Agents Med. Chem.*, **2019**, *19*(15), 1835-1845.
[http://dx.doi.org/10.2174/1871520619666190731155859] [PMID: 31364517]

[69] Gutierrez-Uribe, J.A.; Salinas-Santander, M.; Serna-Guerrero, D.; Serna-Saldivar, S.R.O.; Rivas-Estilla, A.M.; Rios-Ibarra, C.P. Inhibition of MiR31 and MiR92a as oncological biomarkers in RKO colon cancer cells treated with kaempferol-3-O-glycoside isolated from black bean. *J. Med. Food*, **2020**, *23*(1), 50-55.
[http://dx.doi.org/10.1089/jmf.2019.0059] [PMID: 31441682]

[70] Jaramillo Carmona, S.; López, S.; Abia, R.; Rodríguez-Arcos, R.; Jiménez Araujo, A.; Guillén Bejarano, R.; Muriana, F.J.G. Combination of quercetin and kaempferol enhances *in vitro* cytotoxicity on human colon cancer (HCT-116) cells. *Rec. Nat. Prod.*, **2014**, *8*(3), 262-271.

[71] Berger, A.; Venturelli, S.; Kallnischkies, Kaempferol, a new nutrition-derived pan-inhibitor of human histone deacetylases. *J. Nutr. Biochem.*, **2013**, *24*(6), 977-985.
[http://dx.doi.org/10.1016/j.jnutbio.2012.07.001] [PMID: 23159065]

[72] Marfe, G.; Tafani, M.; Indelicato, M.; Sinibaldi-Salimei, P.; Reali, V.; Pucci, B.; Fini, M.; Russo,

M.A. Kaempferol induces apoptosis in two different cell lines *via* Akt inactivation, Bax and SIRT3 activation, and mitochondrial dysfunction. *J. Cell. Biochem.,* **2009**, *106*(4), 643-650. [http://dx.doi.org/10.1002/jcb.22044] [PMID: 19160423]

[73] Allison, S.J.; Milner, J. SIRT3 is pro-apoptotic and participates in distinct basal apoptotic pathways. *Cell Cycle,* **2007**, *6*(21), 2669-2677. [http://dx.doi.org/10.4161/cc.6.21.4866] [PMID: 17957139]

[74] Qiu, W.; Lin, J.; Zhu, Y.; Zhang, J.; Zeng, L.; Su, M.; Tian, Y. Kaempferol modulates DNA methylation and downregulates DNMT3B in bladder cancer. *Cell. Physiol. Biochem.,* **2017**, *41*(4), 1325-1335. [http://dx.doi.org/10.1159/000464435] [PMID: 28278502]

[75] Ma, L.; Feugang, J.M.; Konarski, P.; Wang, J.; Lu, J.; Fu, S.; Ma, B.; Tian, B.; Zou, C.; Wang, Z. *Growth inhibitory effects of quercetin on bladder cancer cell*; Front. Biosci. J. Virtual Libr, **2006**. [http://dx.doi.org/10.2741/1970]

[76] Avila, M.A.; Velasco, J.A.; Cansado, J.; Notario, V. Quercetin mediates the down-regulation of mutant p53 in the human breast cancer cell line MDA-MB468. *Cancer Res.,* **1994**, *54*(9), 2424-2428. [PMID: 8162591]

[77] Kundur, S.; Prayag, A.; Selvakumar, P. Synergistic anticancer action of quercetin and curcumin against triple-negative breast cancer cell lines. *J. Cell. Physiol.,* **2019**, *234*(7), 11103-11118. [http://dx.doi.org/10.1002/jcp.27761] [PMID: 30478904]

[78] Xiao, X.; Shi, D.; Liu, L.; Wang, J.; Xie, X.; Kang, T.; Deng, W. Quercetin suppresses cyclooxygenase-2 expression and angiogenesis through inactivation of P300 signaling. *PLoS One,* **2011**, *6*(8)e22934 [http://dx.doi.org/10.1371/journal.pone.0022934] [PMID: 21857970]

[79] Ruiz, P.A.; Braune, A.; Hölzlwimmer, G.; Quintanilla-Fend, L.; Haller, D. Quercetin inhibits TNF-induced NF-kappaB transcription factor recruitment to proinflammatory gene promoters in murine intestinal epithelial cells. *J. Nutr.,* **2007**, *137*(5), 1208-1215. [http://dx.doi.org/10.1093/jn/137.5.1208] [PMID: 17449583]

[80] Richter, M.; Ebermann, R.; Marian, B. Quercetin-induced apoptosis in colorectal tumor cells: possible role of EGF receptor signaling. *Nutr. Cancer,* **1999**, *34*(1), 88-99. [http://dx.doi.org/10.1207/S15327914NC340113] [PMID: 10453447]

[81] Ranelletti, F.O.; Ricci, R.; Larocca, L.M.; Maggiano, N.; Capelli, A.; Scambia, G.; Benedetti-Panici, P.; Mancuso, S.; Rumi, C.; Piantelli, M. Growth-inhibitory effect of quercetin and presence of type-II estrogen-binding sites in human colon-cancer cell lines and primary colorectal tumors. *Int. J. Cancer,* **1992**, *50*(3), 486-492. [http://dx.doi.org/10.1002/ijc.2910500326] [PMID: 1735617]

[82] Kedhari Sundaram, M.; Hussain, A.; Haque, S.; Raina, R.; Afroze, N. Quercetin modifies 5′CpG promoter methylation and reactivates various tumor suppressor genes by modulating epigenetic marks in human cervical cancer cells. *J. Cell. Biochem.,* **2019**, *120*(10), 18357-18369. [http://dx.doi.org/10.1002/jcb.29147] [PMID: 31172592]

[83] Kang, Y.; Nian, H.; Rajendran, P.; Kim, E.; Dashwood, W.M.; Pinto, J.T.; Boardman, L.A.; Thibodeau, S.N.; Limburg, P.J.; Löhr, C.V.; Bisson, W.H.; Williams, D.E.; Ho, E.; Dashwood, R.H. HDAC8 and STAT3 repress BMF gene activity in colon cancer cells. *Cell Death Dis.,* **2014**, *5*(10), e1476-e1476. [http://dx.doi.org/10.1038/cddis.2014.422] [PMID: 25321483]

[84] Biswas, S.; Reddy, N.D.; Jayashree, B.S.; Rao, C.M. Evaluation of novel 3-hydroxyflavone analogues as HDAC inhibitors against colorectal cancer. *Adv. Pharmacol. Sci.,* **2018**, *2018*, 1-14. [http://dx.doi.org/10.1155/2018/4751806] [PMID: 30687400]

[85] Cai, X.; Fang, Z.; Dou, J.; Yu, A.; Zhai, G. Bioavailability of quercetin: problems and promises. *Curr. Med. Chem.,* **2013**, *20*(20), 2572-2582.

[http://dx.doi.org/10.2174/0929867311320999012O] [PMID: 23514412]

[86] Mukherjee, A.; Mishra, S.; Kotla, N.K.; Manna, K.; Roy, S.; Kundu, B.; Bhattacharya, D.; Das Saha, K.; Talukdar, A. Semisynthetic quercetin derivatives with potent antitumor activity in colon carcinoma. *ACS Omega,* **2019**, *4*(4), 7285-7298.
[http://dx.doi.org/10.1021/acsomega.9b00143]

[87] Alvarez, M.C.; Maso, V.; Torello, C.O.; Ferro, K.P.; Saad, S.T.O. The polyphenol quercetin induces cell death in leukemia by targeting epigenetic regulators of pro-apoptotic genes. *Clin. Epigenetics,* **2018**, *10*(1), 139.
[http://dx.doi.org/10.1186/s13148-018-0563-3] [PMID: 30409182]

[88] Hung, C.H.; Chan, S.H.; Chu, P.M.; Tsai, K.L. Quercetin is a potent anti-atherosclerotic compound by activation of SIRT1 signaling under oxLDL stimulation. *Mol. Nutr. Food Res.,* **2015**, *59*(10), 1905-1917.
[http://dx.doi.org/10.1002/mnfr.201500144] [PMID: 26202455]

[89] Rahnasto-Rilla, M.; Tyni, J.; Huovinen, M.; Jarho, E.; Kulikowicz, T.; Ravichandran, S.; A Bohr, V.; Ferrucci, L.; Lahtela-Kakkonen, M.; Moaddel, R. Natural polyphenols as sirtuin 6 modulators. *Sci. Rep.,* **2018**, *8*(1), 4163.
[http://dx.doi.org/10.1038/s41598-018-22388-5] [PMID: 29515203]

[90] Lerrer, B.; Gertler, A.A.; Cohen, H.Y. The complex role of SIRT6 in carcinogenesis. *Carcinogenesis,* **2016**, *37*(2), 108-118.
[http://dx.doi.org/10.1093/carcin/bgv167] [PMID: 26717993]

[91] Heger, V.; Tyni, J.; Hunyadi, A.; Horáková, L.; Lahtela-Kakkonen, M.; Rahnasto-Rilla, M. Quercetin based derivatives as sirtuin inhibitors. *Biomed. Pharmacother.,* **2019**, *111*, 1326-1333.
[http://dx.doi.org/10.1016/j.biopha.2019.01.035] [PMID: 30841446]

[92] Raj, U.; Kumar, H.; Varadwaj, P.K. Molecular docking and dynamics simulation study of flavonoids as BET bromodomain inhibitors. *J. Biomol. Struct. Dyn.,* **2017**, *35*(11), 2351-2362.
[http://dx.doi.org/10.1080/07391102.2016.1217276] [PMID: 27494802]

[93] Prieto-Martínez, F.; Medina-Franco, J. Flavonoids as putative epi-modulators: insight into their binding mode with BRD4 bromodomains using molecular docking and dynamics. *Biomolecules,* **2018**, *8*(3), 61.
[http://dx.doi.org/10.3390/biom8030061] [PMID: 30041464]

[94] Dhananjayan, K. Molecular docking study characterization of rare flavonoids at the Nac-binding site of the first bromodomain of BRD4 (BRD4 BD1). *J. Cancer Res.,* **2015**, •••, 1-15.

[95] Xu, X.; Peng, W.; Liu, C.; Li, S.; Lei, J.; Wang, Z.; Kong, L.; Han, C. Flavone-based natural product agents as new lysine-specific demethylase 1 inhibitors exhibiting cytotoxicity against breast cancer cells *in vitro. Bioorg. Med. Chem.,* **2019**, *27*(2), 370-374.
[http://dx.doi.org/10.1016/j.bmc.2018.12.013] [PMID: 30552007]

[96] Sakurai, M.; Rose, N.R.; Schultz, L.; Quinn, A.M.; Jadhav, A.; Ng, S.S.; Oppermann, U.; Schofield, C.J.; Simeonov, A. A miniaturized screen for inhibitors of Jumonji histone demethylases. *Mol. Biosyst.,* **2010**, *6*(2), 357-364.
[http://dx.doi.org/10.1039/B912993F] [PMID: 20094655]

[97] Basu Mallik, S.; Pai, A.; Shenoy, R.R.; Jayashree, B.S. Novel flavonol analogues as potential inhibitors of JMJD3 histone demethylase—A study based on molecular modelling. *J. Mol. Graph. Model.,* **2017**, *72*, 81-87.
[http://dx.doi.org/10.1016/j.jmgm.2016.12.002] [PMID: 28064082]

[98] Shukla, S.; Gupta, S. Apigenin: a promising molecule for cancer prevention. *Pharm. Res.,* **2010**, *27*(6), 962-978.
[http://dx.doi.org/10.1007/s11095-010-0089-7] [PMID: 20306120]

[99] Imran, M.; Rauf, A.; Abu-Izneid, T. Luteolin, a flavonoid, as an anticancer agent: A review. *Biomed.*

Pharmacother., **2019**, *112*108612
[http://dx.doi.org/10.1016/j.biopha.2019.108612] [PMID: 30798142]

[100] Mani, R.; Natesan, V. Chrysin: Sources, beneficial pharmacological activities, and molecular mechanism of action. *Phytochemistry,* **2018**, *145*, 187-196.
[http://dx.doi.org/10.1016/j.phytochem.2017.09.016] [PMID: 29161583]

[101] Ozbey, U.; Attar, R.; Romero, M.A. Apigenin as an effective anticancer natural product: Spotlight on TRAIL, WNT/β-catenin, JAK-STAT pathways, and microRNAs. *J. Cell. Biochem.,* **2018**.
[PMID: 30278099]

[102] Ganai, S.A. Plant-derived flavone Apigenin: The small-molecule with promising activity against therapeutically resistant prostate cancer. *Biomed. Pharmacother.,* **2017**, *85*, 47-56.
[http://dx.doi.org/10.1016/j.biopha.2016.11.130] [PMID: 27930986]

[103] Mak, P.; Leung, Y.K.; Tang, W.Y.; Harwood, C.; Ho, S.M. Apigenin suppresses cancer cell growth through ERbeta. *Neoplasia,* **2006**, *8*(11), 896-904.
[http://dx.doi.org/10.1593/neo.06538] [PMID: 17132221]

[104] Tseng, T.H.; Chien, M.H.; Lin, W.L. Inhibition of MDA-MB-231 breast cancer cell proliferation and tumor growth by apigenin through induction of G2/M arrest and histone H3 acetylation-mediated p21 $^{WAF1/CIP1}$ expression. *Environ. Toxicol.,* **2017**, *32*(2), 434-444.
[http://dx.doi.org/10.1002/tox.22247] [PMID: 26872304]

[105] Pandey, M.; Kaur, P.; Shukla, S.; Abbas, A.; Fu, P.; Gupta, S. Plant flavone apigenin inhibits HDAC and remodels chromatin to induce growth arrest and apoptosis in human prostate cancer cells: *In vitro* and *in vivo* study. *Mol. Carcinog.,* **2012**, *51*(12), 952-962.
[http://dx.doi.org/10.1002/mc.20866] [PMID: 22006862]

[106] Lascano, S.; Lopez, M.; Arimondo, P.B. Natural products and chemical biology tools: alternatives to target epigenetic mechanisms in cancers. *Chem. Rec.,* **2018**, *18*(12), 1854-1876.
[http://dx.doi.org/10.1002/tcr.201800133] [PMID: 30537358]

[107] Scafuri, B.; Bontempo, P.; Altucci, L.; De Masi, L.; Facchiano, A. Molecular docking simulations on histone deacetylases (HDAC)-1 and -2 to investigate the flavone binding. *Biomedicines,* **2020**, *8*(12), 568.
[http://dx.doi.org/10.3390/biomedicines8120568] [PMID: 33291755]

[108] Hu, Y.; Wu, F.; Liu, Y.; Zhao, Q.; Tang, H. DNMT1 recruited by EZH2-mediated silencing of miR-484 contributes to the malignancy of cervical cancer cells through MMP14 and HNF1A. *Clin. Epigenetics,* **2019**, *11*(1), 186.
[http://dx.doi.org/10.1186/s13148-019-0786-y] [PMID: 31810492]

[109] Paredes-Gonzalez, X.; Fuentes, F.; Su, Z.Y.; Kong, A.N.T. Apigenin reactivates Nrf2 anti-oxidative stress signaling in mouse skin epidermal JB6 P + cells through epigenetics modifications. *AAPS J.,* **2014**, *16*(4), 727-735.
[http://dx.doi.org/10.1208/s12248-014-9613-8] [PMID: 24830944]

[110] Tamir, J. V. *Curr. Med. Chem.,* **2014**, *11*(10), 1333-1343.

[111] Collins, B.M.; McLachlan, J.A.; Arnold, S.F. The estrogenic and antiestrogenic activities of phytochemicals with the human estrogen receptor expressed in yeast. *Steroids,* **1997**, *62*(4), 365-372.
[http://dx.doi.org/10.1016/S0039-128X(96)00246-2] [PMID: 9090797]

[112] Thangavel, P.; Puga-Olguín, A.; Rodríguez-Landa, J.F.; Zepeda, R.C. Genistein as potential therapeutic candidate for menopausal symptoms and other related diseases. *Molecules,* **2019**, *24*(21), 3892.
[http://dx.doi.org/10.3390/molecules24213892] [PMID: 31671813]

[113] Guo, A.J.; Choi, R.C.; Zheng, K.Y.; Chen, V.P.; Dong, T.T.; Wang, Z.T.; Vollmer, G.; Lau, D.T.; Tsim, K.W. Kaempferol as a flavonoid induces osteoblastic differentiation *via* estrogen receptor signaling. *Chin. Med.,* **2012**, *7*(1), 10.

[http://dx.doi.org/10.1186/1749-8546-7-10] [PMID: 22546174]

[114] Hsieh, C.Y.; Santell, R.C.; Haslam, S.Z.; Helferich, W.G. Estrogenic effects of genistein on the growth of estrogen receptor-positive human breast cancer (MCF-7) cells *in vitro* and *in vivo*. *Cancer Res.*, **1998**, *58*(17), 3833-3838.
[PMID: 9731492]

[115] Allred, C.D.; Allred, K.F.; Ju, Y.H.; Virant, S.M.; Helferich, W.G. Soy diets containing varying amounts of genistein stimulate growth of estrogen-dependent (MCF-7) tumors in a dose-dependent manner. *Cancer Res.*, **2001**, *61*(13), 5045-5050.
[PMID: 11431339]

[116] Rietjens, I.M.C.M.; Sotoca, A.M.; Vervoort, J.; Louisse, J. Mechanisms underlying the dualistic mode of action of major soy isoflavones in relation to cell proliferation and cancer risks. *Mol. Nutr. Food Res.*, **2013**, *57*(1), 100-113.
[http://dx.doi.org/10.1002/mnfr.201200439] [PMID: 23175102]

[117] Petrakis, N.L.; Barnes, S.; King, E.B.; Lowenstein, J.; Wiencke, J.; Lee, M.M.; Miike, R.; Kirk, M.; Coward, L. Stimulatory influence of soy protein isolate on breast secretion in pre- and postmenopausal women. *Cancer Epidemiol. Biomarkers Prev.*, **1996**, *5*(10), 785-794.
[PMID: 8896889]

[118] Khan, S.A.; Chatterton, R.T.; Michel, N. Soy isoflavone supplementation for breast cancer risk reduction: a randomized phase II trial. *Cancer Prev. Res. (Phila.)*, **2012**, *5*(2), 309-319.
[http://dx.doi.org/10.1158/1940-6207.CAPR-11-0251] [PMID: 22307566]

[119] Hargreaves, D.F.; Potten, C.S.; Harding, C.; Shaw, L.E.; Morton, M.S.; Roberts, S.A.; Howell, A.; Bundred, N.J. Two-week dietary soy supplementation has an estrogenic effect on normal premenopausal breast. *J. Clin. Endocrinol. Metab.*, **1999**, *84*(11), 4017-4024.
[http://dx.doi.org/10.1210/jc.84.11.4017] [PMID: 10566643]

[120] Cheng, G.; Wilczek, B.; Warner, M.; Gustafsson, J.Å.; Landgren, B.M. Isoflavone treatment for acute menopausal symptoms. *Menopause*, **2007**, *14*(3), 468-473.
[http://dx.doi.org/10.1097/GME.0b013e31802cc7d0] [PMID: 17290160]

[121] Sartippour, M.R.; Rao, J.Y.; Apple, S.; Wu, D.; Henning, S.; Wang, H.; Elashoff, R.; Rubio, R.; Heber, D.; Brooks, M.N. A pilot clinical study of short-term isoflavone supplements in breast cancer patients. *Nutr. Cancer*, **2004**, *49*(1), 59-65.
[http://dx.doi.org/10.1207/s15327914nc4901_8] [PMID: 15456636]

[122] Adlercreutz, H. Phytoestrogens: epidemiology and a possible role in cancer protection. *Environ. Health Perspect.*, **1995**, *103* Suppl. 7, 103-112.
[PMID: 8593855]

[123] Torrens-Mas, M.; Roca, P. Phytoestrogens for cancer prevention and treatment. *Biology (Basel)*, **2020**, *9*(12), 427.
[http://dx.doi.org/10.3390/biology9120427] [PMID: 33261116]

[124] Shen, J.C.; Klein, R.D.; Wei, Q.; Guan, Y.; Contois, J.H.; Wang, T.T.Y.; Chang, S.; Hursting, S.D. Low-dose genistein induces cyclin-dependent kinase inhibitors and G1 cell-cycle arrest in human prostate cancer cells. *Mol. Carcinog.*, **2000**, *29*(2), 92-102.
[http://dx.doi.org/10.1002/1098-2744(200010)29:2<92::AID-MC6>3.0.CO;2-Q] [PMID: 11074606]

[125] Onozawa, M.; Fukuda, K.; Ohtani, M.; Akaza, H.; Sugimura, T.; Wakabayashi, K. Effects of soybean isoflavones on cell growth and apoptosis of the human prostatic cancer cell line LNCaP. *Jpn. J. Clin. Oncol.*, **1998**, *28*(6), 360-363.
[http://dx.doi.org/10.1093/jjco/28.6.360] [PMID: 9730149]

[126] Zhou, J.R.; Gugger, E.T.; Tanaka, T.; Guo, Y.; Blackburn, G.L.; Clinton, S.K. Soybean phytochemicals inhibit the growth of transplantable human prostate carcinoma and tumor angiogenesis in mice. *J. Nutr.*, **1999**, *129*(9), 1628-1635.
[http://dx.doi.org/10.1093/jn/129.9.1628] [PMID: 10460196]

[127] Adjakly, M.; Ngollo, M.; Boiteux, J-P.; Bignon, Y-J.; Guy, L.; Bernard-Gallon, D. Genistein and daidzein: different molecular effects on prostate cancer. *Anticancer Res.*, **2013**, *33*(1), 39-44. [PMID: 23267126]

[128] Almasan, A.; Ashkenazi, A. Apo2L/TRAIL: apoptosis signaling, biology, and potential for cancer therapy. *Cytokine Growth Factor Rev.*, **2003**, *14*(3-4), 337-348. [http://dx.doi.org/10.1016/S1359-6101(03)00029-7] [PMID: 12787570]

[129] Kazi, A.; Daniel, K.G.; Smith, D.M.; Kumar, N.B.; Dou, Q.P. Inhibition of the proteasome activity, a novel mechanism associated with the tumor cell apoptosis-inducing ability of genistein. *Biochem. Pharmacol.*, **2003**, *66*(6), 965-976. [http://dx.doi.org/10.1016/S0006-2952(03)00414-3] [PMID: 12963483]

[130] Jadhav, R.; Santucci-Pereira, J.; Wang, Y. DNA methylation targets influenced by bisphenol A and/or genistein are associated with survival outcomes in breast cancer patients. *Genes (Basel),* **2017**, *8*(5), 144. [http://dx.doi.org/10.3390/genes8050144] [PMID: 28505145]

[131] Xie, Q.; Bai, Q.; Zou, L.Y. Genistein inhibits DNA methylation and increases expression of tumor suppressor genes in human breast cancer cells. *Genes Chromosomes Cancer,* **2014**, *53*(5), 422-431. [http://dx.doi.org/10.1002/gcc.22154] [PMID: 24532317]

[132] Romagnolo, D.F.; Donovan, M.G.; Papoutsis, A.J.; Doetschman, T.C.; Selmin, O.I. Genistein prevents BRCA1 CpG methylation and proliferation in human breast cancer cells with activated aromatic hydrocarbon receptor. *Curr. Dev. Nutr.,* **2017**, *1*(6)e000562 [http://dx.doi.org/10.3945/cdn.117.000562] [PMID: 29955703]

[133] Magdinier, F.; Ribieras, S.; Lenoir, G.M.; Frappart, L.; Dante, R. Down-regulation of BRCA1 in human sporadic breast cancer; analysis of DNA methylation patterns of the putative promoter region. *Oncogene,* **1998**, *17*(24), 3169-3176. [http://dx.doi.org/10.1038/sj.onc.1202248] [PMID: 9872332]

[134] Donovan, M.G.; Selmin, O.I.; Doetschman, T.C.; Romagnolo, D.F. Epigenetic activation of BRCA1 by genistein *in vivo* and triple negative breast cancer cells linked to antagonism toward aryl hydrocarbon receptor. *Nutrients,* **2019**, *11*(11), 2559. [http://dx.doi.org/10.3390/nu11112559] [PMID: 31652854]

[135] Wu, Q.; Odwin-Dacosta, S.; Cao, S.; Yager, J.D.; Tang, W. Estrogen down regulates COMT transcription *via* promoter DNA methylation in human breast cancer cells. *Toxicol. Appl. Pharmacol.,* **2019**, *367*, 12-22. [http://dx.doi.org/10.1016/j.taap.2019.01.016] [PMID: 30684530]

[136] Paul, B.; Li, Y.; Tollefsbol, T. The effects of combinatorial genistein and sulforaphane in breast tumor inhibition: role in epigenetic regulation. *Int. J. Mol. Sci.,* **2018**, *19*(6), 1754. [http://dx.doi.org/10.3390/ijms19061754] [PMID: 29899271]

[137] Sundaram, M.K.; Ansari, M.Z.; Al Mutery, A.; Ashraf, M.; Nasab, R.; Rai, S.; Rais, N.; Hussain, A. Genistein induces alterations of epigenetic modulatory signatures in human cervical cancer cells. *Anticancer. Agents Med. Chem.,* **2018**, *18*(3), 412-421. [http://dx.doi.org/10.2174/1871520617666170918142114] [PMID: 28925878]

[138] Kovacs, J.J.; Murphy, P.J.M.; Gaillard, S.; Zhao, X.; Wu, J.T.; Nicchitta, C.V.; Yoshida, M.; Toft, D.O.; Pratt, W.B.; Yao, T.P. HDAC6 regulates Hsp90 acetylation and chaperone-dependent activation of glucocorticoid receptor. *Mol. Cell,* **2005**, *18*(5), 601-607. [http://dx.doi.org/10.1016/j.molcel.2005.04.021] [PMID: 15916966]

[139] Karsli-Ceppioglu, S.; Ngollo, M.; Adjakly, M.; Dagdemir, A.; Judes, G.; Lebert, A.; Boiteux, J.P.; Penault-LLorca, F.; Bignon, Y.J.; Guy, L.; Bernard-Gallon, D. Genome-wide DNA methylation modified by soy phytoestrogens: role for epigenetic therapeutics in prostate cancer? *OMICS,* **2015**, *19*(4), 209-219. [http://dx.doi.org/10.1089/omi.2014.0142] [PMID: 25831061]

[140] Phillip, C.J.; Giardina, C.K.; Bilir, B.; Cutler, D.J.; Lai, Y.H.; Kucuk, O.; Moreno, C.S. Genistein cooperates with the histone deacetylase inhibitor vorinostat to induce cell death in prostate cancer cells. *BMC Cancer,* **2012**, *12*(1), 145.
[http://dx.doi.org/10.1186/1471-2407-12-145] [PMID: 22494660]

[141] Fang, M.Z.; Chen, D.; Sun, Y.; Jin, Z.; Christman, J.K.; Yang, C.S. Reversal of hypermethylation and reactivation of p16INK4a, RARbeta, and MGMT genes by genistein and other isoflavones from soy. *Clin. Cancer Res.,* **2005**, *11*(19), 7033-7041.
[http://dx.doi.org/10.1158/1078-0432.CCR-05-0406] [PMID: 16203797]

[142] Wang, L.S.; Stoner, G.D. Anthocyanins and their role in cancer prevention. *Cancer Lett.,* **2008**, *269*(2), 281-290.
[http://dx.doi.org/10.1016/j.canlet.2008.05.020] [PMID: 18571839]

[143] Kresty, L.A.; Mallery, S.R.; Stoner, G.D. Black raspberries in cancer clinical trials: Past, present and future. *J. Berry Res.,* **2016**, *6*(2), 251-261.
[http://dx.doi.org/10.3233/JBR-160125] [PMID: 27594930]

[144] Wang, L.S.; Kuo, C.T.; Cho, S.J. Black raspberry-derived anthocyanins demethylate tumor suppressor genes through the inhibition of DNMT1 and DNMT3B in colon cancer cells. *Nutr. Cancer,* **2013**, *65*(1), 118-125.
[http://dx.doi.org/10.1080/01635581.2013.741759] [PMID: 23368921]

[145] Kuo, H.C.D.; Wu, R.; Li, S.; Yang, A.Y.; Kong, A.N. Anthocyanin delphinidin prevents neoplastic transformation of mouse skin JB6 P+ cells: epigenetic re-activation of Nrf2-ARE pathway. *AAPS J.,* **2019**, *21*(5), 83.
[http://dx.doi.org/10.1208/s12248-019-0355-5] [PMID: 31254216]

[146] Jeong, M.H.; Ko, H.; Jeon, H. Delphinidin induces apoptosis *via* cleaved HDAC3-mediated p53 acetylation and oligomerization in prostate cancer cells. *Oncotarget,* **2016**, *7*(35), 56767-56780.
[http://dx.doi.org/10.18632/oncotarget.10790] [PMID: 27462923]

[147] Escaffit, F.; Vaute, O.; Chevillard-Briet, M. Cleavage and cytoplasmic relocalization of histone deacetylase 3 are important for apoptosis progression. *Mol. Cell. Biol.,* **2007**, *27*(2), 554-567.
[http://dx.doi.org/10.1128/MCB.00869-06] [PMID: 17101790]

[148] Natarajan, T.; Anandhi, M.; Aiswarya, D.; Ramkumar, R.; Kumar, S.; Perumal, P. Idaein chloride induced p53 dependent apoptosis in cervical cancer cells through inhibition of viral oncoproteins. *Biochimie,* **2016**, *121*, 13-20.
[http://dx.doi.org/10.1016/j.biochi.2015.11.008] [PMID: 26586108]

[149] Karthi, N.; Karthiga, A.; Kalaiyarasu, T. Exploration of cell cycle regulation and modulation of the DNA methylation mechanism of pelargonidin: Insights from the molecular modeling approach. *Comput. Biol. Chem.,* **2017**, *70*, 175-185.
[http://dx.doi.org/10.1016/j.compbiolchem.2017.08.002] [PMID: 28950208]

[150] Seong, A.R.; Yoo, J.Y.; Choi, K. Delphinidin, a specific inhibitor of histone acetyltransferase, suppresses inflammatory signaling *via* prevention of NF-κB acetylation in fibroblast-like synoviocyte MH7A cells. *Biochem. Biophys. Res. Commun.,* **2011**, *410*(3), 581-586.
[http://dx.doi.org/10.1016/j.bbrc.2011.06.029] [PMID: 21683061]

[151] Khan, N.; Mukhtar, H. Tea polyphenols for health promotion. *Life Sci.,* **2007**, *81*(7), 519-533.
[http://dx.doi.org/10.1016/j.lfs.2007.06.011] [PMID: 17655876]

[152] Del Rio, D.; Rodriguez-Mateos, A.; Spencer, J.P.E.; Tognolini, M.; Borges, G.; Crozier, A. Dietary (poly)phenolics in human health: structures, bioavailability, and evidence of protective effects against chronic diseases. *Antioxid. Redox Signal.,* **2013**, *18*(14), 1818-1892.
[http://dx.doi.org/10.1089/ars.2012.4581] [PMID: 22794138]

[153] Stalmach, A.; Troufflard, S.; Serafini, M.; Crozier, A. Absorption, metabolism and excretion of Choladi green tea flavan-3-ols by humans. *Mol. Nutr. Food Res.,* **2009**, *53*(S1) Suppl. 1, S44-S53.

[http://dx.doi.org/10.1002/mnfr.200800169] [PMID: 18979506]

[154] Chen, D.; Wang, C.Y.; Lambert, J.D.; Ai, N.; Welsh, W.J.; Yang, C.S. Inhibition of human liver catechol-O-methyltransferase by tea catechins and their metabolites: Structure–activity relationship and molecular-modeling studies. *Biochem. Pharmacol.,* **2005**, *69*(10), 1523-1531. [http://dx.doi.org/10.1016/j.bcp.2005.01.024] [PMID: 15857617]

[155] Wu, A.H.; Tseng, C-C.; Van Den Berg, D.; Yu, M.C. Tea intake, COMT genotype, and breast cancer in Asian-American women. *Cancer Res.,* **2003**, *63*(21), 7526-7529. [PMID: 14612555]

[156] Lee, W.J.; Shim, J.Y.; Zhu, B.T. Mechanisms for the inhibition of DNA methyltransferases by tea catechins and bioflavonoids. *Mol. Pharmacol.,* **2005**, *68*(4), 1018-1030. [http://dx.doi.org/10.1124/mol.104.008367] [PMID: 16037419]

[157] Fang, M.Z.; Wang, Y.; Ai, N.; Hou, Z.; Sun, Y.; Lu, H.; Welsh, W.; Yang, C.S. Tea polyphenol (---epigallocatechin-3-gallate inhibits DNA methyltransferase and reactivates methylation-silenced genes in cancer cell lines. *Cancer Res.,* **2003**, *63*(22), 7563-7570. [PMID: 14633667]

[158] Khan, M.A.; Hussain, A.; Sundaram, M.K.; Alalami, U.; Gunasekera, D.; Ramesh, L.; Hamza, A.; Quraishi, U. (−)-Epigallocatechin-3-gallate reverses the expression of various tumor-suppressor genes by inhibiting DNA methyltransferases and histone deacetylases in human cervical cancer cells. *Oncol. Rep.,* **2015**, *33*(4), 1976-1984. [http://dx.doi.org/10.3892/or.2015.3802] [PMID: 25682960]

[159] Palii, S.S.; Van Emburgh, B.O.; Sankpal, U.T.; Brown, K.D.; Robertson, K.D. DNA methylation inhibitor 5-Aza-2′-deoxycytidine induces reversible genome-wide DNA damage that is distinctly influenced by DNA methyltransferases 1 and 3B. *Mol. Cell. Biol.,* **2008**, *28*(2), 752-771. [http://dx.doi.org/10.1128/MCB.01799-07] [PMID: 17991895]

[160] Pandey, M.; Shukla, S.; Gupta, S. Promoter demethylation and chromatin remodeling by green tea polyphenols leads to re-expression of GSTP1 in human prostate cancer cells. *Int. J. Cancer,* **2010**, *126*(11), NA. [http://dx.doi.org/10.1002/ijc.24988] [PMID: 19856314]

[161] Jones, P.A.; Gonzalgo, M.L. Altered DNA methylation and genome instability: A new pathway to cancer? *Proc. Natl. Acad. Sci. USA,* **1997**, *94*(6), 2103-2105. [http://dx.doi.org/10.1073/pnas.94.6.2103] [PMID: 9122155]

[162] Saldanha, S.N.; Kala, R.; Tollefsbol, T.O. Molecular mechanisms for inhibition of colon cancer cells by combined epigenetic-modulating epigallocatechin gallate and sodium butyrate. *Exp. Cell Res.,* **2014**, *324*(1), 40-53. [http://dx.doi.org/10.1016/j.yexcr.2014.01.024] [PMID: 24518414]

[163] Choi, K.C.; Jung, M.G.; Lee, Y.H. Epigallocatechin-3-gallate, a histone acetyltransferase inhibitor, inhibits EBV-induced B lymphocyte transformation *via* suppression of RelA acetylation. *Cancer Res.,* **2009**, *69*(2), 583-592. [http://dx.doi.org/10.1158/0008-5472.CAN-08-2442] [PMID: 19147572]

[164] Meeran, S. M.; Patel, S. N.; Chan, T.-H.; Tollefsbol, T. O. A novel prodrug of epigallocatechin---gallate: differential epigenetic HTERT repression in human breast cancer cells. *Cancer Prev. Res. (Phila. Pa.).,* **2011**, *4*(9), 1243-1254.

[165] Lam, W.H.; Kazi, A.; Kuhn, D.J. A potential prodrug for a green tea polyphenol proteasome inhibitor: evaluation of the peracetate ester of (−)-epigallocatechin gallate [(−)-EGCG]. *Bioorg. Med. Chem.,* **2004**, *12*(21), 5587-5593. [http://dx.doi.org/10.1016/j.bmc.2004.08.002] [PMID: 15465336]

[166] Stresemann, C.; Brueckner, B.; Musch, T.; Stopper, H.; Lyko, F. Functional diversity of DNA methyltransferase inhibitors in human cancer cell lines. *Cancer Res.,* **2006**, *66*(5), 2794-2800. [http://dx.doi.org/10.1158/0008-5472.CAN-05-2821] [PMID: 16510601]

[167] de Boer, V.C.J.; de Goffau, M.C.; Arts, I.C.W.; Hollman, P.C.H.; Keijer, J. SIRT1 stimulation by polyphenols is affected by their stability and metabolism. *Mech. Ageing Dev.,* **2006**, *127*(7), 618-627. [http://dx.doi.org/10.1016/j.mad.2006.02.007] [PMID: 16603228]

[168] Medina-Franco, J.L.; López-Vallejo, F.; Kuck, D.; Lyko, F. Natural products as DNA methyltransferase inhibitors: a computer-aided discovery approach. *Mol. Divers.,* **2011**, *15*(2), 293-304.
[http://dx.doi.org/10.1007/s11030-010-9262-5] [PMID: 20697809]

[169] Zaveri, N.T. Synthesis of a 3,4,5-trimethoxybenzoyl ester analogue of epigallocatechin-3-gallate (EGCG): a potential route to the natural product green tea catechin, EGCG. *Org. Lett.,* **2001**, *3*(6), 843-846.
[http://dx.doi.org/10.1021/ol007000o] [PMID: 11263896]

[170] Waleh, N.S.; Chao, W-R.; Bensari, A.; Zaveri, N.T. Novel D-ring analog of epigallocatechin-3-gallate inhibits tumor growth and VEGF expression in breast carcinoma cells. *Anticancer Res.,* **2005**, *25*(1A), 397-402.
[PMID: 15816564]

[171] Valcic, S.; Muders, A.; Jacobsen, N.E.; Liebler, D.C.; Timmermann, B.N. Antioxidant chemistry of green tea catechins. Identification of products of the reaction of (-)-epigallocatechin gallate with peroxyl radicals. *Chem. Res. Toxicol.,* **1999**, *12*(4), 382-386.
[http://dx.doi.org/10.1021/tx990003t] [PMID: 10207128]

[172] Rensburg, H.; van, ; Heerden, P. S.; van, ; Ferreira, D. *Enantioselective synthesis of flavonoids.,* **1997**.

[173] Wan, S.B.; Ping Dou, Q.; Chan, T.H. Regiospecific and enantioselective synthesis of methylated metabolites of tea catechins. *Tetrahedron,* **2006**, *62*(25), 5897-5904.
[http://dx.doi.org/10.1016/j.tet.2006.04.010]

[174] Anderson, J.C.; Grounds, H.; Reeves, S.; Taylor, P.W. Improved synthesis of structural analogues of (−)-epicatechin gallate for modulation of staphylococcal β-lactam resistance. *Tetrahedron,* **2014**, *70*(21), 3485-3490.
[http://dx.doi.org/10.1016/j.tet.2014.03.052] [PMID: 24876661]

[175] Yang, Z.; Xiao, F.; Zhang, Y.; Wu, Z.; Zheng, X. Asymmetric synthesis of chiral flavan-3-ols. *Nat. Prod. Res.,* **2019**, *33*(20), 2995-3010.
[http://dx.doi.org/10.1080/14786419.2018.1509337] [PMID: 30521402]

[176] Landis-Piwowar, K.R.; Wan, S.B.; Wiegand, R.A.; Kuhn, D.J.; Chan, T.H.; Dou, Q.P. Methylation suppresses the proteasome-inhibitory function of green tea polyphenols. *J. Cell. Physiol.,* **2007**, *213*(1), 252-260.
[http://dx.doi.org/10.1002/jcp.21124] [PMID: 17477351]

[177] Romanov-Michailidis, F.; Viton, F.; Fumeaux, R.; Lévèques, A.; Actis-Goretta, L.; Rein, M.; Williamson, G.; Barron, D. Epicatechin B-ring conjugates: first enantioselective synthesis and evidence for their occurrence in human biological fluids. *Org. Lett.,* **2012**, *14*(15), 3902-3905.
[http://dx.doi.org/10.1021/ol3016463] [PMID: 22799566]

[178] Hayes, C.J.; Whittaker, B.P.; Watson, S.A.; Grabowska, A.M. Synthesis and preliminary anticancer activity studies of C4 and C8-modified derivatives of catechin gallate (CG) and epicatechin gallate (ECG). *J. Org. Chem.,* **2006**, *71*(26), 9701-9712.
[http://dx.doi.org/10.1021/jo061740e] [PMID: 17168588]

[179] Ikeda, M.; Ueda-Wakagi, M.; Hayashibara, K.; Kitano, R.; Kawase, M.; Kaihatsu, K.; Kato, N.; Suhara, Y.; Osakabe, N.; Ashida, H. Substitution at the C-3 position of catechins has an influence on the binding affinities against serum albumin. *Molecules,* **2017**, *22*(2), 314.
[http://dx.doi.org/10.3390/molecules22020314] [PMID: 28218710]

[180] Park, K.D.; Lee, S.G.; Kim, S.U.; Kim, S.H.; Sun, W.S.; Cho, S.J.; Jeong, D.H. Anticancer activity of 3-O-acyl and alkyl-(−)-epicatechin derivatives. *Bioorg. Med. Chem. Lett.,* **2004**, *14*(20), 5189-5192.

[http://dx.doi.org/10.1016/j.bmcl.2004.07.063] [PMID: 15380225]

[181] Kumar, D.; Harshavardhan, S.J.; Chirumarry, S.; Poornachandra, Y.; Jang, K.; Kumar, C.G.; Yoon, Y-J.; Zhao, B-X.; Miao, J-Y.; Shin, D-S. Design, synthesis *in vitro* anticancer activity and docking studies of (-)-catechin derivatives. *Bull. Korean Chem. Soc.,* **2015**, *36*(2), 564-570.

[182] Dasgupta, A.; Klein, K. Herbal and other dietary supplements that are antioxidants.*Antioxidants in Food, Vitamins and Supplements*; Dasgupta, A.; Klein, K., Eds.; Elsevier: San Diego, **2014**, pp. 295-315.
[http://dx.doi.org/10.1016/B978-0-12-405872-9.00016-1]

[183] Sandur, S.K.; Pandey, M.K.; Sung, B.; Ahn, K.S.; Murakami, A.; Sethi, G.; Limtrakul, P.; Badmaev, V.; Aggarwal, B.B. Curcumin, demethoxycurcumin, bisdemethoxycurcumin, tetrahydrocurcumin and turmerones differentially regulate anti-inflammatory and anti-proliferative responses through a ROS-independent mechanism. *Carcinogenesis,* **2007**, *28*(8), 1765-1773.
[http://dx.doi.org/10.1093/carcin/bgm123] [PMID: 17522064]

[184] Tuorkey, M. Curcumin a potent cancer preventive agent: Mechanisms of cancer cell killing. *Interv. Med. Appl. Sci.,* **2014**, *6*(4), 139-146.
[http://dx.doi.org/10.1556/imas.6.2014.4.1] [PMID: 25598986]

[185] Srivastava, R.K.; Chen, Q.; Siddiqui, I.; Sarva, K.; Shankar, S. Linkage of curcumin-induced cell cycle arrest and apoptosis by cyclin-dependent kinase inhibitor p21(/WAF1/CIP1). *Cell Cycle,* **2007**, *6*(23), 2953-2961.
[http://dx.doi.org/10.4161/cc.6.23.4951] [PMID: 18156803]

[186] Ono, M.; Higuchi, T.; Takeshima, M.; Chen, C.; Nakano, S. Differential anti-tumor activities of curcumin against Ras- and Src-activated human adenocarcinoma cells. *Biochem. Biophys. Res. Commun.,* **2013**, *436*(2), 186-191.
[http://dx.doi.org/10.1016/j.bbrc.2013.05.071] [PMID: 23726918]

[187] Yoshino, M.; Haneda, M.; Naruse, M.; Htay, H.H.; Tsubouchi, R.; Qiao, S.L.; Li, W.H.; Murakami, K.; Yokochi, T. Prooxidant activity of curcumin: copper-dependent formation of 8-hydroxy--'-deoxyguanosine in DNA and induction of apoptotic cell death. *Toxicol. In Vitro,* **2004**, *18*(6), 783-789.
[http://dx.doi.org/10.1016/j.tiv.2004.03.009] [PMID: 15465643]

[188] Hasima, N.; Aggarwal, B. Targeting proteasomal pathways by dietary curcumin for cancer prevention and treatment. *Curr. Med. Chem.,* **2014**, *21*(14), 1583-1594.
[http://dx.doi.org/10.2174/09298673113206660135] [PMID: 23834173]

[189] He, M.; Li, Y.U.; Zhang, L.I. Curcumin suppresses cell proliferation through inhibition of the Wnt/β-catenin signaling pathway in medulloblastoma. *Oncol. Rep.,* **2014**, *32*(1), 173-180.
[http://dx.doi.org/10.3892/or.2014.3206] [PMID: 24858998]

[190] Han, S.S.; Chung, S.T.; Robertson, D.A.; Ranjan, D.; Bondada, S. Curcumin causes the growth arrest and apoptosis of B cell lymphoma by downregulation of egr-1, c-myc, bcl-XL, NF-kappa B, and p53. *Clin. Immunol.,* **1999**, *93*(2), 152-161.
[http://dx.doi.org/10.1006/clim.1999.4769] [PMID: 10527691]

[191] Moragoda, L.; Jaszewski, R.; Majumdar, A.P. Curcumin induced modulation of cell cycle and apoptosis in gastric and colon cancer cells. *Anticancer Res.,* **2001**, *21*(2A), 873-878.
[PMID: 11396178]

[192] Teiten, M.H.; Dicato, M.; Diederich, M. Curcumin as a regulator of epigenetic events. *Mol. Nutr. Food Res.,* **2013**, *57*(9), 1619-1629.
[http://dx.doi.org/10.1002/mnfr.201300201] [PMID: 23754571]

[193] Balasubramanyam, K.; Varier, R.A.; Altaf, M.; Swaminathan, V.; Siddappa, N.B.; Ranga, U.; Kundu, T.K. Curcumin, a novel p300/CREB-binding protein-specific inhibitor of acetyltransferase, represses the acetylation of histone/nonhistone proteins and histone acetyltransferase-dependent chromatin transcription. *J. Biol. Chem.,* **2004**, *279*(49), 51163-51171.

[http://dx.doi.org/10.1074/jbc.M409024200] [PMID: 15383533]

[194] Reed, S.; Quelle, D. p53 Acetylation: regulation and consequences. *Cancers (Basel),* **2014**, *7*(1), 30-69.
[http://dx.doi.org/10.3390/cancers7010030] [PMID: 25545885]

[195] Shankar, S.; Srivastava, R. Involvement of Bcl-2 family members, phosphatidylinositol 3′-kinase/AKT and mitochondrial p53 in curcumin (diferulolylmethane)-induced apoptosis in prostate cancer. *Int. J. Oncol.,* **2007**, *30*(4), 905-918.
[http://dx.doi.org/10.3892/ijo.30.4.905] [PMID: 17332930]

[196] Yun, J.-M.; Jialal, I.; Devaraj, S. *Epigenetic regulation of high glucose-induced proinflammatory cytokine production in monocytes by curcumin.,* **2010**.
[http://dx.doi.org/10.1096/fasebj.24.1_supplement.1030.9]

[197] Neckers, L.; Trepel, J.; Lee, S.; Chung, E.J.; Lee, M.J.; Jung, Y-J.; Marcu, M. Curcumin is an inhibitor of p300 histone acetylatransferase. *Med. Chem.,* **2006**, *2*(2), 169-174.
[http://dx.doi.org/10.2174/157340606776056133] [PMID: 16787365]

[198] Chen, Y.; Shu, W.; Chen, W.; Wu, Q.; Liu, H.; Cui, G. Curcumin, both histone deacetylase and p300/CBP-specific inhibitor, represses the activity of nuclear factor kappa B and Notch 1 in Raji cells. *Basic Clin. Pharmacol. Toxicol.,* **2007**, *101*(6), 427-433.
[http://dx.doi.org/10.1111/j.1742-7843.2007.00142.x] [PMID: 17927689]

[199] Lee, S.J.; Krauthauser, C.; Maduskuie, V.; Fawcett, P.T.; Olson, J.M.; Rajasekaran, S.A. Curcumin-induced HDAC inhibition and attenuation of medulloblastoma growth *in vitro* and *in vivo*. *BMC Cancer,* **2011**, *11*(1), 144.
[http://dx.doi.org/10.1186/1471-2407-11-144] [PMID: 21501498]

[200] Bora-Tatar, G.; Dayangaç-Erden, D.; Demir, A.S.; Dalkara, S.; Yelekçi, K.; Erdem-Yurter, H. Molecular modifications on carboxylic acid derivatives as potent histone deacetylase inhibitors: Activity and docking studies. *Bioorg. Med. Chem.,* **2009**, *17*(14), 5219-5228.
[http://dx.doi.org/10.1016/j.bmc.2009.05.042] [PMID: 19520580]

[201] Shu, L.; Khor, T.O.; Lee, J.H.; Boyanapalli, S.S.S.; Huang, Y.; Wu, T.Y.; Saw, C.L.L.; Cheung, K.L.; Kong, A.N.T. Epigenetic CpG demethylation of the promoter and reactivation of the expression of Neurog1 by curcumin in prostate LNCaP cells. *AAPS J.,* **2011**, *13*(4), 606-614.
[http://dx.doi.org/10.1208/s12248-011-9300-y] [PMID: 21938566]

[202] Young, M.D.; Willson, T.A.; Wakefield, M.J.; Trounson, E.; Hilton, D.J.; Blewitt, M.E.; Oshlack, A.; Majewski, I.J. ChIP-seq analysis reveals distinct H3K27me3 profiles that correlate with transcriptional activity. *Nucleic Acids Res.,* **2011**, *39*(17), 7415-7427.
[http://dx.doi.org/10.1093/nar/gkr416] [PMID: 21652639]

[203] Li, W.; Su, Z.Y.; Guo, Y. Curcumin derivative epigenetically reactivates Nrf2 antioxidative stress signaling in mouse prostate cancer TRAMP C1 cells. *Chem. Res. Toxicol.,* **2018**, *31*(2), 88-96.
[http://dx.doi.org/10.1021/acs.chemrestox.7b00248] [PMID: 29228771]

[204] Du, L.; Xie, Z.; Wu, L.; Chiu, M.; Lin, J.; Chan, K.K.; Liu, S.; Liu, Z. Reactivation of RASSF1A in breast cancer cells by curcumin. *Nutr. Cancer,* **2012**, *64*(8), 1228-1235.
[http://dx.doi.org/10.1080/01635581.2012.717682] [PMID: 23145775]

[205] Abusnina, A.; Keravis, T.; Yougbaré, I.; Bronner, C.; Lugnier, C. Anti-proliferative effect of curcumin on melanoma cells is mediated by PDE1A inhibition that regulates the epigenetic integrator UHRF1. *Mol. Nutr. Food Res.,* **2011**, *55*(11), 1677-1689.
[http://dx.doi.org/10.1002/mnfr.201100307] [PMID: 22045655]

[206] Parashar, G.; Parashar, N.C.; Capalash, N. Curcumin causes promoter hypomethylation and increased expression of FANCF gene in SiHa cell line. *Mol. Cell. Biochem.,* **2012**, *365*(1-2), 29-35.
[http://dx.doi.org/10.1007/s11010-012-1240-z] [PMID: 22297615]

[207] Liu, Z.; Xie, Z.; Jones, W.; Pavlovicz, R.E.; Liu, S.; Yu, J.; Li, P.; Lin, J.; Fuchs, J.R.; Marcucci, G.;

Li, C.; Chan, K.K. Curcumin is a potent DNA hypomethylation agent. *Bioorg. Med. Chem. Lett.*, **2009**, *19*(3), 706-709.
[http://dx.doi.org/10.1016/j.bmcl.2008.12.041] [PMID: 19112019]

[208] Khor, T.O.; Keum, Y.S.; Lin, W.; Kim, J.H.; Hu, R.; Shen, G.; Xu, C.; Gopalakrishnan, A.; Reddy, B.; Zheng, X.; Conney, A.H.; Kong, A.N.T. Combined inhibitory effects of curcumin and phenethyl isothiocyanate on the growth of human PC-3 prostate xenografts in immunodeficient mice. *Cancer Res.*, **2006**, *66*(2), 613-621.
[http://dx.doi.org/10.1158/0008-5472.CAN-05-2708] [PMID: 16423986]

[209] Mansouri, K.; Rasoulpoor, S.; Daneshkhah, A.; Abolfathi, S.; Salari, N.; Mohammadi, M.; Rasoulpoor, S.; Shabani, S. Clinical effects of curcumin in enhancing cancer therapy: A systematic review. *BMC Cancer,* **2020**, *20*(1), 791.
[http://dx.doi.org/10.1186/s12885-020-07256-8] [PMID: 32838749]

[210] Sharma, R.A.; Steward, W.P.; Gescher, A.J. Pharmacokinetics and pharmacodynamics of curcumin. *Adv. Exp. Med. Biol.*, **2007**, *595*, 453-470.
[http://dx.doi.org/10.1007/978-0-387-46401-5_20] [PMID: 17569224]

[211] Fuchs, J.R.; Pandit, B.; Bhasin, D.; Etter, J.P.; Regan, N.; Abdelhamid, D.; Li, C.; Lin, J.; Li, P.K. Structure–activity relationship studies of curcumin analogues. *Bioorg. Med. Chem. Lett.*, **2009**, *19*(7), 2065-2069.
[http://dx.doi.org/10.1016/j.bmcl.2009.01.104] [PMID: 19249204]

[212] Somsakeesit, L.; Senawong, T.; Kumboonma, P.; Saenglee, S.; Samankul, A.; Senawong, G.; Yenjai, C.; Phaosiri, C. Influence of side-chain changes on histone deacetylase inhibitory and cytotoxicity activities of curcuminoid derivatives. *Bioorg. Med. Chem. Lett.*, **2020**, *30*(11)127171
[http://dx.doi.org/10.1016/j.bmcl.2020.127171] [PMID: 32273215]

[213] Iranshahi, M.; Chini, M.G.; Masullo, M. Can small chemical modifications of natural pan-inhibitors modulate the biological selectivity? The case of curcumin prenylated derivatives acting as HDAC or MPGES-1 inhibitors. *J. Nat. Prod.*, **2015**, *78*(12), 2867-2879.
[http://dx.doi.org/10.1021/acs.jnatprod.5b00700] [PMID: 26588603]

[214] Kumboonma, P.; Senawong, T.; Saenglee, S.; Senawong, G.; Somsakeesit, L.; Yenjai, C.; Phaosiri, C. New histone deacetylase inhibitors and anticancer agents from Curcuma longa. *Med. Chem. Res.*, **2019**, *28*(10), 1773-1782.
[http://dx.doi.org/10.1007/s00044-019-02414-5]

[215] Simoni, D.; Rizzi, M.; Rondanin, R. Antitumor effects of curcumin and structurally β-diketone modified analogs on multidrug resistant cancer cells. *Bioorg. Med. Chem. Lett.*, **2008**, *18*(2), 845-849.
[http://dx.doi.org/10.1016/j.bmcl.2007.11.021] [PMID: 18039573]

[216] Liang, G.; Shao, L.; Wang, Y.; Zhao, C.; Chu, Y.; Xiao, J.; Zhao, Y.; Li, X.; Yang, S. Exploration and synthesis of curcumin analogues with improved structural stability both *in vitro* and *in vivo* as cytotoxic agents. *Bioorg. Med. Chem.*, **2009**, *17*(6), 2623-2631.
[http://dx.doi.org/10.1016/j.bmc.2008.10.044] [PMID: 19243951]

[217] Yadav, B.; Taurin, S.; Rosengren, R.J.; Schumacher, M.; Diederich, M.; Somers-Edgar, T.J.; Larsen, L. Synthesis and cytotoxic potential of heterocyclic cyclohexanone analogues of curcumin. *Bioorg. Med. Chem.*, **2010**, *18*(18), 6701-6707.
[http://dx.doi.org/10.1016/j.bmc.2010.07.063] [PMID: 20728364]

[218] Zhou, D.Y.; Ding, N.; Du, Z.Y.; Cui, X.X.; Wang, H.; Wei, X.C.; Conney, A.H.; Zhang, K.; Zheng, X. Curcumin analogues with high activity for inhibiting human prostate cancer cell growth and androgen receptor activation. *Mol. Med. Rep.*, **2014**, *10*(3), 1315-1322.
[http://dx.doi.org/10.3892/mmr.2014.2380] [PMID: 25060817]

[219] Fioravanti, R.; Tomassi, S.; Di Bello, E.; Romanelli, A.; Plateroti, A.M.; Benedetti, R.; Conte, M.; Novellino, E.; Altucci, L.; Valente, S.; Mai, A. Properly substituted cyclic bis-(2-bromobenzylidene) compounds behaved as dual p300/CARM1 inhibitors and induced apoptosis in cancer cells. *Molecules,*

2020, *25*(14), 3122.
[http://dx.doi.org/10.3390/molecules25143122] [PMID: 32650558]

[220] Jeandet, P.; Bessis, R.; Sbaghi, M.; Meunier, P. Production of the phytoalexin resveratrol by grapes as a response to botrytis attack under natural conditions. *J. Phytopathol.,* **1995**, *143*(3), 135-139. [http://dx.doi.org/10.1111/j.1439-0434.1995.tb00246.x]

[221] Jeandet, P.; Sbaghi, M.; Bessis, R.; Meunier, P. The potential relationship of stilbene (resveratrol) synthesis to anthocyanin content in grape berry skins. *VITIS - J. Grapevine Res.,* **1995**, *34*(2), 91-91.

[222] Talhi, O.; Pinto, D.C.G.A.; Silva, A.M.S. The French paradox at tea time: from antioxidant flavonoids and stilbenes toward bio-inspired synthetic derivatives.*Recent advances in redox active plant and microbial products: from basic chemistry to widespread applications in medicine and agriculture*; Jacob, C.; Kirsch, G.; Slusarenko, A.; Winyard, P.G.; Burkholz, T., Eds.; Springer Netherlands: Dordrecht, **2014**, pp. 149-189.
[http://dx.doi.org/10.1007/978-94-017-8953-0_6]

[223] Elattar, T.M.; Virji, A.S. The effect of red wine and its components on growth and proliferation of human oral squamous carcinoma cells. *Anticancer Res.,* **1999**, *19*(6B), 5407-5414.
[PMID: 10697569]

[224] Rimando, A.M.; Cuendet, M.; Desmarchelier, C.; Mehta, R.G.; Pezzuto, J.M.; Duke, S.O. Cancer chemopreventive and antioxidant activities of pterostilbene, a naturally occurring analogue of resveratrol. *J. Agric. Food Chem.,* **2002**, *50*(12), 3453-3457.
[http://dx.doi.org/10.1021/jf0116855] [PMID: 12033810]

[225] Pezzuto, J.M. Resveratrol as an inhibitor of carcinogenesis. *Pharm. Biol.,* **2008**, *46*(7-8), 443-573.
[http://dx.doi.org/10.1080/13880200802116610]

[226] Chiou, Y.S.; Tsai, M.L.; Nagabhushanam, K.; Wang, Y.J.; Wu, C.H.; Ho, C.T.; Pan, M.H. Pterostilbene is more potent than resveratrol in preventing azoxymethane (AOM)-induced colon tumorigenesis *via* activation of the NF-E2-related factor 2 (Nrf2)-mediated antioxidant signaling pathway. *J. Agric. Food Chem.,* **2011**, *59*(6), 2725-2733.
[http://dx.doi.org/10.1021/jf2000103] [PMID: 21355597]

[227] Mohar, D.S.; Malik, S. The Sirtuin System: The Holy Grail of Resveratrol? *J. Clin. Exp. Cardiolog.,* **2012**, *3*(11), 216.
[http://dx.doi.org/10.4172/2155-9880.1000216] [PMID: 23560248]

[228] Potente, M.; Ghaeni, L.; Baldessari, D. SIRT1 controls endothelial angiogenic functions during vascular growth. *Genes Dev.,* **2007**, *21*(20), 2644-2658.
[http://dx.doi.org/10.1101/gad.435107] [PMID: 17938244]

[229] Wang, S.; Wang, X.; Yan, J. Resveratrol inhibits proliferation of cultured rat cardiac fibroblasts: Correlated with NO–cGMP signaling pathway. *Eur. J. Pharmacol.,* **2007**, *567*(1-2), 26-35.
[http://dx.doi.org/10.1016/j.ejphar.2007.04.023] [PMID: 17499237]

[230] Karaman Mayack, B.; Sippl, W.; Ntie-Kang, F. Natural products as modulators of Sirtuins. *Molecules,* **2020**, *25*(14), 3287.
[http://dx.doi.org/10.3390/molecules25143287] [PMID: 32698385]

[231] Beher, D.; Wu, J.; Cumine, S.; Kim, K.W.; Lu, S.C.; Atangan, L.; Wang, M. Resveratrol is not a direct activator of SIRT1 enzyme activity. *Chem. Biol. Drug Des.,* **2009**, *74*(6), 619-624.
[http://dx.doi.org/10.1111/j.1747-0285.2009.00901.x] [PMID: 19843076]

[232] Pacholec, M.; Bleasdale, J.E.; Chrunyk, B. SRT1720, SRT2183, SRT1460, and resveratrol are not direct activators of SIRT1. *J. Biol. Chem.,* **2010**, *285*(11), 8340-8351.
[http://dx.doi.org/10.1074/jbc.M109.088682] [PMID: 20061378]

[233] Cao, D.; Wang, M.; Qiu, X.; Liu, D.; Jiang, H.; Yang, N.; Xu, R.M. Structural basis for allosteric, substrate-dependent stimulation of SIRT1 activity by resveratrol. *Genes Dev.,* **2015**, *29*(12), 1316-1325.

[http://dx.doi.org/10.1101/gad.265462.115] [PMID: 26109052]

[234] Kumar, A.; Levenson, A.S. Chapter 8 - Epigenetic mechanisms of resveratrol and its analogs in cancer prevention and treatment. In Epigenetics of cancer prevention; Bishayee, A., Bhatia, D., Eds.; Translational Epigenetics; Academic Press , **2019**; 8, pp. 169-186.

[235] Venturelli, S.; Berger, A.; Böcker, A. Resveratrol as a pan-HDAC inhibitor alters the acetylation status of histone [corrected] proteins in human-derived hepatoblastoma cells. *PLoS One,* **2013**, *8*(8)e73097 [http://dx.doi.org/10.1371/journal.pone.0073097] [PMID: 24023672]

[236] Kai, L.; Samuel, S.K.; Levenson, A.S. Resveratrol enhances p53 acetylation and apoptosis in prostate cancer by inhibiting MTA1/NuRD complex. *Int. J. Cancer,* **2010**, *126*(7), NA. [http://dx.doi.org/10.1002/ijc.24928] [PMID: 19810103]

[237] Dhar, S.; Kumar, A.; Li, K.; Tzivion, G.; Levenson, A.S. Resveratrol regulates PTEN/Akt pathway through inhibition of MTA1/HDAC unit of the NuRD complex in prostate cancer. *Biochim. Biophys. Acta Mol. Cell Res.,* **2015**, *1853*(2), 265-275. [http://dx.doi.org/10.1016/j.bbamcr.2014.11.004] [PMID: 25447541]

[238] Dhar, S.; Kumar, A.; Zhang, L.; Rimando, A.M.; Lage, J.M.; Lewin, J.R.; Atfi, A.; Zhang, X.; Levenson, A.S. Dietary pterostilbene is a novel MTA1-targeted chemopreventive and therapeutic agent in prostate cancer. *Oncotarget,* **2016**, *7*(14), 18469-18484. [http://dx.doi.org/10.18632/oncotarget.7841] [PMID: 26943043]

[239] Li, K.; Dias, S.J.; Rimando, A.M.; Dhar, S.; Mizuno, C.S.; Penman, A.D.; Lewin, J.R.; Levenson, A.S. Pterostilbene acts through metastasis-associated protein 1 to inhibit tumor growth, progression and metastasis in prostate cancer. *PLoS One,* **2013**, *8*(3)e57542 [http://dx.doi.org/10.1371/journal.pone.0057542] [PMID: 23469203]

[240] Butt, N.A.; Kumar, A.; Dhar, S. Targeting MTA 1/ HIF -1 α signaling by pterostilbene in combination with histone deacetylase inhibitor attenuates prostate cancer progression. *Cancer Med.,* **2017**, *6*(11), 2673-2685. [http://dx.doi.org/10.1002/cam4.1209] [PMID: 29024573]

[241] Medina-Aguilar, R.; Pérez-Plasencia, C.; Marchat, L.A. Methylation landscape of human breast cancer cells in response to dietary compound resveratrol. *PLoS One,* **2016**, *11*(6)e0157866 [http://dx.doi.org/10.1371/journal.pone.0157866] [PMID: 27355345]

[242] Lubecka, K.; Kurzava, L.; Flower, K. Stilbenoids remodel the DNA methylation patterns in breast cancer cells and inhibit oncogenic NOTCH signaling through epigenetic regulation of MAML2 transcriptional activity. *Carcinogenesis,* **2016**, *37*(7), 656-668. [http://dx.doi.org/10.1093/carcin/bgw048] [PMID: 27207652]

[243] Kala, R.; Shah, H.N.; Martin, S.L.; Tollefsbol, T.O. Epigenetic-based combinatorial resveratrol and pterostilbene alters DNA damage response by affecting SIRT1 and DNMT enzyme expression, including SIRT1-dependent γ-H2AX and telomerase regulation in triple-negative breast cancer. *BMC Cancer,* **2015**, *15*(1), 672. [http://dx.doi.org/10.1186/s12885-015-1693-z] [PMID: 26459286]

[244] Liu, T.; Liu, P.Y.; Marshall, G.M. The critical role of the class III histone deacetylase SIRT1 in cancer. *Cancer Res.,* **2009**, *69*(5), 1702-1705. [http://dx.doi.org/10.1158/0008-5472.CAN-08-3365] [PMID: 19244112]

[245] Gao, Y.; Tollefsbol, T. Combinational proanthocyanidins and resveratrol synergistically inhibit human breast cancer cells and impact epigenetic–mediating machinery. *Int. J. Mol. Sci.,* **2018**, *19*(8), 2204. [http://dx.doi.org/10.3390/ijms19082204] [PMID: 30060527]

[246] Papoutsis, A.J.; Borg, J.L.; Selmin, O.I.; Romagnolo, D.F. BRCA-1 promoter hypermethylation and silencing induced by the aromatic hydrocarbon receptor-ligand TCDD are prevented by resveratrol in MCF-7 Cells. *J. Nutr. Biochem.,* **2012**, *23*(10), 1324-1332. [http://dx.doi.org/10.1016/j.jnutbio.2011.08.001] [PMID: 22197621]

[247] Papoutsis, A.J.; Selmin, O.I.; Borg, J.L.; Romagnolo, D.F. Gestational exposure to the AhR agonist 2,3,7,8-tetrachlorodibenzo- *p* -dioxin induces BRCA-1 promoter hypermethylation and reduces BRCA-1 expression in mammary tissue of rat offspring: Preventive effects of resveratrol. *Mol. Carcinog.*, **2015**, *54*(4), 261-269.
[http://dx.doi.org/10.1002/mc.22095] [PMID: 24136580]

[248] Zhu, W.; Qin, W.; Zhang, K.; Rottinghaus, G.E.; Chen, Y.C.; Kliethermes, B.; Sauter, E.R. Trans-resveratrol alters mammary promoter hypermethylation in women at increased risk for breast cancer. *Nutr. Cancer,* **2012**, *64*(3), 393-400.
[http://dx.doi.org/10.1080/01635581.2012.654926] [PMID: 22332908]

[249] Aldawsari, F.S.; Aguayo-Ortiz, R.; Kapilashrami, K.; Yoo, J.; Luo, M.; Medina-Franco, J.L.; Velázquez-Martínez, C.A. Resveratrol-salicylate derivatives as selective DNMT3 inhibitors and anticancer agents. *J. Enzyme Inhib. Med. Chem.*, **2016**, *31*(5), 695-703.
[http://dx.doi.org/10.3109/14756366.2015.1058256] [PMID: 26118420]

[250] Duan, Y.C.; Guan, Y.Y.; Zhai, X.Y. Discovery of resveratrol derivatives as novel LSD1 inhibitors: Design, synthesis and their biological evaluation. *Eur. J. Med. Chem.*, **2017**, *126*, 246-258.
[http://dx.doi.org/10.1016/j.ejmech.2016.11.035] [PMID: 27888721]

[251] Mazué, F.; Colin, D.; Gobbo, J.; Wegner, M.; Rescifina, A.; Spatafora, C.; Fasseur, D.; Delmas, D.; Meunier, P.; Tringali, C.; Latruffe, N. Structural determinants of resveratrol for cell proliferation inhibition potency: Experimental and docking studies of new analogs. *Eur. J. Med. Chem.*, **2010**, *45*(7), 2972-2980.
[http://dx.doi.org/10.1016/j.ejmech.2010.03.024] [PMID: 20395019]

[252] Karki, S.S.; Bhutle, S.R.; Sahoo, S.; Reddy, R.; Balzarini, J.; De Clercq, E.; Darji, S.Y. Synthesis and biological evaluation of some stilbene derivatives. *Med. Chem. Res.*, **2011**, *20*(8), 1349-1356.
[http://dx.doi.org/10.1007/s00044-010-9484-1]

[253] Stefański, T.; Mikstacka, R.; Kurczab, R.; Dutkiewicz, Z.; Kucińska, M.; Murias, M.; Zielińska-Przyjemska, M.; Cichocki, M.; Teubert, A.; Kaczmarek, M.; Hogendorf, A.; Sobiak, S. Design, synthesis, and biological evaluation of novel combretastatin A-4 thio derivatives as microtubule targeting agents. *Eur. J. Med. Chem.*, **2018**, *144*, 797-816.
[http://dx.doi.org/10.1016/j.ejmech.2017.11.050] [PMID: 29291446]

[254] Roberti, M.; Pizzirani, D.; Simoni, D.; Rondanin, R.; Baruchello, R.; Bonora, C.; Buscemi, F.; Grimaudo, S.; Tolomeo, M. Synthesis and biological evaluation of resveratrol and analogues as apoptosis-inducing agents. *J. Med. Chem.*, **2003**, *46*(16), 3546-3554.
[http://dx.doi.org/10.1021/jm030785u] [PMID: 12877593]

[255] Mayhoub, A.S.; Marler, L.; Kondratyuk, T.P.; Park, E.J.; Pezzuto, J.M.; Cushman, M. Optimizing thiadiazole analogues of resveratrol *versus* three chemopreventive targets. *Bioorg. Med. Chem.*, **2012**, *20*(1), 510-520.
[http://dx.doi.org/10.1016/j.bmc.2011.09.031] [PMID: 22115839]

[256] Mayhoub, A.S.; Marler, L.; Kondratyuk, T.P.; Park, E.J.; Pezzuto, J.M.; Cushman, M. Optimization of thiazole analogues of resveratrol for induction of NAD(P)H:quinone reductase 1 (QR1). *Bioorg. Med. Chem.*, **2012**, *20*(24), 7030-7039.
[http://dx.doi.org/10.1016/j.bmc.2012.10.006] [PMID: 23142320]

[257] Mayhoub, A.S.; Marler, L.; Kondratyuk, T.P.; Park, E.J.; Pezzuto, J.M.; Cushman, M. Optimization of the aromatase inhibitory activities of pyridylthiazole analogues of resveratrol. *Bioorg. Med. Chem.*, **2012**, *20*(7), 2427-2434.
[http://dx.doi.org/10.1016/j.bmc.2012.01.047] [PMID: 22386564]

[258] Ertas, M.; Sahin, Z.; Berk, B.; Yurttas, L.; Biltekin, S.N.; Demirayak, S. Pyridine-substituted thiazolylphenol derivatives: Synthesis, modeling studies, aromatase inhibition, and antiproliferative activity evaluation. *Arch. Pharm. (Weinheim),* **2018**, *351*(3-4)1700272
[http://dx.doi.org/10.1002/ardp.201700272] [PMID: 29522642]

[259] Belluti, F.; Fontana, G.; Bo, L.D.; Carenini, N.; Giommarelli, C.; Zunino, F. Design, synthesis and anticancer activities of stilbene-coumarin hybrid compounds: Identification of novel proapoptotic agents. *Bioorg. Med. Chem.*, **2010**, *18*(10), 3543-3550.
[http://dx.doi.org/10.1016/j.bmc.2010.03.069] [PMID: 20409723]

[260] Herrera-R, A.; Castrillón, W.; Otero, E.; Ruiz, E.; Carda, M.; Agut, R.; Naranjo, T.; Moreno, G.; Maldonado, M.E.; Cardona-G, W. Synthesis and antiproliferative activity of 3- and 7-styrylcoumarins. *Med. Chem. Res.*, **2018**, *27*(8), 1893-1905.
[http://dx.doi.org/10.1007/s00044-018-2202-0]

[261] De Filippis, B.; De Lellis, L.; Florio, R.; Ammazzalorso, A.; Amoia, P.; Fantacuzzi, M.; Giampietro, L.; Maccallini, C.; Amoroso, R.; Veschi, S.; Cama, A. Synthesis and cytotoxic effects on pancreatic cancer cells of resveratrol analogs. *Med. Chem. Res.*, **2019**, *28*(7), 984-991.
[http://dx.doi.org/10.1007/s00044-019-02351-3]

[262] Srivastava, V.; Lee, H. Synthesis and bio-evaluation of novel quinolino-stilbene derivatives as potential anticancer agents. *Bioorg. Med. Chem.*, **2015**, *23*(24), 7629-7640.
[http://dx.doi.org/10.1016/j.bmc.2015.11.007] [PMID: 26602827]

[263] Wei, Q.; Li, J.; Tang, F.; Yin, Y.; Zhao, Y.; Yao, Q. Synthesis and biological evaluation of novel 2-arylvinyl-substituted naphtho[2,3- d]imidazolium halide derivatives as potent antitumor agents. *Eur. J. Med. Chem.*, **2018**, *144*, 504-516.
[http://dx.doi.org/10.1016/j.ejmech.2017.12.008] [PMID: 29288947]

[264] Nakahara, T.; Takeuchi, M.; Kinoyama, I. YM155, a novel small-molecule survivin suppressant, induces regression of established human hormone-refractory prostate tumor xenografts. *Cancer Res.*, **2007**, *67*(17), 8014-8021.
[http://dx.doi.org/10.1158/0008-5472.CAN-07-1343] [PMID: 17804712]

[265] Orsini, F.; Verotta, L.; Klimo, K.; Gerhäuser, C. Synthesis of resveratrol derivatives and *in vitro* screening for potential cancer chemopreventive activities. *Arch. Pharm. (Weinheim)*, **2016**, *349*(6), 414-427.
[http://dx.doi.org/10.1002/ardp.201600022] [PMID: 27159630]

[266] Martí-Centelles, R.; Falomir, E.; Murga, J.; Carda, M.; Marco, J.A. Inhibitory effect of cytotoxic stilbenes related to resveratrol on the expression of the VEGF, hTERT and c-Myc genes. *Eur. J. Med. Chem.*, **2015**, *103*, 488-496.
[http://dx.doi.org/10.1016/j.ejmech.2015.09.014] [PMID: 26402726]

[267] Martí Centelles, R.; Murga, J.; Falomir, E.; Carda, M.; Marco, J.A. Synthesis and biological evaluation of imines structurally related to resveratrol as dual inhibitors of VEGF protein secretion and HTERT gene expression. *Nat. Prod. Commun.*, **2017**, *12*(5)1934578X1701200
[http://dx.doi.org/10.1177/1934578X1701200514] [PMID: 30496679]

[268] Zhang, W.; Sviripa, V.; Kril, L.M. Fluorinated N,N-dialkylaminostilbenes for Wnt pathway inhibition and colon cancer repression. *J. Med. Chem.*, **2011**, *54*(5), 1288-1297.
[http://dx.doi.org/10.1021/jm101248v] [PMID: 21291235]

[269] Yoo, K.M.; Kim, S.; Moon, B.K.; Kim, S.S.; Kim, K.T.; Kim, S.Y.; Choi, S.Y. Potent inhibitory effects of resveratrol derivatives on progression of prostate cancer cells. *Arch. Pharm. (Weinheim)*, **2006**, *339*(5), 238-241.
[http://dx.doi.org/10.1002/ardp.200500228] [PMID: 16619281]

[270] Ma, J.; Li, J.; Tian, Y.S. Synthesis and bioactivity evaluation of 2,3-diaryl acrylonitrile derivatives as potential anticancer agents. *Bioorg. Med. Chem. Lett.*, **2017**, *27*(1), 81-85.
[http://dx.doi.org/10.1016/j.bmcl.2016.11.025] [PMID: 27887843]

[271] Alam, M.S.; Nam, Y.J.; Lee, D.U. Synthesis and evaluation of (Z)-2,3-diphenylacrylonitrile analogs as anti-cancer and anti-microbial agents. *Eur. J. Med. Chem.*, **2013**, *69*, 790-797.
[http://dx.doi.org/10.1016/j.ejmech.2013.08.031] [PMID: 24113364]

[272] Madadi, N.R.; Penthala, N.R.; Ketkar, A.; Eoff, R.L.; Trujullo-Alonso, V.; Guzman, M.L.; Crooks, P.A. Synthesis and evaluation of 2-naphthaleno trans-stilbenes and cyanostilbenes as anticancer agents. *Anticancer. Agents Med. Chem.*, **2018**, *18*(4), 556-564. [http://dx.doi.org/10.2174/1871521409666170412115703] [PMID: 28403783]

[273] Sale, S.; Verschoyle, R.D.; Boocock, D. Pharmacokinetics in mice and growth-inhibitory properties of the putative cancer chemopreventive agent resveratrol and the synthetic analogue trans 3,4,5,4′-tetramethoxystilbene. *Br. J. Cancer,* **2004**, *90*(3), 736-744. [http://dx.doi.org/10.1038/sj.bjc.6601568] [PMID: 14760392]

[274] Bandyopadhyay, A.; Gao, J. Targeting biomolecules with reversible covalent chemistry. *Curr. Opin. Chem. Biol.,* **2016**, *34*, 110-116. [http://dx.doi.org/10.1016/j.cbpa.2016.08.011] [PMID: 27599186]

[275] Marier, J.F.; Vachon, P.; Gritsas, A.; Zhang, J.; Moreau, J.P.; Ducharme, M.P. Metabolism and disposition of resveratrol in rats: extent of absorption, glucuronidation, and enterohepatic recirculation evidenced by a linked-rat model. *J. Pharmacol. Exp. Ther.,* **2002**, *302*(1), 369-373. [http://dx.doi.org/10.1124/jpet.102.033340] [PMID: 12065739]

SUBJECT INDEX

A

B

C

D

E

F

G

H

I

J

K

L

M

N

O

P

Q

R

S

Made in United States
North Haven, CT
04 November 2026

21719573R00288